Renal Dysfunction : Mechanisms Involved in Fluid and Solute Imbalance

16.95
NET

Renal Dysfunction : Mechanisms Involved in Fluid and Solute Imbalance

Heinz Valtin, M.D., *Andrew C. Vail Professor and Chairman of Physiology, Dartmouth Medical School; Consultant Nephrologist, Dartmouth-Hitchcock Medical Center, Hanover, New Hampshire*

Little, Brown and Company : Boston

First Edition

Library of Congress Catalog Card No. 78-61277

ISBN 0-316-89553-9 (C)
ISBN 0-316-89554-7 (P)

Printed in the United States of America

HAL

The cover design, representing two kidneys on a background of the world, is based on the official emblem of the V International Congress of Nephrology, Mexico City, 1972. The symbol is used with the kind permission of Dr. Herman Villareal, President of the Congress.

To

Eva W. Valtin

Foreword from the Series Editor

The goal of the Little, Brown Physiopathology Series is to provide textbooks that describe and illustrate the scientific foundations underlying the current practice of clinical medicine. The concept of this series developed from curricular changes that occurred in many medical schools during the early 1970s. These changes resulted in increased emphasis in the teaching of normal and abnormal human biology, usually to second year medical students, as the bridge between the traditional basic science courses and the clinical clerkships. A need exists for textbooks in this "bridge" area.

Each book in this series will deal with a different medical subspecialty. Each book will aim to provide a clear and solid discussion of the basic scientific concepts and principles on which the clinical subspecialty is built. This discussion will include selected aspects of normal and abnormal physiology, biochemistry, morphology, cell biology, and so on, as appropriate. The discussion of the basic science material will usually be presented in the context of the approach to the study of clinical material. Major clinical phenomena and disease processes will, in turn, be analyzed in terms of normal and abnormal human biology. Thus, the books will try to show how the art of modern clinical medicine involves firm scientific knowledge and the scientific approach in order to be effective.

Although designed for second year medical students, this series will, we hope, be useful as well to more advanced students and practitioners as a readable and up-to-date review of the scientific basis for clinical practice in a given area.

DeWitt S. Goodman, M.D.
Tilden-Weger-Bieler Professor
Department of Medicine
Columbia University College
of Physicians and Surgeons

Preface

This book embodies my conviction of what medical education should be. During the three or four years that medical students are with us, we should strive to exemplify a scientific approach to clinical problems. Accordingly, three major phases should be identifiable in a medical curriculum: teaching the principles of basic science; applying these principles to the understanding and, hence, logical management of disease; and a clinical experience. The last of these phases, like the first two, should concentrate on principles; clear and thorough examples of a logical approach to clinical problems (even if only a few) should take precedence over experience with the myriad of diseases. The three phases can be taught either in sequence or almost conjointly. Whatever the means, however, the aim of medical education should be the mastery of a scientific principle of approach that will allow a physician to handle logically, correctly, and *safely* even those diseases with which he or she may not have had previous experience. Obviously, practical experience is also important, but while some of that experience can be gained in medical school, the major opportunity for it should be provided in subsequent training.

This volume has been written to serve as a textbook for the second of the phases listed above. As such, the book concentrates on the analysis of disease processes in nephrology, and it deliberately stops short of clinical descriptions of specific diseases. Armed with an understanding of the mechanisms involved, a student can then proceed to reading more clinically oriented material, much of which is cited in the selected references at the end of each chapter. This material has been chosen with three purposes in mind: (1) to list some classical contributions, (2) to cite pertinent investigations, and (3) to provide standard text references and up-to-date review articles.

In order to illustrate how the didactic material can be applied to patients, each chapter ends with a series of problems, most of which are based on clinical histories. Detailed answers to these problems appear in a separate section at the end of this book.

This work has been written as a sequel to my first book, *Renal Function: Mechanisms Preserving Fluid and Solute Balance in Health.* Although each volume is meant to be complete in itself, in some instances the present work can be used to complement the first. Thus, a number of topics that are often considered in courses on renal physiology – for example, the renin-angiotensin-aldosterone system, the action of antidiuretic hormone, and the interaction among phosphate, calcium, and vitamin D – are more thoroughly described in this book than in the first. Throughout, I have tried to take up topics in the context of their pertinence to nephrology. For that reason, phosphate, calcium, and vitamin D are discussed not as separate entities but in the chapter on chronic renal failure; the renin-angiotensin-aldosterone system in the chapter on hypertension; and dialysis under acute and chronic renal failure.

I originally conceived this book as an independent sequel to my first volume on normal renal function. But when, in the planning stages, I spoke with Dr. DeWitt Goodman, the editor of Little, Brown's Physiopathology Series, it immediately became evident that our ideas on that subject coincided so precisely that we decided the present work should be written for that series. I am very pleased indeed by that decision.

I welcome criticism about this textbook from my colleagues, be they students, teachers, or clinicians.

H. V.

Acknowledgments

Many persons have helped in this project. In naming them, I live in fear of having forgotten someone. Only that individual will spot the inadvertent oversight, and he or she will do me a great favor in bringing the omission to my attention so that I can correct it.

If the material presented in this book is found to be largely free of error, the credit must go to colleagues who checked the text for me. Each chapter was reviewed by at least one person who is expert in the topic of that chapter. Because my request for these reviews was invariably an imposition on very busy people, I shall here acknowledge these individuals by name: Jerome P. Kassirer, John F. Seely, Howard S. Frazier, William B. Schwartz, Carl W. Gottschalk, Richard L. Tannen, Michael J. Dunn, Charles R. Scriver, Gary L. Robertson, Paul H. Stern, Gilbert H. Mudge, Douglas R. Wilson, Laurence E. Earley, and Neal S. Bricker.

In addition, I received advice and help from many people at Dartmouth Medical School: Gilbert H. Mudge, Paul H. Stern, Brian R. Edwards, S. Marsh Tenney, Eugene E. Nattie, Peter K. Spiegel, Harte C. Crow, V. Peter Semogas, Frederick M. Appleton, Howard H. Green, William G. North, Frederick T. LaRochelle, Jr., Robert C. Charman, William J. Lancaster, O. Ross McIntyre, John E. Lawe, Herbert L. Bonkowsky, Arthur Naitove, and Douglas J. Segan.

Grace E. McCann diligently typed the manuscript and Ethel B. Garrity helped with proofreading and editorial chores. The illustrations were executed by Valma and Henry Page, Kathleen M. McCarthy, and Hathorn-Olson. The staff of Dana Biomedical Library at Dartmouth provided space, a cheerful atmosphere, and much help. I particularly want to acknowledge the help of the superb staff at Little, Brown and Company, led by Fred Belliveau and Lin Richter; they understand authors. Anne N. Merian thoughtfully guided the book through production, and the exquisite taste of Clifton Gaskill is responsible for its design.

Finally, I am indebted to many investigators and publishers for permission to reproduce their work. I trust that due recognition has been accorded in the legends to the figures and tables.

H. V.

Contents

Renal Dysfunction : Mechanisms Involved in Fluid and Solute Imbalance

1 : Balance: The Steady State

Clinical Nephrology

In this book, I shall illustrate a scientific approach to the interpretation and logical management of some major disease *processes* in clinical nephrology. Since the approach involves the application of basic principles, an understanding of renal, water, and electrolyte physiology is assumed. In this sense, I consider my earlier book, *Renal Function,* to be a companion piece to the present text. Nevertheless, the present work is meant to be self-contained, and some concepts and illustrations from the first book will therefore be repeated in this volume.

The area of clinical nephrology, despite the name that seems to restrict it to the kidneys, encompasses not only diseases of the kidneys but also disorders of fluid and solute balance. This extension no doubt arises because the kidneys usually provide the "final common pathway" through which fluid and solute balance is regulated. Yet, like many biological regulatory systems, the mechanisms preserving fluid and solute balance – and hence those responsible for fluid and solute *im*balance – involve not only the kidneys but many other organs as well. One cannot deal with a problem of water balance without taking into account the possible contributory role of the antidiuretic hormone (ADH or vasopressin) that is produced in the brain, nor a problem of Na^+ balance without considering aldosterone, nor a problem of H^+ balance without thinking about respiration. In this textbook, problems of balance are taken up first and renal disorders later. One reason for this sequence is my conviction that renal dysfunction – for example, acute and chronic renal failure – can be understood better if the concept of balance has been mastered.

Concept of Balance

The terms *balance* and *steady state* are synonymous. Both refer to a state of equilibrium of a biological system in which the total input of a given substance into that system (both exogenous and endogenous) equals the total output from that system. At any one time, this system might be in balance for one substance, say H_2O or calories, while it is out of balance for another substance, such as K^+ or H^+. In clinical nephrology we usually specify the balance we are talking about, whether it be balance for H_2O, Na^+, K^+, Cl^-, H^+, HCO_3^-, N, or any of the other substances in the body. Furthermore, we *usually* refer to a 24-hour period; that is, we speak of the *daily* output of the given substance being equal to the daily intake plus endogenous production of that substance. Finally, in the parlance of clinical nephrology, we often, but not necessarily, imply that the person is in balance on a normal intake and normal endogenous production of the given substance.

Positive Balance Versus Negative Balance

When a subject or a patient is in *im*balance, the total output of a given substance does not equal the sum of its intake plus production. If the sum exceeds the output, the individual is in *positive balance;* if the sum is less than the output, he is in *negative balance.* Thus, if a patient's daily intake of Na^+ is greater than the total output of this ion, the patient gains Na^+ and is said to be in positive Na^+ balance; conversely, if the daily intake of Na^+ is less than the output, the patient loses Na^+ and is in negative Na^+ balance.

Clinical Criteria of Fluid and Solute Balance

Body Weight. In a patient who is eating adequately, a change in H_2O balance will be reflected by a change in body weight. If the patient drinks more fluid than he excretes and if his caloric intake balances his caloric expenditure, the excess fluid intake must be reflected — gram per gram — in a gain of body weight; the reverse holds for a patient who is drinking less fluid than he excretes. The body weight will quite accurately reflect an acute (48- to 72-hour) change in H_2O balance, even in a patient who is not eating. During more prolonged periods of fasting, about 250 g per day in an adult patient must be subtracted from the total weight loss to obtain an estimate of H_2O loss; this subtraction accounts for the loss in body weight that is due to catabolism of endogenous fats and proteins.

As a means of assessing H_2O balance, the simple test of weighing the patient on the same scales once or twice daily is far simpler, less expensive, and often more accurate than either measuring the intake and output of fluid or using cumbersome dilution techniques. This fact cannot be overemphasized, and the usefulness of measuring body weight in dealing with problems of fluid and solute balance will be repeatedly referred to in this text.

Plasma or Serum Concentration. Let us consider another common criterion of the steady state: the plasma or serum Na^+ concentration. The normal range for this variable is about 136 to 146 mEq per liter. (The difference between plasma and serum is the absence of the blood-clotting proteins from the latter; this difference has a negligible influence on the Na^+ concentration and is therefore ordinarily ignored.) The concentration of a given solute is the amount of the solute divided by the volume of the solvent. The determinants of the plasma Na^+ concentration are therefore the amount of Na^+ in the plasma and the plasma volume, which is mainly H_2O (about 92 percent). A person who is in balance for Na^+ and H_2O by definition excretes the same amount of these two substances that he ingests and produces endogenously during a 24-hour period. Hence, over that period of time, the amount of both Na^+ and H_2O in the plasma compartment will remain stable and therefore so will the plasma Na^+ concentration. For these reasons, a stable plasma Na^+ concentration reflects the balanced state.

Note that the presence of a normal plasma Na^+ concentration is not an essential condition for balance. Many patients with an abnormal, say low, plasma Na^+ concentration attain a new steady state. This point is considered further in relation to the syndrome of inappropriate ADH secretion (SIADH), discussed below (Fig. 1-3) and in Chapter 2.

Obviously, a steady state could be judged as well by a stable concentration for any of the solutes in plasma (Fig. 1-1) or by the concentration of all the solutes combined. The latter, known as the *osmolality,* is a function of the *number* of discrete particles in solution, regardless of their mass, charge, or size. Which concentration the physician pays the greatest attention to is determined by which balance he is concerned about. If he is worried about the patient's H_2O balance, he will watch the body weight and the plasma Na^+ concentration or the serum osmolality; if he is concerned about H^+ balance, he will follow mainly the plasma HCO_3^- concentration or the pH; and there are many other examples.

Clinical Tests Are Estimates

The determinants of the plasma Na^+ concentration are not quite as simple as they were described above. In the clinical laboratory, plasma or serum Na^+ concentration is measured on the whole plasma or whole serum, not just on that part of the plasma or serum that is H_2O. To the extent, therefore, that the nonaqueous portion of plasma or serum may change, the volume of the plasma or serum (and hence the Na^+ concentration) may change, even when the body is in balance for Na^+ and H_2O. The solutes that can thus alter the Na^+ concentration are mainly proteins, fats, and carbohydrates. When these solutes are present in the plasma in amounts sufficient to alter the Na^+ concentration, they usually reflect a severe disease state to which the physician will have been alerted, for example, multiple myeloma, hypercholesterolemia, or diabetes mellitus (see Problem 3-1 and Table 3-4).

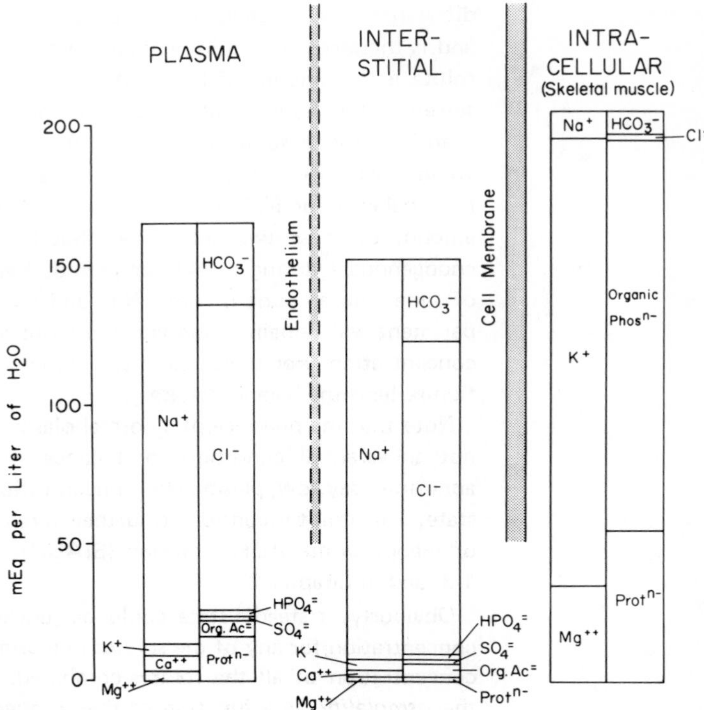

Figure 1-1

The main solute constituents of the major body-fluid compartments. The concentrations are expressed as chemical equivalents to emphasize that the compartments are made up mainly of electrolytes and that within any one space, the total negative charges are neutralized by the positive charges.

The values depicted for the intracellular fluid are rough approximations at best. They reflect current estimates for skeletal muscle, but since some cells have unique composition, these estimates are not precisely representative of all intracellular fluid. Furthermore, the extent to which some intracellular ions are bound or ionized is not known, so that the equivalences for such ions, as well as for organic phosphates and proteins, are also approximations. Despite these limitations, however, the diagram serves to emphasize important and typical differences between intracellular and extracellular fluid. Organic phosphates include the adenosine phosphates (AMP, ADP, and ATP), glycerophosphate, and creatine phosphate. Modified from J. L. Gamble, *Chemical Anatomy, Physiology and Pathology of Extracellular Fluid* (6th ed.). Cambridge, Mass.: Harvard University Press, 1954.

A second source of possible error arises because Na^+ and H_2O are not confined exclusively to the plasma compartment (Fig. 1-1). One cannot be sure, therefore, that because the entire body is in balance for Na^+ and H_2O there will be no change in the amount of Na^+ and of H_2O in the plasma compartment (see Concept of External and Internal Balance, below). Usually, however, this is the case. Even in diseases in which internal shifts of solute and water occur, a new steady state is attained that is analogous to the one that will be shown in Figure 1-3.

Most clinical tests do in fact yield estimates, rather than precise measurements, of the function that is being assessed. In a research setting, one can determine Na^+ balance rather precisely by measuring all dietary intake of Na^+ as well as all the output of this ion, not only in urine but also in the stool and other secretions such as sweat. One also can rather accurately determine H_2O balance through the use of the dilution principle, which involves injection of a foreign substance such as antipyrine, heavy H_2O (D_2O), or tritiated H_2O (HTO). Such methods, however, require hospitalization of the patient on a special ward, the injection of foreign compounds, and the use of specially trained personnel and expensive equipment. The simpler clinical tests yield values that are often nearly as accurate; in any case, they are precise enough for the diagnosis and treatment of clinical problems. Thus, for the sake of low cost, convenience, and safety for the patient, the clinical test often represents a slight compromise in precision and specificity.

Concept of External and Internal Balance

In most of the preceding discussion, we dealt with body H_2O as if it were contained in a single, homogeneous pool, and with solutes such as Na^+ as if they were distributed evenly throughout a single space. Actually, of course, H_2O is apportioned among three major compartments — intracellular, interstitial, and plasma — and several minor (transcellular) compartments (Fig. 1-2). Its distribution in these spaces is not homogeneous. Furthermore, solutes (e.g., proteins, Na^+, K^+, and H^+) are distributed even less uniformly among these compartments (Fig. 1-1). Nevertheless, in the steady state during health, the normally uneven distribution of these substances is maintained. That is the tacit assumption when considering balance, as we did above; the body is taken to be a unit (i.e., a "black box") and we consider only what has entered the body plus what has been produced by it and what has left it during a given interval of time. This concept of balance, that is, when the body is considered as a black box, is known as *external balance.*

In many disease processes, there are alterations in the proportions in which H_2O and solutes are normally distributed among the various body-fluid compartments. For example, in some

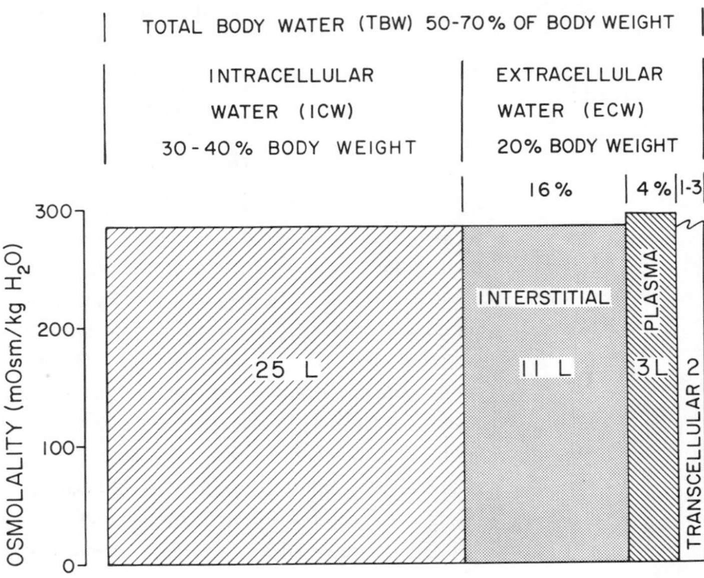

Figure 1-2
Approximate sizes of the major body-fluid compartments, expressed both as percentages of body weight and in mean absolute values for an adult human being who weighs 70 kg (154 pounds). The normal values among individuals vary considerably, and thus no one value should be taken too rigidly; a good rule of thumb to remember is "20, 40, 60," referring to the percentage of the body weight that is constituted by extracellular, intracellular, and total body water, respectively. The plasma has a slightly higher osmolality than the intracellular and interstitial compartments; this small difference can be ignored when dealing with problems of fluid balance. From H. Valtin, *Renal Function: Mechanisms Preserving Fluid and Solute Balance in Health.* Boston: Little, Brown, 1973.

forms of K^+ deficiency, there is a selective shift of H^+ from the extracellular to the intracellular compartment (see Fig. 4-2); similarly, in primary disturbances of H^+ balance, K^+ often moves from one compartment to the other (also Fig. 4-2). Consideration of such shifts within the body constitutes the topic of *internal balance.* Disturbances of internal balance can occur without a disruption of external balance. More commonly, however, the two happen simultaneously, especially as a disease process evolves.

Steady State in Disease

Frequently in disease a new steady state is reached in which external balance is normal while, at the same time, both the volume and composition of some or all of the fluid compartments are maintained at abnormal values (Fig. 1-3). (A second example of the attainment of a new steady state in disease is discussed as part of Problem 1-1, for which a detailed answer is given in the section, Answers to Problems, following the text.)

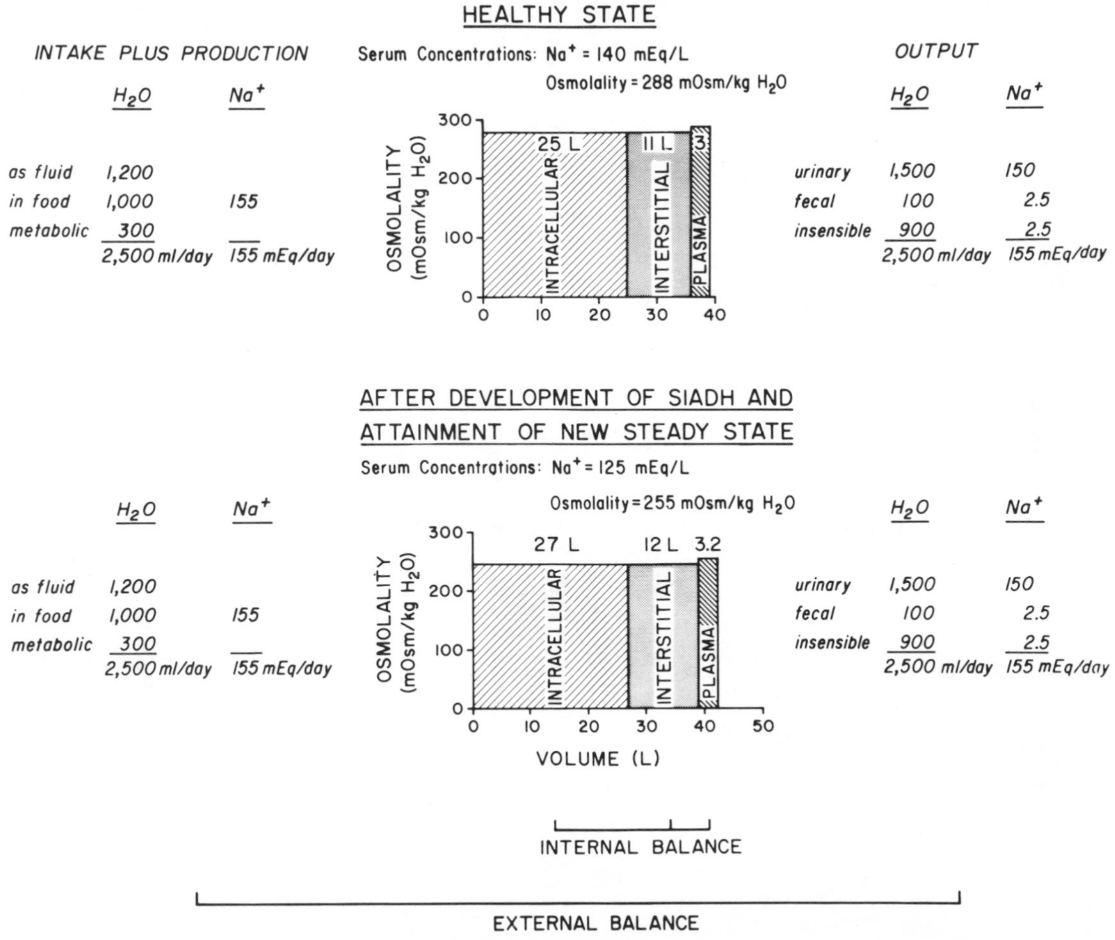

Figure 1-3
Dynamics for the development of a new steady state in the syndrome of inappropriate secretion of antidiuretic hormone (SIADH). Data based in part on J. R. Jaenike and C. Waterhouse, *J. Clin. Endocrinol. Metab.* 21:231, 1961.

HEALTHY STATE

Serum Concentrations: Na^+ = 140 mEq/L
Osmolality = 288 mOsm/kg H_2O

INTAKE PLUS PRODUCTION

	H_2O	Na^+
as fluid	1,200	
in food	1,000	155
metabolic	300	
	2,500 ml/day	155 mEq/day

OSMOLALITY (mOsm/kg H_2O): 300, 200, 100, 0
INTRACELLULAR 25 L; INTERSTITIAL 11 L; PLASMA 3
0 10 20 30 40

OUTPUT

	H_2O	Na^+
urinary	1,500	150
fecal	100	2.5
insensible	900	2.5
	2,500 ml/day	155 mEq/day

AFTER DEVELOPMENT OF SIADH AND ATTAINMENT OF NEW STEADY STATE

Serum Concentrations: Na^+ = 125 mEq/L
Osmolality = 255 mOsm/kg H_2O

	H_2O	Na^+
as fluid	1,200	
in food	1,000	155
metabolic	300	
	2,500 ml/day	155 mEq/day

OSMOLALITY (mOsm/kg H_2O): 300, 200, 100, 0
INTRACELLULAR 27 L; INTERSTITIAL 12 L; PLASMA 3.2
0 10 20 30 40 50
VOLUME (L)

	H_2O	Na^+
urinary	1,500	150
fecal	100	2.5
insensible	900	2.5
	2,500 ml/day	155 mEq/day

INTERNAL BALANCE

EXTERNAL BALANCE

In the healthy state a person is in both external and internal balance (Fig. 1-3). He consumes 2,500 ml of H_2O per day: 1,200 ml as liquid, 1,000 ml in food, and 300 ml from aerobic metabolism. He also excretes 2,500 ml of H_2O each day: 1,500 ml as urine, 100 ml in stool, and 900 ml as insensible loss (i.e., loss that is not perceived, as by evaporation from breath and skin). His intake of Na^+ is 155 mEq per day, and he excretes 155 mEq: 150 mEq in the urine and about 2.5 mEq each in stool and by insensible means. He is thus in external balance for H_2O and Na^+, and the volume and composition of his fluid compartments are stable at normal values.

As this person develops the syndrome of inappropriate secretion of antidiuretic hormone (SIADH, in Chap. 2), he goes into positive H_2O balance; that is, the total loss of H_2O from his body is less than the sum of H_2O intake plus endogenous H_2O production. In the example illustrated in Figure 1-3, the patient retained a total of 3 liters of solute-free H_2O over a period of perhaps eight days. Because the membranes separating the major fluid compartments (Fig. 1-1) are freely permeable to H_2O, this extra H_2O was distributed throughout the compartments in proportion to their original sizes; the approximate increase in the volume of each compartment is shown in the lower half of Figure 1-3. During the development of SIADH, there is also a slight loss of Na^+, amounting, in the example illustrated, to a cumulative total of about 110 mEq.

After seven to ten days, many patients reach a new steady state. External balance for H_2O and Na^+ is reestablished, the daily total output of these substances again equaling their intake and production. There is also internal balance, for both the volume and composition of the fluid compartments are stable. Note, however, that in the new steady state, some major variables are at abnormal levels: the serum Na^+ concentration and serum osmolality are low, the fluid compartments are expanded, and the osmolality of the compartments is abnormally low.

Summary

When an individual is in *balance* — that is, in the steady or equilibrium state — the intake plus the endogenous production of a given substance over a period of time equals the output of that substance during the same interval. When the sum of intake plus production of a substance exceeds its output, the individual is in *positive balance* for that substance; when the sum is less than the output, the individual is in *negative balance.* The substance for which balance is determined must be specified — for example, H_2O balance, H^+ balance, or nitrogen balance — and it is possible for an individual to be simultaneously in negative balance for one or more substances and in positive balance for others.

In clinical practice, the balanced state is usually judged by the stability of some parameter such as the body weight (H_2O balance), the serum Na^+ concentration (Na^+ balance and/or H_2O balance), the body temperature (caloric balance), or the arterial pH (H^+ balance).

External balance means a state in which the sum of intake and endogenous production of a substance equals the output of that substance, regardless of how the substance is distributed among the various body-fluid compartments. *Internal balance* refers to shifts of H_2O or solutes from one body-fluid compartment to another. During the development of an illness (i.e., during the acute state, usually lasting from a few hours to a few days), a patient is frequently in both external and internal *im*balance. In chronic diseases, the patient is often in both external and internal balance, but in a "new" steady state in which both the volume and composition of some or all of the body-fluid compartments — and hence the body weight or certain serum concentrations — may be abnormal.

Problem 1-1

Note: The answers to this and subsequent problems are given in a special section at the end of the text.

In the clinical laboratory, serum concentrations of phosphate are usually reported as milligrams of inorganic phosphorus per 100 ml of serum (often referred to as *mg percent* or *mg per deciliter*). A test on a patient in renal failure is reported as 6.2 mg/dl.

Express this value in millimoles and milliequivalents of phosphate per liter of serum. (For atomic and molecular weights, see Appendix, Table 1-7.)

Why is the serum concentration of phosphate elevated in renal failure? (*Hint:* Recall how phosphate is normally handled by the kidneys, and consider how the filtered load of phosphate — that is, the product of glomerular filtration rate (GFR) times the plasma phosphate concentration (P_{Phos}) — is changed as the GFR is decreased. Then think of the effect of these changes on the balance for phosphate.)

Problem 1-2

Why does a blood urea nitrogen concentration (BUN) of 14 mg/100 ml contribute 5 mOsm/kg H_2O to the plasma osmolality (Table 1-2)? Why does a blood glucose concentration of 80 mg/100 ml contribute 4 mOsm/kg H_2O?

Appendix

In clinical nephrology, the physician frequently *assumes* normal values in calculating fluid and solute balance. These assumptions are usually rounded off and thus may deviate slightly from the true average. Common examples include a serum Na^+ concentration of 140 mEq per liter, total body water equal to 60 percent of body weight, and a normal plasma osmolality of 300 mOsm/kg H_2O. It is the purpose of this appendix to provide a single place where nearly all the normal values used in this text are assembled.

Several of the following tables list ranges as well as mean values. This has been done in order to emphasize that for many parameters, there is a wide range of normality. Nevertheless, when a given datum must be assumed, it is usually safe to choose the average value listed.

Probably the most important *exception* to the safe use of many of the "normal" values listed below applies to pediatric nephrology. For example, the volume of extracellular fluid decreases during the first year of life from about 45 percent to about 25 percent of body weight. Such changes are even more striking in premature infants. The special values for pediatrics have not been listed in this appendix, because the principles are by and large not different from those in adult nephrology; only specific values may be different, and then mainly during the first year of life. The special considerations that apply to pediatric nephrology can be found in the references that have been listed at the end of this chapter.

Table 1-1
Normal plasma, serum, or blood concentrations in adults*

Substance	Range	Average Value Usually Quoted in Treating Patients	Comments
Alcohol (ethanol)	0	0	Illegal for driving: 100 to 150 mg/100 ml Intoxicated: 250 to 400 mg/100 ml Stuporous: >350 mg/100 ml
Barbiturates	0	0	Levels seen in coma: phenobarbital, about 11 mg/100 ml; most other barbiturates, 2 to 4 mg/100 ml
Bicarbonate	24 to 30 mMoles/L[a]	24 mEq/L[b]	[a]Venous plasma [b]Arterial plasma, which is now commonly sampled in patients with problems of H^+ balance
Calcium	4.5 to 5.5 mEq/L	10 mg/100 ml	Approximately 50% is bound to serum proteins
Chloride	96 to 106 mEq/L	100 mEq/L	
Creatinine	0.7 to 1.5 mg/100 ml	1.2 mg/100 ml	
Doriden (glutethimide)	0	0	A nonbarbiturate sedative that is sometimes used in suicide attempts. Levels seen in coma: >1 to 2 mg/100 ml
Glucose	70 to 100 mg/100 ml	80 mg/100 ml[c]	[c]Determined in the fasting state; so-called fasting blood sugar (FBS)
Hematocrit (Hct)	40% to 50%	45%	Also frequently called packed cell volume (PCV)
Lactic acid	0.6 to 1.8 mEq/L	—	
Lipids:			
Cholesterol	135 to 270 mg/100 ml	—	
Triglycerides	50 to 150 mg/100 ml	—	
Lithium	0	0	Used in the treatment of manic-depressive disorders. Effective level, about 1.5 to 2.0 mEq/L; toxic level, >2.5 mEq/L. Lithium can cause nephrogenic diabetes insipidus (see Chap. 13)
Magnesium	1.6 to 2.2 mEq/L	2 mEq/L	
Osmolality	280 to 295 mOsm/kg H_2O	287 mOsm/kg H_2O[d]	[d]A value of 300 is often used because it is a round figure that is easy to remember. This approximation does not introduce important quantitative error in most computations for evaluation of fluid and solute balance

(Continued)

Table 1-1 (Continued)

Substance	Range	Average Value Usually Quoted in Treating Patients	Comments
Oxygen saturation (arterial)	96% to 100%	—	
PCO_2 (arterial)	37 to 43 mm Hg	40 mm Hg	
PO_2 (arterial)	75 to 100 mm Hg	—	While breathing room air. Value varies with age
pH (arterial)	7.37 to 7.42	7.40	
Phosphate[e]	2 to 3 mEq/L	3.5 mg/100 ml	[e]Measured as phosphorus. The exact concentration of phosphate in milliequivalents per liter depends on pH of plasma. See Answer to Problem 1-1
Potassium	3.5 to 5.5 mEq/L	4.5 mEq/L	
Protein (total)	6 to 8 g/100 ml	7 g/100 ml	
Albumin[f]	4 to 5 g/100 ml	—	[f]Proportions of albumin and the various globulins, expressed as percentages of total protein, are now commonly measured by paper electrophoresis
Globulin[f]	2 to 3 g/100 ml	—	
Salicylate	0	0[g]	[g]Therapeutic, 20 to 25 mg/100 ml; toxic >30 mg/100 ml
Sodium	136 to 146 mEq/L	140 mEq/L	
Urea nitrogen (BUN)	9 to 18 mg/100 ml	12 mg/100 ml[h]	[h]Measured as the nitrogen contained in urea. Since urea diffuses freely into cells, values for serum, plasma, or whole blood are nearly identical (BUN = blood urea nitrogen). Average value varies with diet; BUN of 18 mg/100 ml may be normal or may reflect considerable reduction in renal function (see Chap. 8)
Uric acid	3 to 7 mg/100 ml	5 mg/100 ml	

*Some values are different in children; see text (Appendix).

Table 1-2
Determinants of plasma osmolality

Cations	mEq/L	mMoles/L	Anions	mEq/L	mMoles/L
Na^+	140	140	Cl^-	100	100
K^+	4	4.5	HCO_3^-	26	26
Ca^{2+}	5	2.5	HPO_4^{2-}	2	1
Mg^{2+}	2	1	SO_4^{2-}	1	0.5
			Organic acids	7	3.5
			Proteins	15	3
Totals:	151	148.0		151	134.0

Blood urea nitrogen (BUN) of 14 mg/100 ml contributes 5 mOsm/kg H_2O
Blood glucose of 80 mg/100 ml contributes 4 mOsm/kg H_2O
Total calculated osmolality = 148 + 134 + 5 + 4 = 291 mOsm/kg H_2O
Rule of thumb: $2[Na^+]$ = plasma osmolality

Table 1-2 contains several approximations, which, however, do not introduce important quantitative errors: (1) the equivalances of phosphates, organic acids, and proteins vary, but reasonable average values are listed; (2) similarly, because there are several organic acids and different proteins, their molar concentrations represent averages; (3) finally, the molar concentrations have been converted to milliosmoles per kilogram of water without correcting for the difference between liters of solution and kilograms of solvent or for dissociation of the compounds. To the extent that a molecule of NaCl is not completely dissociated into an ion of Na^+ and one of Cl^-, the molecule contributes less than two discrete particles to the solution; hence, 100 mMoles of NaCl per liter is somewhat less (by about 5 percent) than 200 mOsm/kg H_2O. The osmotic coefficient that corrects for this effect varies not only for each compound but also with the concentration of that compound. The corrections may be ignored, however, since even without them, the calculated osmolality of plasma falls within the normal range (Table 1-1) as determined by measuring the freezing-point depression of many samples of normal plasma.

The rule of thumb — two times plasma Na^+ concentration equals plasma osmolality — yields an estimate that usually falls within ±10 mOsm/kg H_2O of the true value as measured with an osmometer. This estimate is sufficiently accurate for the vast majority of clinical purposes. The reason that the rule of thumb works is that Na^+ and its attendant anions (mainly Cl^- and HCO_3^-) normally account for at least 90 percent of the osmotically active particles in plasma. Even a near-lethal doubling of the K^+ concentration (i.e., to 8 mEq per liter) would increase the plasma osmolality by only 1 percent.

A change in the concentration of certain solutes besides Na^+, Cl^-, and HCO_3^- can importantly alter the plasma osmolality. These other solutes mainly include lipids, urea, and sugar (see Chap. 3), but the physician is usually alerted to these possible exceptions to the rule of thumb by his knowing that the patient has hyperlipidemia, renal failure, or diabetes mellitus. Furthermore, BUN and blood sugar have often been measured as part of a routine screening procedure, so corrections for these solutes can be applied in calculating the plasma osmolality.

Table 1-3
Normal urinary concentrations in adult humans whose diet includes protein

Urinary *concentration* depends not only on the rate of excretion of a particular solute but also on the amount of the solvent (i.e., urine) that is excreted. Since the excretion of both solute and solvent can vary greatly depending on their intake, the normal concentrations have wide ranges, and a single average value is almost meaningless

Urine output is normally 1 to 1.5 liters per day. Therefore, the range of the normal rate of urinary excretion of a particular substance can be quickly estimated as being from the concentration of the substance listed below to about 1.5 times that concentration

Substance	Range	Comments
Ammonium	30 to 50 mEq/L	
Calcium	5 to 12 mEq/L	Normal excretion is 150 mg (7.5 mEq) per day or less
Chloride	50 to 130 mEq/L	
Creatinine	6 to 20 mMoles/L	Daily production of creatinine depends primarily on skeletal muscle mass. Since this mass varies greatly among individuals, so does the normal urinary excretion of creatinine: children, >8 mg; women, 9 to 27 mg; men, 16 to 32 mg per kilogram of body weight per day
Glucose	≈ 0	About 15 to 130 mg of glucose may be normally excreted per day. This amount, however, is not detected by routine tests, which are sensitive to about 1,000 mg of glucose per liter of urine
Magnesium	2 to 18 mEq/L	
Organic acids (total)	10 to 25 mMoles/L	These acids have different valences, depending on the compound and the urinary pH; the molar concentration listed assumes an average valence of minus two
Citric acid[a]	0.5 to 7 mMoles/L	[a]The sum of these three acids does not equal the above total, because there are other organic acids in urine
Lactic acid[a]	1 to 7 mMoles/L	
Uric acid[a]	0.5 to 6.0 mMoles/L	
Osmolality	500 to 800 mOsm/kg H_2O	A random sample is likely to have an osmolality in the range indicated. However, a healthy person may show a urine osmolality of less than 100 mOsm/kg H_2O if he has drunk large amounts of fluid or up to 1,400 mOsm/kg H_2O if he is dehydrated

(Continued)

Table 1-3 (Continued)

Substance	Range	Comments
pH	5.0 to 7.0	
Phosphate	20 to 40 mMoles/L	Measured as phosphorus; excretion rates are usually expressed in grams per day, and the average normal value is 1 g per day
Potassium	20 to 70 mEq/L	
Protein	≈ 0	Healthy persons excrete small amounts of protein, the normal value being less than 150 mg per day. This amount usually cannot be detected by routine tests, which are sensitive to about 100 mg per liter
Sodium	50 to 130 mEq/L	
Specific gravity	1.015 to 1.022	See comment regarding osmolality. A healthy person may have a range of urine specific gravity from about 1.001 to 1.030 or slightly higher
Sulfate	30 to 45 mEq/L	
Titratable acid (T.A.)	10 to 40 mEq/L	Usually expressed as daily excretion, for which the normal range is 20 to 40 mEq per day
Urea	10 to 20 g/L	Usually measured as urea nitrogen, for which the range would be about 5 to 10 g per liter

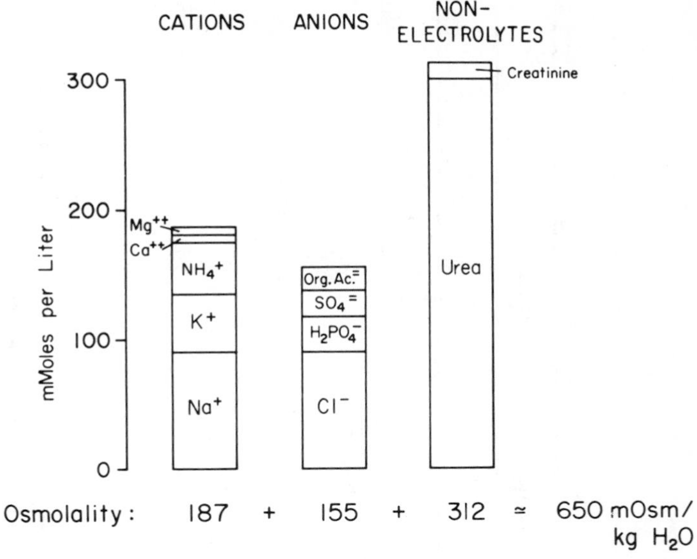

Figure 1-4
Determinants of the urine osmolality. The major constituents of normal urine at their average concentrations have been taken from Table 1-3. Note that the determinants of the urine osmolality differ strikingly from those of plasma (Table 1-2): (1) urea accounts for about 40 percent of urine osmolality, whereas it contributes less than 2 percent to the osmolality of normal plasma, and (2) Na^+, with its attendant anions, usually makes up less than one-third of the urine osmolality, while it constitutes 95 percent or more of normal plasma osmolality. Therefore, a simple rule of thumb cannot be applied to urine.

There are two means of estimating urine osmolality, provided that abnormal solutes (e.g., glucose, glycerol, or contrast media used in radiology) are not present in the urine in large amounts.

1. The sum,

   $$\text{Urea concentration} + 2(Na^+ + K^+ \text{ concentrations})$$

   will usually come within 15 percent of the urine osmolality.

2. The urine specific gravity (S.G.) will yield an estimate within ±200 mOsm per kilogram H_2O of the true osmolality as measured in an osmometer (see Figs. 2-2 and 11-A). Perhaps surprisingly, this estimate is sufficiently close to be useful in most clinical problems. Many nephrologists use the following estimates, interpolating linearly for the specific gravities not listed:

Measured Urine Specific Gravity	Estimated Urine Osmolality (mOsm/kg H_2O)
1.010	300
1.020	700
1.030	1,100

Figure from H. Valtin, ***Renal Function: Mechanisms Preserving Fluid and Solute Balance in Health.*** Boston: Little, Brown, 1973.

Table 1-4
Daily volumes and concentrations of major electrolytes in gastrointestinal secretions, diarrhea, and sweat

	Volume (liters/day)	Electrolyte Concentration (mEq/L)				
		Na^+	K^+	H^+	Cl^-	HCO_3^-
Saliva: Mean	1.5	30	20	—	31	15
(Range)[a]		(20 to 46)	(16 to 23)	—	(24 to 44)	(12 to 18)
Gastric juice	2.5	50	10	90	110	0
		(30 to 90)	(4 to 12)	—	(52 to 124)	—
Bile	0.5	140	5	—	105	40
		(120 to 170)	(3 to 12)	—	(80 to 120)	(30 to 50)
Pancreatic juice	0.7	140	5	—	60	90
		(113 to 153)	(3 to 7)	—	(54 to 95)	(70 to 110)
Small intestine	1.5	120	5	—	110	35
		(72 to 158)	(4 to 7)	—	(70 to 127)	(20 to 40)
Diarrhea	1.0 to 1.5[b]	130	10	—	95	20
		(120 to 140)	(5 to 15)	—	(90 to 100)	(15 to 30)
Sweat	0 to 3.0[b]	50	5	—	50	0
		(18 to 97)	(1 to 15)	—	(18 to 97)	—

[a]In many clinical situations (e.g., vomiting, diarrhea, or surgical drainage of intestinal secretions) volume and electrolyte concentrations are not determined. In lieu of precise measurements, the physician then proceeds to treat the patient on the basis of estimates. The mean values listed serve as a useful guide for such estimates; normal ranges are also given in order to emphasize that there is wide variability.

[b]May be greater.

Data compiled from M. G. Rosenfeld (ed.), *Manual of Medical Therapeutics* (22nd ed.). Boston: Little, Brown, 1977; J. L. Gamble, *Chemical Anatomy, Physiology, and Pathology of Extracellular Fluid* (6th ed.). Cambridge, Mass.: Harvard University Press, 1954; A. I. Arieff, in M. H. Maxwell and C. R. Kleeman (eds.), *Clinical Disorders of Fluid and Electrolyte Metabolism* (2nd ed.). New York: McGraw-Hill, 1972.

Table 1-5
Miscellaneous normal values for adult humans not given in preceding figures and tables

	Average Value	Comments
Anion gap	13 mEq/L	Anion gap = $[Na^+] - ([Cl^-] + [HCO_3^-])$ Normal range: 10 to 16 mEq/L
Body surface area	1.73 meter^2	
Body weight	70 kg	
Chloride:		
Total body	2,400 mEq	
Exchangeable	2,000 mEq	Refers to the amount of Cl^- that is readily miscible with ingested or administered Cl^-
Creatinine, daily rise during acute renal failure	2.5 mg/100 ml	At normal metabolic rate
Fluid volumes:	—	For ranges, see Fig. 1-2
Total body water (TBW)	60% of body weight	
Intracellular water (ICW)	40% of body weight	Often abbreviated as ICF (intracellular fluid)
Extracellular water (ECW)	20% of body weight	Often abbreviated as ECF (extracellular fluid)
Plasma	4% of body weight	Not calculated separately in most clinical problems but usually considered as the single space of extracellular fluid
Interstitial fluid	16% of body weight	
Glomerular filtration rate (GFR)	125 ml/min	
$[H^+]$ of arterial plasma	40 nEq/L	A rule of thumb that yields a rough estimate of $[H^+]$ within the range compatible with survival is $[H^+] = 25\ PCO_2/[HCO_3^-]$. Note that units are nanoequivalents per liter
Lean tissue balance:		
On basis of nitrogen	30 g wet tissue per gram N balance	Assumes (1) no parenteral administration of protein and (2) steady-state excretion of nitrogen
Ratio of potassium to nitrogen	3 mEq K^+ per gram N balance	When either a positive or negative balance shows a ratio of about this value, it may be assumed that lean tissue — mainly protein in muscle, but also in connective tissue and solution — is being either formed or broken down, respectively

(Continued)

Table 1-5 (Continued)

	Average Value	Comments
Protein	1 g N per 6 g protein	
pK:		Selected list of some common physiological compounds
Acetic acid	4.7	
Acetoacetic acid	3.8	
Ammonia	9.2	At 25°C
β-hydroxybutyric acid	4.8	
Creatinine	5.0	
Lactic acid	3.9	
Oxyhemoglobin	6.7	
Phosphoric acid	6.8	Refers to HPO_4^{2-}: $H_2PO_4^-$; phosphoric acid has two other pKs
Reduced hemoglobin	7.9	
Potassium:		
Total body	3,500 mEq	Refers to the total amount of K^+ present in the body
Exchangeable	3,000 mEq	Refers to the amount of K^+ that is readily miscible with ingested or administered K^+
Sodium:		
Total body	5,000 mEq	
Exchangeable	3,000 mEq	Much of the nonexchangeable Na^+ is in bone
Urea, daily rise during acute renal failure	20 mg/100 ml	At normal metabolic rate
Water content of tissues:		
Bone	25%	
Fat	20%	
Muscle	80%	
Plasma	92%	

Table 1-6
Average daily balance (amount per day) for water and some major solutes
Data for an adult human under normal environmental conditions who is eating a normal diet containing protein

Substance	Intake		Output		
	Oral	Metabolic	Urinary	Fecal	Insensible
Water (ml):					
As fluid	1,200	300	1,500	100	900
In food	1,000	—	—	—	—
Sodium (mEq)	155	—	150	2.5	2.5
Potassium (mEq)	75	—	70	5	—
Chloride (mEq)	155	—	150	2.5	2.5
Nitrogen (g)	10	—	9	1	—
Acid (mEq):					
Nonvolatile	—	50	50	—	—
Volatile	—	14,000	—	—	14,000

INTAKE PLUS ENDOGENOUS PRODUCTION ml/day		OUTPUT ml/day	
Water as fluid	1,200	Urine	1,500
Water in food	1,000	Insensible	900
Water of oxidation	300	Respiratory 400	
		Skin 500	

Internal Cycling of Gastrointestinal Fluid	Secreted		Reabsorbed
Saliva	1,500		
Gastric juice	2,500		
Bile	500		
Pancreatic juice	700		
Intestinal juice	3,000		
	8,200	–	8,100

= Water in stool 100

FLUID BALANCE 2,500 ... 2,500

Figure 1-5
Average turnover of fluid (milliliters per day) of a healthy adult human who is moderately active in a temperate environment. Note that although normally nearly all the gastrointestinal secretions are reabsorbed, in disease states such as vomiting or diarrhea, these secretions can quickly lead to negative fluid balance, as well as to negative balance of electrolytes (Table 1-4). Modified from J. A. F. Stevenson, in W. S. Yamamoto and J. R. Brobeck (eds.), *Physiological Controls and Regulations.* Philadelphia: Saunders, 1965.

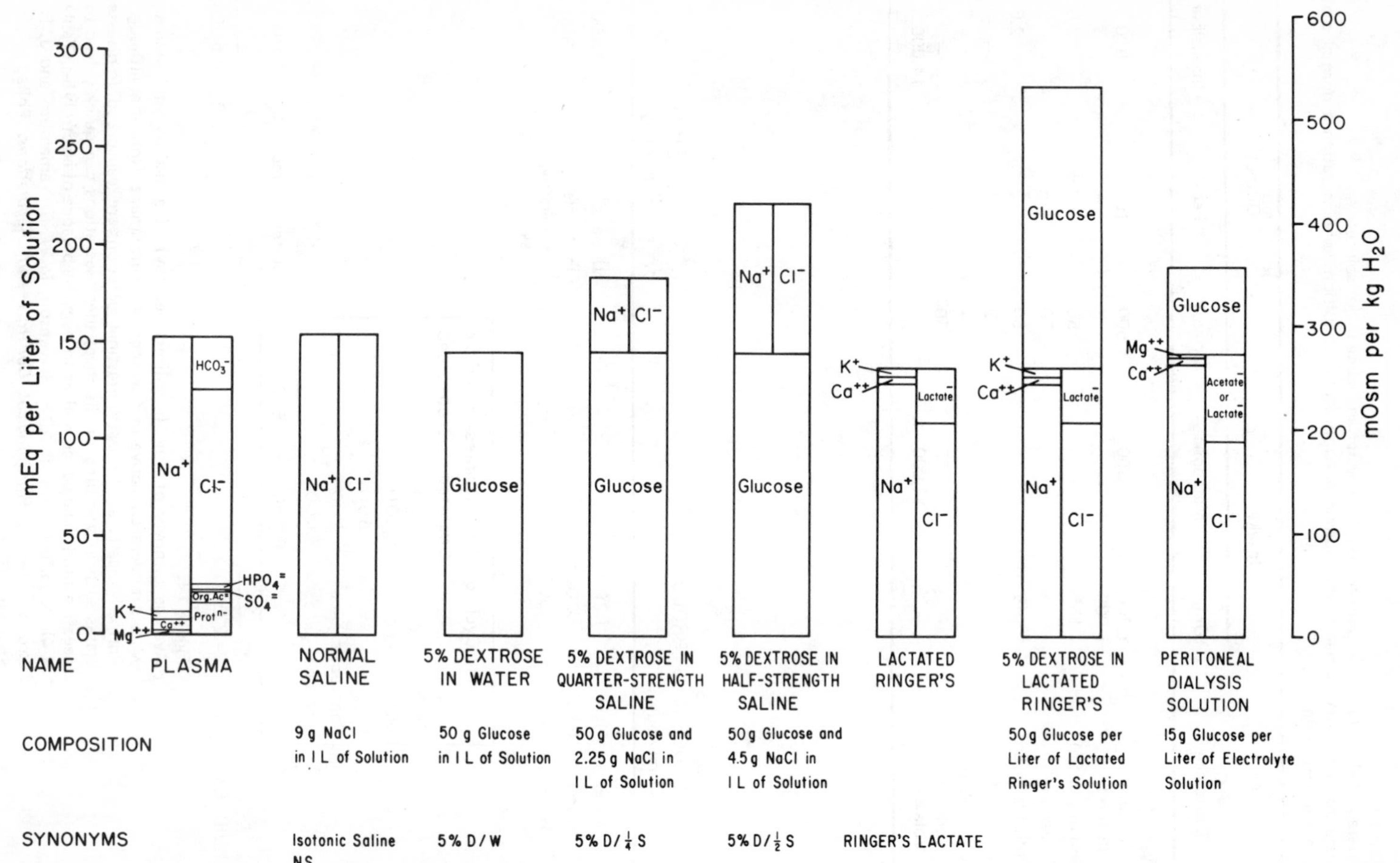

mEq per Liter of Solution
0
50
100
150
200
250
300
mOsm per kg H_2O
0
100
200
300
400
500
600
NAME
COMPOSITION
SYNONYMS
PLASMA
Na^+
K^+
Mg^{++}
Ca^{++}
HCO_3^-
Cl^-
Org. Ac.
Prot^{n-}
$HPO_4^=$
$SO_4^=$
NORMAL SALINE
Na^+
Cl^-
9 g NaCl in 1 L of Solution
Isotonic Saline NS
5% DEXTROSE IN WATER
Glucose
50 g Glucose in 1 L of Solution
5% D/W
5% DEXTROSE IN QUARTER-STRENGTH SALINE
Na^+
Cl^-
Glucose
50 g Glucose and 2.25 g NaCl in 1 L of Solution
5% D/¼ S
5% DEXTROSE IN HALF-STRENGTH SALINE
Na^+
Cl^-
Glucose
50 g Glucose and 4.5 g NaCl in 1 L of Solution
5% D/½ S
LACTATED RINGER'S
K^+
Ca^{++}
Na^+
Lactate$^-$
Cl^-
RINGER'S LACTATE
5% DEXTROSE IN LACTATED RINGER'S
Glucose
K^+
Ca^{++}
Na^+
Lactate$^-$
Cl^-
50 g Glucose per Liter of Lactated Ringer's Solution
PERITONEAL DIALYSIS SOLUTION
Glucose
Mg^{++}
Ca^{++}
Na^+
Acetate$^-$ or Lactate$^-$
Cl^-
15 g Glucose per Liter of Electrolyte Solution

(a)

SOLUTIONS USED OCCASIONALLY OR RARELY

SOLUTION	DEXTROSE g per L of solution	Na^+	K^+	Ca^{++}	Cl^-	ALCOHOL ml per L of solution	Approximate OSMOLALITY mOsm/kg H_2O
		—mEq per L	of solution—				
10% Dextrose	100						548
20% Dextrose	200						1096
5% Dextrose in 5% Alcohol	50					50	1361
5% Dextrose in 0.9% NaCl	50	154			154		565
10% Dextrose in 0.9% NaCl	100	154			154		839
Ringer's Solution		147	4	5	156		295
0.45% NaCl		77			77		146
5% NaCl		856			856		1617

(b)

CONCENTRATED SOLUTIONS USED AS ADDITIVES

NAME	VOLUME OF COMMERCIAL AMPULE ml	CONCENTRATION per ml	COMMENTS
Ammonium chloride	30	3 mEq NH_4^+[a]	Always diluted before use. Used as an acidifying agent, net effect being addition of HCl.
Calcium chloride	10	1.4 mEq Ca^{++}	
Calcium gluconate	10	0.5 mEq Ca^{++}	
Glucose, 50%	50	0.5 g dextrose	
Magnesium sulfate	2	4.1 mEq Mg^{++}	
Mannitol	50	0.25 g mannitol	
Potassium chloride	10	2 mEq K^+	Always diluted before use.
Potassium phosphate	30	2 mEq K^+	Always diluted before use.
Sodium acetate	30	3 mEq acetate	Used as an alkalinizing agent, acetate being metabolized to bicarbonate.
Sodium bicarbonate	50	1 mEq HCO_3^-	
Sodium chloride	40	2.5 mEq Na^+	Always diluted before use.
Sodium lactate	20	2.5 mEq lactate	Used as an alkalinizing agent, lactate being metabolized to bicarbonate.

(c) [a] Ion listed is the one for which solution is given to patient.

Figure 1-6
Composition of various parenteral solutions. The ones that are most commonly used in many hospitals are illustrated by the bar graphs (a). For comparison, the composition of normal plasma is given in the bar graph on the left. Other solutions that are also available commercially, but used only occasionally or rarely, have been listed in the box on the left (b). The commercial forms of various concentrated solutions are given in the box on the right (c); note that their concentrations are expressed *per milliliter,* which emphasizes the fact that most of these solutions must be diluted prior to use.

Table 1-7
Atomic and molecular weights of substances commonly dealt with in clinical nephrology

Substance	Symbol	Atomic or Molecular Weight*
Albumin	–	60,000
Aluminum	Al	27
Bromine	Br	80
Calcium	Ca	40
Carbon	C	12
Chlorine	Cl	35
Chromium	Cr	52
Citric acid	–	192
Copper	Cu	64
Creatinine	–	113
Ethanol	–	46
Glucose	–	180
Hydrogen	H	1
Inulin	–	~5,000
Iodine	I	127
Iron	Fe	56
Lactic acid	–	90
Lithium	Li	7
Magnesium	Mg	24
Manganese	Mn	55
Mannitol	–	182
Mercury	Hg	201
Nitrogen	N	14
Oxygen	O	16
p-Aminohippuric acid (PAH)	–	194
Phosphorus	P	31
Potassium	K	39
Sodium	Na	23
Sulfur	S	32
Urea	–	60
Uric acid	–	158

*Rounded off at least to nearest unit.

Selected References

General

Bergner, P. E., and Lushbaugh, C. C. (eds.). *Compartments, Pools, and Spaces in Medical Physiology.* Oak Ridge, Tenn.: U.S. Atomic Energy Commission, 1967.

Black, D. A. K. (ed.). *Renal Disease* (3rd ed.). Oxford, Eng.: Blackwell, 1972.

Bland, J. H. *Clinical Recognition and Management of Disturbances of Body Fluids* (2nd ed.). Philadelphia: Saunders, 1956.

Brenner, B. M., and Rector, F. C., Jr. (eds.). *The Kidney.* Philadelphia: Saunders, 1976.

Deane, N. Methods of Study of Body Water Compartments. In A. C. Corcoran (ed.), *Methods in Medical Research,* vol. 5. Chicago: Year Book, 1952.

de Wardener, H. E. *The Kidney: An Outline of Normal and Abnormal Structure and Function* (4th ed.). Edinburgh: Churchill/Livingstone, 1973.

Dick, D. A. T. *Cell Water.* Washington, D.C.: Butterworth, 1966.

Elkinton, J. R., and Danowski, T. S. *The Body Fluids.* Baltimore: Williams & Wilkins, 1955.

Fischer, J. E. (ed.). *Total Parenteral Nutrition.* Boston: Little, Brown, 1976.

Gamble, J. L. *Chemical Anatomy, Physiology and Pathology of Extracellular Fluid* (6th ed.). Cambridge, Mass.: Harvard University Press, 1954.

Hamburger, J., Richet, G., Crosnier, J., Funck-Brentano, J. L., Antoine, B., Ducrot, H., Mery, J. P., and deMontera, H. *Nephrology.* Philadelphia: Saunders, 1968.

Heptinstall, R. H. *Pathology of the Kidney* (2nd ed.). Boston: Little, Brown, 1976.

Kurtzman, N. A. (ed.). Symposium on renal pathophysiology. *Arch. Intern. Med.* 131:779, 1973.
This symposium includes, among others, the following topics: excretion of Na^+ and edema, disorders of urinary concentration and dilution, excretion of phosphate and calcium, renin, aldosterone, excretion of K^+, acute renal failure, and erythropoietin.

Maxwell, M. H., and Kleeman, C. R. (eds.). *Clinical Disorders of Fluid and Electrolyte Metabolism* (2nd ed.). New York: McGraw-Hill, 1972.

Moore, F. D. *Metabolic Care of the Surgical Patient.* Philadelphia: Saunders, 1959.

Moore, F. D., and Ball, M. R. *The Metabolic Response to Surgery.* Springfield, Ill.: Thomas, 1952.

Papper, S. *Clinical Nephrology* (2nd ed.). Boston: Little, Brown, 1978.

Peters, J. P. *Body Water: The Exchange of Fluids in Man.* Springfield, Ill.: Thomas, 1935.

Rose, B. D. *Clinical Physiology of Acid-Base and Electrolyte Disorders.* New York: McGraw-Hill, 1977.

Rosenfeld, M. G. (ed.). *Manual of Medical Therapeutics* (22nd ed.). Boston: Little, Brown, 1977.

Schrier, R. W. (ed.). *Renal and Electrolyte Disorders.* Boston: Little, Brown, 1976.

Smith, H. W. *The Evolution of the Kidney* (Porter Lectures, Series 9). Lawrence, Kans.: University of Kansas Press, 1943.

Smith, H. W. *The Kidney: Structure and Function in Health and Disease.* New York: Oxford University Press, 1951.

Strauss, M. B. *Body Water in Man: The Acquisition and Maintenance of Body Fluids.* Boston: Little, Brown, 1957.

Strauss, M. B., and Welt, L. G. (eds.). *Diseases of the Kidney* (2nd ed.). Boston: Little, Brown, 1971.

Valtin, H. *Renal Function: Mechanisms Preserving Fluid and Solute Balance in Health.* Boston: Little, Brown, 1973.

Welt, L. G. *Clinical Disorders of Hydration and Acid-Base Equilibrium* (2nd ed.). Boston: Little, Brown, 1959.

Wesson, L. G. *Physiology of the Human Kidney.* New York: Grune & Stratton, 1969.

Widdowson, E. M., and Dickerson, J. W. T. Chemical Composition of the Body. In C. L. Comar and F. Bronner (eds.), *Mineral Metabolism,* vol. 2, part A. New York: Academic, 1964.

Balance

Drenick, E. J. The Effects of Acute and Prolonged Fasting and Refeeding on Water, Electrolyte, and Acid-Base Metabolism. In M. H. Maxwell and C. R. Kleeman (eds.), *Clinical Disorders of Fluid and Electrolyte Metabolism* (2nd ed.). New York: McGraw-Hill, 1972.

Gamble, J. L. *Physiological Information Gained from Studies on the Life Raft Ration.* Harvey Lectures, Series 42. Lancaster, Pa.: Science Press, 1947, pp. 247-273.

Jaenike, J. R., and Waterhouse, C. The renal response to sustained administration of vasopressin and water in man. *J. Clin. Endocrinol. Metab.* 21:231, 1961.

Loeb, R. F., Atchley, D. W., Richards, D. W., Jr., Benedict, E. M., and Driscoll, M. E. On the mechanism of nephrotic edema. *J. Clin. Invest.* 11:621, 1932.

This work included, for purposes of control, one of the earliest and most complete balance studies on a healthy young man. The study lasted 45 days, during which the subject ate identical meals, with "... never any return of food to the kitchen...."

Moore, F. D., and Brennan, M. F. Intravenous feeding. *N. Engl. J. Med.* 287:862, 1972.

Newburgh, L. H., Johnston, M. W., Lashmet, F. H., and Sheldon, J. M. Further experiences with the measurement of heat production from insensible loss of weight. *J. Nutr.* 13:203, 1937.

Normal Values

Arieff, A. I. Principles of Parenteral Therapy. In M. H. Maxwell and C. R. Kleeman (eds.), *Clinical Disorders of Fluid and Electrolyte Metabolism* (2nd ed.). New York: McGraw-Hill, 1972.

Castleman, B. J. (ed.). Case records of the Massachusetts General Hospital. Normal laboratory values. *N. Engl. J. Med.* 290:39, 1974.

Chattaway, F. W., Hullin, R. P., and Odds, F. C. The variability of creatinine excretion in normal subjects, mental patients and pregnant women. *Clin. Chim. Acta* 26:567, 1969.

Conn, H. F. (ed.). *Current Therapy 1973.* Philadelphia: Saunders, 1973.

Conn, R. B. Clinical laboratories: Profit center, production industry or patient-care resource? *N. Engl. J. Med.* 298:422, 1978.

Davidsohn, I., and Henry, J. B. (eds.). *Todd-Sanford Clinical Diagnosis by Laboratory Methods* (15th ed.). Philadelphia: Saunders, 1974.

Diem, K. (ed.). *Documenta Geigy. Scientific Tables* (6th ed.). Ardsley, N.Y.: Geigy Pharmaceuticals, 1968.

An exceptionally useful and extensive compilation of data — from both the biological and physical sciences — that have been assembled especially for the medical practitioner and the biomedical investigator.

Edelman, I. S., and Leibman, J. Anatomy of body water and electrolytes. *Am. J. Med.* 27:256, 1959.

Faulkner, W. R., King, J. W., and Damm, H. C. (eds.). *Handbook of Clinical Laboratory Data* (2nd ed.). Cleveland: Chemical Rubber Co., 1968.

Francke, D. E. (ed.). *Handbook of I.V. Additive Reviews.* Cincinnati: Drug Intelligence Publications, 1973.

Hays, R. M. Dynamics of Body Water and Electrolytes. In M. H. Maxwell and C. R. Kleeman (eds.), *Clinical Disorders of Fluid and Electrolyte Metabolism* (2nd ed.). New York: McGraw-Hill, 1972.

Krupp, M. A., and Chatton, M. J. *Current Medical Diagnosis and Treatment.* Los Altos, Calif.: Lange, 1977.

This work has a useful appendix for ready reference.

Lancet Editorial. Microbiological hazards of intravenous infusions. *Lancet* 1:543, 1974.

Moore, F. D., Oleson, K. H., McMurrey, J. D., Parker, H. V., Ball, M. R., and Boyden, C. M. *The Body Cell Mass and Its Supporting Environment: Body Composition in Health and Disease.* Philadelphia: Saunders, 1963.

Page, L. B., and Culver, P. J. (eds.). *A Syllabus of Laboratory Examinations in Clinical Diagnosis: Critical Evaluation of Laboratory Procedures in the Study of the Patient.* Cambridge, Mass.: Harvard University Press, 1960.

Rosenfeld, M. G. (ed.). *Manual of Medical Therapeutics* (22nd ed.). Boston: Little, Brown, 1977.

Scully, R. E., McNeely, B. U., and Galdabini, J. J. Normal reference laboratory values. *N. Engl. J. Med.* 298:34, 1978.

Wallach, J. *Interpretation of Diagnostic Tests: A Handbook Synopsis of Laboratory Medicine* (2nd ed.). Boston: Little, Brown, 1974.

Winkelstein, J. A. (ed.). *The Harriet Lane Handbook: A Manual for Pediatric House Officers* (6th ed.). Chicago: Year Book, 1972.

Young, D. S. Standardized reporting of laboratory data. The desirability of using SI units. *N. Engl. J. Med.* 290:368, 1974.

Pediatric Nephrology

Edelmann, C. M., Jr. (ed.). *Pediatric Kidney Disease.* Boston: Little, Brown, 1978.

Edelmann, C. M., Jr., and Barnett, H. L. Pediatric Nephrology. In M. B. Strauss and L. G. Welt (eds.), *Diseases of the Kidney,* vol. 2 (2nd ed.). Boston: Little, Brown, 1971.

Holliday, M. A. Body Fluid Physiology During Growth. In M. H. Maxwell and C. R. Kleeman (eds.), *Clinical Disorders of Fluid and Electrolyte Metabolism* (2nd ed.). New York: McGraw-Hill, 1972.

James, J. A. *Renal Disease in Childhood* (2nd ed.). St. Louis: Mosby, 1972.

Klaus, M. H., and Fanaroff, A. A. (eds.). *Care of the High-Risk Neonate.* Philadelphia: Saunders, 1973.

McCrory, W. W. *Developmental Nephrology.* Cambridge, Mass.: Harvard University Press, 1972.

Winters, R. W. (ed.). *The Body Fluids in Pediatrics: Medical, Surgical, and Neonatal Disorders of Acid-Base Status, Hydration, and Oxygenation.* Boston: Little, Brown, 1973.

2 : Disorders of H_2O Balance. Antidiuretic Hormone (ADH)

In all biological systems tested thus far, H_2O appears to move passively in response to osmotic differences set up by the active transport of solutes. It is not surprising, therefore, that H_2O movement commonly follows that of solute, as in the formation of edema (see Chap. 3). Nevertheless, passive transport of H_2O can be regulated independently of the transport of solute through the action of antidiuretic hormone (ADH or vasopressin). This chapter deals mainly with abnormalities of H_2O balance arising from irregularities of ADH.

Regulation of ADH Secretion

The classic studies of E. B. Verney elucidated some of the major mechanisms that regulate the secretion of ADH from the posterior pituitary gland. Verney worked with trained, unanesthetized dogs in which he had previously exteriorized loops of the common carotid arteries.

Verney's results are illustrated in Figure 2-1a. Within 60 to 90 minutes after receiving an oral load of H_2O, the dogs excreted large amounts of hyposmotic urine. This water diuresis could be abruptly interrupted by infusing a bolus of hyperosmotic solution into the exteriorized carotid loop, but not if the posterior pituitary gland had been removed. If posterior pituitary extract was given to an hypophysectomized animal, the water diuresis was also interrupted. On the basis of these results, Verney proposed the scheme outlined in Figure 2-1b. When an individual is deprived of H_2O, the continued obligatory excretion of H_2O renders his plasma hyperosmotic. This change stimulates secretion of ADH from the posterior pituitary gland, possibly through the intermediation of osmoreceptors. The resulting high concentration of ADH in the blood then increases the permeability to H_2O of the distal renal tubules and collecting ducts, so that antidiuresis ensues.

Conversely, when the individual drinks a large amount of dilute fluid, his plasma becomes hyposmotic. This presumably sets off the opposite chain of events, leading to a decreased concentration of ADH in the blood, decreased H_2O permeability of the distal tubules and collecting ducts, and water diuresis.

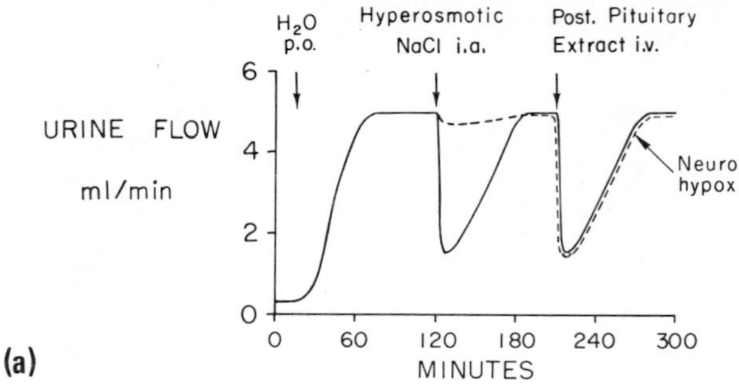

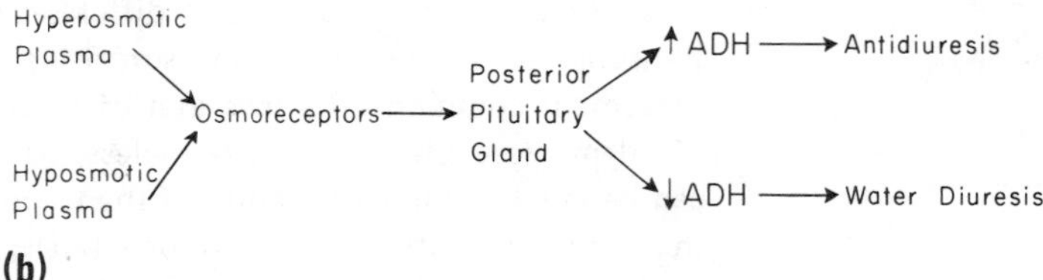

Figure 2-1
(a) Summary of some of the important results obtained on unanesthetized dogs by E. B. Verney (*Proc. R. Soc. Lond. [Biol.]* 135:25, 1947). Solid line graph represents results on a dog prior to removal of the neurohypophysis; the dashed line represents results on the same dog after neurohypophysectomy. *p.o.* = per os (by mouth); *i.a.* = intra-arterially (into the exteriorized loop of the common carotid artery); *i.v.* = intravenously.

(b) Chain of events whereby changes in plasma osmolality regulate antidiuretic hormone (ADH) secretion and hence urine flow. Although many other factors — e.g., drugs, alcohol, or extracellular fluid volume — can also affect ADH secretion, the osmoreceptor system is probably the major mechanism for regulating water balance.

From H. Valtin, *Renal Function: Mechanisms Preserving Fluid and Solute Balance in Health.* Boston: Little, Brown, 1973.

Ordinarily, the osmoreceptor system is probably the major mechanism for regulating the secretion of ADH. Other factors, however, can also play a role (e.g., drugs, alcohol, and extracellular fluid volume), and they sometimes alter the influence of osmolality on the secretion of ADH.

Thirst

In addition to the regulation of ADH secretion, another important regulator of H_2O balance is thirst. Normally, when a subject is deprived of H_2O, thirst is stimulated and the resultant increased intake of fluid tends to correct the deficit; the converse change of events tends to correct a positive balance of H_2O.

Deficiency of ADH and Diabetes Insipidus (D.I.)

The term *diabetes insipidus* is derived from the Greek *diabainein,* meaning "to pass through," and from the Latin *insipidus,* meaning "not savory." The term thus refers to the passing through the body of tasteless fluid. Freely translated, it refers to the passage of large amounts of hyposmotic (hence, tasteless) fluid which, according to the experiments of Verney, can be due to one of three fundamental causes: (1) chronic and excessive ingestion of fluid, leading to constant inhibition of ADH secretion from the posterior pituitary gland; (2) hypothalamic failure, involving a defect in the production or release of ADH from the hypothalamo-neurohypophyseal system; or (3) a renal defect, manifested by deficient renal H_2O reabsorption despite ample amounts of ADH in the blood. All three causes — and hence three types of diabetes insipidus — occur in humans, and they can be distinguished by the so-called *Hickey-Hare test,* which is a clinical application of the experiments of Verney.

It must be emphasized that if a patient presents himself to his doctor with a chief complaint of excessive thirst and urination, the most probable diagnosis is diabetes mellitus. Once this disease has been excluded through appropriate tests, however, an effort must be made to identify which type of diabetes insipidus the patient has.

Types of Diabetes Insipidus

The Hickey-Hare test (Fig. 2-2) is in effect a repetition of Verney's experiments. When the presence of a high rate of urine flow has been established, the patient's plasma is rendered hyperosmotic through an intravenous infusion of 2.5% NaCl (having an osmolality of about 850 mOsm/kg H_2O). If the patient responds *promptly* by decreasing the urine flow and increasing the urine osmolality or urine specific gravity, it may be concluded not only that his hypothalamo-neurohypophyseal system can release ADH appropriately, but also that his kidneys can respond to the hormone. Hence, this patient has *primary polydipsic diabetes insipidus;* it is "primary" in the sense that the initial event leading to excessive urine flow is the drinking of large amounts of fluid. Most clinicians do not classify this entity as diabetes insipidus and usually refer to it as compulsive water drinking or psychogenic polydipsia. However, according to the meaning of the term as discussed above, the condition should properly be considered a form of diabetes insipidus. (*Note:* Patients with partial hypothalamic diabetes insipidus — see Figure 2-3 — will also decrease urine flow and increase urine osmolality in response to hypertonic NaCl; thus, the distinction between primary polydipsic and partial hypothalamic diabetes insipidus often cannot be as sharply drawn as is implied in the above description.)

If the patient does not decrease urine flow in response to hyperosmotic NaCl, he is then given an injection of ADH. If he now

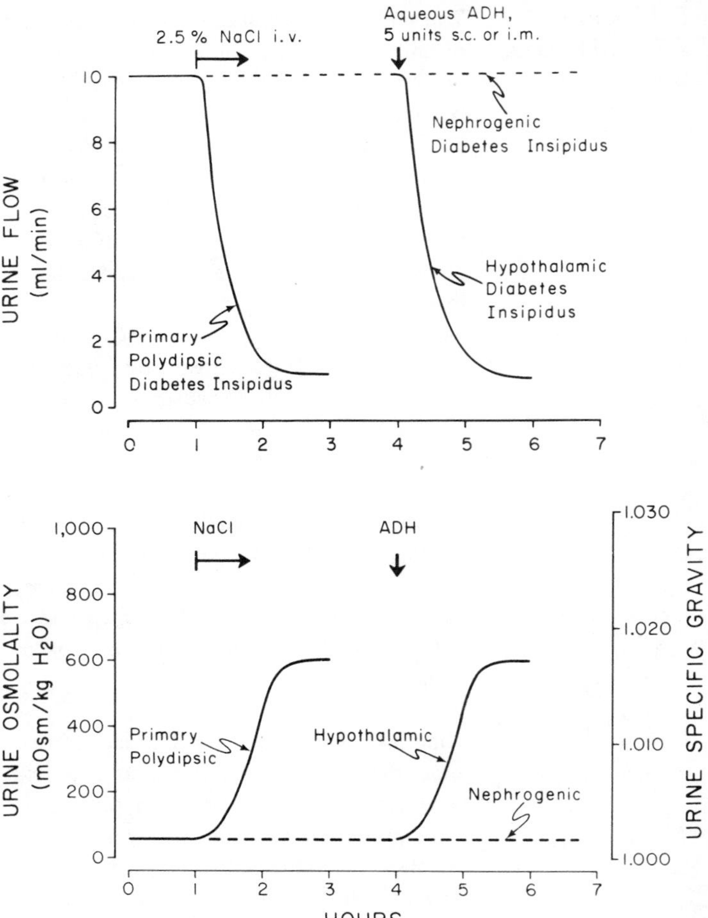

Figure 2-2
Hickey-Hare test, used to differentiate the major types of diabetes insipidus. The lower graph shows the approximate relationship between the specific gravity and the osmolality of normal urine (see also Fig. 11-A, Answer to Problem 11-1). *i.v.* = intravenously; *s.c.* = subcutaneously; *i.m.* = intramuscularly.

decreases urine flow and increases urine concentration, it may be deduced that he has a hypothalamic (but not a renal) defect; he is therefore said to have *hypothalamic diabetes insipidus.* Finally, if he does not respond to exogenous ADH, the abnormality must be in the kidneys, and he is said to have *nephrogenic diabetes insipidus.*

Modification of the Hickey-Hare Test. Many physicians prefer to render the patient's plasma hyperosmotic by withdrawing drinking fluid, rather than through an infusion of hyperosmotic

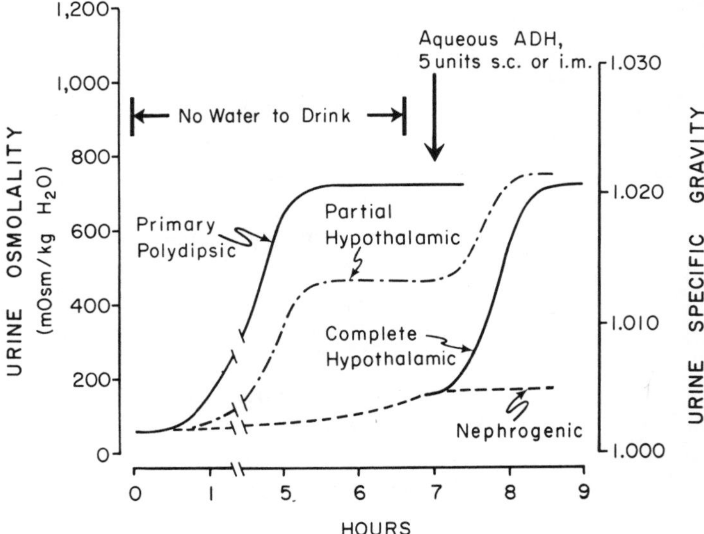

Figure 2-3
The so-called water deprivation test for differentiating the major types of diabetes insipidus (D.I.). In this modification of the Hickey-Hare test, the plasma is rendered hyperosmotic by withdrawing drinking fluid rather than by infusing hyperosmotic NaCl. The means for discriminating partial hypothalamic D.I. from primary polydipsic D.I. are also illustrated: in the latter, water deprivation results in maximal urine osmolality for that patient and exogenous ADH will not further raise the value, whereas in partial hypothalamic D.I., exogenous ADH will raise the urine osmolality beyond the value achieved by water deprivation alone.

NaCl. Typical results are shown in Figure 2-3 (the details of this variation are discussed in several of the references listed at the end of this chapter and will not be given here, mainly because the modification does not alter the principles that underlie the Hickey-Hare test). The modification does, however, embody several concepts of patient care that are worth stressing.

Giving exogenous compounds to patients, especially intravenously, should be avoided whenever possible. An infusion of hyperosmotic NaCl, for example, can lead to undesirable circulatory overload. Beyond that, patients with primary polydipsic diabetes insipidus, be it psychological or somatic in origin, often have intense thirst. They may therefore suffer greatly if not allowed to drink (see Problem 13-2), and patients with either the hypothalamic or nephrogenic form may have such a high obligatory urine output that they may quickly become dangerously dehydrated as well as very thirsty. For these reasons, the so-called water deprivation test should be started in the morning so that the patient can be under constant observation and the test be terminated if necessary. An additional reason is that the patient must be watched for illicit drinking; sometimes the thirst is so compelling that the patient drinks water from the flower vases. The simplest and most reliable means of preventing dangerous dehydration is to weigh the patient hourly on the same scales. A weight loss amounting to 3 percent of the original body weight will lead to an increase in plasma osmolality of about 15 mOsm/kg H_2O (see Problem 2-1), which is ample to stimulate the hypothalamo-neurohypophyseal system maximally. Therefore, the test need not be continued beyond this point, and it should always be terminated when 5 percent of the initial body weight has been lost. For analogous reasons, it is both unnecessary and possibly dangerous to carry out fluid restriction on a polyuric patient whose plasma osmolality exceeds 300 mOsm/kg H_2O while he is drinking ad libitum.

Pitfalls. When plasma osmolality is increased in normal subjects either by infusing hyperosmotic NaCl or by withholding drinking fluid, their urinary concentration rises to an osmolality of at least 800 to 1,000 mOsm/kg H_2O, or a specific gravity of about 1.025. Note that the rise in urinary concentration is less in primary polydipsic diabetes insipidus (Figs. 2-2 and 2-3). The reason for this diminished response is that the interstitial osmolality in the renal medulla is lower in H_2O diuresis than in antidiuresis; consequently, when H_2O permeability is suddenly increased through the release of endogenous ADH, fluid in the collecting duct is osmotically equilibrated against a lower interstitial osmolality than ordinarily obtains in prolonged states of antidiuresis (see Chap. 13, under Decreased Corticopapillary Gradient Versus Decreased Water Permeability).

This phenomenon can lead to difficulty in differentiating primary polydipsic from partial hypothalamic diabetes insipidus. Many patients with the latter disease have only a partial deficiency of ADH. Therefore, as drinking fluid is withheld from them, some ADH is released from the hypothalamo-neurohypophyseal system and their urine osmolality may rise to an intermediate level of 500 to 600 mOsm/kg H_2O (Fig. 2-3). The question then arises whether this intermediate level reflects the blunted response of primary polydipsic diabetes insipidus (which is due to a decreased interstitial osmolality in the face of a supramaximal plasma concentration of ADH), or whether it reflects a less than maximal plasma concentration of ADH that has prevented full osmotic equilibration with the interstitium. The question can sometimes be answered by giving exogenous ADH on top of dehydration: the patient with primary polydipsic diabetes insipidus will show no further rise in urine osmolality, whereas one with incomplete hypothalamic diabetes insipidus will show an increase of at least 50 mOsm/kg H_2O and often much more, because the exogenous ADH will further augment the H_2O permeability of the distal tubules and collecting ducts.

Despite the logic that underlies the Hickey-Hare and the water deprivation tests, these procedures cannot always distinguish one form of D.I. from another. The differential diagnosis can be aided by measuring ADH in plasma or urine (Fig. 2-4). Note that by this criterion, the hypothalamic form (even when partial) is clearly distinguished from primary polydipsic diabetes insipidus (Fig. 2-4a), and if the plasma concentration of ADH is considered in relation to the urine osmolality in the same patient, nephrogenic diabetes insipidus can be separated from the other types. The measurement of ADH by radioimmunoassay, especially in plasma, is a difficult procedure that currently is performed accurately in only a few laboratories. It seems likely, however, that this aid will soon become available more routinely.

Causes and Treatment of Diabetes Insipidus

Primary Polydipsic D.I. The causes of this form of D.I. are listed in Table 2-1. Note that with the possible exception of primary polydipsic D.I. in man, all three forms of this disease may be either acquired or hereditary. The fact that hereditary primary polydipsic D.I. exists in other species (e.g., mice and rabbits) suggests that the hereditary form may also some day be identified in man. In humans, primary polydipsic D.I. is usually considered to be psychogenic, as is implied in its more common appellations of compulsive water drinking or psychogenic polydipsia; certainly, however, the possibility of a somatic cause for this disorder has not been ruled out. It must be stressed that when psychogenic, the compulsive drinking may be an important compensatory mechanism for the patient. Therefore, telling such a patient that all he has to do to correct the situation is to drink less is likely to be as naive and ineffectual as giving the same advice to an alcoholic. Rather, sympathetic psychiatric help will be needed.

Hypothalamic D.I. The acquired causes of hypothalamic D.I. are listed in Table 2-1 in order of decreasing occurrence. Drug therapy is thus far most satisfactory for this type of diabetes insipidus. The missing hormone, vasopressin, can be given in its native form or in a variety of synthetic analogues. The latter look particularly promising, not only because they need not be injected, but also because they have a very specific antidiuretic (as opposed to vasopressor) action and a relatively long-lasting effect of nearly 24 hours. The main advantage of chlorpropamide is that, unlike the vasopressins, which are inactivated by gastrointestinal enzymes, it can be taken orally.

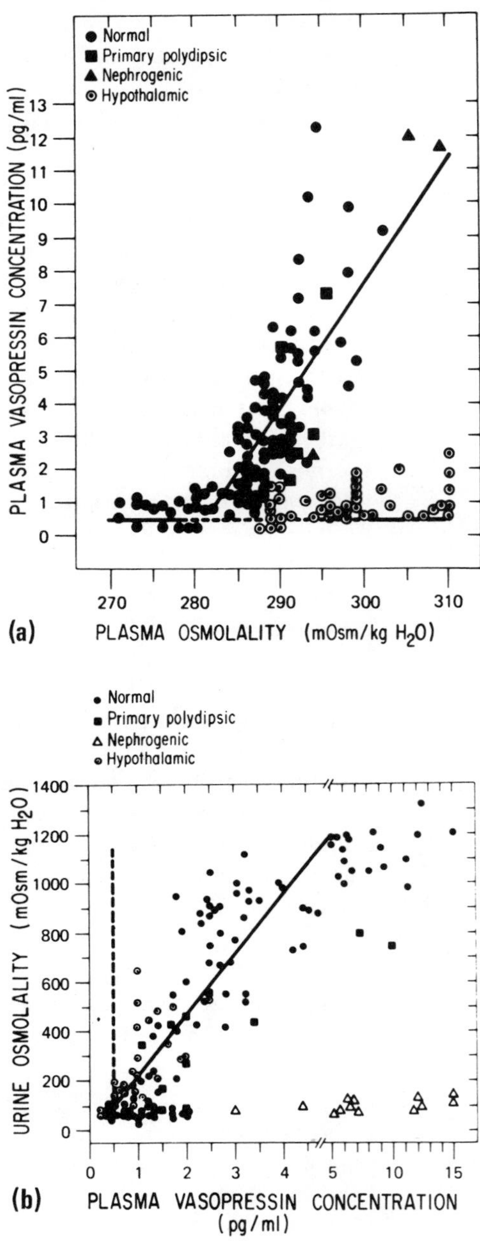

Figure 2-4

(a) Plasma concentration of vasopressin (ADH) when plasma osmolality is raised in normal subjects and in patients with the three forms of diabetes insipidus. The same type of relationships could be shown if urinary excretion of ADH were plotted against plasma osmolality.

(b) The urine osmolality achieved by a subject or patient at a given plasma concentration of ADH. The dashed lines (a) denote the minimal plasma concentration of ADH that can be detected by the assay.

Modified from G. L. Robertson et al., *J. Clin. Invest.* 52:2340, 1973.

Table 2-1
Causes and treatment of diabetes insipidus (D.I.)

Type of D.I. (synonyms)	Causes	Treatment
1. Primary polydipsic diabetes insipidus (compulsive water drinking; psychogenic polydipsia)	Acquired 1. Emotional 2. Nonpsychogenic (?); e.g., tumors or other lesions causing chronic stimulation of the thirst center(?)	Psychiatric
	Hereditary (?); described in species other than man but not yet in man	
2. Hypothalamic diabetes insipidus (diabetes insipidus; true diabetes insipidus)	Acquired 1. Unknown (idiopathic) 2. Neoplastic 3. Traumatic; e.g., auto accidents 4. Neurosurgical procedures 5. Nonneoplastic; e.g., histiocytosis X, sarcoidosis, syphilis, Sheehan's syndrome, encephalitis, leukemia, and others	Amelioration or elimination of the primary lesion if possible. Various drugs: ADH or one of its synthetic analogues; chlorpropamide (potentiates cellular effect of ADH and hence can be used only in partial hypothalamic D.I.)
	Hereditary	Same as for "Acquired"
3. Nephrogenic diabetes insipidus (vasopressin-resistant diabetes insipidus)	Acquired; e.g., drugs, hypokalemia, hypercalcemia, sickle-cell anemia, and other causes (see Chap. 13)	Withdrawal of the offending agent or correction of the primary disorder
	Hereditary	Unsatisfactory in most instances; however, the following are used: 1. Adequate fluid intake at all times 2. Thiazide diuretics 3. Reduction of protein and NaCl intake and hence of renal solute output

Nephrogenic D.I. The causes of nephrogenic diabetes insipidus are given in Table 2-1 and are discussed in detail in Chapter 13. Many of the acquired forms can be cured, especially if the cause is discovered in time. The hereditary form is very rare, and its treatment remains unsatisfactory. In such patients, it is therefore of the utmost importance to maintain adequate fluid intake at all times in order to prevent severe dehydration and brain damage. Some reduction in urine flow (about 50 percent) can be achieved by two means. One is through the seemingly paradoxical use of the thiazide diuretics. The mechanism of their *anti*diuretic action remains unknown; it may involve NaCl depletion, increased reabsorption of isosmotic fluid in the proximal tubules, and decreased production of free H_2O in the early distal tubules (see discussion of hyponatremia in heart failure under Conditions that Mimic SIADH, below, and Answer to Problem 13-1). The other means of reducing urine flow is to reduce dietary solute intake and thereby renal solute excretion. It follows from the relationship,

$$U_{Osm} = \text{amount of solute/urine volume}$$

that for any given ability to concentrate the urine, there is a direct correlation between the amount of solute and the amount of H_2O that must be excreted by the kidneys. In the steady state, the rate of renal solute excretion is determined by the amount of solute ingested, mainly proteins and NaCl. Therefore, the urine flow can be decreased appreciably by limiting the intake of these solutes.

Surfeit of ADH and the Syndrome of Inappropriate ADH Secretion (SIADH)

This condition was discussed in Chapter 1 (see Steady State in Disease). As shown in Figure 1-3, SIADH is characterized by a low plasma Na^+ concentration and by its almost invariable concomitant, a low plasma osmolality (Table 1-2). The name of the syndrome refers to *inappropriate* secretion of ADH, because the normal response to a low plasma osmolality is an inhibition of ADH release (Fig. 2-1b), whereas in SIADH, the low plasma osmolality is associated with increased secretion of ADH.

Chain of Events in SIADH

The causal sequence in the development of SIADH is shown in Figure 2-5. The syndrome develops when a sustained, normal or high plasma concentration of ADH is accompanied by a normal or high fluid intake. This combination makes it impossible for the kidneys to excrete enough solute-free H_2O for the individual to remain in H_2O balance; that is, the patient goes into positive H_2O balance, which expands all the body-fluid compartments, including the extracellular space. These events can suffice to ex-

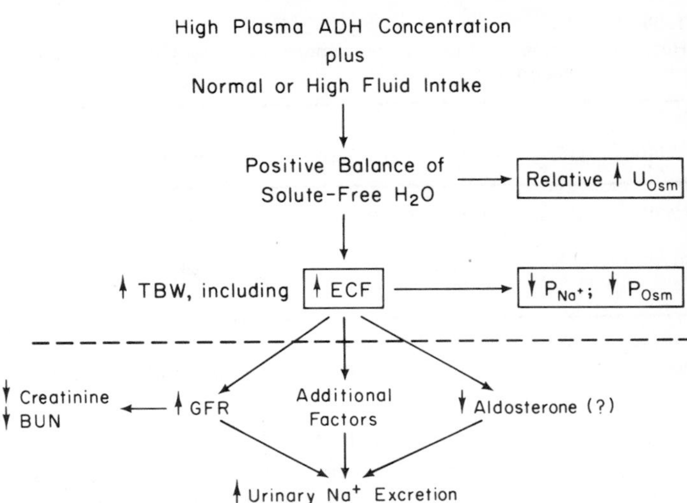

Figure 2-5
Chain of events leading to the syndrome of inappropriate ADH secretion (SIADH). The major findings that are invariably present are enclosed in boxes. The events below the dashed line are often seen in SIADH, but not invariably, especially not after the new steady state has been reached.

plain the hallmarks of SIADH: (1) expansion of the extracellular fluid volume, which leads to dilution of the body Na^+ and hence to a decrease in the plasma Na^+ concentration and plasma osmolality, and (2) retention of free H_2O by the kidneys, which leads to an increase in the urine osmolality. The urine osmolality need not be hyperosmotic compared to plasma, but it must be relatively hyperosmotic, "relative" either with respect to the degree of hyposmolality of the plasma (in the face of which one would expect a maximally dilute urine of 50 to 75 mOsm/kg H_2O) or with respect to the H_2O balance. The latter point is illustrated in Table 2-2. In health, a person may be in H_2O balance when he consumes 400 mOsmoles of solute daily and excretes urine having an osmolality of 500 mOsm/kg H_2O. As this person develops SIADH, he may still consume the same amount of solute per day, but he will now have a high intake of fluid, which, because of the high plasma concentration of ADH, he cannot excrete completely. Dissolving 400 mOsmoles of solute in 1,800 ml of urinary H_2O yields a urine osmolality of 222 mOsm/kg H_2O; thus, even though this patient excretes hyposmotic urine, he is in positive H_2O balance. That is why we speak of a *relative* increase in urine osmolality, that is, high in relation to the H_2O balance or the plasma osmolality.

The events depicted beneath the horizontal dashed line in Figure 2-5 usually occur during the development of SIADH, but they are not necessarily observed when the new steady state

Table 2-2
Retention of free H_2O in the syndrome of inappropriate ADH secretion (SIADH) despite hyposmolality of the urine

State	Daily Intake (per day)	Urine Flow (ml/day)	U_{Osm} (mOsm/kg H_2O)	H_2O Balance (ml/day)
Healthy	400 mOsmoles 800 ml H_2O*	800	500	0
SIADH	400 mOsmoles 2,000 ml H_2O*	1,800	222	+200

*Intake minus insensible loss and minus H_2O in stool.
Modified from F. C. Bartter and W. B. Schwartz. *Am. J. Med.* 42:790, 1967.

is reached (Fig. 1-3). Expansion of the extracellular fluid volume often leads to an increase in the glomerular filtration rate (GFR), a decrease in the plasma concentration of aldosterone, as well as a number of other changes; the latter may be hormonal or physical, such as decreased plasma oncotic pressure and increased hydrostatic pressure in the peritubular capillaries (see Chap. 3 for detailed discussion). All these consequences of expanding the extracellular space would be expected to lead to increased urinary Na^+ excretion, which usually contributes to the development of the low plasma Na^+ concentration in SIADH. It should be emphasized, however, that the low plasma Na^+ concentration reflects mainly the dilution of nearly normal amounts of Na^+ by an excess of free H_2O. When a very low plasma Na^+ concentration develops (< 115 mEq per liter), neither H_2O retention, increased Na^+ excretion, nor their combined effect can fully account for the hyponatremia. In such instances, the concept of internal imbalance must be invoked; it has been postulated that "osmotic inactivation" of some intracellular solute(s) — for example, by binding — causes a decrease of intracellular osmolality and a consequent shift of H_2O into the extracellular space, thereby further diluting the extracellular Na^+.

Experimental Evidence for the Chain of Events in SIADH. All the changes depicted in Figure 2-5 have been shown to occur in patients with SIADH. The changes are not necessarily concurrent, nor is each change necessarily seen in all patients. Probably the best experimental evidence is provided by the reproduction of the entire sequence in normal subjects when they are given high doses of ADH at the same time that they consume large amounts of liquid.

Diagnostic Criteria for SIADH

The major findings in this syndrome can be predicted from its pathogenesis (Fig. 2-5) and include the following: (1) hyponatremia and corresponding hyposmolality of the plasma; (2) a urine osmolality that is inappropriately high, although not necessarily hyperosmotic with respect to the plasma; (3) evidence for the expansion of the body-fluid compartments, which is usually reflected by a gain of body weight; and (4) absence of certain other diseases that can also cause retention of free H_2O and hyponatremia (e.g., adrenal or thyroid insufficiency and renal, cardiac, or hepatic failure; see below). In regard to points (3) and (4), it should be emphasized that SIADH cannot be diagnosed if there is evidence of volume contraction, not only because such contraction causes *appropriate* release of ADH, but more importantly because the treatment of SIADH – namely, fluid restriction (see next section) – would be contraindicated if contraction exists. A number of additional findings are helpful, *but not essential,* to the diagnosis: (1) a medical history suggesting one of the causes of SIADH (Table 2-3); this is not essential, because in some cases of SIADH – that is, so-called idiopathic – no cause can be identified; (2) decreased plasma concentrations of creatinine and urea (BUN), which, in the face of normal production of these compounds, must follow an increase in GFR (see Chap. 8); and (3) increased urinary Na^+ excretion. The last change is seen during the development of the syndrome but not necessarily in the new steady state (Fig. 1-3), when by definition the output of Na^+ equals its intake. Thus, in the new steady state, if the patient has a low Na^+ intake, the urinary excretion of Na^+ will be low, and vice versa if the patient is on a high Na^+ intake.

The last point raises the question of the usefulness – or, more accurately, of the futility – of measuring the urinary Na^+ excretion as it is routinely done with hospitalized patients. Often, the Na^+ concentration is measured on a random, so-called spot, urine sample. Such a test, of course, does not determine a rate of excretion, but only a concentration value, which is usually meaningless because it can vary so widely depending on the patient's Na^+ and fluid intake during the several hours before the urine was voided (see title of Table 1-3). But even the determination of the urinary Na^+ excretion over a 24-hour period is ordinarily not helpful, not only because it is extremely difficult to obtain an accurate collection of urine in a routine hospital ward, but also because the rate of urinary Na^+ excretion will be a function of the patient's intake of Na^+ and not usually of his disease process.

Causes and Treatment of SIADH

The syndrome has been associated with a large variety of disorders, mainly those involving the lungs and the central nervous system (Table 2-3). The number of causes increases almost weekly as the ectopic production of hormones by various tumors

Table 2-3
Disorders associated with the syndrome of inappropriate ADH secretion (SIADH)

1. Lungs
   - Tuberculosis
   - Pneumonia
   - Carcinoma
   - Others
2. Central nervous system
   - Meningitis
   - Abscess
   - Tumors
   - Acute intermittent porphyria
   - Head injuries
   - Encephalitis
   - Subarachnoid hemorrhage
   - Psychogenic illness
   - Others
3. Other tumors
   - Duodenal carcinoma
   - Pancreatic carcinoma
   - Thymoma
   - Others
4. Drugs
   - Chlorpropamide
   - Vincristine or cyclophosphamide
   - Carbamazepine
   - Clofibrate
   - Others

Modified from F. C. Bartter and W. B. Schwartz. *Am. J. Med.* 42:790, 1967.

and the antidiuretic action of various drugs are continually reported. In some of the conditions, there probably exists truly inappropriate secretion of ADH from the hypothalamo-neurohypophyseal system; this mechanism would be suspected in many lesions of the central nervous system, with the administration of certain drugs, and perhaps in the case of certain lesions of the lungs, where it might operate through the intermediation of volume receptors. In other conditions, especially tumors, there appears to be autonomous production of arginine-vasopressin or a similar polypeptide having antidiuretic activity. In still others, as with drug-induced SIADH, the syndrome may be due not to the secretion of endogenous ADH but to an ADH-like effect of the drug. Chlorpropamide, for example, probably acts on the renal tubules by potentiating the antidiuretic action of even very small amounts of ADH.

Treatment follows logically from knowledge of the pathogenesis. If the underlying cause can be identified (Table 2-3), it should, of course, be attended to; if successful, this will reduce or eliminate sustained antidiuretic activity. In the meantime, since the major cause of SIADH is retention of H_2O (Fig. 2-5), the syndrome can usually be corrected by the simple measure of restricting liquid intake. In most adult patients, limiting drinking fluids to 800 ml per day will suffice. The adequacy of the restriction can be most easily gauged by following the body weight; if the patient gained weight (i.e., H_2O) during the development of SIADH, then he must lose weight (i.e., H_2O) during its correction. Giving Na^+ is usually illogical, unnecessary, and useless. Most patients will not have sustained a large deficit of body Na^+. Beyond that, any additional Na^+ given to such patients will be quickly excreted, not only because the patient is in the new steady state, but also because the pathogenic mechanisms that promote increased urinary Na^+ excretion (Fig. 2-5) will remain – or be aggravated by further expansion of the extracellular compartment – until fluid restriction has been instituted.

Some patients with SIADH manifest predominantly neurological symptoms, even when the cause of the syndrome does not involve the central nervous system. The patients may have anorexia, nausea, and vomiting, they may become irritable and show personality changes and neurological signs (e.g., altered tendon reflexes), and they may lapse into coma and have convulsions. These symptoms reflect "water intoxication," and they probably result from the hyposmolality of plasma and the consequent internal imbalance for H_2O; as a rule, the more severe the hyponatremia, the more intense the symptoms. Since some of the consequences of H_2O intoxication are serious or even fatal, patients with very low plasma Na^+ concentrations (e.g., < 115 mEq per liter) require therapeutic measures in addition to fluid restriction. The hyposmolality of the extracellular fluid causes an osmotic shift of H_2O into the intracellular compartment. This shift and the resultant swelling occur in most body cells; the shift may be partly ameliorated by a loss of solute from the cells, including those of the brain. Nevertheless, the shift of H_2O may be least tolerable in the cells of the brain, which get compressed against the inexpansible cranium. In order to relieve the neurological signs and symptoms, therefore, fairly rapid reversal of the cellular swelling should be brought about. This can be accomplished by giving the patient an intravenous infusion of hyperosmotic NaCl, which quickly raises the osmolality of the extracellular fluid and thereby withdraws H_2O from the cells.

Conditions that Mimic SIADH

A number of diseases are often accompanied by hyponatremia. Since this is the abnormality that usually makes a physician first think of SIADH, these diseases enter into the differential diagnosis of the syndrome. Some occur much more commonly than

SIADH; in order of approximate decreasing frequency, they are *heart failure* (especially when combined with the use of *diuretics*), *liver failure, renal failure, adrenal insufficiency,* and *myxedema* (Table 3-3).

Until the plasma concentration of ADH can be measured more routinely than is now possible, it will not be known to what extent ADH is involved in mimicking the syndrome in these disease states. In some of the conditions, ADH is at least not *essential* to mimicking the syndrome. Basic to this fact is the finding that renal retention of solute-free H_2O can occur even in the absence of ADH. One possible chain of events by which this might be brought about is shown in Figure 2-6. The most essential element is probably increased reabsorption of NaCl in the proximal tubules. This process results in decreased delivery of NaCl to the loops of Henle and early distal tubules, which may lead in turn to decreased reabsorption of NaCl from these segments. It is mainly in these portions of the nephron that the process of reabsorbing electrolytes to the virtual exclusion of H_2O generates solute-free H_2O. Hence, decreased reabsorption of NaCl from the ascending limbs and early distal tubules will decrease the production of free H_2O and thereby its excretion.

It is not known to what extent these mechanisms may be causative in the various disease states listed above; certainly

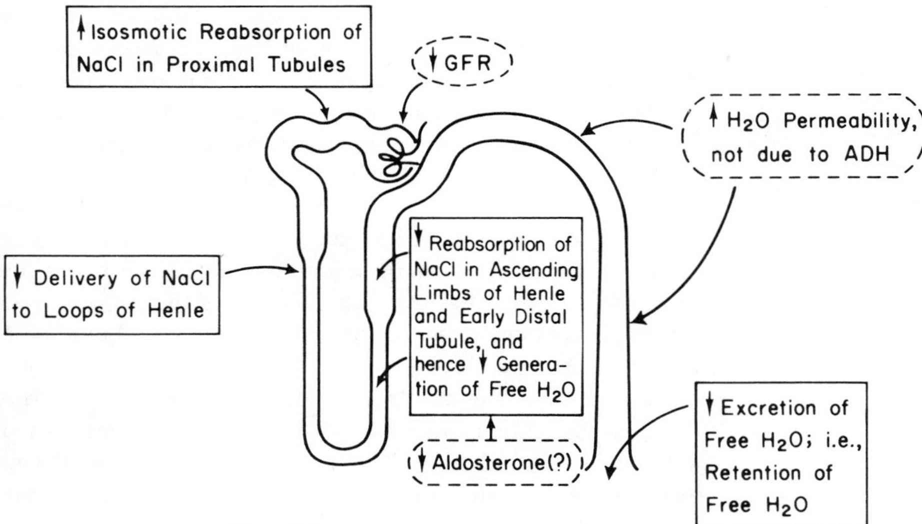

Figure 2-6
Possible chain of events whereby solute-free H_2O might be retained in disease states that mimic the syndrome of inappropriate ADH secretion (SIADH). The elements that *may* be common to all such disease states are outlined in boxes; those that contribute under some conditions are enclosed by dashed rings.

they vary in detail. A decrease in GFR, which reduces the filtered load of NaCl, may contribute to decreased delivery of electrolytes to the ascending limbs and beyond in some conditions, but not in others. A decrease in the plasma concentration of aldosterone may contribute to diminished electrolyte reabsorption from the ascending limbs or beyond in adrenal insufficiency, but probably not in heart and liver failure. And increased H_2O permeability of the distal tubules and collecting ducts (due to the absence of adrenal steroids and not necessarily to the presence of ADH) may be involved in adrenal insufficiency, but not in the other conditions listed. Suffice it to say that the presence of these disease states must be ruled out when a diagnosis of SIADH is made.

Types of Volume Contraction and Volume Expansion

The state of losing fluid from the body is often loosely called dehydration. This is an inadequate term, because it does not specify the composition of the fluid that was lost, that is, whether it was isosmotic, hyposmotic, or hyperosmotic with respect to plasma. The term overhydration has the same shortcoming. In order to overcome this inexactness, six terms are used to classify changes in the body fluid volumes. These terms and their meaning are listed in Table 2-4, and the changes in the volume and osmolality of the body-fluid compartments are shown in Figure 2-7.

Three types of contraction and three types of expansion are recognized: *isosmotic, hyperosmotic,* and *hyposmotic.* The change in volume, whether it be expansion or contraction, describes *only the extracellular volume* and not necessarily the intracellular volume (Table 2-4). The osmolality values are those of the extracellular volume, but since in the steady state the extracellular and intracellular fluids are in osmotic equilibrium, these values also describe the osmolality of the intracellular compartment. Each change described in Table 2-4 refers to the *new steady state* that is attained after the perturbation has occurred.

Isosmotic Contraction. The classic example is seen in cholera, in which the stool, being composed chiefly of the chloride and bicarbonate salts of Na^+ and K^+, approaches isosmolality. Initially the fluid is lost from the plasma, and this loss is largely replenished from the interstitial space because of a change in Starling forces. Therefore, the entire extracellular compartment contracts, but since the loss is isosmotic, there will be no major change in the osmolality of extracellular fluid, and hence no shift of H_2O in or out of the intracellular space will occur. The

Table 2-4
Classification of imbalances of body fluids and associated changes in volume and composition

Type of Imbalance	Clinical Examples	Changes in Volume		Changes in Extracellular Concentrations			
		ECF*	ICF*	Na^+	Protein	Osmolality	Hct*
Isosmotic contraction	Cholera	↓	0	0	↑	0	↑
Hyperosmotic contraction	Man lost at sea or in desert Fever	↓	↓	↑	↑	↑	0
Hyposmotic contraction	Adrenal insufficiency	↓	↑	↓	↑	↓	↑
Isosmotic expansion	Edema	↑	0	0	↓	0	↓
Hyperosmotic expansion	NaCl poisoning	↑	↓	↑	↓	↑	↓
Hyposmotic expansion	Syndrome of inappropriate ADH secretion (SIADH)	↑	↑	↓	↓	↓	0

*ECF = extracellular fluid; ICF = intracellular fluid; Hct = hematocrit.

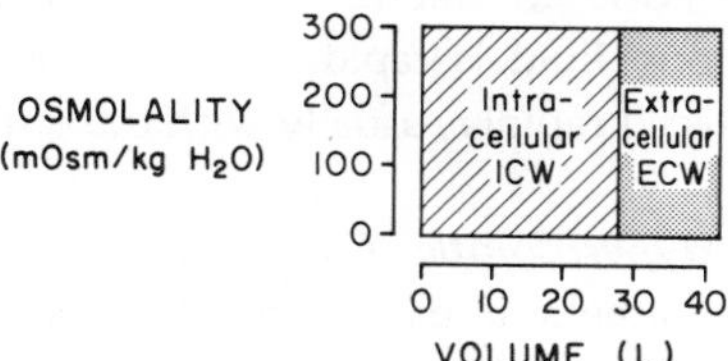

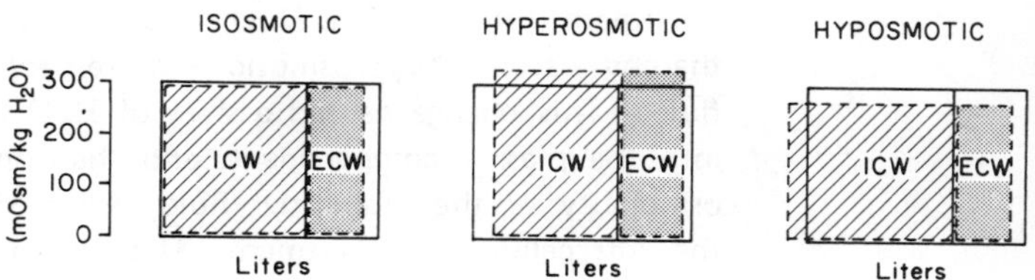

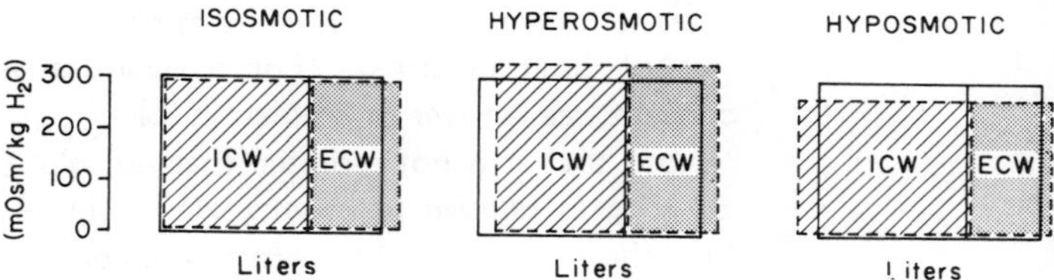

Figure 2-7
Types of contraction and expansion of the body-fluid compartments. The plasma and the interstitial fluid are here portrayed as a single extracellular compartment, and the slightly higher osmolality of plasma compared to that of interstitial and intracellular fluid (see Fig. 1-2) is ignored. In each diagram, the healthy state is drawn in solid lines, and it is contrasted with the new steady state in disease, which is delineated by the dashed lines. This type of portrayal, known as a ***Darrow-Yannet diagram,*** was introduced by these two workers in a classic contribution on this subject (*J. Clin. Invest.* 14:266, 1935).

final result will be a reduction in the volume of the extracellular fluid, but no change in its osmolality; that is, isosmotic contraction takes place.

The Na^+ concentration of choleraic stool is nearly the same as that in plasma (Table 1-4); therefore, the plasma Na^+ concentration does not change appreciably even though large amounts of stool and Na^+ are being lost. Plasma protein, however, increases in concentration as the extracellular volume is decreased, because the protein is not lost in the stool. Similarly, the hematocrit (Hct) increases, because there is essentially no blood in choleraic stool.

Inasmuch as the fluid loss in isosmotic contraction comes from the extracellular space and is not shared by the intracellular compartment, circulatory deficiency sets in earlier than in hyperosmotic contraction (see below). Hence, when the loss of isosmotic fluid is rapid, as it is in cholera, the volume must be replaced rapidly, usually with 0.9% (isosmotic) NaCl.

Hyperosmotic Contraction. In the purest form, this state represents a deficit of H_2O but not of solute, which occurs mainly when the insensible loss is high. In persons lost at sea or in the desert or in patients with fever, even when they are not sweating profusely, much H_2O is evaporated from the skin and the breath (Fig. 1-5). This H_2O came first from the plasma, which thereby became hyperosmotic with respect to the other body fluids. This change caused a shift of H_2O from the interstitial into the plasma compartment, and the consequent rise in the osmolality of the interstitial fluid caused H_2O to flow out of the intracellular compartment. That is, in hyperosmotic contraction, the volume of all the major fluid compartments is decreased, and if the deficit is one of H_2O without solute, the reduction of the intracellular and extracellular compartments bears a direct, quantitative relation to their sizes before the loss of fluid occurred. (For a quantitative treatment of this concept, see Answer to Problem 3-3.)

Note that it is not essential that no solute whatsoever be lost. So long as *relative to normal plasma* more H_2O than solute is lost, the result will be hyperosmotic contraction. The concentrations of all the major solutes, such as plasma Na^+ and protein, will rise. The Hct, however, would theoretically not change. Erythrocytes contract or swell with increases or decreases, respectively, in the osmolality of the plasma, and since the H_2O movement in or out of the cells is quantitatively related to the change in osmolality, the volume of packed cells after centrifugation will theoretically change in direct proportion to the reduction or expansion of the plasma volume.

Hyposmotic Contraction. This state results from a loss of solute in excess of H_2O, *relative to normal plasma.* The classic clinical example is demonstrated in adrenal insufficiency (Addison's disease), in which the solute lost is mainly NaCl. Since this compound comes almost exclusively from the extracellular compartment, the osmolality within that space will fall. Consequently, H_2O will shift from the extracellular into the intracellular space. The result (Table 2-4 and Fig. 2-7) will be contraction of the extracellular space but expansion of the intracellular compartment. The extracellular Na^+ concentration, and hence extracellular osmolality, will fall, but the protein concentration will rise, since protein has not been depleted. The Hct will also rise, partly because H_2O has moved into the erythrocytes. In contrast to the situation in pure hyperosmotic contraction, the Hct rises because the plasma is reduced in volume, not by the loss of H_2O only (which would result in a *proportional* shift of H_2O out of erythrocytes), but principally by the loss of solute (which is not followed by a similar shift of H_2O).

Isosmotic Expansion. This state is exemplified by one of the most common clinical signs of fluid imbalance, edema. In this state (discussed further in Chap. 3), there is a positive external balance of what is essentially a solution of NaCl that is isosmotic with normal plasma. Since both Na^+ and Cl^- are almost exclusively extracellular solutes, the retained solution is added to the extracellular compartment. Inasmuch as an isosmotic solution is being added to normal plasma, there is no change in the osmolality of the extracellular fluid, and hence no shift of H_2O in or out of the intracellular space occurs. The result is a selective enlargement of the extracellular compartment (Fig. 2-7), with a consequent decrease in the Hct and plasma protein concentration (Table 2-4).

Hyperosmotic Expansion. This state results from a positive external balance of extracellular solute in excess of H_2O, "excess" again being defined in relation to normal plasma. The situation arises perhaps most commonly in the treatment of infant diarrhea when the mother, advised to give the baby supplementary table salt, is overly zealous in her care. Since hyperosmotic NaCl is being given, the plasma concentrations of Na^+ and Cl^-, and hence the plasma osmolality, will rise. This change causes a shift of H_2O from the intracellular into the extracellular compartment until osmotic equilibrium between the two compartments is reached. In the new steady state, therefore, the extracellular space is expanded, the intracellular is contracted, and the osmolality of both is greater than normal. Inasmuch as no protein or erythrocytes are lost, the serum protein concentration and the Hct are decreased.

Hyposmotic Expansion. A classic clinical example is the syndrome of inappropriate ADH secretion (SIADH), in which there is a positive external balance of H_2O. As described in detail above (under Surfeit of ADH and the Syndrome of Inappropriate ADH Secretion), the retained H_2O is distributed throughout the major fluid compartments, so that both the intracellular and extracellular spaces are expanded. The major solutes are thereby diluted, so the osmolality of both compartments is lower than normal. In analogy with the events seen in pure hyperosmotic contraction, the erythrocytes enlarge in direct proportion to the amount of extra H_2O being retained in the extracellular compartment; consequently, in the slightly hypothetical, "pure" situation in which the change in balance is limited to H_2O, the Hct does not change.

Summary

In mammals, disorders of H_2O balance can arise from irregularities in the plasma concentration of antidiuretic hormone (vasopressin or ADH), from conditions that mimic such irregularities, or from abnormal output or intake of H_2O and salt.

Deficits of ADH in the plasma or renal defects that block or lessen the action of ADH will cause diabetes insipidus (D.I.). Three forms of this disorder are recognized: (1) primary polydipsic D.I., in which excessive drinking dilutes the plasma and thereby chronically inhibits the secretion of endogenous ADH; (2) hypothalamic D.I., in which some defect in the hypothalamoneurohypophyseal system decreases or prevents the production or release of ADH; and (3) nephrogenic D.I., in which a defect within the kidneys precludes a normal antidiuretic response to ADH, even though the plasma concentration of the hormone is normal or high. The three forms can be distinguished by means of the Hickey-Hare test (or some modification thereof), which represents a direct application of the classic, physiological experiments of E. B. Verney.

An excess of ADH in the plasma, when combined with a normal or high fluid intake, will usually result in a positive H_2O balance, because the kidneys will be unable to excrete enough solute-free H_2O. The classic clinical example of this state is the syndrome of inappropriate ADH secretion (SIADH). In this syndrome, the retention of H_2O leads to (1) dilution of the plasma Na^+, and hence an abnormally low plasma osmolality, and (2) a relatively high urine osmolality, when a minimal value would normally be predicted on the basis of the low plasma osmolality. During the development of SIADH, but not necessarily in the new steady state attained, increased urinary excretion of Na^+ may contribute to the hyponatremia. The syndrome may also be caused by other substances that have an ADH-like, antidiuretic effect (e.g., polypeptide analogues of arginine-vasopressin or certain drugs).

Usually the first sign that alerts a physician to the possible existence of SIADH is hyponatremia. Therefore, a number of diseases that are commonly accompanied by hyponatremia enter into the differential diagnosis of SIADH. In order of approximate decreasing frequency, these diseases are heart failure, liver failure, renal failure, adrenal insufficiency, and myxedema. It is possible that the main mechanism(s) leading to the retention of free H_2O

in these conditions may reside within the kidneys and may not necessarily involve high plasma concentrations of ADH.

Although the terms dehydration and overhydration literally refer to a loss or surfeit of H_2O, they are often used in clinical parlance to denote a change in the balance of body *fluids,* that is, H_2O plus solute. It is more accurate, and hence more useful, to describe disorders of fluid balance as *volume contraction* or *volume expansion* and to modify these terms with adjectives that describe the state of the extracellular fluid after the perturbation has occurred. There are six types of fluid imbalance: isosmotic contraction, hyperosmotic contraction, hyposmotic contraction, isosmotic expansion, hyperosmotic expansion, and hyposmotic expansion. Although these terms describe the final state of the extracellular compartment, changes also occur in the intracellular space in all but the isosmotic disturbances. The changes in both compartments are shown in Table 2-4 and Figure 2-7.

The dynamics leading to the various states of fluid imbalance can be logically predicted from a knowledge of the type of fluid that is lost from or gained by the body. For example, when H_2O is lost in excess of solute (relative to normal plasma), extracellular solutes are concentrated. The consequent rise in extracellular osmolality causes a shift of H_2O from the intracellular into the extracellular compartment that continues until osmotic equilibrium between the two compartments has been restored. The new steady state will be characterized by *hyperosmotic contraction of the extracellular space;* in this type of contraction, but not in others, similar changes will have occurred in the intracellular fluid.

Problem 2-1

A water deprivation test is run on an adult patient who weighs 75 kg. Drinking fluid is withheld until the patient has lost 3 percent of the initial weight. Assuming that the plasma osmolality and the plasma Na^+ concentration were 290 mOsm/kg H_2O and 140 mEq per liter, respectively, at the beginning of the test, what should be the approximate values for these two concentrations after the weight has been lost?

Make the following assumptions in solving this problem: (1) all the weight loss represents loss of fluid; (2) only H_2O, and no solute, has been lost; and (3) total body water (TBW), intracellular water (ICW), and extracellular water (ECW) equal 60, 40, and 20 percent of body weight, respectively.

Problem 2-2

Loss of fluid through sweat is a hypotonic loss (see Table 1-4); that is, it leads to hyperosmotic contraction (Table 2-4). Why then do athletes apparently benefit from ingesting salt tablets? Why does this practice not lead to further hypertonicity of the extracellular fluid?

Problem 2-3 "Water, water every where, nor any drop to drink." Was Coleridge right; that is, should a castaway at sea drink seawater, or should he not?

Selected References

General

Adolph, E. F., and Associates. *Physiology of Man in the Desert.* New York: Interscience, 1947.

Andersson, B., and McCann, S. M. Drinking, antidiuresis and milk ejection from electrical stimulation within the hypothalamus of the goat. *Acta Physiol. Scand.* 35:191, 1955.

Andreoli, T. E., Grantham, J. J., and Rector, F. C., Jr. (eds.). *Disturbances in Body Fluid Osmolality.* Bethesda, Md.: American Physiological Society, 1977.
This volume contains many useful articles on topics ranging from the cellular action of ADH to the clinical syndromes of water imbalance.

Epstein, A. N., Kissileff, H. R., and Stellar, E. *The Neuropsychology of Thirst: New Findings and Advances in Concepts.* Washington, D.C.: Winston, 1973.

Gamble, J. L. *Companionship of Water and Electrolytes in the Organization of Body Fluids.* Stanford, Calif.: Stanford University Press, 1951.

Gauer, O. H., Henry, J. P., and Behn, C. The regulation of extracellular fluid volume. *Annu. Rev. Physiol.* 32:547, 1970.

Hays, R. M., and Levine, S. D. Pathophysiology of Water Metabolism. In B. M. Brenner and F. C. Rector, Jr. (eds.), *The Kidney.* Philadelphia: Saunders, 1976.

Jamison, R. L., and Maffly, R. H. The urinary concentrating mechanism. *N. Eng. J. Med.* 295:1059, 1976.

Maffly, R. H. The Body Fluids: Volume, Composition, and Physical Chemistry. In B. M. Brenner and F. C. Rector, Jr. (eds.), *The Kidney.* Philadelphia: Saunders, 1976.

Massry, S. G., and Coburn, J. W. Clinical Physiology of Heat Exposure. In M. H. Maxwell and C. R. Kleeman (eds.), *Clinical Disorders of Fluid and Electrolyte Metabolism* (2nd ed.). New York: McGraw-Hill, 1972.

Maxwell, M. H., and Kleeman, C. R. (eds.). *Clinical Disorders of Fluid and Electrolyte Metabolism* (2nd ed.). New York: McGraw-Hill, 1972.

Mudge, G. H., and Welt, L. G. Agents Affecting Volume and Composition of Body Fluids. In L. S. Goodman and A. Gilman (eds.), *The Pharmacological Basis of Therapeutics* (5th ed.). New York: Macmillan, 1974.

Schmidt-Nielsen, K. *Desert Animals: Physiological Problems of Heat and Water.* London: Oxford University Press, 1964.

Schrier, R. W. (ed.). Symposium on water metabolism. *Kidney Int.* 10:1, 1976.
Another useful and up-to-date compendium covering both basic science and clinical aspects of water balance.

Schrier, R. W., and Berl, T. Nonosmolar factors affecting renal water excretion. *N. Engl. J. Med.* 292:81 and 141, 1975.

Valtin, H. *Renal Function: Mechanisms Preserving Fluid and Solute Balance in Health.* Boston: Little, Brown, 1973. Chap. 8.

Wolf, A. V. *Thirst: Physiology of the Urge to Drink and Problems of Water Lack.* Springfield, Ill.: Thomas, 1958.

Antidiuretic Hormone (ADH)

Andreoli, T. E., and Schafer, J. A. Mass transport across cell membranes: The effects of antidiuretic hormone on water and solute flows in epithelia. *Annu. Rev. Physiol.* 39:451, 1976.

Berde, B. (ed.). Neurohypophysial Hormones and Similar Polypeptides. In *Handbook of Experimental Pharmacology,* vol. 23. Berlin: Springer, 1968.

Champion, H. R., Caplan, Y. H., Baker, S. P., Long, W. B., Benner, C., Cowley, R. A., Fisher, R., and Gill, W. Alcohol intoxication and serum osmolality. *Lancet* 1:1402, 1975.

Dousa, T. P. Cellular action of antidiuretic hormone in nephrogenic diabetes insipidus. *Proc. Staff Meetings Mayo Clin.* 49:188, 1974.

Dunn, F. L., Brennan, T. J., Nelson, A. E., and Robertson, G. L. The role of blood osmolality and volume in regulating vasopressin secretion in the rat. *J. Clin. Invest.* 52:3212, 1973.

Dunn, M. J., and Hood, V. L. Prostaglandins and the kidney. *Am. J. Physiol.* 233:F 169, 1977.

Gauer, O. H., and Henry, J. P. Circulatory basis of fluid volume control. *Physiol. Rev.* 43:423, 1963.

Grantham, J. J. Action of Antidiuretic Hormone in the Mammalian Kidney. In K. Thurau (ed.), *Kidney and Urinary Tract Physiology.* Baltimore: University Park Press, 1974.

Harris, G. W., and Donovan, B. T. (eds.). *The Pituitary Gland,* vol. 3. *Pars Intermedia and Neurohypophysis.* Berkeley: University of California Press, 1966.

Heller, H. (ed.). *The Neurohypophysis.* London: Butterworth, 1957.

Johnson, J. A., Zehr, J. E., and Moore, W. W. Effects of separate and concurrent osmotic and volume stimuli on plasma ADH in sheep. *Am. J. Physiol.* 218:1273, 1970.

Knobil, E., and Sawyer, W. H. (eds.). *Handbook of Physiology,* Section 7, The Pituitary Gland and Its Neuroendocrine Control, vol. 4, part 1. Washington, D.C.: American Physiological Society, 1974.

Manning, M., Balaspiri, L., Acosta, M., and Sawyer, W. H. Solid phase synthesis of [1-deamino,4-valine]-8-D-arginine-vasopressin (DVDAVP), a highly potent and specific antidiuretic agent possessing protracted effects. *J. Med. Chem.* 16:975, 1973.

Robertson, G. L., Mahr, E. A., Athar, S., and Sinha, T. Development and clinical application of a new method for the radioimmunoassay of arginine vasopressin in human plasma. *J. Clin. Invest.* 52:2340, 1973.

Robinson, A. G. DDAVP in the treatment of central diabetes insipidus. *N. Engl. J. Med.* 294:507, 1976.

Robinson, A. G., and Loeb, J. N. Ethanol ingestion — commonest cause of elevated plasma osmolality? *N. Engl. J. Med.* 284:1253, 1971.

de Rubertis, F. R., Michelis, M. F., Beck, N., Field, J. B., and Davis, B. B. "Essential" hypernatremia due to ineffective osmotic and intact volume regulation of vasopressin secretion. *J. Clin. Invest.* 50:97, 1971.

Sawyer, W. H., Acosta, M., Balaspiri, L., Judd, J., and Manning, M. Structural changes in the arginine vasopressin molecule that enhance antidiuretic activity and specificity. *Endocrinology* 94:1106, 1974.

Sawyer, W. H., and Manning, M. Synthetic analogs of oxytocin and the vasopressins. *Annu. Rev. Pharmacol. Toxicol.* 13:5, 1973.

Scharrer, E., and Scharrer, B. Hormones produced by neurosecretory cells. *Recent Prog. Horm. Res.* 10:183, 1954.

Schwartz, I. L., and Schwartz, W. B. (eds.). Symposium on antidiuretic hormones. *Am. J. Med.* 42:651, 1967.

This symposium is dedicated to Dr. Vincent du Vigneaud, who was the first person to synthesize a polypeptide hormone (oxytocin) and who, a few years later, also succeeded in synthesizing vasopressin. The symposium is a useful source of information on the antidiuretic hormones, covering topics such as their chemistry, evolution, release, biosynthesis, bioassay, metabolism, and mode of action, as well as the clinical entities of diabetes insipidus and the syndrome of inappropriate secretion of antidiuretic hormone (SIADH).

Szczepańska-Sadowska, E. The activity of the hypothalamo-hypophysial antidiuretic system in conscious dogs: II. Role of the left vasosympathetic trunk. *Pflügers Arch. Eur. J. Physiol.* 335:147, 1972.

Valtin, H., Stewart, J., and Sokol, H. W. Genetic Control of the Production of Posterior Pituitary Principles. In E. Knobil and W. H. Sawyer (eds.), *Handbook of Physiology,* Section 7, The Pituitary Gland and Its Neuroendocrine Control, vol. 4, part 1. Washington, D.C.: American Physiological Society, 1974.

Verney, E. B. The antidiuretic hormone and the factors which determine its release. *Proc. R. Soc. Lond. [Biol.]* 135:25, 1947.

du Vigneaud, V. Trail of sulfur research: From insulin to oxytocin. *Science* 123:967, 1956.

Diabetes Insipidus and Related Disorders

Barlow, E. D., and de Wardener, H. E. Compulsive water drinking. *Q. J. Med.* 28:235, 1959.

Berndt, W. O., Miller, M., Kettyle, W. M., and Valtin, H. Potentiation of the antidiuretic effect of vasopressin by chlorpropamide. *Endocrinology* 86:1028, 1970.

Coggins, C. H., and Leaf, A. Diabetes insipidus. *Am. J. Med.* 42:807, 1967.

Crawford, J. D., and Bode, H. H. Disorders of the Posterior Pituitary in Children. In L. I. Gardner (ed.), *Endocrine and Genetic Diseases of Childhood and Adolescence* (2nd ed.). Philadelphia: Saunders, 1975.

Crawford, J. D., and Kennedy, G. C. Chlorothiazid in diabetes insipidus. *Nature* 183:891, 1959.

Dashe, A. M., Cramm, R. E., Crist, C. A., Habener, J. F., and Solomon, D. H. A water deprivation test for the differential diagnosis of polyuria. *J. A. M. A.* 185:699, 1963.

de Wardener, H. E. Polyuria . *J. Chronic Dis.* 11:199, 1960.

Dingman, J. F., Benirschke, K., and Thorn, G. W. Studies of neurohypophyseal function in man: Diabetes insipidus and psychogenic polydipsia. *Am. J. Med.* 23:226, 1957.

Earley, L. E. Chlorpropamide antidiuresis. *N. Engl. J. Med.* 284:103, 1971.

Edwards, C. R. W., Kitau, M. J., Chard, T., and Besser, G. M. Vasopressin analogue DDAVP in diabetes insipidus: Clinical and laboratory studies. *Br. Med. J.* 2:375, 1973.

Fischer, C., Ingram, W. R., and Ranson, S. W. *Diabetes Insipidus and the Neuro-Hormonal Control of Water Balance: A Contribution to the Structure and Function of the Hypothalamico-Hypophyseal System.* Ann Arbor, Mich.: Edwards, 1938.

Forrest, J. N., Jr., Cohen, A. D., Torretti, J., Himmelhoch, J. M., and Epstein, F. H. On the mechanism of lithium-induced diabetes insipidus in man and rat. *J. Clin. Invest.* 53:1115, 1974.

Harrington, A. R., and Valtin, H. Impaired urinary concentration after vasopressin and its gradual correction in hypothalamic diabetes insipidus. *J. Clin. Invest.* 47:502, 1968.

Hickey, R. C., and Hare, K. The renal excretion of chloride and water in diabetes insipidus. *J. Clin. Invest.* 23:768, 1944.

Hollinshead, W. H. The interphase of diabetes insipidus. *Proc. Mayo Clin.* 39:92, 1964.

Kleeman, C. R. Water Metabolism. In M. H. Maxwell and C. R. Kleeman (eds.), *Clinical Disorders of Fluid and Electrolyte Metabolism* (2nd ed.). New York: McGraw-Hill, 1972.

Lozada, E. S., Gouaux, J., Franki, N., Appel, G. B., and Hays, R. M. Studies of the mode of action of the sulfonylureas and phenylacetamides in enhancing the effect of vasopressin. *J. Clin. Endocrinol. Metab.* 34:704, 1972.

Miller, M., Dalakos, T., Moses, A. M., Fellerman, H., and Streeten, D. H. P. Recognition of partial defects in antidiuretic hormone secretion. *Ann. Intern. Med.* 73:721, 1970.

Miller, M., and Moses, A. M. Mechanism of chlorpropamide action in diabetes insipidus. *J. Clin. Endocrinol. Metab.* 30:488, 1970.

Orloff, J., and Burg, M. G. Vasopressin-resistant Diabetes Insipidus. In M. B. Strauss and L. G. Welt (eds.), *Diseases of the Kidney* (2nd ed.). Boston: Little, Brown, 1971.

ten Bensel, R. W., and Peters, E. R. Progressive hydronephrosis, hydroureter, and dilatation of the bladder in siblings with congenital nephrogenic diabetes insipidus. *J. Pediatr.* 77:439, 1970.

Thomas, W. C., Jr. Diabetes insipidus. *J. Clin. Endocrinol. Metab.* 17:565, 1957.

Valtin, H. Hereditary Diabetes Insipidus: Lessons Learned from Animal Models. In C. Gual (ed.), *Progress in Endocrinology.* Amsterdam: Excerpta Medica Foundation, 1969, p. 321.

Valtin, H., and Green, H. H. Diabetes Insipidus. In H. F. Conn and R. B. Conn, Jr. (eds.), *Current Therapy.* Philadelphia: Saunders, 1974.

Zweig, S. M., Ettinger, B., and Earley, L. E. Mechanism of antidiuretic action of chlorpropamide in the mammalian kidney. *Am. J. Physiol.* 221:911, 1971.

SIADH and Related Disorders

Abbrecht, P. H., and Malvin, R. L. Effects of GFR and renal plasma flow on urine osmolarity. *Am. J. Physiol.* 201:754, 1961.

Bartter, F. C., and Schwartz, W. B. The syndrome of inappropriate secretion of antidiuretic hormone. *Am. J. Med.* 42:790, 1967.

Bell, N. H., Schedl, H. P., and Bartter, F. C. An explanation for abnormal water retention and hypoosmolality in congestive heart failure. *Am. J. Med.* 36:351, 1964.

Berliner, R. W., and Davidson, D. G. Production of hypertonic urine in the absence of pituitary antidiuretic hormone. *J. Clin. Invest.* 36:1416, 1957.

DiScala, V. A., and Kinney, M. J. Effects of myxedema on the renal diluting and concentrating mechanism. *Am. J. Med.* 50:325, 1971.

Farber, M. O., Bright, T. P., Strawbridge, R. A., Robertson, G. L., and Manfredi, F. Impaired water handling in chronic obstructive lung disease. *J. Lab. Clin. Med.* 85:41, 1975.

Forrest, J. N., Jr. Lithium inhibition of cAMP-mediated hormones: A caution. *N. Engl. J. Med.* 292:423, 1975.

Forrest, J. N., Jr., Cox, M., Hong, C., Morrison, G., Bia, M., and Singer, I. Superiority of demeclocycline over lithium in the treatment of chronic syndrome of inappropriate secretion of antidiuretic hormone. *N. Engl. J. Med.* 298:173, 1978.

George, J. M., Capen, C. C., and Phillips, A. S. Biosynthesis of vasopressin in vitro and ultrastructure of a bronchogenic carcinoma. *J. Clin. Invest.* 51:141, 1972.

Green, H. H., Harrington, A. R., and Valtin, H. On the role of antidiuretic hormone in the inhibition of acute water diuresis in adrenal insufficiency and the effects of gluco- and mineralocorticoids in reversing the inhibition. *J. Clin. Invest.* 49:1724, 1970.

Harrington, A. R. Hyponatremia due to sodium depletion in the absence of vasopressin. *Am. J. Physiol.* 222:768, 1972.

Kinney, M. J., Stein, R. M., and DiScala, V. A. The polyuria of paroxysmal atrial tachycardia. *Circulation* 50:429, 1974.

Kleeman, C. R. Water Metabolism. In M. H. Maxwell and C. R. Kleeman (eds.), *Clinical Disorders of Fluid and Electrolyte Metabolism* (2nd ed.). New York: McGraw-Hill, 1972.

Klein, L. A., Rabson, A. S., and Worksman, J. In vitro synthesis of vasopressin by lung tumor cells. *Surg. Forum* 20:231, 1969.

Langgård, H., and Smith, W. O. Self-induced water intoxication without predisposing illness: Report of two cases. *N. Engl. J. Med.* 266:378, 1962.

Leaf, A., Bartter, F. C., Santos, R. F., and Wrong, O. Evidence in man that urinary electrolyte loss induced by pitressin is a function of water retention. *J. Clin. Invest.* 32:868, 1953.

Levinsky, N. G., Davidson, D. G., and Berliner, R. W. Changes in urine concentration during prolonged administration of vasopressin and water. *Am. J. Physiol.* 196:451, 1959.

Moses, A. M., and Miller, M. Drug-induced dilutional hyponatremia. *N. Engl. J. Med.* 291:1234, 1974.

Nicholson, R. G., and Feldman, W. Hyponatremia in association with vincristine therapy. *Can. Med. Assoc. J.* 106:356, 1972.

Padfield, P. L., Morton, J. J., Brown, J. J., Lever, A. F., Robertson, J. I. S., Wood, M., and Fox, R. Plasma arginine vasopressin in the syndrome of antidiuretic hormone excess associated with bronchogenic carcinoma. *Am. J. Med.* 61:825, 1976.

Sawyer, W. H. Pharmacological characteristics of the antidiuretic principle in a bronchogenic carcinoma from a patient with hyponatremia. *J. Clin. Endocrinol. Metab.* 27:1497, 1967.

Schedl, H. P., and Bartter, F. C. An explanation for and experimental correction of the abnormal water diuresis in cirrhosis. *J. Clin. Invest.* 39:248, 1960.

Schrier, R. W. New treatments for hyponatremia. *N. Engl. J. Med.* 298: 214, 1978.

Schrier, R. W., and Berl, T. Hyponatremia and related disorders. *Kidney* 7:1, 1974.

Schwartz, W. B., Bennett, W., Curelop, S., and Bartter, F. C. A syndrome of renal sodium loss and hyponatremia probably resulting from inappropriate secretion of antidiuretic hormone. *Am. J. Med.* 23:529, 1957.

Ufferman, R. C., and Schrier, R. W. Importance of sodium intake and mineralocorticoid hormone in the impaired water excretion in adrenal insufficiency. *J. Clin. Invest.* 51:1639, 1972.

Weissman, P. N., Shenkman, L., and Gregerman, R. I. Chlorpropamide hyponatremia. Drug-induced inappropriate antidiuretic-hormone activity. *N. Engl. J. Med.* 284:65, 1971.

White, M. G., and Fetner, C. D. Treatment of the syndrome of inappropriate secretion of antidiuretic hormone with lithium carbonate. *N. Engl. J. Med.* 292:390, 1975.

Types of Fluid Imbalance

Arieff, A. I., and Kleeman, C. R. Studies on mechanisms of cerebral edema in diabetic comas: Effects of hyperglycemia and rapid lowering of plasma glucose in normal rabbits. *J. Clin. Invest.* 52:571, 1973.

Finberg, L. Hypernatremic (hypertonic) dehydration in infants. *N. Engl. J. Med.* 289:196, 1973.

Finberg, L., Kiley, J., and Luttrell, C. N. Mass accidental salt poisoning in infancy. *J. A. M. A.* 184:187, 1963.

Fulop, M., Tannenbaum, H., and Dreyer, N. Ketotic hyperosmolar coma. *Lancet* 2:635, 1973.

Holliday, M. A. Body Fluid Physiology During Growth. In M. H. Maxwell and C. R. Kleeman (eds.), *Clinical Disorders of Fluid and Electrolyte Metabolism* (2nd ed.). New York: McGraw-Hill, 1972.

Holliday, M. A., Kalayci, M. N., and Harrah, J. Factors that limit brain volume changes in response to acute and sustained hyper- and hyponatremia. *J. Clin. Invest.* 47:1916, 1968.

Tyler, F. H. Hyperosmolar coma. *Am. J. Med.* 45:485, 1968.

3 : Disorders of Na^+ Balance. Edema

Importance of Na^+ Balance

Among the variables that a normal organism keeps constant are the osmolality and volume of the extracellular fluid. Inasmuch as Na^+ and its attendant anions are by far the most abundant particles in this fluid, the concentration of Na^+ within it reflects the extracellular osmolality under most conditions (Table 1-2). Yet, perhaps surprisingly, the plasma concentration of Na^+ is usually *not* determined as much by the Na^+ balance as it is by H_2O balance, which was discussed in the preceding chapter. For example, hyperosmotic contraction and hyposmotic expansion – that is, imbalances predominantly of H_2O – are more common clinical causes of hypernatremia and hyponatremia (Table 2-4) than are imbalances of Na^+, at least in adult medicine. This fact embodies an important lesson that is too often forgotten: In the majority of adult patients, hypernatremia and hyponatremia reflect an imbalance of H_2O that is relatively greater than the imbalance of Na^+.

The *volume* of the extracellular fluid, however, depends critically on the balance of Na^+. The regulatory responses to changes in the intake of H_2O set in very rapidly (Figs. 2-1 and 2-3); hence, the plasma Na^+ concentration and osmolality are normally kept constant. It then follows from the relationship

$$\text{Concentration} = \frac{\text{Amount of solute}}{\text{Volume of solvent}} \qquad (3\text{-}1)$$

that the amount of Na^+ (and its attendant anions) mainly determines the size of the extracellular compartment (Fig. 2-7 and Table 2-4). One component of this compartment is the plasma (Fig. 1-2), and therein lies the importance of Na^+ balance: A *positive* balance will lead to an expansion of the plasma volume, which may eventuate in cardiac failure, and a *negative* Na^+ balance results in contraction of the plasma volume, which may lead to circulatory insufficiency.

In health, Na^+ balance is regulated primarily or exclusively by the kidneys. For example, of the 155 mEq of Na^+ that may be ingested daily by a healthy, adult human (Table 1-6), about 150 mEq is excreted in the urine, and this amount is carefully adjusted from day to day to conform to variations in the intake of Na^+. In this chapter we will review the mechanisms that are thought to govern Na^+ balance in health, and we will then examine how disturbances of the normal regulatory factors lead to surfeits or deficits of Na^+.

Regulation of Na^+ Balance in Health

Time Course

The time course for the attainment of Na^+ balance when the intake of Na^+ is changed abruptly varies with the prior history of Na^+ intake. In Figure 3-1, the first seven days depict the control situation; the person ingests 150 mEq of Na^+ each day, excretes virtually all of it in the urine, and is therefore in balance. The diagram for day 4 shows how the balance over a 24-hour period is actually achieved. If a normal subject ingests the daily allowance of 150 mEq of Na^+ in four equal portions, virtually all the ingested Na^+ will be excreted during each ensuing 6-hour period. There will be slight positive or negative balances during any one 6-hour period (which are due mainly to diurnal variations), but the cumulative balance for the 24-hour period will be zero.

When the dietary intake of Na^+ is suddenly doubled from a normal of 150 mEq per day to 300 mEq, balance can be attained by the second day. On the first day of doubling the dietary intake, the subject excretes only about 75 mEq of Na^+ more than in the control situation. Since he ingested 300 mEq but excreted only 225 mEq, he is in positive Na^+ balance; this excess Na^+ *would* lead to an increase in plasma osmolality were it not for the fact that it causes thirst. If the person drinks sufficient H_2O to maintain normal plasma osmolality, then, for a net positive Na^+ balance of 75 mEq, he will retain 0.5 liter of H_2O. This would be reflected in a weight gain of 0.5 kg, or less than 1 percent of the control weight.

Thus, the adjustment to a change in Na^+ intake, when superimposed on a healthy person in balance *on a normal Na^+ intake,* is relatively rapid, a matter of a few hours to a day. The adjustment is slower when the increment of Na^+ is given to a healthy subject who has been on a low intake of Na^+. This point is illustrated by the graph for days 29 through 34 in Figure 3-1. On days 26 through 28, the subject is in balance, ingesting and excreting approximately 10 mEq of Na^+ daily. When the intake of Na^+ is increased by nearly 150 mEq per day, the subject excretes only about one-half the increased load, the same response

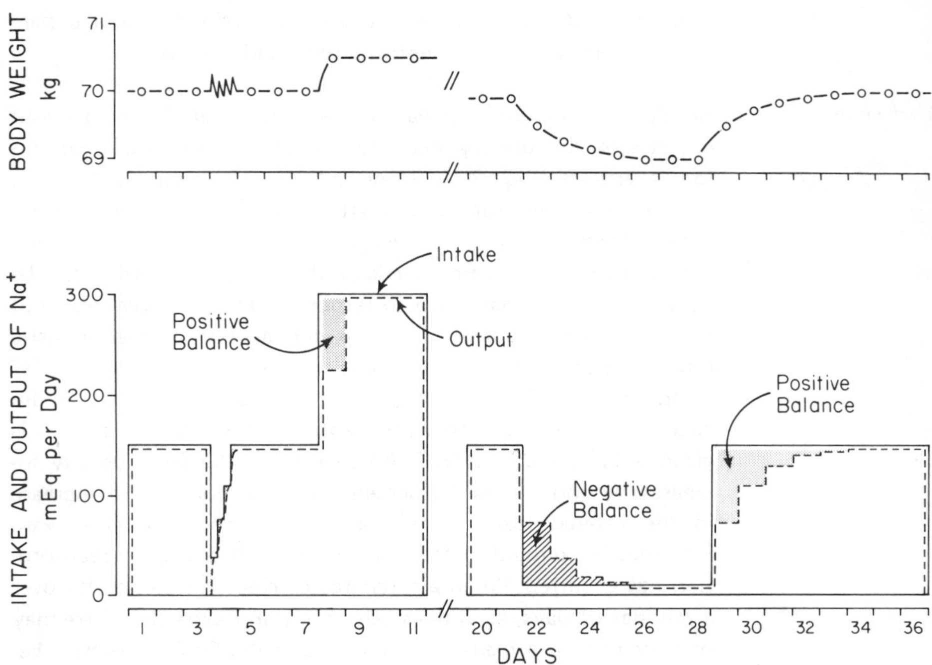

Figure 3-1
Responses of a normal person to sudden changes in Na^+ (Cl^-) intake (solid lines). The "output" (dashed lines) plotted here is the urinary excretion of Na^+, which normally amounts to more than 95 percent of the total Na^+ excretion (see Table 1-6). Note (1) that body weight is an excellent indicator of balance and (2) that the time course for the attainment of balance depends on the prior history of Na^+ intake. For day 4, the ordinate for Na^+ should read "mEq per 6 Hours," rather than "mEq per Day." Adapted from M. B. Strauss et al., *Arch. Intern. Med.* 102:527, 1958; L. E. Earley, in M. H. Maxwell and C. R. Kleeman (eds.), *Clinical Disorders of Fluid and Electrolyte Metabolism* (2nd ed.). New York: McGraw-Hill, 1972, p. 95.

as on day 8. In contrast to the earlier situation, however, it now takes him an additional three to five days to attain balance. During the days of adjustment, there is a cumulative, positive Na^+ balance of about 150 mEq. As before, this is accompanied by sufficient H_2O intake to maintain a normal plasma osmolality; that is, 1 liter of isosmotic NaCl is retained, and this is reflected in a weight gain of 1 kg. A similar, relatively slow adjustment occurs when the dietary intake of Na^+ (Cl^-) is reduced to 10 mEq, as on day 22.

The reasons for the differences in time course are not fully understood, mainly because all the mechanisms for the renal regulation of Na^+ balance are not yet clear (see below). However, whether the full compensation takes a few hours, as on day 4 in Figure 3-1, or several days, as from days 29 to 34, the important point is that in health, balance is reestablished with remarkable precision and with sufficient rapidity to prevent serious expansion or contraction of the extracellular fluid volume.

Mechanisms

Multiple mechanisms appear to be involved in bringing about changes in the urinary excretion of Na^+ as the intake of this ion is altered (Fig. 3-1). They fall into two major categories: (1) changes in the rate of glomerular filtration and hence in the filtered load of Na^+ (GFR · P_{Na^+}) and (2) changes in the tubular reabsorption of Na^+. For the sake of simplicity, we will describe here the changes that occur in response to an *increased* intake of Na^+; generally, changes that are similar but in the opposite direction occur when Na^+ intake is curtailed.

Increased GFR. Measurement of the GFR (e.g., by inulin clearance) is accurate to within about ±10%. When a subject is given a large load of NaCl intravenously, the GFR usually increases by more than 10 percent, and the consequent increase in the filtered load of Na^+ can easily account for the extra Na^+ that is excreted in the urine, even if no change in reabsorption has occurred. When a surcharge of NaCl is given orally over a number of days, as in the study shown in Figure 3-1, there may or may not be a *measurable* increase in the GFR. However, because the rate at which Na^+ is filtered into the tubular system is so high compared to the rate at which Na^+ is excreted, even an unmeasurable increase in GFR could account for the extra Na^+ that is excreted. The following example illustrates this point.

In the study shown in Figure 3-1, as the intake of Na^+ (Cl^-) was doubled during days 8 through 11, an additional 150 mEq of Na^+ was excreted each day. Since there are 1,440 minutes in a day, this extra excretion amounts to 0.104 mEq per minute. If, during the control period when the Na^+ intake was 150 mEq per day, the person had a normal GFR of 125 ml per minute, his filtered load of Na^+ was 125 ml/min × 0.140 mEq/ml = 17.5 mEq per minute. If, during the period of increased Na^+ intake, the GFR increased by just 1 percent to 126.3 ml per minute — a change that cannot be measured with confidence — then the filtered load of Na^+ would have increased to 126.3 ml/min × 0.140 mEq/ml = 17.7 mEq per minute; that is, the increment in the amount of Na^+ that is filtered would be nearly two times greater than the extra Na^+ (0.104 mEq per minute) that is excreted. For these reasons, it may be difficult or impossible to gauge the contribution of an increased GFR to the greater urinary Na^+ excretion during salt loading.

The mechanisms whereby an increased intake of Na^+ raises the GFR are not fully known. They probably involve changes in the Starling forces across the glomerular capillaries (e.g., increased hydrostatic pressure within these capillaries resulting from a higher systemic blood pressure or changes in the resistances at the afferent or efferent arterioles), decreased plasma oncotic pressure, and increased flow of plasma through the glomerular capillaries.

Decreased Tubular Reabsorption. An increased intake of Na^+ diminishes the release of *aldosterone* from the adrenal cortex and thus lowers the plasma concentration of this hormone. This effect could contribute importantly to decreased tubular reabsorption of Na^+ during salt loading. The sites in the nephron where aldosterone acts have not been conclusively identified; they include the distal tubules and collecting ducts, as well as possibly the thick ascending limbs of Henle.

The classic experiments of H. E. de Wardener and his associates, published in 1961, have shown conclusively that there are mechanisms besides an increase in GFR and a decrease in aldosterone that play a role in the renal response to a surfeit of Na^+. These additional factors are *nonaldosterone effects* that also decrease the tubular reabsorption of Na^+; they appear to act not only on the proximal tubules, but also on the more distal portions of the nephron. Although the existence of all the additional factors has not yet been irrefutably demonstrated, these factors may include a change in the plasma concentration of a *natriuretic hormone;* a change in the *hemodynamics and rate of glomerular filtration of single nephrons* (sGFR as distinct from GFR, which refers to the glomerular filtration rate of all nephrons combined); and a change in the *Starling forces across the peritubular capillaries.*

The natriuretic hormone, if it exists, would presumably act in a manner opposite to that of aldosterone; that is, in the presence of the hormone, tubular reabsorption of Na^+ would be inhibited. Despite a tremendous amount of work in numerous laboratories, the source of the hormone, its nature, its mode and site of action, and its very existence remain in doubt.

It is now well established that functionally as well as anatomically, the kidney consists of at least two types of nephron, the *superficial cortical nephron* and the *juxtamedullary nephron.* The glomerular filtration rate of a single nephron (sGFR) is considerably lower in a superficial cortical than in a juxtamedullary nephron, and the two types also differ in the behavior of their peritubular blood flow, which probably plays an important role in the tubular reabsorption of Na^+ (see below). Furthermore, the juxtamedullary nephron has a longer proximal tubule and a much longer loop of Henle than does the superficial cortical nephron. These latter characteristics have given rise to the notion that juxtamedullary nephrons may conserve Na^+ more avidly than superficial cortical nephrons. Juxtamedullary nephrons have therefore been dubbed "relative salt savers" and superficial cortical nephrons, "relative salt losers."

Consistent with this notion are observations (by some, though not by all, investigators) that both the blood supply and sGFR of "salt-wasting" superficial cortical nephrons are increased in response to an imposed Na^+ load, while the blood flow and sGFR may be simultaneously decreased in the "salt-saving" juxtamedullary nephrons. This phenomenon – called *redistribution of renal blood flow and single-nephron filtration rate* – occurs in the opposite direction in pathological states (e.g., congestive heart failure) that are associated with abnormal retention of Na^+.

Figure 3-2 depicts a possible scheme whereby changes in the Starling forces across peritubular capillaries might effect an increased excretion of Na^+ when a Na^+ load is given. The critical proposed changes are an increase in the hydrostatic pressure and a decrease in the plasma oncotic pressure within the peritubular capillaries. These changes might come about directly as a result of increased systemic arterial pressure and expansion of the extracellular fluid volume, as well as possibly indirectly through a postulated decrease in vascular resistance at the efferent arterioles. Such decreased resistance would permit greater transmission of the systemic arterial pressure into the peritubular capillaries; it would also decrease the filtration fraction, thereby leaving more plasma in the postglomerular vessels and diluting the proteins in the postglomerular blood. (The right combination of increased arterial pressure – that is, renal perfusing pressure – and decreased resistance in the efferent arterioles could lead simultaneously to an increased GFR and to a decreased filtration fraction; the scheme depicted in Figure 3-2 therefore does not contradict the mechanism involving an increased GFR that was invoked earlier.) As a result of the changes in two major Starling forces, the fluid uptake into the peritubular capillaries would be decreased. Net Na^+ reabsorption might then be diminished secondarily through a number of possible changes within the intercellular spaces: for example, differences in diffusion distances for Na^+, in concentration gradients, or in permeabilities for Na^+. These possible effects have not yet been identified.

Volume Receptors. At the beginning of this chapter, we emphasized that the importance of Na^+ balance lies in the preservation of a normal extracellular fluid volume, not in the preservation of a normal extracellular concentration of Na^+. It is not surprising, therefore, that the renal mechanisms described above should be triggered by changes in the volume of extracellular fluid, not by changes in plasma Na^+ concentration. Two examples illustrate this point: First, in the syndrome of inappropriate ADH secretion (SIADH), increased urinary Na^+ excretion occurs in the face of a low serum Na^+ concentration but an expanded extracellular fluid volume (Fig. 2-5 and Table 2-4).

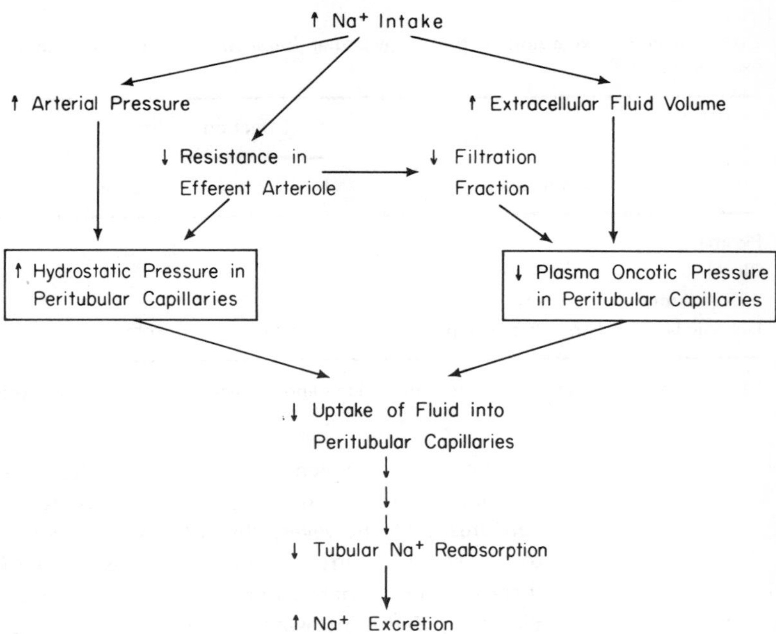

Figure 3-2
Proposed scheme whereby increased Na^+ intake might lead to increased Na^+ excretion through changes in Starling forces across the peritubular capillaries. Modified from L. E. Earley and T. M. Daugharty, *N. Engl. J. Med.* 281:72, 1969. Reproduced from H. Valtin, *Renal Function: Mechanisms Preserving Fluid and Solute Balance in Health.* Boston: Little, Brown, 1973.

Second, the classic experiment for investigating the regulation of Na^+ balance involves expanding the extracellular fluid volume with isotonic saline, which does not alter the normal serum Na^+ concentration. Investigators have therefore tried to locate receptors that sense changes in the volume of the extracellular fluid (or some derivative of that volume, such as flow, pressure, composition, or oxygen consumption) and then transmit a message to the kidneys. Despite an extensive search, the site(s) of these receptors remains obscure, and only some general principles are understood.

Ultimately, the importance of maintaining a normal extracellular fluid volume may be the preservation of a normal intravascular volume and hence the prevention of heart failure or of shock. From such teleological reasoning, one would predict that the expansion of the intravascular space should be the critical variable that determines an increase in Na^+ excretion. As shown in Table 3-1, however, this is not necessarily true. Whether or not an increase in the intravascular volume leads to augmented Na^+ excretion depends on the agent that is used to expand this

Table 3-1
Effect of equal expansion of the intravascular (plasma) volume by various agents on the renal excretion of Na^+

Agent (given intravenously)	Effect on Volume		Effect on Renal Na^+ Excretion*
	Intravascular*	Interstitial*	
Plasma	+++	+	++
Blood	+++	+	0 to -
30% Albumin	+++	-	0 to -
Isotonic NaCl or Ringer's solution	+++	+++	++++

*Semiquantitative estimate; range: minus sign denotes decrease, ++++ signifies the greatest increase.

volume. The intravenous infusion of plasma, which enlarges predominantly the intravascular space, leads to a rather large natriuresis. If, however, the intravascular volume is expanded to an equal extent through the transfusion of whole blood, there may be no natriuresis or even a decrease in Na^+ excretion. Similarly, if the intravascular space is expanded equally with a hyperosmotic solution of albumin (which contracts the interstitial space), there again is no change or a decrease in Na^+ excretion. By far the largest increase in Na^+ excretion follows the enlargement of the intravascular space with isotonic NaCl or Ringer's solution (for composition of solutions, see Fig. 1-6), which simultaneously and proportionally expands the interstitial space as well. These differences in the renal response to equal increases in the intravascular volume might be attributable not only to the concurrent changes in the interstitial volume, but also to changes in the concentration of substances other than Na^+; for example, the infusion of plasma decreases the hematocrit, which does not change when whole blood is transfused.

Although the evidence for volume perception is clear, the location of the receptors is completely unsettled. The brain, the heart (especially the atria), the veins, the arteries, and other anatomical structures have all been suggested, but the experimental evidence for any of these sites is equivocal. In fact, there may not be an extrarenal site for volume perception, and receptors as anatomical entities may not exist. It is possible that a change in volume is sensed within the kidneys themselves (e.g., through a change in hemodynamics or the composition of the perfusing blood) and that such signals, singly or in combination, are translated into responses by the various renal mechanisms for the excretion of Na^+ that were described above.

Thus, numerous factors normally come into play when a load of Na^+ (Cl^-) is given: the recognition of a change in volume or composition of the extracellular fluid, an increased GFR, decreased aldosterone levels, a redistribution of the sGFR and of the peritubular blood flow between the two types of nephron, changes in Starling forces, and possibly an increase in the plasma concentration of a natriuretic hormone. It is not known whether any one of these factors is paramount; in fact, different combinations of these effects may be active and may predominate under different experimental conditions. In any case, it seems likely that one or more of the multiple factors that operate in health is prevented from exerting its full influence in pathological disturbances of Na^+ balance, and we will now analyze such disturbances from that point of view.

Surfeit of Na^+: Edema

Edema may be defined as an abnormal expansion of the interstitial fluid compartment. It may be sharply localized, as in a minor inflammation, or generalized, as in heart failure. In the latter instance, but usually not in the former, it reflects a positive Na^+ balance, and it is one of the most common clinical signs. The pathogenesis of edema may be simple and well understood, as in certain forms of localized edema, or very complex and not yet fully defined, as in most forms of generalized edema.

Localized Edema

The pathogenesis of most forms of localized edema can be adequately explained on the basis of a change in the Starling forces that govern the exchange of fluid between plasma and the interstitium. These forces are related as in the following expression:

$$\dot{q} = K_f[(P_c - P_t) - (\pi_p - \pi_t)] \tag{3-2}$$

where $\dot{q}$ = rate of fluid movement across the capillary wall

K_f = the filtration coefficient, which is proportional not only to the capillary permeability per unit of surface area, but also to the total surface area of the capillary bed

P_c = the intracapillary hydrostatic pressure

P_t = the tissue turgor pressure

π_p = the plasma oncotic pressure

π_t = the interstitial oncotic pressure

Inflammation or Localized Hypersensitivity. These conditions are accompanied by vasodilatation, which augments fluid movement out of the capillary mainly by increasing P_c and K_f. The latter is raised partly because new capillaries may open up in the affected area, partly because the capillaries are dilated, and partly because the permeability of the capillary walls to solutes may be increased. The last often includes permeability to proteins; in that case, a decrease in π_p and an increase in π_t will also contribute to the greater $\dot{q}$. Thus, the cardinal signs of localized inflammation – redness, heat, and swelling – can be explained on the basis of vasodilatation and the consequent alterations in Starling forces.

Lymphatic Obstruction. In health, some protein filters across the capillary walls into the interstitial space. This protein is ordinarily returned to the intravascular space via the lymphatic channels. When these channels are obstructed (as in filariasis) or obliterated (as following radical resection of the lymph nodes), the filtered protein remains within the interstitial space of the affected area, thereby raising π_t and lowering π_p. The result (see Eq. 3-2) is an increased $\dot{q}$, which is manifested clinically as edema. A common example is the swelling of an arm after a radical mastectomy and dissection of the regional lymph nodes (Fig. 3-3b).

Venous Obstruction. Partial obstruction of the veins commonly occurs in inflammation of these vessels, which is called thrombophlebitis. This condition often affects a leg, and it is characterized by warmth, redness, and tender swelling of the affected extremity. The signs result partly from inflammation, as explained above, but predominantly from the rise in the intracapillary hydrostatic pressure, P_c, that is consequent upon an increase in venous pressure.

Generalized Edema

Certain prevalent pathological states – notably congestive heart failure, cirrhosis of the liver, and the nephrotic syndrome – are accompanied by widespread swelling of most interstitial spaces. Although the formation of edematous fluid in these states cannot be explained simply on the basis of shifts in the balance of Starling forces, the distribution of the excess fluid probably can.

Characteristic Distribution. In most (but not all) forms of *congestive heart failure,* a point is reached when the myocardium responds to an increased diastolic volume with a decreased force of contraction, rather than an increased force, as it would in health. The consequences of such failure are a damming of blood proximal to the heart and an increase in venous pressure, which is transmitted to the capillaries and is ultimately manifested as increased P_c. When the problem is primarily so-called right-sided heart failure, the edema appears predominantly in dependent portions of the body, where hydrostatic venous pressures resulting from the erect posture are greatest. Typically, the swelling is seen in the feet and ankles and in front of the tibia and sacrum; it is described in clinical jargon as "ankle" edema or "pretibial" or "presacral" edema (Fig. 3-3a). When the failure involves primarily the left side of the heart, the damming of blood may be principally in the pulmonary veins, with a consequent increase in hydrostatic pressure within the pulmonary capillaries. The result will then be "pulmonary" edema, an often dramatic event in which an expansion of the interstitial spaces around the alveoli leads to extreme shortness of breath.

Disease of the liver often leads to scarring or "cirrhosis" of the hepatic tissue and an increase in the hydrostatic pressure within portal vessels, so-called cirrhosis with portal hypertension. There is then often a selective damming of blood proximal to the liver and an increase of hydrostatic pressure preferentially within the splanchnic capillaries. This effect, coupled with transudation of fluid directly from the damaged liver, leads to the formation of edematous fluid within the abdominal cavity. Such collection of fluid, called *ascites,* is thus typical of hepatic failure (Fig. 3-3c).

Many disorders of the kidneys, notably the nephrotic syndrome, are accompanied by increased urinary excretion of protein. When the proteinuria is sufficiently great to eventuate in a decrease in the plasma concentration of protein, known as *hypoproteinemia,* the resultant reduction in plasma oncotic pressure (π_p) is found in virtually all capillaries, so the edema becomes distributed throughout the body. It may be especially prominent in areas that have a particularly low tissue turgor pressure (P_t). Thus, the dramatic, generalized swelling of the nephrotic syndrome typically involves a tremendous enlargement of the scrotum and of the face, especially of the subcutaneous tissues surrounding the eyes, which are often so distended that the eyes are shut (Fig. 3-3d). Facial swelling in such patients is especially prominent in the morning when the effect of increased hydrostatic pressure in the head, which follows the supine position, is added to the decreased intracapillary plasma oncotic pressure.

Pathogenesis. The explanations cited above to account for the characteristic distribution of generalized edema are inadequate to account for its pathogenesis. This statement is based on numerous observations that the generalized edemas of cardiac, hepatic, or renal failure are not *necessarily* accompanied by the changes that were invoked above. Thus, absolute cardiac output is normal or even increased in certain types of heart failure, so the postulated damming of blood behind the heart (the so-called backward failure theory) may not be present; not all patients with hepatic failure and edema have portal hypertension; and there are some nephrotic patients who have no edema even though their plasma protein concentrations are as low as or lower than those of other nephrotic patients who show massive edema. Rather, the essential

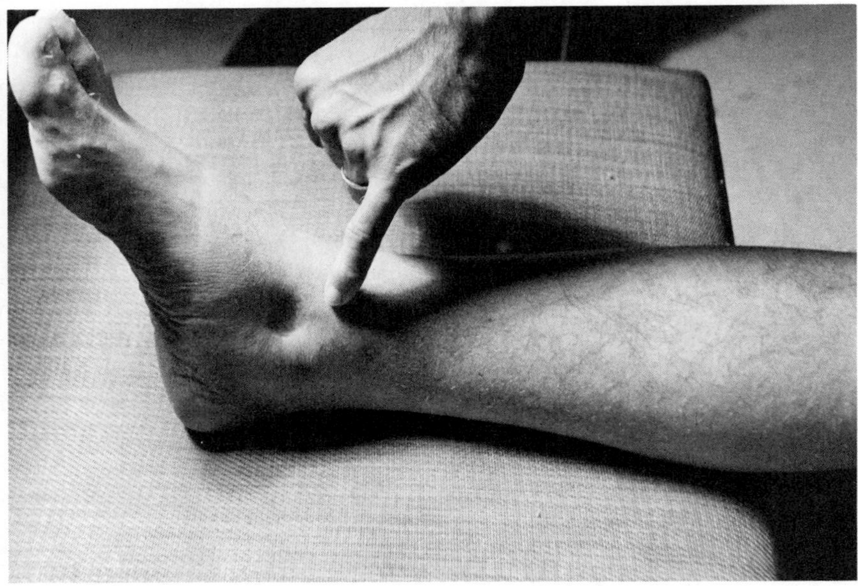

(a)

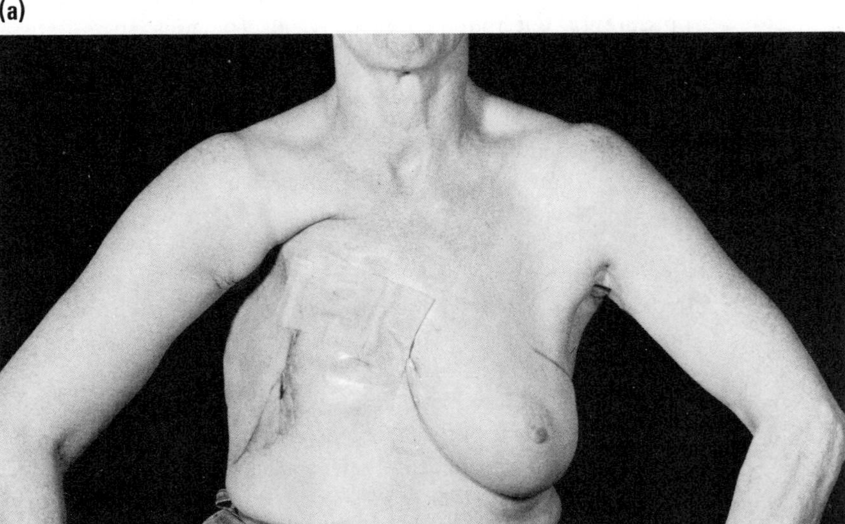

(b)

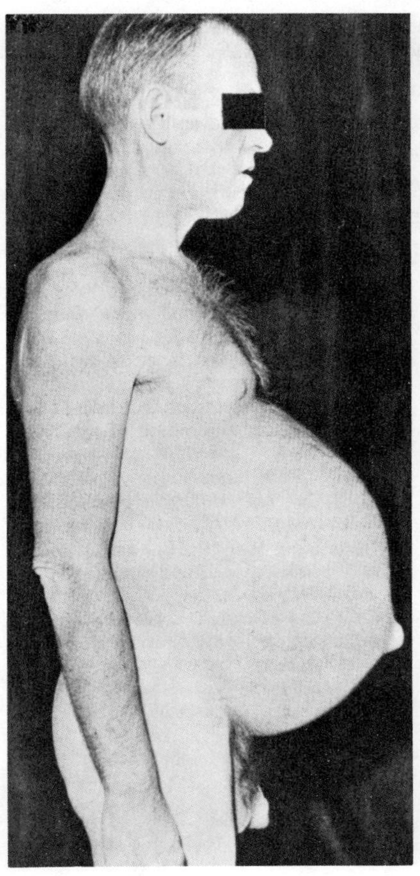

(c)

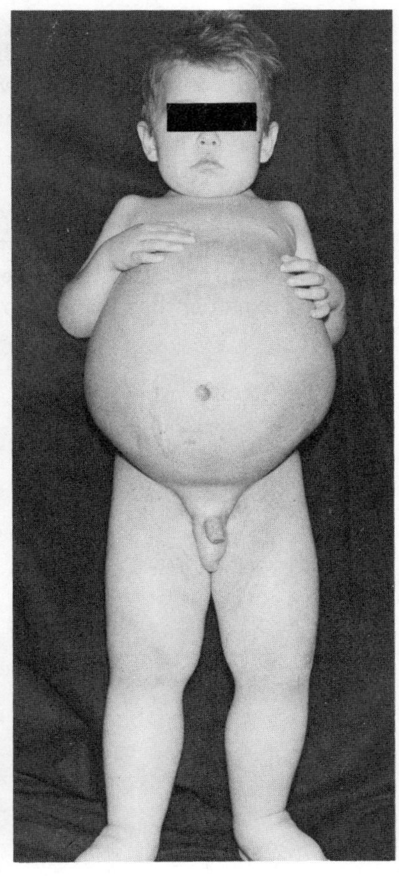

(d)

Figure 3-3
Typical distribution of edema in various disorders.

(a) "Pitting" of ankle and pretibial edema in congestive heart failure.

(b) Localized edema in an arm following mastectomy and dissection of regional lymph nodes.

(c) Ascites in cirrhosis with portal hypertension. From M. J. Orloff, *Ann. N.Y. Acad. Sci.* 170:213, 1970.

(d) Generalized swelling in the nephrotic syndrome.

element for the formation of generalized edema appears to be an abnormal *renal retention of Na^+ (Cl^-)* and H_2O. This fact is shown in Figure 3-4 for the case of cardiac failure. It should be emphasized that although the renal retention is essential, it is not necessarily the primary event.

Figure 3-4 contrasts the response of a normal subject with that of a patient to sudden, identical loads of Na^+, given orally as NaCl. Both subjects had been on low Na^+ intakes of 10 mEq per day during the four days before the test. Whereas the healthy person reached a new steady state within about five days (see also Fig. 3-1), the patient was unable to increase urinary Na^+ excretion until about the seventh day after the load was imposed.

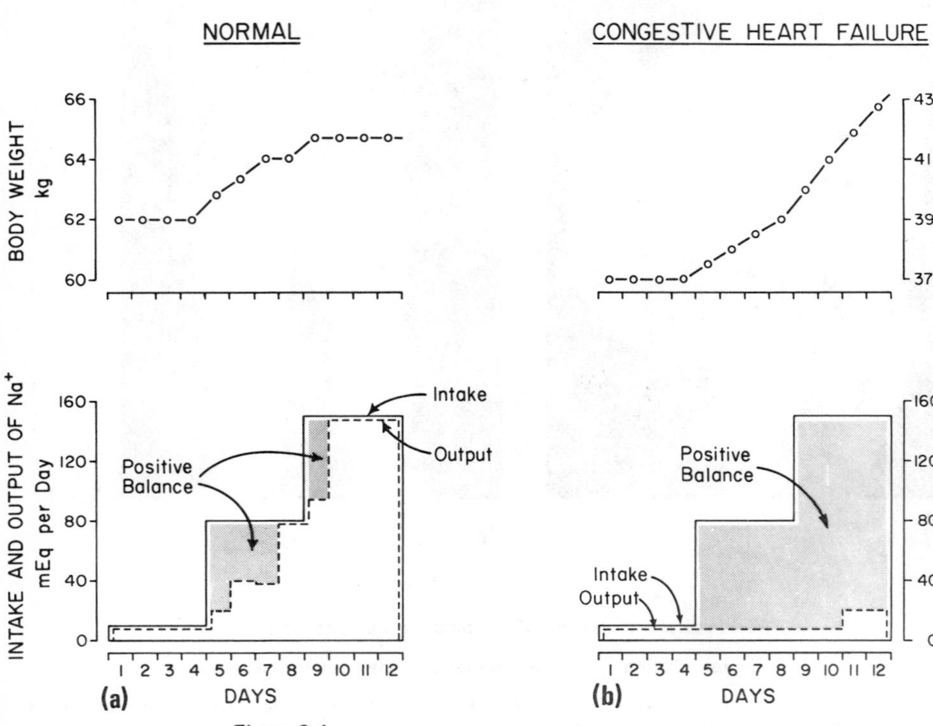

Figure 3-4
Responses of (a) a healthy subject and (b) a patient with congestive heart failure to equal increments in the intake of Na^+. Both subjects were in the steady state on a low Na^+ intake on the first four days. The response of the normal subject was similar to that depicted in Figure 3-1, reaching a new steady state within five days. In contrast, the patient with congestive heart failure was virtually unable to excrete the Na^+ load and accumulated a positive balance of nearly 6 liters of isosmotic NaCl. The cause of the heart failure in this patient was leakage of the mitral valve. Five months after alleviation of the failure through surgical replacement of the mitral valve, the patient responded to Na^+ loading in a manner identical to that of the normal subject. Modified from E. Braunwald et al., *Circulation* 32:223, 1965.

Even then, the patient excreted far less Na^+ than the daily intake; by the eighth day after first increasing the intake, the patient had not yet reached a new steady state, and by this time he had a cumulative positive balance of about 6 liters of isosmotic NaCl, as reflected by a weight gain of about 6 kg. Similar, sluggish renal excretion of a Na^+ load can be demonstrated in the edematous states that are associated with hepatic and renal diseases.

The mechanisms that lead to the renal retention of Na^+ in generalized edema have not been fully clarified. A number of major elements – for example, decreased cardiac output, decreased plasma volume, decreased GFR, increased aldosterone levels, a change in Starling forces, redistribution of the sGFR, and others – can be identified *at certain times in certain disease states.* There are, however, notable exceptions: The plasma volume and the cardiac output are sometimes normal or increased in major edematous states (as in the cardiac failure of anemia, hyperthyroidism, and beriberi); the GFR may not be decreased in cardiac or hepatic failure or in the nephrotic syndrome with marked edema; patients with aldosterone-secreting tumors are not usually edematous; and so on. Largely because of such exceptions, attempts to identify a major factor or factors that can be held responsible for renal Na^+ retention in all major edematous states have thus far failed. One possible unifying scheme is presented in Figure 3-5.

The theory illustrated in Figure 3-5 proposes that the common pathway that ultimately leads to renal retention of Na^+ is inadequate circulation. Inasmuch as the main purpose of maintaining normal Na^+ balance is presumably to preserve a normal plasma volume and thereby to sustain a circulation that is adequate to metabolic needs, it has been tempting to regard a decreased plasma volume as a factor that is common to the major edematous states. However, the first exception cited above (i.e., that some generalized edema is associated with a normal or increased plasma volume) plus the importance of the interstitial space in the regulation of Na^+ excretion (Table 3-1) make such a simple solution untenable. Nevertheless, in view of the paramount role of volume perception in the normal regulation of Na^+ excretion (see Volume Receptors, p. 62), the idea persists that some abnormality of volume initiates the events that lead to abnormal renal Na^+ retention. The theory therefore proposes that common to all major edematous states is a decrease in the *effective* extracellular volume; that is, the theory states that when cardiac, hepatic, or renal failure is accompanied by generalized edema, the kidneys act *as if* the extracellular fluid volume were contracted.

The concept of effective volume is not merely a fanciful inven-

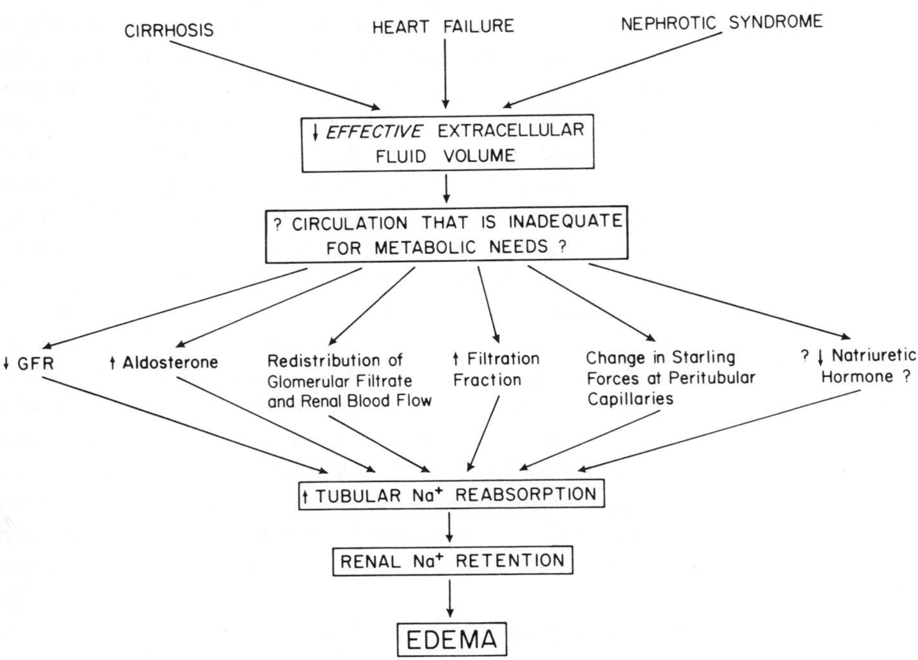

Figure 3-5
Possible scheme for the pathogenesis of generalized edema. Although many of the elements depicted here have been identified as playing a role in some forms of edema, it must be emphasized that the diagram presents a *theory,* that the chain of events is not necessarily as shown here, and that a single, unifying schema that operates in all forms of generalized edema might not exist.

tion to hide ignorance; rather, it is supported by certain observations regarding the normal regulation of Na^+ excretion. For example, when healthy man changes from the upright to the recumbent position, Na^+ excretion is increased. Such changes in posture probably do not alter the total volume of extracellular fluid, but they do change its distribution. Similarly, when an arteriovenous fistula is first closed, Na^+ excretion is increased, even though the total volume of extracellular fluid is not modified.

As was true for volume perception in the healthy state, so too in disease, the site(s) for sensing effective volume is unknown. The volume or some derivative thereof (e.g., flow, pressure, or composition) may be sensed somehow within the kidneys themselves. By whatever means the message is perceived, it may then elicit one or more of the many changes — within the kidneys or outside them — that culminate in the decreased urinary excretion of Na^+ (Fig. 3-5).

It should be emphasized that the scheme presented in Figure 3-5 is hypothetical. It is not even clear whether the sequence of events is necessarily as indicated. In some instances, the renal changes shown in the bottom half of the figure *may* be the initial event, and a decrease in effective volume may follow secondarily from Na^+ retention and a consequent rise in intracapillary hydrostatic pressure. Such *may* be the case in certain primary renal diseases (e.g., acute glomerulonephritis) or in so-called forward cardiac failure, in which the damming of blood and increased venous pressure are viewed as the consequences, not as the causes, of Na^+ retention. The word "may" has been italicized to emphasize that some experts disagree with this view. It could finally turn out that a single, unifying pathway for the formation of generalized edema does not exist, but that the various mechanisms shown in Figure 3-5 predominate at different times and operate in different combinations, depending on the underlying disease that causes the edema.

Treatment. In addition to efforts to correct the primary disease process, the use of diuretics constitutes the major mode of therapy for generalized edema (these agents are discussed in Chap. 7). Although logically diuretics might be taken up in the next chapter, the subject is postponed because the use of diuretics can cause disorders of K^+ and H^+ balance, which will be better understood if those topics are considered first.

In most patients with generalized edema, the intake of Na^+ is restricted, usually to about 35 mEq per day or less. The rationale for such treatment is well illustrated in Figure 3-4b: Salt restriction enables the patient with congestive heart failure to be in Na^+ balance with an extracellular fluid volume that is smaller by 2 to 6 liters than it would be on a normal intake of NaCl.

Deficit of Na^+

Figure 3-6 shows the sequence of events that ensues during progressive Na^+ deficiency in healthy persons. The experiment was reported in 1936 by R. A. McCance, who induced extreme Na^+ deficits in himself and two medical students by eating a diet very low in NaCl and through frequent periods of extreme and uncomfortable sweating in a hot box. The latter maneuver was necessary, because normal kidneys can conserve Na^+ so avidly that it is difficult or impossible to effect a large negative Na^+ balance by dietary restriction alone (Fig. 3-1). Intake of H_2O as desired was maintained throughout the experiment.

Two variables have been plotted in Figure 3-6: the loss or gain in Na^+ and the loss or gain in body weight. (The latter reflects almost entirely changes in body fluids, because the subject's caloric intake was normal, and he showed but a small negative balance for nitrogen.) The scales for Na^+ and for body weight have been so adjusted that a change of 140 mEq of Na^+ corresponds to a change of 1 kg of body weight, that is, a change of

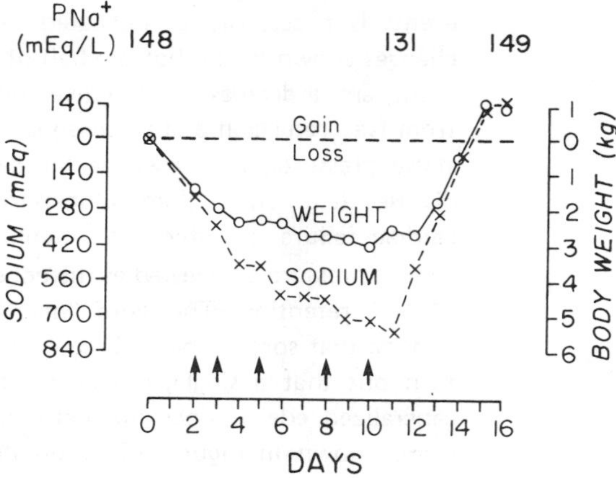

Figure 3-6
Changes in body weight and Na^+ balance during Na^+ depletion (days 1 through 11) and Na^+ repletion (days 12 through 16) in adult man. The ordinate scales have been adjusted so that a change of 140 mEq in Na^+ balance corresponds to a change of 1 liter in H_2O balance; hence, when the symbols for the two balances coincide, isosmotic fluid has been lost or gained. Each arrow denotes a two-hour period that the subject spent in a sweat box. Modified from R. A. McCance, *Proc. R. Soc. Lond. [Biol.]* 119:245, 1936.

approximately 1 liter of body fluid. Hence, as long as the symbols for Na^+ are superimposed on those for body weight, isosmotic fluid will have been lost or gained. This situation held during the first two days of Na^+ depletion; since an isosmotic solution of NaCl was lost, the plasma osmolality remained normal except for the slight rise due to the concentration of plasma proteins. Then, however, as periodic sweating (indicated by the arrows in the figure) was continued through the tenth day, relatively more Na^+ than H_2O was lost. This represents an important adjustment for survival. Had this much Na^+, amounting to about 25 percent of the total exchangeable Na^+ (Table 1-5), been lost isosmotically – that is, with sufficient H_2O to render the lost fluid isosmotic with plasma – the body weight would have decreased by 5.5 kg, reflecting a loss of body fluid of 5.5 liters. Furthermore, since an isosmotic loss would come entirely from the extracellular compartment (Table 2-4 and Fig. 2-7), this compartment would have been contracted by about 40 percent, and shock would have supervened. This dire consequence was prevented by the loss of relatively more Na^+ than H_2O, as the divergence of the two slopes shows. Consequently, only about 2.5 liters (instead of 5.5 liters) of fluid was lost, and vital functions were maintained. Since between days 2 and 11 relatively more Na^+ than H_2O was lost, the plasma concentration of Na^+ – and hence the osmolality of the body fluids – was lowered from 148 mEq to 131 mEq per liter.

During the recovery period when the subject gradually replenished the Na^+ deficit, Na^+ was at first retained in excess of H_2O, and from day 13 onward, fluid was again retained isosmotically. The subject for whom data are shown in Figure 3-6 slightly overshot the replenishment, but this was not true of the other subject, who sustained an equally great deficit of Na^+. The third subject replenished a smaller deficit more quickly by ingesting 1,200 mEq of Na^+ and much H_2O within a few hours, and she regained normal body weight overnight.

This classic experiment has been interpreted to reflect a priority in the maintenance of two constants, osmolality and volume. Plasma osmolality — and hence the osmolality of all body fluids — is regulated first, even at the sacrifice of a change in the volume of body fluids. At the point, however, where normal plasma osmolality could be preserved only at so great a reduction in volume that survival is threatened, the volume is upheld, but now at the price of a reduction in osmolality.

The mechanisms that bring about the selective retention of H_2O — such as those operating in the above experiment between days 2 and 11 — are not yet fully understood. Although the plasma concentrations of ADH may be high at this point, it seems clear that ADH is not essential to the H_2O retention. This has been shown in a strain of rats that cannot produce ADH; when such animals are subjected to Na^+ depletion, they manifest selective H_2O retention and develop hyponatremia, just like control animals that can secrete ADH. It is possible that the free H_2O is retained principally by the mechanisms outlined in Figure 2-6; that is, when Na^+ depletion has led to a critical reduction in body fluids, the GFR may be decreased, and the chain of events that leads to diminished generation of free H_2O is set into motion.

Clinical Causes of Na^+ Depletion

Table 3-2 lists the causes of Na^+ deficiency in their approximate order of frequency, which actually represents a guess. This order will depend not only on the type of medical practice (i.e., whether pediatric, surgical, or medical) but also on the geographic location and the time of year. Thus, in countries where cholera is fairly common, diarrhea may be the major cause of Na^+ depletion, and certain severe infant diarrheas are more common during the summer than at other seasons.

The amount of Na^+ that is lost in various biological fluids can be considerable. Several liters per day may be excreted in severe diarrhea, during vigorous diuretic therapy, or with surgical drainage. If not replaced, such losses can quickly produce a deficit amounting to 20 percent or more of the total exchangeable Na^+ (Tables 1-4 and 1-5).

Table 3-2
Clinical conditions possibly associated with a deficiency of total body Na^+, listed in approximate order of frequency. For electrolyte composition of the various eliminated fluids, see Table 1-4

Disorder	Comments
Severe diarrhea	Especially in infants
Prolonged vomiting	
Diuresis	Especially with "high-ceiling" diuretics (see Chap. 7)
Surgical drainage of intestinal fluids	
Salt restriction in chronic renal failure	See Chap. 10
Frequent abdominal paracentesis	Performed for the relief of ascites
Severe sweating	
Adrenal insufficiency	The complex of symptoms in this condition cannot be ascribed simply to Na^+ depletion, but probably reflects, at least in part, deficiency of some specific actions of the adrenocortical hormones

Most patients in chronic renal failure are in balance on a normal intake of Na^+ (Chap. 10). When the intake is either increased or decreased, however, the patient may take a long time to re-establish balance, just as does the patient in congestive heart failure (Fig. 3-4). A serious deficit of Na^+ can therefore develop during the interval between the time that salt intake is first restricted and the diseased kidneys finally adjust by avidly reabsorbing Na^+.

The Meaning of Hyponatremia and Hypernatremia

We end this chapter by reemphasizing the important dictum that we stated at its beginning: that although in most adult patients aberrations in the plasma concentration of Na^+ reflect imbalances of both Na^+ and H_2O, the latter predominates. That is, most hyponatremia results from the retention of H_2O *relative* to Na^+, and hypernatremia results from the loss of H_2O *relative* to Na^+. The term "relative" connotes that the absolute change in H_2O balance may be positive, as in the hyponatremia of SIADH, or negative, as in Na^+ depletion (Fig. 3-6); in both instances, however, an excess of H_2O over Na^+ has diluted the Na^+ in the plasma. The dictum carries an inference that is too often forgotten at the bedside: that in most instances the hyponatremia or hypernatremia should be corrected by altering the water intake more than the Na^+ intake. In practice, both measures are carried out simultaneously, but the change in balance that one strives for is usually greater for H_2O than for Na^+. Because hyponatremia is encountered much more frequently than hypernatremia, the following discussion will be limited to the former.

The causes of hyponatremia are listed in Table 3-3. It was pointed out in Chapter 2 (see Conditions that Mimic SIADH) that the commonest causes of hyponatremia are cardiac, hepatic, and renal failure. These conditions are often accompanied by generalized edema, and hence by the use of diuretics which tend to aggravate the hyponatremia. (The possible mechanisms whereby these pathological states and the use of diuretics lead to retention of free H_2O and decreased plasma Na^+ concentration are shown in Figure 2-6.) The fact that hyponatremia is most commonly encountered in edematous patients whose total body Na^+ is increased emphasizes the importance of not treating such patients by giving Na^+, since this measure could worsen or precipitate cardiac failure.

Acute dilutional hyponatremia is seen immediately after vigorous diuretic therapy or after the removal of large volumes of ascites through abdominal paracentesis. These therapeutic measures often make patients very thirsty, and if such patients satiate their thirst very rapidly, their tendency to hold on to H_2O can lead to hyponatremia.

The mechanisms that lower the plasma Na^+ concentration in SIADH were discussed in Chapter 2. The evolution of hyponatremia during Na^+ deficiency (Fig. 3-6) emphasizes that even when the precipitating event is a lack of Na^+, a low plasma Na^+ concentration does not develop until a dilutional component has been added. Inasmuch as normal osmolality is first preserved at the sacrifice of volume (through day 2), the appearance of hyponatremia during Na^+ deficiency signals a potentially dangerous contraction of the extracellular fluid volume.

The term "essential" is used in clinical jargon to denote an inherent or fundamental property; in most instances, the term is used when the cause of a given disorder is not known. In this sense, so-called essential hyponatremia is sometimes seen in very ill, often terminal patients. These individuals maintain their plasma Na^+ concentration and plasma osmolality at an abnor-

Table 3-3
Causes of hyponatremia, listed in approximate order of frequency for adults

Heart failure
Liver failure
Kidney failure
Diuretic therapy
Acute dilutional hyponatremia
Syndrome of inappropriate ADH secretion (SIADH)
Na^+ deficiency
Essential hyponatremia

mally low value, even though they respond normally to imposed loads of H_2O or Na^+. It has been postulated, therefore, that the "osmostat" in these patients is set at a new level, and in the absence of a more precisely identified cause, the resetting has been attributed to a general dysfunction of cells in very ill patients.

Pseudohyponatremia

It was pointed out in Chapter 1 (see Clinical Tests Are Estimates) that in the clinical laboratory, the plasma concentration of Na^+ is measured on whole plasma, not the plasma H_2O in which the Na^+ is actually dissolved. When certain plasma solutes (e.g., proteins and lipids) are increased in disease, the total volume of plasma may be increased enough to lead to an abnormally low plasma Na^+ concentration as reported by the clinical laboratory. Under these conditions, however, neither the amount of Na^+ nor the amount of H_2O in the plasma is changed, and the Na^+ concentration, when expressed *per liter of plasma water,* therefore remains normal. In this sense, the low plasma Na^+ concentration reported by the laboratory is an artifact, and the condition is therefore called *pseudohyponatremia.*

The dynamics of pseudohyponatremia are illustrated in Table 3-4. In health, the plasma volume constitutes about 4 percent of the body weight, which in a person weighing 75 kg (165 pounds) would be 3 liters. In each liter of this whole plasma, there is about 70 g of protein (Table 1-1), and in 3 liters there is therefore about 210 g of protein; that is, approximately 0.2 liter of the 3 liters of whole plasma is occupied by proteins. Since this is the only solute that normally contributes importantly to the total volume of plasma, the plasma H_2O equals 3.0 - 0.2, or 2.8 liters. Phrased differently, 92 to 93 percent of whole plasma is H_2O; hence the plasma H_2O equals 3.0 × 0.92, or 2.8 liters. Assuming a normal plasma Na^+ concentration of

Table 3-4
Dynamics of pseudohyponatremia

State	Total Whole Plasma (liters)	Total Plasma H_2O (liters)	Na^+ Concentration (mEq/L whole plasma)	Na^+ Concentration (mEq/L plasma H_2O)
Health	3	2.8	140	150
Hyperproteinemia	3.2	2.8	131	150
Hyperlipidemia	3.1	2.8	135	150
Hyperglycemia*	3.6	3.4	117	124

*Not pseudohyponatremia, since Na^+ concentration per liter of plasma H_2O is lower than normal (see text).

140 mEq per liter of whole plasma, the total amount of Na^+ in the plasma equals 140 X 3, or 420 mEq. Dividing this total amount, which is dissolved in the plasma H_2O, by 2.8 liters yields a Na^+ concentration of 150 mEq per liter of plasma H_2O.

In certain hyperproteinemic states (e.g., multiple myeloma), the plasma protein concentration may be doubled. Therefore, 0.4 liter must now be added to the normal plasma H_2O volume of 2.8 liters to yield a volume for whole plasma of 3.2 liters. Since neither the amount of Na^+ nor the amount of plasma H_2O has changed, the Na^+ concentration per liter of plasma H_2O remains at 150 mEq. Now, however, dividing the total amount of Na^+, 420 mEq, by 3.2 liters of whole plasma gives the value that will be reported by the clinical laboratory, namely, 131 mEq per liter of whole plasma.

A similar analysis applies to Na^+ concentrations in hyperlipidemia. In health the plasma concentration of lipids (mainly cholesterol and triglycerides) is so low (Table 1-1) that they contribute very little to the volume of whole plasma. In severe hyperlipidemia, however, the lipids may contribute as much as 0.1 liter. Adding this amount and the volume normally occupied by the proteins (0.2 liter) to a total plasma H_2O volume of 2.8 liters gives a total volume for whole plasma of 3.1 liters. Given 420 mEq as the total amount of Na^+ in the plasma, the reported Na^+ concentration will therefore be 135 mEq per liter of whole plasma, even though the Na^+ concentration is still the normal value of 150 mEq per liter of plasma H_2O.

As noted in Table 3-4, the low Na^+ concentration in hyperglycemia is not a pseudohyponatremia, since the Na^+ concentration per liter of plasma H_2O is abnormally low as well. The development of hyponatremia in that circumstance has been described in detail in the answer to Problem 3-1 (see Answers to Problems). Briefly, the large amount of sugar in the plasma provides sufficient osmotic force to cause a shift of H_2O from the intracellular into the extracellular compartment. Consequently, the volume of whole plasma is increased mainly because of the addition of H_2O, not of solute, and hence the concentration of Na^+ is decreased, both per liter of whole plasma and per liter of plasma H_2O. In this regard, the difference between hyperproteinemia and hyperlipidemia, on the one hand, and hyperglycemia on the other is explained by the different sizes of the respective solutes. Proteins and lipids, being relatively large, occupy a quantitatively significant amount of space in whole plasma but add little to its osmolality; in contrast, sugar molecules, being small, occupy a negligible amount of space but raise the osmolality of plasma sufficiently to cause an internal shift of H_2O.

These examples emphasize that laboratory reports of hyponatremia do not necessarily reflect an external imbalance of H_2O or Na^+, nor even necessarily an internal imbalance. In most patients, the disease that is causing the hyperproteinemia, hyperlipidemia, or hyperglycemia is sufficiently evident that these causes of hyponatremia are detected.

Summary

The primary importance of Na^+ balance is that it determines the size of the extracellular fluid compartment, one portion of which is the plasma. When Na^+ balance is positive, there is danger that overexpansion of the plasma volume will lead to cardiac failure; when Na^+ balance is negative, severe contraction of the plasma volume may eventuate in shock.

A surfeit of Na^+ is often reflected by generalized edema, which is an abnormal expansion of the interstitial space. The most common causes of edema are certain types of cardiac, hepatic, and renal failure. The pathogenesis of generalized edema is not fully understood, but it probably involves the perception of an inadequate ***effective*** extracellular fluid volume, either within or outside of the kidneys, plus one or more mechanisms, mainly intrarenal, that lead to decreased urinary excretion of Na^+. These mechanisms may involve a decreased GFR, increased plasma concentration of aldosterone, a shift of the glomerular filtrate away from salt-wasting superficial cortical nephrons and toward salt-saving juxtamedullary nephrons, increased filtration fraction, changes in Starling forces at the peritubular capillary, and possibly the inhibition of a natriuretic hormone (see Fig. 3-5). The importance of some of these mechanisms – and in some cases, even their existence – has not yet been conclusively demonstrated; it is possible that they function at different intensities and in different combinations, depending on the disease that is responsible for the generalized edema.

The major forms of generalized edema are distributed in a characteristic manner, which can be explained on the basis of a change in Starling forces across the walls of systemic capillaries (Fig. 3-3). In right-sided heart failure, the edema appears mainly in dependent portions of the body; in left-sided heart failure, the edema is often most marked in the lungs (so-called pulmonary edema). In cirrhosis with portal hypertension, the edematous fluid accumulates primarily within the peritoneal cavity (so-called ascites). And in renal failure, edema appears in all parts of the body, most characteristically in tissues with poor turgor, such as the scrotum and periorbital areas.

Edema may also be localized, as in inflammation and in lymphatic or venous obstruction. In contrast to generalized edema, localized edema does not usually reflect a positive Na^+ balance, but rather it is due to a change in Starling forces within a confined area.

In patients, a deficit of Na^+ occurs most commonly with severe diarrhea or prolonged vomiting, with the use of potent diuretics, and with surgical drainage of the intestine (Table 3-2). During the initial period of Na^+ depletion, the osmolality of the plasma, and hence of all the body fluids, is maintained at or near the normal value; inevitably, this maintenance of osmolality entails a reduction in extracellular fluid volume. At the point where further preservation of normal osmolality might so encroach on the extracellular volume that survival is threatened, the maintenance of fluid volume takes precedence, but now necessarily at the price of decreased osmolality and hyponatremia (Fig. 3-6). The mechanisms that lead to renal retention of solute-free H_2O during the latter stages of Na^+ depletion may be intrinsic to the kidneys (as outlined in Fig. 2-6), and they may or may not require major hormonal changes, such as an increase in the plasma concentration of ADH.

In most adult patients, hyponatremia reflects an imbalance of both Na^+ and H_2O, but predominantly of the latter. That is, whether the total body Na^+ is low (as in Na^+ depletion) or high (as in edematous states), the net result is *relative* retention of H_2O and dilution of the Na^+; an analogous situation applies to hypernatremia. Pseudohyponatremia – a relatively rare occurrence that is seen during severe hyperproteinemia or hyperlipidemia – is an artifact and is not due to an imbalance of either H_2O or Na^+. In uncontrolled diabetes mellitus with high plasma concentrations of glucose, the hyponatremia reflects mainly an internal imbalance in which H_2O has shifted from the intracellular into the extracellular space (see Problem 3-1).

Problem 3-1

A 52-year-old male patient has diabetes mellitus. When checked by his physician, the patient was feeling well and the disease appeared to be in good control, as reflected by the absence of glucose in his urine and by a blood glucose concentration of 126 mg/100 ml; he weighed 70 kg at this time. Two weeks later, he consulted his doctor because he had a severe cold. He had experienced some polyuria and increased thirst, he now weighed 69 kg, he had a fever of 39°C, and his urine contained sugar. His physician concluded that with the intercurrent illness, the patient's diabetes mellitus was no longer under control. He therefore admitted the patient to the hospital, where the blood glucose concentration was found to be 756 mg/100 ml and the serum Na^+ concentration, 133 mEq per liter. The blood urea nitrogen (BUN) concentration was normal at this time.

Can you account for the low serum Na^+ concentration on the

Table 3-5
Development of hyponatremia during uncontrolled diabetes mellitus

					Plasma Concentration		
State	Body Weight (kg)	TBW* (liters)	ICW* (liters)	ECW* (liters)	Glucose (mg/100 ml)	Osmolality (mOsm/kg)	Na^+ (mEq/L)
"Healthy"	70	42	28	14	126	300	140
Hypothetical transient state	69	41			"126" (hypothetical)		
New steady state	69	41			756		

*TBW = total body water; ICW = intracellular water; ECW = extracellular water.

basis of the hyperglycemia, or must you invoke additional mechanisms? That is, what serum Na^+ concentration would be predicted on a basis of the shift of H_2O from the intracellular to the extracellular space that results from the rise in plasma osmolality due to the high glucose concentration? (*Hint:* Utilize Table 3-5 to solve this problem and assume a transient state in which 1 liter of H_2O without solute was lost before the blood sugar rose.)

Problem 3-2 What is a normal dietary intake of sodium for a normal adult human? How much sodium is contained in the salt-poor or low-salt diet that is prescribed for many patients? Express your answer as grams, millimoles, and milliequivalents per day.

Problem 3-3 A mother brings her 9-month-old infant to the emergency department. She says that the baby has had diarrhea for three days. During this time, she has tried to feed the child formula with added salt, but his appetite has been very poor and he has managed to keep down very little of what he has eaten. The mother thinks that the baby has lost weight.

On admission, the child weighs 7 kg. He had been seen one week earlier in a routine checkup, when he weighed 8 kg. The baby's skin and mucous membranes are very dry. The doctor therefore surmises that the patient has lost approximately 1 liter of fluid and that the major problem is some form of contraction of the body fluids (Table 2-4). A plasma Na^+ concentration is determined immediately and is found to be 160 mEq per liter.

In order to analyze the problem fully and to treat the baby properly, the doctor wants to know whether the high plasma Na^+ concentration is due entirely to a loss of H_2O in relative excess of Na^+ (Table 1-4), or whether overzealous feeding of NaCl by the mother has also contributed to the high plasma Na^+ concentration. Answer these questions by completing Table 3-6.

Table 3-6
Sequential analysis for the cause of hypernatremia in infant diarrhea

State	Body Weight (kg)	Volume of Body Fluids			
		TBW* (ml)	ICW* (ml)	ECW* (ml)	P_{Na^+} (mEq/L)
Healthy	8	5,600	3,200	2,400	140
Hypothetical loss of 1 liter H_2O	7				
Hypothetical loss of 1 liter isotonic NaCl	7				
Actual loss	7				160

*TBW = total body water; ICW = intracellular water; ECW = extracellular water.

Problem 3-4

A 47-year-old woman was brought to the emergency room because she had had a generalized seizure at home, following which she had remained confused. The main abnormal result reported by the laboratory was a serum Na^+ concentration of 112 mEq per liter. Specifically, the patient had a normal blood concentration of glucose, a normal neurological examination, and no history of grand mal epilepsy. It was thought likely that the convulsion was due to "water intoxication" and that the hyponatremia should therefore be corrected quickly.

If it is desired to raise the plasma Na^+ concentration to 132 mEq per liter, how much 5% NaCl solution should be infused intravenously? The patient weighs 53 kg.

Selected References

General

Barger, A. C., and Herd, J. A. Renal Vascular Anatomy and Distribution of Blood Flow. In J. Orloff and R. W. Berliner (eds.), *Handbook of Physiology,* Section 8, Renal Physiology. Washington, D.C.: American Physiological Society, 1973.

Berliner, R. W. (chairman). Neural control of body salt and water (Physiology Society Symposium). *Fed. Proc.* 27:1127, 1968.

Bourgoignie, J. J., Hwang, K. H., Espial, C., Klahr, S., and Bricker, N. S. A natriuretic factor in the serum of patients with chronic uremia. *J. Clin. Invest.* 51:1514, 1972.

Bresler, E. H. The problem of the volume component of body fluid homeostasis. *Am. J. Med. Sci.* 232:93, 1956.

Cotlove, E., and Hogben, C. A. M. Chloride. In C. L. Comar and F. Bronner (eds.), *Mineral Metabolism,* vol. 2, part B. New York: Academic, 1962.

Earley, L. E., and Daugharty, T. M. Sodium metabolism. *N. Engl. J. Med.* 281:72, 1969.

Forbes, G. B. Sodium. In C. L. Comar and F. Bronner (eds.), *Mineral Metabolism,* vol. 2, part B. New York: Academic, 1962.

Laragh, J. H., and Sealey, J. E. The Renin-Angiotensin-Aldosterone Hormonal System and Regulation of Sodium, Potassium, and Blood Pressure Homeostasis. In J. Orloff and R. W. Berliner (eds.), *Handbook of Physiology,* Section 8, Renal Physiology. Washington, D.C.: American Physiological Society, 1973.

Möhring, J., and Möhring, B. Evaluation of sodium and potassium balance in rats. *J. Appl. Physiol.* 33:688, 1972.

Muldowney, F. P., and Williams, R. T. Clinical disturbances in serum sodium and potassium in relation to alteration in total exchangeable sodium, exchangeable potassium and total body water. *Am. J. Med.* 35:768, 1964.

Orloff, J., and Burg, M. Kidney. *Annu. Rev. Physiol.* 33:83, 1971.
This review contains a short section on the regulation of sodium excretion which, although written a number of years ago, presents a lucid and often amusing summary of the complex problem(s) of sodium balance.

Seldin, D. W. (chairman). The Physiology of Diuretic Agents. *Ann. N.Y. Acad. Sci.* 139:275, 1966.
This record of an international symposium contains much useful information, not only on diuretics but also on the mechanisms of Na^+ balance in health and disease.

Sharp, G. W. G., and Leaf, A. Effects of Aldosterone and Its Mechanism of Action on Sodium Transport. In J. Orloff and R. W. Berliner (eds.), *Handbook of Physiology,* Section 8, Renal Physiology. Washington, D.C.: American Physiological Society, 1973.

Vander, A. J. Control of renin release. *Physiol. Rev.* 47:359, 1967.

Walser, M. Sodium Excretion. In C. Rouiller and A. F. Muller (eds.), *The Kidney,* vol. 3. New York: Academic, 1971.

Na^+ Balance in Health

August, J. T., Nelson, D. H., and Thorn, G. W. Response of normal subjects to large amounts of aldosterone. *J. Clin. Invest.* 37:1549, 1958.

Bartoli, E., and Earley, L. E. The relative contributions of reabsorptive rate and redistributed nephron filtration rate to changes in proximal tubular fractional reabsorption during acute saline infusion and aortic constriction in the rat. *J. Clin. Invest.* 50:2191, 1971.

Bennett, C. M. Effect of extracellular volume expansion upon sodium reabsorption in the distal nephron of dogs. *J. Clin. Invest.* 52:2548, 1973.

Blythe, W. B., D'Avila, D., Gitelman, H. J., and Welt, L. G. Further evidence for a humoral natriuretic factor. *Circ. Res.* 28 [Suppl. 2]: II-21, 1971.

de Wardener, H. E., Mills, I. H., Clapham, W. F., and Hayter, C. J. Studies on the efferent mechanism of the sodium diuresis which follows the administration of intravenous saline in the dog. *Clin. Sci.* 21:249, 1961.

Earley, L. E. Sodium Metabolism. In M. H. Maxwell and C. R. Kleeman (eds.), *Clinical Disorders of Fluid and Electrolyte Metabolism* (2nd ed.). New York: McGraw-Hill, 1972.

Earley, L. E., Humphreys, M. H., and Bartoli, E. Capillary circulation as a regulator of sodium reabsorption and excretion. *Circ. Res.* 31 [Suppl. 2]: II-1, 1972.

Earley, L. E., and Schrier, R. W. Intrarenal Control of Sodium Excretion by Hemodynamic and Physical Factors. In J. Orloff and R. W. Berliner (eds.), *Handbook of Physiology,* Section 8, Renal Physiology. Washington, D.C.: American Physiological Society, 1973.

Gertz, K. H., and Boylan, J. H. Glomerular-Tubular Balance. In J. Orloff and R. W. Berliner (eds.), *Handbook of Physiology,* Section 8, Renal Physiology. Washington, D.C.: American Physiological Society, 1973.

Hollenberg, N. K., Epstein, M., Guttmann, R. D., Conroy, M., Basch, R. I., and Merrill, J. P. Effect of sodium balance on intrarenal distribution of blood flow in normal man. *J. Appl. Physiol.* 28:312, 1970.

Klahr, S., and Rodriguez, H. J. Natriuretic hormone. *Nephron* 15:387, 1975.

Knox, F. G., Schneider, E. G., Willis, L. R., Strandhoy, J. W., and Ott, C. E. Effect of volume expansion on sodium excretion in the presence and absence of increased delivery from superficial proximal tubules. *J. Clin. Invest.* 52:1642, 1973.

Leaf, A., Couter, W. T., and Newburgh, L. H. Some effects of variation in sodium intake and of different sodium salts in normal subjects. *J. Clin. Invest.* 28:1082, 1949.

Lynch, R. E., Schneider, E. G., Willis, L. R., and Knox, F. G. Absence of mineralocorticoid-dependent sodium reabsorption in dog proximal tubule. *Am. J. Physiol.* 223:40, 1972.

Mulrow, P. J., and Boyd, J. E. Hormonal Effects on Water and Electrolyte Metabolism, Excluding Divalent Cations and Neurohypophyseal Hormones. In M. H. Maxwell and C. R. Kleeman (eds.), *Clinical Disorders of Fluid and Electrolyte Metabolism* (2nd ed.). New York: McGraw-Hill, 1972.

Nizet, A., Godon, J. P., and Mahieu, P. Quantitative excretion of water and sodium load by isolated dog kidney: Autonomous renal response to blood dilution factors. *Pflügers Arch. Eur. J. Physiol.* 304:30, 1968.

Posternak, L., Brunner, H. R., Gavras, H., and Brunner, D. B. Angiotensin II blockade in normal man: Interaction of renin and sodium in maintaining blood pressure. *Kidney Int.* 11:197, 1977.

Stein, J. H., and Reineck, H. J. Effect of alterations in extracellular fluid volume on segmental sodium transport. *Physiol. Rev.* 55:127, 1975.

Wills, L. R., Schneider, E. G., Lynch, R. E., and Knox, F. G. Effect of chronic alteration of sodium balance on reabsorption by proximal tubule of the dog. *Am. J. Physiol.* 223:34, 1972.

Wright, F. S., Brenner, B. M., Bennett, C. M., Keimowitz, R. I., Berliner, R. W., Schrier, R. W., Verroust, P. J., de Wardener, H. E., and Holzgreve, H. Failure to demonstrate a hormonal inhibitor of proximal sodium reabsorption. *J. Clin. Invest.* 48:1107, 1969.

Volume Perception

Bartter, F. C., and Gann, D. S. On the hemodynamic regulation of the secretion of aldosterone. *Circulation* 21:1016, 1960.

Bartter, F. C., Liddle, G. W., Duncan, L. E., Jr., Barber, J. K., and Delea, C. The regulation of aldosterone secretion in man: The role of fluid volume. *J. Clin. Invest.* 35:1306, 1956.

Chapman, L. W., and Henry, J. P. The role of cardiac receptors in fluid balance. *Physiologist* 16:194, 1973.

Epstein, F. H. Renal excretion of sodium and the concept of a volume receptor. *Yale J. Biol. Med.* 29:282, 1956.

Epstein, F. H., Post, R. S., and McDowell, M. The effect of an arteriovenous fistula on renal hemodynamics and electrolyte excretion. *J. Clin. Invest.* 32:233, 1953.

Goetz, K. L., Bond, G. C., and Bloxham, D. D. Atrial receptors and renal function. *Physiol. Rev.* 55:157, 1975.

Lawrence, M., Ledsome, J. R., and Mason, J. M. The time course of the diuretic response to left atrial distension. *Q. J. Exp. Physiol.* 58:219, 1973.

Lindheimer, M. D., Lalone, R. C., and Levinsky, N. G. Evidence that an acute increase in glomerular filtration has little effect on sodium excretion in the dog unless extracellular volume is expanded. *J. Clin. Invest.* 46:256, 1967.

Opava-Stitzer, S., and Malvin, R. L. Right atrium and renal sodium excretion. *Am. J. Physiol.* 228:184, 1975.

Paintal, A. S. A study of right and left atrial receptors. *J. Physiol.* 120: 596, 1953.

Smith, H. W. Salt and water volume receptors. An exercise in physiologic apologetics. *Am. J. Med.* 23:623, 1957.

deTorrente, A., Robertson, G. L., McDonald, K. M., and Schrier, R. W. Mechanism of diuretic response to increased left atrial pressure in the anesthetized dog. *Kidney Int.* 8:355, 1975.

Welt, L. G. Volume receptors. *Circulation* 21:1002, 1960.

Edema

Barger, A. C. Renal hemodynamic factors in congestive heart failure. *Ann. N.Y. Acad. Sci.* 139:276, 1966.

Bourgoignie, J. J., Hwang, K. H., Espinel, C., Klahr, S., and Bricker, N. S. A natriuretic factor in the serum of patients with chronic uremia. *J. Clin. Invest.* 51:1514, 1972.

Braunwald, E., Plauth, W. H., and Morrow, A. G. A method for the detection and quantification of impaired sodium excretion. Results of an oral sodium tolerance test in normal subjects and in patients with heart disease. *Circulation* 32:223, 1965.

Cannon, P. J. The kidney in heart failure. *N. Engl. J. Med.* 296:26, 1977.

Chaimovitz, C., Szylman, P., Alroy, G., and Better, O. S. Mechanism of increased renal tubular sodium reabsorption in cirrhosis. *Am. J. Med.* 52:198, 1972.

Davis, J. O. The mechanisms of salt and water retention in cardiac failure. *Hosp. Pract.* 5:63, 1970.

Hayslett, J. P., Kashgarian, M., Bensch, K. G., Spargo, B. H., Freedman, L. R., and Epstein, F. H. Clinicopathological correlations in the nephrotic syndrome due to primary renal disease. *Medicine* (Baltimore) 52:93, 1973.

Lancet Editorial. Hereditary angioneurotic oedema. *Lancet* 1:1044, 1973.

Laragh, J. H. Pathophysiology of Edema. In R. W. Winters (ed.), *The Body Fluids in Pediatrics.* Boston: Little, Brown, 1973.

Möhring, J., and Möhring, B. Reevaluation of DOCA escape phenomenon. *Am. J. Physiol.* 223:1237, 1972.

Perera, G. A., and Blood, D. W. Disturbance in salt and water metabolism in hypertension. *Am. J. Med.* 1:602, 1946.

Schreiner, G. E. The Nephrotic Syndrome. In M. B. Strauss and L. G. Welt (eds.), *Diseases of the Kidney* (2nd ed.). Boston: Little, Brown, 1971.

Sheffer, A. L., Austen, K. F., and Rosen, F. S. Tranexamic acid therapy in hereditary angioneurotic edema. *N. Engl. J. Med.* 287:452, 1972.

Stumpe, K. O., Lowitz, H. -S., and Ochwadt, B. Function of juxtamedullary nephrons in normotensive and chronically hypertensive rats. *Pflügers Arch. Eur. J. Physiol.* 313:43, 1969.

Welt, L. G. Edema. In M. M. Wintrobe et al. (eds.), *Harrison's Principles of Internal Medicine* (7th ed.). New York: McGraw-Hill, 1974, p. 176.

Weston, R. E. Pathogenesis and Treatment of Edema with Special Reference to Use of Diuretics. In M. H. Maxwell and C. R. Kleeman (eds.), *Clinical Disorders of Fluid and Electrolyte Metabolism* (2nd ed.). New York: McGraw-Hill, 1972.

Na^+ Deficiency and Excess

Calvin, M. E., Knepper, R., and Robertson, W. O. Salt poisoning. *N. Engl. J. Med.* 270:625, 1964.

Finberg, L. Hypernatremic (hypertonic) dehydration in infants. *N. Engl. J. Med.* 289:196, 1973.

Finberg, L., Kiley, J., and Luttrell, C. N. Mass accidental salt poisoning in infancy. *J.A.M.A.* 184:187, 1963.

McCance, R. A. Experimental sodium chloride deficiency in man. *Proc. R. Soc. Lond. [Biol.]* 119:245, 1936.
This paper simply, clearly, and briefly describes a meticulous balance study that has become a classic.

Strauss, M. B., Lamdin, E., Smith, W. P., and Bleifer, D. J. Surfeit and deficit of sodium: A kinetic concept of sodium excretion. *Arch. Intern. Med.* 102:527, 1958.

Volpe, J. Neonatal intracranial hemorrhage — Iatrogenic etiology? *N. Engl. J. Med.* 291:43, 1974.

Hyponatremia and Hypernatremia

Berl, T., Anderson, R. J., McDonald, K. M., and Schrier, R. W. Clinical disorders of water metabolism. *Kidney Int.* 10:117, 1976.

Edelman, I. S., Leibman, J., O'Meara, M. P., and Birkenfeld, L. W. Interrelations between serum sodium concentration, serum osmolarity and total exchangeable sodium, total exchangeable potassium, and total body water. *J. Clin. Invest.* 37:1236, 1958.

Finberg, L. Hypernatremic (hypertonic) dehydration in infants. *N. Engl. J. Med.* 289:196, 1973.

Finberg, L. Diarrheal Dehydration. In R. W. Winters (ed.), *The Body Fluids in Pediatrics.* Boston: Little, Brown, 1973.

Gault, M. H., Dixon, M. E., Doyle, M., and Cohen, W. M. Hypernatremia, azotemia, and dehydration due to high-protein tube feeding. *Ann. Intern. Med.* 68:778, 1968.

Harrington, A. R. Hyponatremia due to sodium depletion in the absence of vasopressin. *Am. J. Physiol.* 222:768, 1972.

Humphries, J. O., Hinman, E. J., Bernstein, L., and Walker, W. G. Effect of artificial pacing of the heart on cardiac and renal function. *Circulation* 36:717, 1967.

Jaenike, J. R., and Waterhouse, C. Body fluid alterations during the development of and recovery from hyponatremia in heart failure. *Am. J. Med.* 26:862, 1959.

Leaf, A. The clinical and physiologic significance of the serum sodium concentration. *N. Engl. J. Med.* 267:24 and 77, 1962.

Maffly, R. H., and Edelman, I. S. The Role of Sodium, Potassium and Water in the Hypo-osmotic States of Heart Failure. In C. K. Friedberg (ed.), *Heart, Kidney, and Electrolytes.* New York: Grune & Stratton, 1962.

Miles, A. I., and Needle, M. A. Fixed hyponatremia with normal responses to varying salt and water intakes. *N. Engl. J. Med.* 284:26, 1971.

Orloff, J., and Burg, M. B. The Pathogenesis of Hyponatremia in Congestive Heart Failure. In C. K. Friedberg (ed.), *Heart, Kidney, and Electrolytes.* New York: Grune & Stratton, 1962.

Ross, E. J., and Christie, S. B. M. Hypernatremia. *Medicine* (Baltimore) 48:441, 1969.

4 : Disorders of K^+ Balance

Potassium is the most abundant cation within cells (Fig. 1-1), and it plays a major role in some vital processes, most notably in the functioning of excitable tissues and of many enzyme systems. For this reason, and because internal and external imbalances of K^+ are rather common in patients, the specific consequences of K^+ deficit or excess will be discussed in many subsequent chapters: K^+ depletion and hypokalemia accompanying acid-base disturbances (Chap. 6), diuretic-induced K^+ deficiency (Chap. 7), hyperkalemia during acute renal failure (Chap. 9), K^+ depletion in renal tubular acidosis (Chap. 12), and hypokalemic nephropathy (Chap. 13). The present chapter will be limited to the discussion of some general principles of K^+ imbalance that can be applied to the analysis of clinical disorders.

Distribution of K^+ in the Body

One obvious consequence of the K^+ concentration, $[K^+]$, being very low in the extracellular fluid (ECF) and very high within intracellular fluid (ICF) is that virtually all the total body K^+ is found within the cells (Fig. 4-1). In addition to the roughly 65 mEq of K^+ in the plasma and interstitial fluid, approximately 65 mEq is also found in dense connective tissue and cartilage and in that part of bone that is not cellular. Even taking this further quantity into account, however, extracellular K^+ accounts for only about 5 percent of the total body K^+. By far the greatest part of intracellular K^+ is found in skeletal muscles, not because muscle cells necessarily have a higher K^+ concentration than other cells, but because muscles constitute far and away the largest portion (about 75 percent) of cellular tissue, often referred to as *lean tissue mass.* Although the explanation for the accumulation of K^+ by cells is not fully settled, most workers believe that it involves active transport across the cell membrane. This transport may or may not be coupled to the active extrusion of Na^+ from cells; even if it is coupled, however, a simple one-to-one exchange of K^+ for Na^+ does not seem to occur in many circumstances.

Figure 4-1 shows the two tissues that, after muscle, contain

INTAKE (mEq/day)		DISTRIBUTION		OUTPUT (mEq/day)	
		Intracellular	Extracellular		
Diet	100	$[K^+] \simeq$ 125 mEq/kg tissue	$[K^+] \simeq$ 4 mEq/L	Urine	92
		Muscle 3,000 mEq		Stool	8
		Skin and sub-cut. tissue 500			
		RBC 250			
		3,750 mEq	65 mEq		
	100	← EXTERNAL K^+ BALANCE (mEq/day) →			100

Figure 4-1
Dynamics of K^+ balance in a healthy adult human. The distribution of K^+ is superimposed on the relative sizes of the intracellular and extracellular compartments. All values are approximate; normal dietary intake of K^+ can vary from 50 to 150 mEq per day. Adapted from D. A. K. Black, in M. H. Maxwell and C. R. Kleeman (eds.), *Clinical Disorders of Fluid and Electrolyte Metabolism* (2nd ed.). New York: McGraw-Hill, 1972.

the most K^+. The K^+ content of erythrocytes may be important when giving blood transfusions. As blood is stored, erythrocytes die, and this process may release enough K^+ into the transfused plasma to raise its $[K^+]$ to more than 20 mEq per liter, that is, about four times greater than the normal plasma concentration.

K^+ Balance

External Balance

Dietary intake of K^+ in a healthy adult averages about 100 mEq per day (Fig. 4-1); it can normally range between 50 and 150 mEq per day. Most of the daily K^+ excretion occurs through the kidneys, which are the primary regulators of external K^+ balance. An appreciable amount of K^+, however, is excreted in the stool, even under healthy circumstances. Whether the dietary intake of K^+ is normal or abnormally low or high, 80 to 90 percent of the filtered K^+ is reabsorbed in the proximal tubules and loops of Henle. External balance of K^+ is regulated in the distal tubules and collecting ducts, where the handling of K^+ can vary from net reabsorption during a period of low K^+ intake to net secretion during one of high K^+ intake.

As a general rule, normal kidneys respond quickly to high intakes of K^+ but sluggishly to low intakes. Large loads of K^+ (100 to 200 mEq) can be excreted in the urine within hours, and, with adaptation, several hundred milliequivalents can be excreted per day. In contrast, three to four weeks may be required before the kidneys respond fully to a low K^+ intake by reabsorbing the ion so avidly that virtually no K^+ appears in the urine. The reasons for these differences are not clear; changes in the production of aldosterone probably play a role in the slow adaptation and during prolonged alterations of intake.

It must be borne in mind, especially in disease, that the renal excretion of K^+ is governed by a number of factors besides the K^+ intake. Other things being equal, K^+ excretion is increased by a concurrent high intake of Na^+, alkalosis, excess adrenal mineralocorticoids, or increased urine flow, especially when induced by major diuretic drugs. Changes of these factors in the opposite direction generally decrease the renal excretion of K^+.

Internal Balance

Shifts of K^+ between the extracellular and intracellular compartments occur fairly commonly in clinical medicine, and they can play a large role in governing the concentration of K^+ in plasma. The major conditions under which such shifts occur are shown in Figure 4-2.

During K^+ deficiency of whatever cause (Table 4-1), the plasma concentration of K^+ tends to be low. This change favors a greater than normal efflux of K^+ out of cells. Reciprocally, Na^+ enters the cells, but ordinarily not in a one-to-one ratio; usually, about

PRIMARY MOVEMENT OF K^+

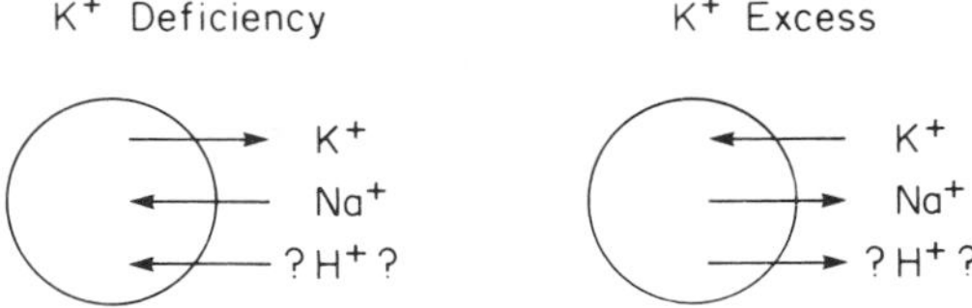

PRIMARY MOVEMENT OF H^+

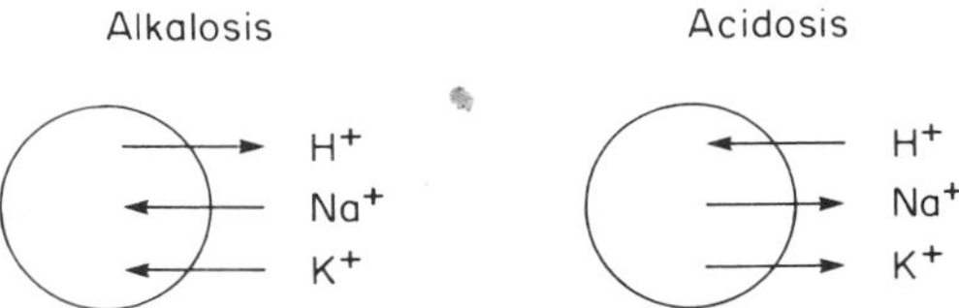

Figure 4-2
Reciprocal movement of K^+, Na^+, and, in some instances, H^+ between the intracellular and extracellular compartments. The circles represent body cells surrounded by extracellular fluid, and the arrows indicate the direction of ion migration *after* a given disturbance has been established. In acidosis, for example, a relatively high concentration of H^+ in the extracellular fluid favors net movement of H^+ into the cells; reciprocally, Na^+ and K^+ move out of cells. It is not settled whether H^+ ions participate in the shifts during primary imbalances of K^+; in most clinical situations, however, it is assumed that they do.

two Na^+ ions enter the cells for every three K^+ ions leaving them. Despite a great deal of work, there is no agreement on what cations besides Na^+ enter the cells. Some believe it to be basic amino acids (e.g., lysine), but the more popular view is that it is H^+. If the latter is correct, one would predict an increase in the intracellular concentration of H^+. The obstacle to settling the issue has been largely the difficulty of measuring intracellular pH. Some workers have recorded decreased intracellular pH during K^+ depletion; others have not. Even if H^+ does enter the cells under these conditions, however, the magnitude of this shift is unlikely to account for all the "missing" cations, for the deficit of intracellular $[K^+]$ is reckoned in milliequivalents per liter whereas the increase in intracellular $[H^+]$ would be on the order of nanoequivalents per liter, or one-millionth the concentration of K^+. Depletion of K^+ is in fact associated with *extracellular* alkalosis, although the cause may be more a matter of increased renal excretion of H^+ (Chap. 6, under Metabolic Alkalosis, and Fig. 6-1) than of the internal imbalance suggested in Figure 4-2. Suffice it to say that many phenomena observed in K^+ depletion can be visualized as consequences of the events depicted in Figure 4-2, and physicians therefore find the concept useful, even if they will eventually have to abandon it should further experimental evidence disprove it.

Experimental evidence to support the proposed events shown for K^+ excess is even poorer. This is partly because, as mentioned earlier, normal kidneys readily excrete extra K^+, and partly because hyperkalemia is an emergent, often lethal, situation, so large surfeits of total body K^+ rarely occur. Again, however, the diagram in Figure 4-2 portrays a useful concept for managing patients.

There is more solid evidence for the events occurring during acid-base disturbances (Fig. 4-2). The reciprocal movements of H^+ in one direction and of Na^+ and K^+ in the other occur because a large portion of a deficit or excess of acid is buffered within the cells. Thus, in alkalosis, the low extracellular concentration of H^+ promotes movement of H^+ out of the cells. This H^+, which was "released" from intracellular buffers, is replaced by Na^+ or K^+, as shown in the following reactions during metabolic alkalosis due to a loss of HCl:

Interstitial Fluid		*Cells*
$Na^+ + Cl^- \leftrightharpoons Cl^- + H^+$	←	H^+
Na^+	→	$Na^+ + Prot^- \rightleftharpoons H\text{-}Prot$ (or organic phosphates)
$K^+ + Cl^- \leftrightharpoons Cl^- + H^+$	←	H^+
K^+	→	$K^+ + Prot^- \rightleftharpoons H\text{-}Prot$ (or organic phosphates)

These reactions proceed in the opposite direction during acidosis. One would predict from the diagrams in Figure 4-2 that alkalosis would be associated with a decrease in serum K^+ concentration and acidosis with an increase. This does occur, even in the face of deficits or excesses of total body K^+ (Fig. 4-3). It follows that the serum K^+ concentration may be a poor guide to the total body stores of K^+; this point is discussed next.

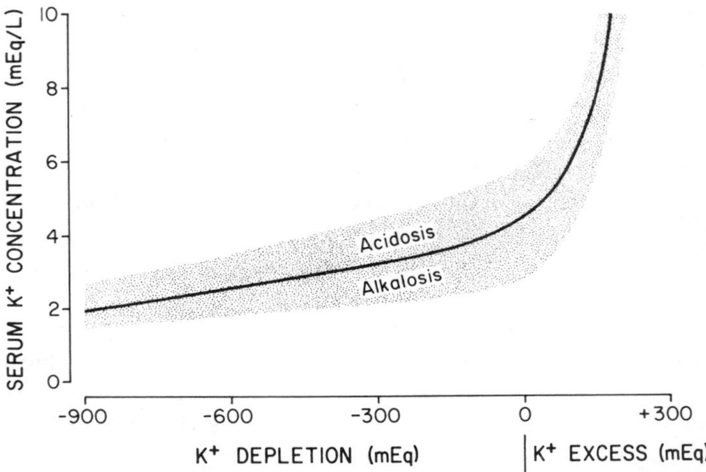

Figure 4-3
Approximate relationship between changes in total body K^+ and the serum concentration of K^+ in an adult. The graph should not be interpreted as being quantitatively precise, because the serum K^+ concentration is influenced by several factors besides the total body K^+. These factors include the status of adrenal mineralocorticoids, the concurrent intake of NaCl, the H^+ balance, and whether the change is acute or chronic. The graph does, however, emphasize several points: (1) the H^+ balance has an important influence on the serum K^+ concentration; (2) given a history of K^+ *depletion,* the serum K^+ concentration will be a rough gauge of the degree of negative balance; and (3) increases in total body K^+ are rare and minimal, and hyperkalemia usually reflects an acute imbalance between the exogenous or endogenous load of K^+ and the ability of the kidneys to excrete the load. Adapted from W. B. Schwartz and A. S. Relman, *J. Clin. Invest.* 32:258, 1953; F. D. Moore et al., *Metabolism* 5:379, 1955; B. H. Scribner and J. M. Burnell, *Metabolism* 5:468, 1956.

The Meaning of Hypokalemia and Hyperkalemia

The serum K^+ concentration is influenced by a number of factors besides the total amount of K^+ in the body, of which some of the more important have been listed in the legend to Figure 4-3. These factors, most notably the H^+ balance (the influence of which is shown in Figure 4-3), affect the *internal* as well as the external balance (Fig. 4-2), and because the extracellular pool is small (Fig. 4-1), a relatively trivial shift into or out of the large intracellular pool can cause a sizable change in the serum concentration. For these reasons, the serum K^+ concentration may be a poor gauge of the total body K^+. However, if the other factors, especially the concurrent H^+ balance, are kept in mind, then the relationship shown in Figure 4-3 usually holds.

Hypokalemia. The course of the heavy line in Figure 4-3 indicates that the usefulness of the serum K^+ concentration as a guide to total body K^+ is *limited to states of K^+ deficiency.* If the patient has a history of K^+ depletion, then at any given level of acid-base balance there will be a direct correlation between the extent of depletion and the serum K^+ concentration. A useful rule of thumb is that during K^+ depletion, the serum concentration value drops roughly *1 mEq per liter for every 150 mEq deficit in the total body K^+*. It should be noted from Figure 4-3 that this is true only during the early phase of depletion; as more severe deficiency develops, the serum concentration falls less rapidly. The graph also shows that deficits can be considerable. With total body K^+ in a healthy adult amounting to 3,500 to 4,000 mEq (Table 1-5 and Fig. 4-1), a loss of 20 percent of the store is not uncommon (see also Chap. 6, under Metabolic Alkalosis).

Hyperkalemia. Because healthy kidneys can readily excrete large loads of K^+ through efficient tubular secretion, an excess of total body K^+ occurs only when the urinary excretion of the ion is impaired. The classic example is oliguric, acute renal failure (Chap. 9), in which an inability to excrete K^+ is often combined with an increased internal "production" from injured or dying tissue (Problem 4-2). The last point emphasizes that K^+ excess is usually relative, in the sense that it is commonly associated with a decrease in the capacity of the body to hold K^+ rather than with an increase in the total amount of K^+ within the body. A final reason why hyperkalemia usually does not reflect a great excess of total body K^+ is that a high serum K^+ concentration can lead to sudden death from cardiac arrhythmias or cardiac arrest (see Hyperkalemia: K^+ Excess, below). A serum concentration of 7 to 8 mEq of K^+ per liter needs immediate intervention, and a concentration greater than 10 mEq per liter is often fatal. Thus, a patient is likely to die before the cellular tissue can be loaded with K^+.

As a general rule, then, hypokalemia usually reflects a negative external balance of K^+ that is often modified by changes of internal balance; in contrast, hyperkalemia is a poor indicator of external K^+ balance, but rather reflects a diminished ability of the kidneys to excrete K^+ and a decreased cellular mass to hold the K^+.

K^+ Deficiency

Any wasting disease in which the lean tissue mass is reduced will be accompanied by a decrease in total body K^+. Such conditions, however, are not ordinarily considered to represent K^+ deficiency, because in them the K^+ content *per unit of cell mass* usually remains normal. In clinical usage, *K^+ deficiency* is defined as a decrease in the total body K^+ that is out of proportion to the cell mass.

Causes of K^+ Deficiency

Although it may take three to four weeks for normal kidneys to adapt fully to a low-K^+ diet, a decreased intake of K^+ is not a clinically important cause of K^+ deficiency. Part of the reason for this fact is that nearly all foods contain K^+, so it is virtually impossible to have an oral diet that is free of K^+. Clinically important K^+ deficiency occurs only when the urinary or gastrointestinal excretion of K^+ is abnormally high and exceeds its intake. Of the causes of K^+ deficiency listed in Table 4-1, the first five are fairly common, whereas the last – namely, primary renal disease leading to K^+ wasting – is rarely seen.

Diuretics. The use of certain diuretic agents, mainly the thiazides, furosemide, and ethacrynic acid (Table 7-1), is perhaps the commonest cause of K^+ deficiency. The mechanisms whereby these diuretics produce a marked increase in the urinary excretion of K^+ are not fully understood. They may include an increase of the transepithelial electrical potential difference (P.D.) in the distal tubules and collecting ducts, as well as an increased flow rate of fluid in these nephron segments. These effects are frequently abetted by secondary hyperaldosteronism, which is common in the edematous states for which diuretics are mainly used. Although mercurial diuretics (little used today) also have a "kaliuretic" effect, they do not usually cause severe K^+ depletion. The reason is that the effect of mercurial diuretics is self-limited in that their use leads to metabolic alkalosis, in which state the mercurials become ineffective. Similarly, mannitol does not commonly cause K^+ deficiency, because it is seldom used

Table 4-1
Causes of K^+ deficiency

Causes
Diuretics
Metabolic alkalosis
Metabolic acidosis
Excess adrenal corticosteroids
Hyperaldosteronism
Excess glucocorticoids
Gastrointestinal losses
Diarrhea
Vomiting
Laxatives
Surgical drainage
Villous tumors of colon
Renal disease (e.g., pyelonephritis; Fanconi syndrome; RTA)

over an extended period of time. Another diuretic, triamterene, does not cause kaliuresis, possibly because it reduces the trans-epithelial P.D. in the distal nephron; it is appropriately classified as a K^+-sparing diuretic (Table 7-1).

Diuretic-induced K^+ deficiency is especially important because many edematous patients are treated simultaneously with diuretics and digitalis, and dangerous toxic effects of the latter drug are aggravated in K^+ depletion (see Problem 4-1).

Metabolic Alkalosis. The mechanisms that lead to K^+ deficiency during metabolic alkalosis are described in detail in Chapter 6 (under Metabolic Alkalosis). Usually, the key factor is the increased *urinary* excretion of K^+, even in those instances that involve gastrointestinal losses of K^+ (e.g., vomiting, surgical drainage, or diarrhea, Table 6-5). During metabolic alkalosis, there is an obligatory excretion of HCO_3^-, and one of the cations accompanying the HCO_3^- is K^+ (Fig. 6-1). In some instances (Table 6-5), the increased urinary excretion of K^+ is caused or abetted by primary or secondary hyperaldosteronism. In others, the cause is not yet known; it is possible that the obligatory excretion of HCO_3^- increases the transepithelial P.D. in the distal tubules and collecting ducts, which in turn augments the tubular secretion of K^+ in these segments.

Note that alkalosis leads to K^+ deficiency (also Fig. 6-1) and that the latter, when severe, causes alkalosis (Table 6-5 and Fig. 4-2). This vicious circle is involved in both the generation and maintenance of metabolic alkalosis and has given rise to the expression that "alkalosis begets alkalosis."

Metabolic Acidosis. Several types of metabolic acidosis (Table 6-2) – although notably not that accompanying renal failure – are associated with K^+ depletion. Classic examples are the acidosis of uncontrolled diabetes mellitus and that associated with renal tubular acidosis (RTA, Chap. 12).

In diabetes mellitus, deficient catabolism of carbohydrates leads to increased breakdown of fat and the consequent production of organic acids, mainly β-hydroxybutyric and acetoacetic acids (see Chap. 6, under Uncontrolled Diabetes Mellitus.) The H^+ from these acids is excreted mainly as neutral NH_4^+ salts and partly as titratable acids, including β-hydroxybutyric and acetoacetic acids. However, because of the relatively low pK' of these acids (4.8 and 3.8, respectively) and because of the limitation of renal NH_3 production, not all of the extra H^+ that is produced can be excreted. Hence, much of the filtered anions (e.g., β-hydroxybutyrate and acetoacetate) must be accompanied by cations other than H^+, and one of these is K^+. One reason why K^+ is selectively excreted during diabetic ketoacidosis may be that the abundance of relatively unreabsorbable

β-hydroxybutyrate and acetoacetate increases the transepithelial P.D. and hence the tubular secretion of K^+. A second reason is that diabetic ketoacidosis is invariably accompanied by contraction of the extracellular fluid volume and secondary hyperaldosteronism, which also augments the tubular secretion of K^+. The negative external balance in this type of acidosis is combined with a change of internal balance that promotes a shift of K^+ out of the cells (Fig. 4-2), and it may thus result in a relatively high serum K^+ concentration for the degree of depletion (Fig. 4-3). However, as the diabetic ketoacidosis is treated, K^+ will return into the cells. This migration, plus the already existing K^+ deficiency, can lead to dangerous hypokalemia. For this reason, it is important to give K^+ during the course of treatment for diabetic ketoacidosis (see Chap. 6, under Uncontrolled Diabetes Mellitus).

In renal tubular acidosis (RTA), metabolic acidosis is due either to inadequate reabsorption of filtered HCO_3^- in the proximal tubules or to insufficient H^+ secretion in the distal tubules and collecting ducts (Chap. 12). The latter defect will also lead to increased urinary excretion of HCO_3^-, because for every H^+ ion secreted, an ion of HCO_3^- is reabsorbed. Thus, in either type of RTA, it is the obligatory excretion of HCO_3^- that causes increased excretion of K^+, again possibly because of an increased transepithelial P.D. in the distal tubules and collecting ducts.

Excess Adrenal Corticosteroids. The mechanism by which these hormones cause K^+ depletion probably involves the mineralocorticoid effect, mainly that of aldosterone but also that of glucocorticoids (Table 4-1), which stimulates the secretion of K^+ in the distal tubules and collecting ducts. Whether the increased secretion is due to enhanced peritubular uptake of K^+ by the renal cells or to some other or additional effect is not yet clear. Adequate intake of Na^+ is a prerequisite for the kaliuresis associated with excess adrenal corticosteroids; again, the mechanism of this influence is not known, but it is suspected that it involves an increase of the transepithelial P.D. in the distal tubules and collecting ducts.

Several disease states that are associated with high plasma concentrations of the adrenocortical hormones are listed in Table 6-5. It is not yet clear whether these hormones cause metabolic alkalosis by a direct influence on the tubular secretion of H^+ or by an indirect effect through K^+. In either event, however, the fact that diseases involving hyperactivity of adrenal steroids are listed as causes of both K^+ depletion (Table 4-1) and metabolic alkalosis (Table 6-5) emphasizes the vicious circle referred to earlier, that is, that "alkalosis begets alkalosis."

Gastrointestinal Losses. Table 1-4 shows that the concentration of K^+ in gastrointestinal fluids — especially saliva, gastric juice, and large-intestinal secretions — is equal to or higher than the serum K^+ concentration. It follows that conditions such as vomiting, diarrhea, surgical drainage, and the abuse of laxatives, which in an adult patient can amount to fluid losses of several liters per day, often lead to K^+ deficiency. Although the depletion can occur in the absence of a concomitant metabolic alkalosis, the deficit of K^+ is likely to be more severe if this acid-base disturbance is present. The reason for the greater severity is that in metabolic alkalosis, there are large urinary losses of K^+, even when the cause of the alkalosis is a gastrointestinal disturbance, such as vomiting (see above; also Chap. 6, under Metabolic Alkalosis).

The potential importance of gastrointestinal losses of K^+ is reflected in the utilization of this route for the prevention of hyperkalemia, as in acute renal failure (Chap. 9). When treating this condition, in which hyperkalemia is a threat to life (see below) and which occurs not infrequently in postoperative patients, the attending physician can often utilize surgical drainage tubes already in place or induce diarrhea in order to rid the patient of large amounts of K^+.

Effects of K^+ Deficiency

It was emphasized at the beginning of this chapter that K^+ is a critical element in some vital processes, most notably neuromuscular function and the operation of numerous enzyme systems. It is not surprising, therefore, that the effects of K^+ imbalances are widespread, including, among others, disturbances in H^+ balance, in energy metabolism, and in the ability of the kidneys to concentrate the urine. In this section, however, we shall limit the discussion to the life-threatening effects of K^+ deficiency, namely, those involving neuromuscular irritability.

The excitability of muscles is a function of their resting membrane potential and of their threshold potential. For skeletal muscle, the first has a normal value of about 60 to 70 mV and the second, approximately 30 to 40 mV, the inside of the muscle cell in each instance being negative with respect to the outside. When a muscle is stimulated, its membrane potential is lowered by acetylcholine (depolarization), and when the value of the threshold potential is reached, an action potential is generated, the electrical impulse is transmitted, and the muscle contracts. Any factor that decreases the *difference* between the two potentials will lead to increased neuromuscular excitability; conversely, any process that increases the difference will decrease the excitability.

Because the muscle membrane is highly permeable to K^+,

the major determinant of the resting membrane potential of muscles is the ratio of the K^+ concentration inside the cells to that in the extracellular fluid, $[K^+]_i/[K^+]_e$. As the ratio increases, so does the resting membrane potential (hyperpolarization) and vice versa (depolarization). Because the value of $[K^+]_i$ is so large relative to that of $[K^+]_e$ (see Fig. 4-1), the *ratio* is very sensitive to changes in the latter. Thus, in K^+ deficiency where both $[K^+]_i$ and $[K^+]_e$ decrease (Fig. 4-3), the ratio rises because the change in $[K^+]_e$ is relatively much greater than that of $[K^+]_i$. Consequently, the resting membrane potential increases, the difference between the resting and threshold potentials is greater, and the muscles are less excitable than normally. This chain of events could explain some of the major signs of K^+ deficiency: muscular weakness, sometimes terminating in flaccid paralysis; abnormalities of myocardial contraction and potentiation of digitalis toxicity; adynamic ileus; and, occasionally, paralysis of the muscles of respiration when K^+ depletion is severe.

The importance of the ratio $[K^+]_i/[K^+]_e$ probably also explains why the electrocardiogram (ECG), which reflects myocardial function, is a far better indicator of clinically important K^+ deficiency than is the serum K^+ concentration alone. Changes in the ECG, especially in the precordial leads, are usually monitored in any patient in whom an imbalance of K^+ is suspected. The typical alterations of K^+ deficiency are shown in Figure 4-4b. There are prolongation of the P-R interval, depression of the S-T segment (sometimes with inversion of the T wave), and the appearance of a U wave. The components of the ECG can be correlated with events in the cardiac cycle; for example, the P-R interval reflects the time required for the electrical impulse to be propagated through the atria, the QRS interval measures ventricular depolarization, and the T wave indicates ventricular repolarization. Nevertheless, it would be too simplistic to say that all the changes seen in the ECG during K^+ deficiency reflect decreased excitability of the myocardium. The changes probably are, however, largely a function of $[K^+]_i/[K^+]_e$, and they therefore provide a useful guide to some of the important functional consequences of K^+ deficiency. It must be stressed that these consequences — not only in the myocardium but in other muscles and organ systems as well — cannot be correlated simply with the serum K^+ concentration nor even with the degree of depletion of total body K^+. The effects are also modulated by several other factors (e.g., Na^+, H^+, Mg^{2+}, and Ca^{2+} balance or the presence of cardiac arrhythmias) and by drugs such as the cardiac glycosides.

The cardiac manifestations of digitalis toxicity include inhibi-

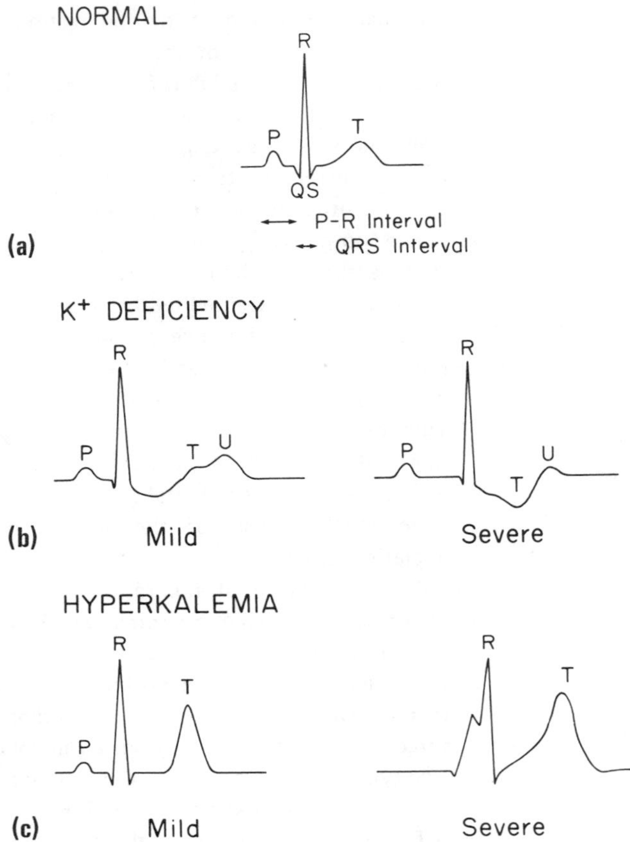

Figure 4-4
Electrocardiogram (ECG), as recorded from a precordial lead, in health (a) and during K^+ deficiency (b) and hyperkalemia (c). In part (b), the heading "K^+ Deficiency" emphasizes a deficit of total body K^+, whereas in (c), the state of K^+ in the blood is stressed by the term "hyperkalemia." This distinction is deliberate, because total body K^+ is usually low when hypokalemia is present, whereas it may be only minimally altered in the face of hyperkalemia (see Fig. 4-3). The patterns shown here are not specific for abnormalities of K^+. Drugs and other ions – notably digitalis and Ca^{2+}, Na^+, Mg^{2+}, and H^+ – can mimic or alter the patterns. Modified from M. J. Goldman, *Principles of Clinical Electrocardiography* (9th ed.). Los Altos, Calif.: Lange Medical Publications, 1976.

tion of Na,K-adenosinetriphosphatase (Na,K-ATPase), reduced excitability, defects in conduction, and arrhythmias. Some of these effects are also seen in K^+ deficiency, and it is not surprising, therefore, that the two conditions – digitalis toxicity and K^+ depletion – can dangerously abet one another. It is important to be constantly alert to this fact, because digitalis and diuretics are so frequently used together in edematous patients, and diuretic therapy is currently perhaps the commonest cause of K^+ deficiency (Table 4-1).

Treatment of K^+ Deficiency

Deficits of total body K^+ may be very large before they are recognized; they often amount to several hundred milliequivalents (Fig. 4-3). Because hyperkalemia can lead to sudden death (see below), a number of precautions must be exercised when correcting the deficits: (1) There must be adequate renal function. The main route for K^+ excretion is renal, and if the urine output is inadequate (as in acute renal failure, Chap. 9), giving K^+ can quickly lead to dangerous hyperkalemia. (2) A slow *rate* of administration is more important than the total amount being given, especially when a parenteral route is used. K^+ is taken up by the cells rather quickly; nevertheless, if it is given too rapidly intravenously, the serum K^+ concentration may rise to lethal levels, especially within the environment of the heart where the intravenously administered K^+ first goes. Therefore, when K^+ is given intravenously, it must be given as a *dilute* solution (usually not greater than 40 mEq per liter; Fig. 1-6), and except under most unusual circumstances, the rate of infusion should not exceed 20 mEq per hour. (3) Because of the dangers of hyperkalemia, replenishment of K^+ by the oral route is preferable to parenteral administration and should be used whenever possible. (4) Finally, the seemingly trite phrase that "prevention is the best treatment" applies especially to K^+ deficiency. Depletion of K^+ is often an insidious process that has many possible causes (Table 4-1), and the physician who wishes to detect it early must be unusually wary. Many conditions that lead to K^+ deficiency — especially the use of diuretics, certain acidotic states (e.g., ketoacidosis and RTA), and certain malabsorption syndromes — are therefore usually treated in part with oral K^+ supplements.

Hyperkalemia: K^+ Excess

We have by now pointed out several times that normal kidneys can excrete a K^+ load efficiently and that the dire consequences of a high serum K^+ concentration usually intervene before the tissues can be loaded with K^+. For these reasons K^+ excess, in the sense of an increase in the total body K^+, is very rare, and this section is therefore more accurately entitled "Hyperkalemia."

Causes of Hyperkalemia

A degree of hyperkalemia that endangers life is seen mainly or solely in the first two conditions among the causes of hyperkalemia listed in Table 4-2. Even the cessation of renal excretion of K^+, as in acute renal failure, does not ordinarily lead to dangerous hyperkalemia if the excessive breakdown of tissues and consequent release of endogenous K^+ is minimized (Chap. 9). Often, however, the very cause of acute renal failure is one like trauma, in which increased breakdown or ischemic hypoxia of tissues occurs; in these instances, marked hyperkalemia is a constant threat.

Table 4-2
Causes of hyperkalemia

Causes of hyperkalemia
Acute (but usually not chronic) renal failure
Injudicious intravenous administration of K^+
Increased tissue breakdown or damage
Trauma; hematomas
Fever; infection; undernourishment
Hypoxia
Poor renal perfusion
Na^+ depletion
Adrenal insufficiency (Addison's disease)
Acidosis
Familial periodic paralysis (adynamia episodica hereditaria)
"Pseudohyperkalemia"
Hemolysis in vitro
Ischemic damage

As discussed above, K^+ should be given intravenously only when the rapid correction of a deficit is essential, only in dilute solution, and only at relatively slow rates. Otherwise, a sudden rise in the serum K^+ concentration, which is "seen" first by the heart, can be fatal.

Poor renal perfusion may elevate the serum K^+ level because of inadequate urinary excretion of the ion, but it is unlikely to lead to extreme hyperkalemia unless severe and prolonged shock is involved, in which case acute renal failure might intervene (Chap. 9). It should be noted (Table 4-2) that adrenal insufficiency raises the serum K^+ level probably more through an indirect effect — that is, through Na^+ depletion, decreased extracellular fluid volume, and poor renal perfusion — than through a direct effect in which the absence of aldosterone decreases the renal tubular secretion of K^+.

Acidosis raises the serum K^+ concentration by a shift in internal balance (Fig. 4-2).

What is perhaps the commonest cause of hyperkalemia is so-called pseudohyperkalemia (Table 4-2). It may result from the hemolysis of erythrocytes and the release of K^+ from them, usually as the blood is drawn from the patient or as the serum is separated in the laboratory. Ischemia of sufficient severity and duration to cause the death of cells is an analogous cause; it may be seen in patients during cardiac arrest or if blood is drawn just after a patient has died. The physician must be aware of these possibilities when evaluating a laboratory report of "hyperkalemia."

Effects of Hyperkalemia

As with K^+ deficiency and hypokalemia, the functional consequences of hyperkalemia probably can be explained through a change in $[K^+]_i/[K^+]_e$, and hence these consequences may involve changes in neuromuscular excitability. In hyperkalemia, however, cardiac arrest frequently occurs before the effects on skeletal striated muscle or intestinal smooth muscle become manifest.

As explained earlier, because $[K^+]_i$ is so much greater than $[K^+]_e$, an equal increment in both will increase $[K^+]_e$ relatively more than $[K^+]_i$, so the ratio will decrease. Consequently, the resting membrane potential falls (i.e., depolarization occurs), and muscles, including the myocardium, become hyperexcitable. In addition, however, hyperkalemia slows the pacemaker and conducting functions of the heart, so the cardiac effects cannot be predicted simply on the basis of hyperexcitability alone. Suffice it to say that hyperkalemia can lead to ventricular arrest or ventricular fibrillation. The importance of the ratio $[K^+]_i/[K^+]_e$ in bringing about these dire changes is suggested by the observation that the sudden rise in $[K^+]_e$ occasioned by an intravenous infusion can lead to serious cardiac disturbances, even though the serum K^+ concentration stays within the normal range. Again, the ECG is therefore a much better premonitor of dangerous hyperkalemia than is the serum K^+ concentration alone.

Typical changes in the electrocardiographic pattern during hyperkalemia are shown in Figure 4-4c. They include tall, peaked T waves in mild elevations; in severe hyperkalemia, such T waves are seen as well as the loss of atrial activity (no P wave) and broadening and disfigurement of the QRS complex.

As in the case of myocardial muscle, one might predict from the fall in $[K^+]_i/[K^+]_e$ that skeletal muscle would also be hyperexcitable in hyperkalemia. However, flaccid paralysis is the more common finding. The probable explanation is that once the resting membrane potential has decreased to the level of the threshold potential, repolarization cannot occur, and the muscle is then no longer excitable. It has been proposed that weakness and flaccid paralysis are seen in both hypokalemia and hyperkalemia because the former leads to hyperpolarization of skeletal muscle while the latter leads to persistent depolarization. This explanation is supported by the findings in two rare diseases, familial periodic paralysis and adynamia episodica hereditaria. In the first, a shift of K^+ into the cells results in hypokalemia, and in the second, a shift of K^+ out of the cells causes hyperkalemia. Both disorders therefore result from abnormalities of internal balance, and both have a mendelian dominant form of inheritance; in fact, the pathogenesis of the disorders may be so similar that some experts now classify both as *familial periodic paralysis.*

Again, it should be stressed that the effects of hyperkalemia are not simply a function of the serum K^+ concentration but are also influenced by other factors, especially by the concurrent balance of Ca^{2+}, Na^+, and H^+.

Treatment of Hyperkalemia

The functional consequences of hyperkalemia (1) are often life-threatening because they involve the heart and (2) result more from an elevation of the serum K^+ concentration than from excess total body K^+. The treatment follows from these premises; various aspects are summarized in Table 4-3.

When the ECG shows signs of severe hyperkalemia (Fig. 4-4c), immediate correction of cardiac function is required. This is accomplished most rapidly by an intravenous infusion of calcium gluconate (Fig. 1-6), which acts strictly by its effect on the heart, not by lowering the serum K^+ concentration or the total body K^+. If myocardial dysfunction is not quite so threatening, a somewhat slower but still rapid measure is to lower the serum K^+ level by causing K^+ to shift into cells. The mechanism by which glucose and insulin accomplish this purpose is thought to be related to the intracellular deposition of glycogen. Alkalinization will serve the same end (Figs. 4-2 and 4-3), and often these modalities are combined in a single intravenous infusion of glucose, insulin, and $NaHCO_3$.

Expansion of the ECF by administration of hypertonic NaCl is usually reserved for those special instances where the hyperkalemia is caused by inadequate renal perfusion (Table 4-2). This measure lowers the serum K^+ concentration by diluting the extracellular K^+ in a greater volume of fluid, and it also possibly increases the renal excretion of K^+.

When the hyperkalemia is relatively mild ($<$6.5 mEq per liter; see Fig. 4-4c) but its progression is likely (as in acute renal fail-

Table 4-3
Treatment of hyperkalemia

Mode of Treatment	Onset of Therapeutic Effect	Effect on P_{K^+}*	Effect on Total Body K^+
Ca^{2+} i.v.*	1 to 5 minutes	None	None
Glucose plus insulin, often with	10 to 15 minutes	↓	None
$NaHCO_3$ i.v.	Within 1 hour	↓	None
Expansion of ECF*	Within 1 hour	↓	Slight ↓
Ion-exchange resin or	Hours	↓	↓
Dialysis	Hours	↓	↓

*P_{K^+} = plasma or serum K^+ concentration; i.v. = intravenously; ECF = extracellular fluid volume.

ure), the use of an ion-exchange resin is an effective therapeutic and preventive measure. One such resin is sodium polystyrene sulfonate (Kayexalate), which exchanges Na^+ for K^+. Its use is often combined with that of an alcohol, sorbitol, which hastens the intestinal excretion of the resin and itself increases the excretion of K^+ by causing diarrhea (Table 1-4). Dialysis, either peritoneal or by machine, also lowers both the serum and the total body K^+, but usually it need not be resorted to if one of the other modes of treatment has been instituted.

Summary

About 95 percent of the total body K^+ is within the cells, most of it in skeletal muscle. External balance of K^+ is regulated by the kidneys, which ordinarily excrete 90 percent or more of the daily intake. The regulation occurs in the distal tubules and collecting ducts, where the net transport of K^+ can vary from avid reabsorption to vigorous secretion. The increase in urinary excretion of K^+ in response to large intakes is usually faster and more completely balanced than the response to a low K^+ intake, which may require weeks to reach full compensation.

The serum or plasma K^+ concentration is governed to an important extent by the internal balance of K^+. Shifts of K^+ either into or out of the large intracellular pool can cause profound hypokalemia or hyperkalemia, respectively. Such shifts are accompanied by reciprocal movements of Na^+ and probably of H^+. Another prominent influence on the serum K^+ concentration is the H^+ balance. During extracellular alkalosis, H^+ shifts out of the cells, and movement of K^+ into the cells tends to lower the plasma K^+ concentration; the opposite changes occur during extracellular acidosis (Fig. 4-3).

In most patients, hypokalemia reflects a decrease in total body K^+. This is not true, however, of hyperkalemia, which is usually due to decreased renal excretion of K^+ and is rarely accompanied by a marked increase in total body K^+. Thus, while it is usually correct to use "K^+ deficiency" and "hypokalemia" synonymously, abnormal increases of K^+ are more accurately termed *hyperkalemia.* Important causes of K^+ deficiency include the use of diuretic drugs, metabolic alkalosis and acidosis, excess adrenal mineralocorticoid effect, and gastrointestinal losses. Hyperkalemia results from acute renal failure (especially when accompanied by increased tissue breakdown), injudicious intravenous administration of K^+, Na^+ depletion and adrenal insufficiency, and internal imbalances occasioned by extracellular acidosis and familial periodic paralysis.

Both K^+ deficiency and hyperkalemia can be life-threatening because of their effects on neuromuscular excitability, including that of the heart. One of the readiest ways of assessing neuromuscular function in patients is the electrocardiogram (ECG); the ECG is therefore used routinely as a premonitor of dangerous K^+ deficiency or hyperkalemia. Important signs of K^+ deficiency include weakness and flaccid paralysis, adynamic ileus, abnormalities of myocardial contraction, and potentiation of digitalis toxicity. Hyperkalemia leads to serious cardiac arrhythmias and sudden death from ventricular arrest or ventricular fibrillation. Although hyperkalemia can also cause flaccid paralysis, dramatic changes in cardiac function usually intervene before the effects on skeletal muscle become manifest.

K^+ deficiency is treated by administering K^+, which should be given cautiously as a dilute solution. Treatment of severe hyperkalemia is often directed first toward reversing dangerous cardiac malfunction (e.g., by Ca^{2+} infusion), and secondarily toward lowering the serum K^+ concentration. Decreasing the total body K^+ (e.g., by using ion-exchange resins or dialysis) is more commonly employed for the prevention of hyperkalemia.

Problem 4-1

For 15 years, a 78-year-old man had been followed by his physician for arteriosclerotic heart disease. His first symptoms had occurred at age 63, when he noted dyspnea on exertion, especially when climbing stairs. Within the next three years, he developed mild, pitting ankle edema (Fig. 3-3a) and some orthopnea; he began to sleep on two pillows instead of his customary one. At that time (i.e., at age 66), his physician put the patient on a low-salt diet (see Answer to Problem 3-2) and gave him digitalis. These measures relieved the patient's symptoms so that he could be physically active. At age 72, the breathlessness and edema had become more severe, and treatment with an oral diuretic, chlorothiazide, was begun. The initial dosage was 0.5 g every third day, and over the next six years (during which time the edema became slowly more severe), the dosage was increased progressively to 1.0 g daily.

During the month prior to a hospital admission at age 78, the patient had experienced symptoms of increasingly severe congestive heart failure. The dyspnea now prevented any physical exertion, and he slept in a room on the ground floor to avoid having to climb stairs. He used three pillows for sleeping, and often preferred to sleep sitting upright in a chair. His feet and ankles were so swollen with edema that he could no longer put on his shoes, and he wore bedroom slippers instead. Although he lost his appetite, he was gaining weight. This course of progressive cardiac failure continued despite adequate digitalization and increasing the chlorothiazide dosage to 2.0 g daily. The patient was therefore admitted to the hospital.

Abnormal findings on admission included a body weight of 84 kg, although the patient reported his normal weight to be 158 pounds (72 kg); moderate dyspnea; severe ankle and pretibial edema; a pulse rate of 92; wet inspiratory rales in the lung bases; an enlarged heart; and a prolonged P-R interval and lowering of the T waves on the ECG. The serum Na^+ concentration was 134 mEq per liter, $[K^+]$ was 3.3 mEq per liter, and $[Cl^-]$ was 92 mEq per liter.

The patient was given another diuretic, furosemide, 40 mg orally, and chlorothiazide administration was stopped but that of digitalis continued. When a diuresis did not ensue, he was given 80 mg of furosemide orally 6 hours after the first dose, and he was placed on a schedule of 80 mg daily. By the third hospital day, he had lost 12 kg. He was now very nauseated and retched frequently. He complained of headache and was drowsy. He felt weak. The ECG showed further prolongation of the P-R interval, an inverted T wave, a prominent U wave, and frequent premature ventricular contractions.

Analyze the patient's course, especially that immediately preceding and following his admission to the hospital. How do you explain the patient's weight gain just before admission, when he had virtually stopped eating? What is the probable interpretation of the patient's symptoms and ECG changes on the third hospital day, and how should treatment have been changed at this time?

Problem 4-2

Acute lymphocytic leukemia was diagnosed in a 9-year-old boy seven weeks prior to the present hospital admission. Treatment at that time with prednisone and vincristine resulted in partial remission; allopurinol was given simultaneously to prevent hyperuricemia (see answer to this problem). Because of relapse of the leukemia, he was referred to the hematology unit of a cancer center.

At the time of admission to the center, the patient was acutely and severely ill. He was pale and lethargic and was bleeding from the nose, the mouth, the bowel, the kidneys, and possibly other sites, such as the spleen and subcutaneous tissues. His spleen and liver were markedly enlarged. He was immediately given an intravenous dose of daunomycin (an antineoplastic agent used in the therapy of this type of leukemia); the administration of prednisone was continued and the dose of allopurinol was increased, but the use of vincristine was stopped. The next morning it was clear that the patient was in oliguric acute renal failure, and by this time the following results had been reported on venous plasma or serum: Na^+ 133 mEq per liter, K^+ 8.0 mEq per liter, Cl^- 89 mEq per liter, HCO_3^- 14 mEq per liter, pH 7.22, BUN 180 mg/100 ml, creatinine 5.1 mg/100 ml, and uric acid 32 mg/100 ml. The ECG showed tall, peaked T waves.

Measures were then promptly instituted to treat the hyperkalemia and acute renal failure (Chap. 9). They included alkalinization with intravenous $NaHCO_3$, intravenous infusion of furosemide (which sometimes increases urine flow in acute renal failure), and cessation of all other fluid intake to prevent overexpansion of the extracellular fluid volume and pulmonary edema. Because of continued bleeding, he was also given one unit of fresh, whole blood. Despite these steps, the patient's course was rapidly downhill. Within 2½ hours, he was comatose and hypotensive (blood pressure, 60/40 mm Hg); his respirations were spasmodic and his heart stopped beating. He had been in the hospital for less than 36 hours.

We have not yet considered some aspects of this patient's illness, such as the acute renal failure (Chap. 9) and the analysis of acid-base status (Chaps. 5 and 6). You should, however, be able to comment intelligently on the causes and treatment of hyperkalemia in this patient.

Selected References

Further references on K^+ are listed in several other chapters in connection with specific causes or consequences of K^+ imbalance, for example, in acid-base disturbances (Chap. 6), with diuretics (Chap. 7), in acute renal failure (Chap. 9), and in discrete renal dysfunctions (Chaps. 12 and 13).

General

Black, D. A. K. Potassium Metabolism. In M. H. Maxwell and C. R. Kleeman (eds.), *Clinical Disorders of Fluid and Electrolyte Metabolism* (2nd ed.). New York: McGraw-Hill, 1972.

Edelman, I. S., and Leibman, J. Anatomy of body water and electrolytes. *Am. J. Med.* 27:256, 1959.

Katz, A. I., and Epstein, F. H. Physiologic role of sodium-potassium-activated adenosine triphosphatase in the transport of cations across biologic membranes. *N. Engl. J. Med.* 278:253, 1968.

Skou, J. C. Enzymatic basis for active transport of Na^+ and K^+ across cell membranes. *Physiol. Rev.* 45:596, 1965.

Tannen, R. L. (ed.). Symposium on potassium homeostasis. *Kidney Int.* 11:389, 1977.
An authoritative, up-to-date collection of papers dealing with both the basic science and the clinical aspects of the subject.

Valtin, H. *Renal Function: Mechanisms Preserving Fluid and Solute Balance in Health.* Boston: Little, Brown, 1973.

Wilde, W. S. Potassium. In C. L. Comar and F. Bronner (eds.), *Mineral Metabolism,* vol. 2, part B. New York: Academic, 1962, p. 73.

Wrong, O., and Metcalfe-Gibson, A. The electrolyte content of faeces. *Proc. R. Soc. Med.* 58:1007, 1965.

Internal Balance

Anderson, H. M., and Mudge, G. H. The effect of potassium on intracellular bicarbonate in slices of kidney cortex. *J. Clin. Invest.* 34:1691, 1955.

Black, D. A. K., and Milne, M. D. Experimental potassium depletion in man. *Clin. Sci.* 11:397, 1952.

Cooke, R. E., Segar, W. E., Cheek, D. B., Coville, F. E., and Darrow, D. C. The extrarenal correction of alkalosis associated with potassium deficiency. *J. Clin. Invest.* 31:798, 1952.

Cotlove, E., Holliday, M. A., Schwartz, R., and Wallace, W. M. Effects of electrolyte depletion and acid-base disturbance on muscle cations. *Am. J. Physiol.* 167:665, 1951.

Darrow, D. C. Tissue water and electrolyte. *Annu. Rev. Physiol.* 6:95, 1944.

Eckel, R. E., Norris, J. E. C., and Pope, C. E., II. Basic amino acids as intracellular cations in K deficiency. *Am. J. Physiol.* 193:644, 1958.

Fenn, W. O., and Cobb, D. M. Potassium equilibrium in muscle. *J. Gen. Physiol.* 17:629, 1934.

Ferrebee, J. W., Parker, D., Carnes, W. H., Gerity, M. K., Atchley, D. W., and Loeb, R. F. Certain effects of desoxycorticosterone. The development of "diabetes insipidus" and the replacement of muscle potassium by sodium in normal dogs. *Am. J. Physiol.* 135:230, 1941.

Giebisch, G., Berger, L., and Pitts, R. F. The extrarenal response to acid-base disturbance of respiratory origin. *J. Clin. Invest.* 34:231, 1955.

Iacobellis, M., Muntwyler, E., and Dodgen, C. L. Free amino acid patterns of certain tissues from potassium and/or protein-deficient rats. *Am. J. Physiol.* 185:275, 1956.

Irvine, R. O. H., Saunders, S. J., Milne, M. D., and Crawford, M. A. Gradients of potassium and hydrogen ion in potassium-deficient voluntary muscle. *Clin. Sci.* 20:1, 1961.

Miller, R. B., Tyson, I., and Relman, A. S. pH of isolated resting skeletal muscle and its relation to potassium content. *Am. J. Physiol.* 204:1048, 1963.

Mudge, G. H., and Hardin, B. Response to mercurial diuretics during alkalosis: A comparison of acute metabolic and chronic hypokalemic alkalosis in the dog. *J. Clin. Invest.* 35:155, 1956.

Orloff, J., Kennedy, T. J., Jr., and Berliner, R. W. The effect of potassium in nephrectomized rats with hypokalemic alkalosis. *J. Clin. Invest.* 32:538, 1953.

Tobin, R. B. Plasma, extracellular and muscle electrolyte responses to acute metabolic acidosis. *Am. J. Physiol.* 186:131, 1956.

K^+ Deficiency

Abrams, W. B., Lewis, D. W., and Bellet, S. The effect of acidosis and alkalosis on the plasma potassium concentration and the electrocardiogram of normal and potassium depleted dogs. *Am. J. Med. Sci.* 222:506, 1951.

Bartter, F. C., Pronove, P., Gill, J. R., Jr., and MacCardle, R. C. Hyperplasia of the juxtaglomerular complex with hyperaldosteronism and hypokalemic alkalosis. A new syndrome. *Am. J. Med.* 33:811, 1962.

Bleich, H. L., Tannen, R. L., and Schwartz, W. B. The induction of metabolic alkalosis by correction of potassium deficiency. *J. Clin. Invest.* 45:573, 1966.

Cannon, P. J., Leeming, J. M., Sommers, S. C., Winters, R. W., and Laragh, J. H. Juxtaglomerular cell hyperplasia and secondary hyperaldosteronism (Bartter's syndrome): A re-evaluation of the pathophysiology. *Medicine* (Baltimore) 47:107, 1968.

Clementsen, H. J. Potassium therapy. A break with tradition. *Lancet* 2:175, 1962.

Conn, J. W. Presidential address, part II. Primary aldosteronism, a new clinical syndrome. *J. Lab. Clin. Med.* 45:3, 1955.

Cort, J. H., and Matthews, H. L. Potassium deficiency in congestive heart failure: Three cases with hyponatraemia, including results of potassium replacement in one case. *Lancet* 1:1202, 1954.

Darrow, D. C. The retention of electrolyte during recovery from severe dehydration due to diarrhea. *J. Pediatr.* 28:515, 1946.

Davidson, C., Burkinshaw, L., McLachlan, M. S. F., and Morgan, D. B. Effect of long-term diuretic treatment on body-potassium in heart-disease. *Lancet* 2:1044, 1976.

de Deuxchaines, C. N., Collet, R. A., Busset, R., and Mach, R. S. Exchangeable potassium in wasting, amyotrophy, heart-disease, and cirrhosis of the liver. *Lancet* 1:681, 1961.

Heppel, L. A. Electrolytes of muscle and liver in potassium-depleted rats. *Am. J. Physiol.* 127:385, 1939.

Holler, J. W. Potassium deficiency occurring during treatment of diabetic acidosis. *J. A. M. A.* 131:1186, 1946.

Klein, R. Periodic Paralysis. In L. I. Gardner (ed.), *Endocrine and Genetic Diseases of Childhood and Adolescence* (2nd ed.). Philadelphia: Saunders, 1975.

Leaf, A., and Santos, R. F. Physiologic mechanisms in potassium deficiency. *N. Engl. J. Med.* 264:335, 1961.

Lown, B., and Levine, H. D. *Atrial Arrhythmias, Digitalis and Potassium.* New York: Landsberger Medical Books, 1958.

Mahler, R. F., and Stanbury, S. W. Potassium-losing renal disease: Renal and metabolic observations on a patient sustaining renal wastage of potassium. *Q. J. Med.* 25:21, 1956.

Moore, F. D., Boling, E. A., Ditmore, H. B., Jr., Sicular, A., Teterick, J. E., Ellison, A. E., Hoye, S. J., and Ball, M. R. Body sodium and potassium. V. The relationship of alkalosis, potassium deficiency and surgical stress to acute hypokalemia in man. *Metabolism* 4:379, 1955.

Read, A. E., Haslam, R. M., Laidlaw, J., and Sherlock, S. Chlorothiazide in control of ascites in hepatic cirrhosis. *Br. Med. J.* 1:963, 1958.

Relman, A. S., and Schwartz, W. B. The effect of DOCA on electrolyte balance in normal man and its relation to sodium chloride intake. *Yale J. Biol. Med.* 24:540, 1952.

Relman, A. S., and Schwartz, W. B. Nephropathy of potassium depletion: Clinical and pathological entity. *N. Engl. J. Med.* 255:195, 1956.

Schwartz, W. B., Levine, H. D., and Relman, A. S. The electrocardiogram in potassium depletion. Its relation to the total potassium deficit and the serum concentration. *Am. J. Med.* 16:395, 1954.

Schwartz, W. B., and Relman, A. S. Metabolic and renal studies in chronic potassium depletion resulting from overuse of laxatives. *J. Clin. Invest.* 32:258, 1953.

Seftel, H. C., and Keu, M. C. Early and intensive potassium replacement in diabetic acidosis. *Diabetes* 15:694, 1966.

Slater, J. D. H., and Nabarro, J. D. N. Clinical experience with chlorothiazide. *Lancet* 1:124, 1958.

Surawicz, B. Relationship between electrocardiogram and electrolytes. *Am. Heart J.* 73:814, 1967.

Talbott, J. H. Periodic paralysis. A clinical syndrome. *Medicine* (Baltimore) 20:85, 1941.

Tannen, R. L. The effect of uncomplicated potassium depletion on urine acidification. *J. Clin. Invest.* 49:813, 1970.

Walker, W. G., Sapir, D. G., Turin, M., and Cheng, J. T. Potassium Homeostasis and Diuretic Therapy. In A. F. Lant and G. M. Wilson (eds.), *Modern Diuretic Therapy in the Treatment of Cardiovascular and Renal Disease.* Amsterdam: Excerpta Medica Foundation, 1973.

Welt, L. G., Hollander, W., Jr., and Blythe, W. B. The consequences of potassium depletion. *J. Chronic Dis.* 11:213, 1960.

Wolff, H. P., Vecsei, P., Krück, F., Roscher, S., Brown, J. J., Düsterdieck, G. O., Lever, A. F., and Robertson, J. I. S. Psychiatric disturbance leading to potassium depletion, sodium depletion, raised plasma-renin concentration, and secondary hyperaldosteronism. *Lancet* 1:257, 1968.

Zierler, K. L., and Andres, R. Movement of potassium into skeletal muscle during spontaneous attack in family periodic paralysis. *J. Clin. Invest.* 36:730, 1957.

Hyperkalemia

Abrams, W. B., Lewis, D. W., and Bellet, S. The effect of acidosis and alkalosis on the plasma potassium concentration and the electrocardiogram of normal and potassium depleted dogs. *Am. J. Med. Sci.* 222:506, 1951.

Bull, G. M., Carter, A. B., and Lowe, K. G. Hyperpotassaemic paralysis. *Lancet* 2:60, 1953.

Drescher, A. N., Talbot, N. B., Meara, P. A., Terry, M., and Crawford, J. D. A study of the effects of excessive potassium intake upon body potassium stores. *J. Clin. Invest.* 37:1316, 1958.

Franklin, S. S., and Maxwell, M. H. Acute Renal Failure. In M. H. Maxwell and C. R. Kleeman (eds.), *Clinical Disorders of Fluid and Electrolyte Metabolism* (2nd ed.). New York: McGraw-Hill, 1972.

Herman, R. H., and McDowell, M. K. Hyperkalemic paralysis (adynamia episodica hereditaria). *Am. J. Med.* 35:749, 1963.

van't Hoff, W. Familial myotonic periodic paralysis. *Q. J. Med.* 31:385, 1962.

Kaplan, N. M. Hyperkalemia and renin deficiency. *N. Engl. J. Med.* 287:611, 1972.

Levinsky, N. G. Management of emergencies — hyperkalemia. *N. Engl. J. Med.* 274:1076, 1966.

Merrill, J. P. Acute Renal Failure. In M. B. Strauss and L. G. Welt (eds.), *Diseases of the Kidney* (2nd ed.). Boston: Little, Brown, 1971.

Posner, J. B., and Jacobs, D. R. Isolated analdosteronism: I. Clinical entity, with manifestations of persistent hyperkalemia, periodic paralysis, salt-losing tendency, and acidosis. *Metabolism* 13:513, 1964.

Schambelan, M., Stockigt, J. R., and Biglieri, E. G. Isolated hypoaldosteronism in adults. A renin-deficiency syndrome. *N. Engl. J. Med.* 287:573, 1972.

Surawicz, B. Relationship between electrocardiogram and electrolytes. *Am. Heart J.* 73:814, 1967.

Surawicz, B., and Gettes, L. S. Two mechanisms of cardiac arrest produced by potassium. *Circ. Res.* 12:415, 1963.

Tannen, R. L., Wedell, E., and Moore, R. Renal adaptation to a high potassium intake. The role of hydrogen ion. *J. Clin. Invest.* 52:2089, 1973.

Wang, P., and Clausen, T. Treatment of attacks in hyperkalaemic familial periodic paralysis by inhalation of salbutamol. *Lancet* 1:221, 1976.

5 : Disorders of H^+ Balance: Useful Tools

Analyzing Clinical Problems

The key to understanding disorders of H^+ balance is to comprehend the interrelationship among three variables in arterial plasma: the concentration of hydrogen ions, $[H^+]$; the partial pressure of carbon dioxide, P_{CO_2}; and the concentration of bicarbonate, $[HCO_3^-]$. This relationship may be given by one form of the Henderson equation,

$$[H^+] = K' \frac{P_{CO_2}}{[HCO_3^-]} \tag{5-1}$$

or it may be expressed as one version of the Henderson-Hasselbalch equation:

$$pH = pK' + \log \frac{[HCO_3^-]}{0.03 P_{CO_2}} \tag{5-2}$$

The derivation of these equations and their usefulness in assessing normal buffering and H^+ balance are discussed in a number of standard texts. I will assume that these concepts, as well as the fundamentals of the renal regulation of H^+ balance, have been mastered and that in this and the following chapter we can therefore proceed directly to applying the basic principles of H^+ balance in health to analyses of H^+ imbalance in disease.

Diagrams and Other Aids

Over the years, numerous aids have been proposed, all designed to help the physician understand problems of H^+ imbalance. Such aids include various diagrams of the Henderson-Hasselbalch equation that yield a designation of the patient's acid-base disturbance (e.g., metabolic acidosis, mixed respiratory alkalosis and metabolic alkalosis, and so on); terms such as "standard bicarbonate," "buffer base," "base excess"; and many others. Although of undoubted utility, these aids have serious shortcomings: (1) All are merely graphical depictions or logical extensions of the Henderson or Henderson-Hasselbalch relationships.

None, therefore, adds a new concept; in fact, the use of the aids *without full understanding* of the above relationships may obscure the dynamics of acid-base disorders. (2) Use of the aids, especially in inexperienced hands, tends to underplay the importance of the history and physical examination of the patient. These two sources of information – especially the history – can lead to the correct diagnosis in the great majority of patients, not only with disorders of H^+ balance but with many other diseases as well. In many instances, laboratory tests should serve mainly to confirm and quantify diagnostic impressions based on the history and physical examination. (3) The "automatic" use of the aids, without concurrent and independent analysis, permits handling of problems in H^+ balance without necessarily understanding the mechanisms involved; such usage may therefore lead to the wrong diagnosis and hence to incorrect treatment. (4) Many of the aids pass through periods of popularity and then fall out of vogue; furthermore, different institutions use different aids. It would therefore be confusing, as well as wasteful of space and time, to describe the several systems that are currently in favor. For all these reasons, I shall not invoke these aids in the body of this chapter.

pH Versus [H⁺]

In recent years a number of experts have advocated the substitution of the hydrogen ion concentration, $[H^+]$, for pH in the handling of patients with disorders of H^+ balance. Some of the major arguments for this view are as follows: (1) It is difficult to handle logarithms, let alone negative logarithms, without the use of log tables or slide rules, which are cumbersome tools at the bedside. (2) Concentrations of all substances in clinical medicine, *except* H^+, are expressed as quantities per unit volume, such as milligrams or milliequivalents per liter. (3) In analyzing the movement of substances across membranes, we commonly consider concentration differences or gradients, which are not immediately apparent from a difference in pH. (4) Because the pH scale is logarithmic, an equal change in pH may reflect unequal changes in H^+ concentration; thus a change in pH from 7.0 to 7.1 represents a change in $[H^+]$ from about 100 to 79 nanoequivalents (nEq) per liter, whereas a change in pH from 7.3 to 7.4 represents only one-half as great a change in $[H^+]$, namely, from 50 to 40 nEq per liter.

Perhaps equally compelling arguments are marshalled by those who advocate the continued use of pH. (1) Unlike that of most other substances in clinical medicine, the concentration of H^+ cannot be measured directly, but is in fact estimated by determining the pH. (2) The modern laboratory now routinely measures or derives – and reports – all three variables of the

Henderson equation (Eq. 5-1) or the Henderson-Hasselbalch equation (Eq. 5-2); this practice eliminates the need for computations involving logarithms at the bedside. (3) Like that of other substances, the biological activity of H^+ is a function of its chemical potential, which is much more closely related to the logarithm of the $[H^+]$ than to the $[H^+]$ itself; therefore, equal changes in pH may more nearly reflect equivalent physiological effects of H^+ than would equal changes in $[H^+]$.

The chemistry of acids and bases continues to be taught with the use of pH. I employed this terminology in my first book, *Renal Function,* when describing H^+ balance in health, and students and physicians still reflexly equate a low pH with acidosis and a high pH with alkalosis. Therefore, I shall utilize the Henderson-Hasselbalch equation in the body of this chapter. For the sake of completeness and illustration, though, the $[H^+]$ corresponding to a given pH is often mentioned.

Useful Tools

In current laboratory practice, disorders of H^+ balance are analyzed by determining the pH and P_{CO_2} of an arterial blood sample, which is obtained anaerobically. In most instances, these two values are then plotted on some diagram or nomogram of the Henderson-Hasselbalch equation (see the appendix at the end of this chapter), so that the value of $[HCO_3^-]$ that satisfies this equation (Eq. 5-2) can be read off or estimated. Many of the diagrams also incorporate a scale for $[H^+]$ so that it, too, can be derived from the two measured values. Finally, the complete analysis usually includes a determination of the arterial P_{O_2} and hematocrit (Hct), because these variables influence the buffering characteristics of blood and because they provide further information about the respiratory system, which plays such an important role, primarily or secondarily, in H^+ balance.

As stated earlier, an automatic use of the diagrams without full understanding of the dynamics of H^+ balance can lead to misinterpretations and incorrect therapy. Many experts in this field therefore prefer to work with the few primary data that the laboratory supplies and individualize the management of the patient. Such individualized analysis, which is facilitated by the four "tools" described below, not only tends to assure full understanding of the problem but also offers the further advantage of providing an independent check on the accuracy of the laboratory reports (see Problem 5-2).

Conversion of pH to $[H^+]$

Table 5-1 lists the pH for arterial plasma over the range that may be encountered in clinical practice. The intervals given are 0.10 unit, except within and near the normal range, where they are

Table 5-1
True and estimated values for hydrogen ion concentration, $[H^+]$, over the range of arterial plasma pH seen in patients

pH	$[H^+]$ (nMoles/L) True	$[H^+]$ (nMoles/L) Estimated*	
6.80	159	100	Too inaccurate to be useful
6.90	126	90	
7.00	100	80	
7.10	79	70	
7.20	63	60	
7.30	50	50	
7.35	45	45	
7.36	44	44	
7.37	43	43	
7.38	42	42	
7.39	41	41	
7.40	40	40	
7.41	39	39	
7.42	38	38	
7.43	37	37	
7.44	36	36	
7.45	35	35	
7.50	32	30	
7.60	25	20	Too inaccurate to be useful
7.70	20	10	
7.80	16	0	

*See text for arithmetical method of estimation.

listed for every 0.01 unit. The "true" values for the corresponding $[H^+]$ were calculated as shown in the example below.

If the activity coefficient for H^+ in plasma is assumed to be unity — which is a very close approximation, since the $[H^+]$ in plasma is extremely low — then, by definition,

$$pH = -\log [H^+]$$

For the normal pH of 7.40,

$$-\log [H^+] = 7.40$$

Therefore,

$$\log [H^+] = -7.40$$

$$= 0.60 - 8.00$$

The antilogarithm of 0.60 = 3.981, and the antilogarithm of -8.00 = 10^{-8}. Thus,

$$[H^+] = 3.981 \times 10^{-8}$$
$$= 39.81 \times 10^{-9}\ Eq/L$$
$$= 39.8 \text{ or } 40\ nEq/L$$

Note the very small units used for $[H^+]$ – nanoequivalents or nanomoles per liter (10^{-9}molar) – as compared to other substances in plasma (e.g., HCO_3^-), which have concentrations in the order of milliequivalents per liter (10^{-3}molar).

Within a rather broad range of pH, the $[H^+]$ can be estimated arithmetically; not only does this obviate the somewhat complicated logarithmic calculations, but, when the rule of thumb given below is used, the estimation requires virtually no computation whatsoever. The estimation is based on two fortuitous relationships: (1) the last two digits of a normal plasma pH of 7.40 – namely, 40 – are the same as a normal $[H^+]$ of 40 nMoles per liter and (2) one can estimate the $[H^+]$ by adding or subtracting 1 nMole per liter for every change in pH of 0.01 unit. Thus, the $[H^+]$ corresponding to a pH of 7.36 can be estimated by adding 4 nMoles per liter to the normal concentration of 40 nMoles per liter. Similarly, in alkalosis, when a pH of 7.50 is given, the $[H^+]$ can be estimated by subtracting 10 nMoles per liter from the normal value of 40 nMoles per liter.

It is clear from inspection of Table 5-1 that the estimates are quite close to the true values between pH 7.10 and 7.50, the errors amounting to 11 and 6 percent, respectively, at these two limits of pH. Below pH 7.10 and above pH 7.50, the estimates are too inaccurate to be useful. In practice, this is not a serious shortcoming, because values do not often fall outside this range. When they do, the physician has the choice of calculating the true $[H^+]$ or looking it up in a reference, such as Table 5-1 or the appendix at the end of this chapter.

Estimation of $[HCO_3^-]$

Estimation of the bicarbonate concentration, $[HCO_3^-]$, from the two values that the laboratory supplies – namely, pH and P_{CO_2} – is often useful for several reasons. (1) It supplies a check on the accuracy of the value for $[HCO_3^-]$ that the laboratory reports, whether the value is derived from the pH and P_{CO_2} or from an independent measurement of total CO_2 on venous blood. (Such checks should not be construed as distrust or disdain for the laboratory; they simply recognize the possibility of human error and emphasize the importance of not treating a patient merely on the basis of a laboratory report.) (2) It permits assessment of the patient's status with respect to the "confidence bands" (see below). (3) It enables calculation of the anion gap (see below), even when a value for $[HCO_3^-]$ has not been given.

The estimate for $[HCO_3^-]$ is based on the Henderson equation (Eq. 5-1), which may be rewritten as

$$[HCO_3^-] = K' \frac{P_{CO_2}}{[H^+]}$$

If $[HCO_3^-]$ is expressed in mMoles per liter, P_{CO_2} in mm Hg, and $[H^+]$ in nMoles per liter, then K' has a value of 23.9; for the sake of simplicity, a value of 25 may be substituted for 23.9. The equation for the estimate is then

$$[HCO_3^-] = 25 \frac{P_{CO_2}}{[H^+]} \qquad (5\text{-}3)$$

For normal arterial plasma – that is, when pH = 7.40 and P_{CO_2} = 40 mm Hg – the method of estimation is as follows. The $[H^+]$ at pH 7.40 is approximated as 40 nMoles per liter (see previous section and Table 5-1). Then,

$$[HCO_3^-] = 25 \frac{40}{40} = 25 \text{ mMoles per liter}$$

This estimate obviously deviates by only 4 percent from the true value of 24 mMoles per liter that satisfies the Henderson-Hasselbalch equation (Eq. 5-2). (By somewhat circular reasoning, this example also shows that it is easy to recall the value of the constant K' by substituting estimates of the normal values for the three variables: $[HCO_3^-]$ = 25, P_{CO_2} = 40, and $[H^+]$ = 40. From Equation 5-3, then, 25 = $K' \times 40/40$.)

In Table 5-2, estimates for $[HCO_3^-]$ in examples of each of the four major acid-base disturbances are compared against the true value of $[HCO_3^-]$ calculated from the Henderson-Hasselbalch equation. The sample computation for the first disturbance listed in Table 5-2 (metabolic alkalosis) is as follows:

1. The pH of 7.55 is converted to $[H^+]$. According to Table 5-1, this pH falls near the range where the usual estimate (40 nMoles/L - 15 nMoles/L) becomes inaccurate. An estimate can be reached by interpolation of the true values listed in Table 5-1, yielding a value of about 28 nMoles per liter.

Table 5-2
True and estimated values for bicarbonate concentration, $[HCO_3^-]$, in four representative disturbances of H^+ balance

Type of Disturbance	Representative Cause of Disturbance	Arterial Plasma: Measured pH	Measured P_{CO_2} (mm Hg)	$[HCO_3^-]$ (mMoles/L) True	$[HCO_3^-]$ (mMoles/L) Estimated*
Metabolic alkalosis	Prolonged vomiting	7.55	44	37.2	39.3
Metabolic acidosis	Chronic renal failure	7.28	32	14.5	15.4
Respiratory alkalosis	Psychogenic hyperventilation	7.48	30	21.6	23.4
Respiratory acidosis	Heroin poisoning	7.10	90	27.0	32.1

*See text for method of estimation.

2. The $[HCO_3^-]$ is then *approximated* using Equation 5-3:

$$[HCO_3^-] = 25\,\frac{P_{CO_2}}{[H^+]}$$

$$= 25\,\frac{44}{28}$$

$$= 39.3 \text{ mMoles/L estimated value}$$

3. The *true* $[HCO_3^-]$ is calculated using the Henderson-Hasselbalch equation (Eq. 5-2) and a pK' of 6.1:

$$pH = 6.1 + \log\frac{[HCO_3^-]}{0.03P_{CO_2}}$$

$$7.55 = 6.1 + \log\frac{[HCO_3^-]}{0.03 \times 44}$$

$$\log\frac{[HCO_3^-]}{1.32} = 1.45$$

$$\frac{[HCO_3^-]}{1.32} = \text{antilog}\,1.45$$

$$= 28.18$$

$$[HCO_3^-] = 28.18 \times 1.32$$

$$= 37.2 \text{ mMoles/L true value}$$

Note that even after using a number of approximations to obtain the estimated [HCO_3^-] of 39.3 mMoles per liter, this estimate differs from the true value by only 6 percent, which is a tolerable discrepancy in the analysis and management of clinical problems.

Confidence Bands

The four *primary disturbances* of H^+ balance are (1) respiratory acidosis, (2) respiratory alkalosis, (3) metabolic acidosis, and (4) metabolic alkalosis. In most instances, these primary disturbances are accompanied by *compensatory responses* that shift the pH toward, but not to, the normal value. A compensatory response involves the system opposite to the one that caused the primary disturbance; thus (1) respiratory acidosis elicits a metabolic response that increases the renal excretion of H^+ and increases the renal reabsorption of HCO_3^-, (2) respiratory alkalosis is usually accompanied by the opposite changes in the renal handling of H^+ and HCO_3^-, (3) metabolic acidosis is compensated for by alveolar hyperventilation, and (4) metabolic alkalosis is often but not invariably accompanied by a respiratory compensation that decreases alveolar ventilation.

Not infrequently, two or more primary disturbances coincide in the same individual; the patient is then said to have a *mixed disturbance* of H^+ balance. For example, a patient may have alveolar hypoventilation from emphysema and protracted vomiting from an obstructed duodenal ulcer; this patient would have a mixed disturbance of respiratory acidosis and metabolic alkalosis. Another patient with emphysema might also have diabetes mellitus that has led to renal failure; if the diabetes mellitus is out of control, this patient might have a mixed disturbance of respiratory acidosis due to emphysema, metabolic acidosis due to uncontrolled diabetes mellitus, plus metabolic acidosis due to renal failure.

The confidence bands (Figs. 5-1 and 5-2) serve two purposes: (1) to distinguish an acute from a chronic respiratory disturbance and (2) to help a physician decide whether a patient probably has a single primary disturbance with a compensatory response or whether the problem is more likely a mixed disorder. Although the confidence bands often cannot, by themselves, decide these issues, they are usually of considerable help, as in the following examples.

1. An arterial blood sample from a patient with emphysema shows a pH of 7.33 and a P_{CO_2} of 68 mm Hg. According to the Henderson-Hasselbalch equation (Eq. 5-2), the [HCO_3^-] in this sample must have been 34 mMoles per liter; alternatively (see the two previous sections or the appendix at the end of this chapter), one can estimate the [H^+] from the pH as being 47 nMoles per

liter and then approximate the $[HCO_3^-]$ as 25 $Pco_2/[H^+]$, or 36.2 mMoles per liter. At least two mechanisms account for this abnormal elevation of HCO_3^-: (a) the hydration of the retained CO_2 and subsequent interaction of H^+ with nonbicarbonate buffers, Buf^-;

$$\begin{array}{c} CO_2 + H_2O \rightleftharpoons H_2CO_3 \rightleftharpoons H^+ + HCO_3^- \\ \qquad\qquad\qquad\qquad + \\ \qquad\qquad\qquad\qquad Buf^- \\ \qquad\qquad\qquad\qquad \updownarrow \\ \qquad\qquad\qquad\qquad H\text{—}Buf \end{array} \qquad (5\text{-}4)$$

and (b) the metabolic compensation for a respiratory acidosis, in which the kidneys excrete more than the normal amount of H^+ and reabsorb more HCO_3^-. The question that the physician needs to answer is whether in a *chronic* primary respiratory disturbance that raises the Pco_2 to 68 mm Hg the above two mechanisms *usually* raise the $[HCO_3^-]$ to about 36 mMoles per liter. Figure 5-1b answers this question affirmatively. The point corresponding to a Pco_2 of 68 mm Hg and a $[HCO_3^-]$ of 36 mMoles per liter falls within the confidence band of chronic (but not of acute) primary respiratory acidosis; the same is true of the point corresponding to a Pco_2 of 68 mm Hg and a pH of 7.33 or a $[H^+]$ of 47 nMoles per liter (Fig. 5-1a). The meaning of the points falling within the confidence bands is that in uncomplicated *chronic* respiratory acidosis, when just the two mechanisms cited above elevate the $[HCO_3^-]$, 95 percent of the values for $[HCO_3^-]$, $[H^+]$, and pH will fall within the span outlined by the band (see Construction of Confidence Bands). Thus, if the patient's history is one of chronic emphysema uncomplicated by other chronic or acute processes, the fact that the points fall within the confidence bands strengthens the physician's impression that he is dealing with the single, primary acid-base disturbance of chronic respiratory acidosis.

2. Suppose that an arterial blood sample from another patient with emphysema also shows the Pco_2 to be elevated to 68 mm Hg but that in this patient, the pH of the same sample is 7.44. By estimation, the $[H^+]$ of this sample would be 36 nMoles per liter (40 nMoles per liter minus 4 nMoles per liter; see also Table 5-1), and the $[HCO_3^-]$ would be 47 mMoles per liter ($25 \times 68/36$). Locating these values on Figure 5-1b shows that they fall outside of the confidence bands for either acute or chronic primary respiratory disturbances. This finding suggests to the physician that he may be dealing either with a laboratory error or with a mixed disturbance. He can best decide between these alternatives *on the basis of the patient's history.* The patient in question was in fact

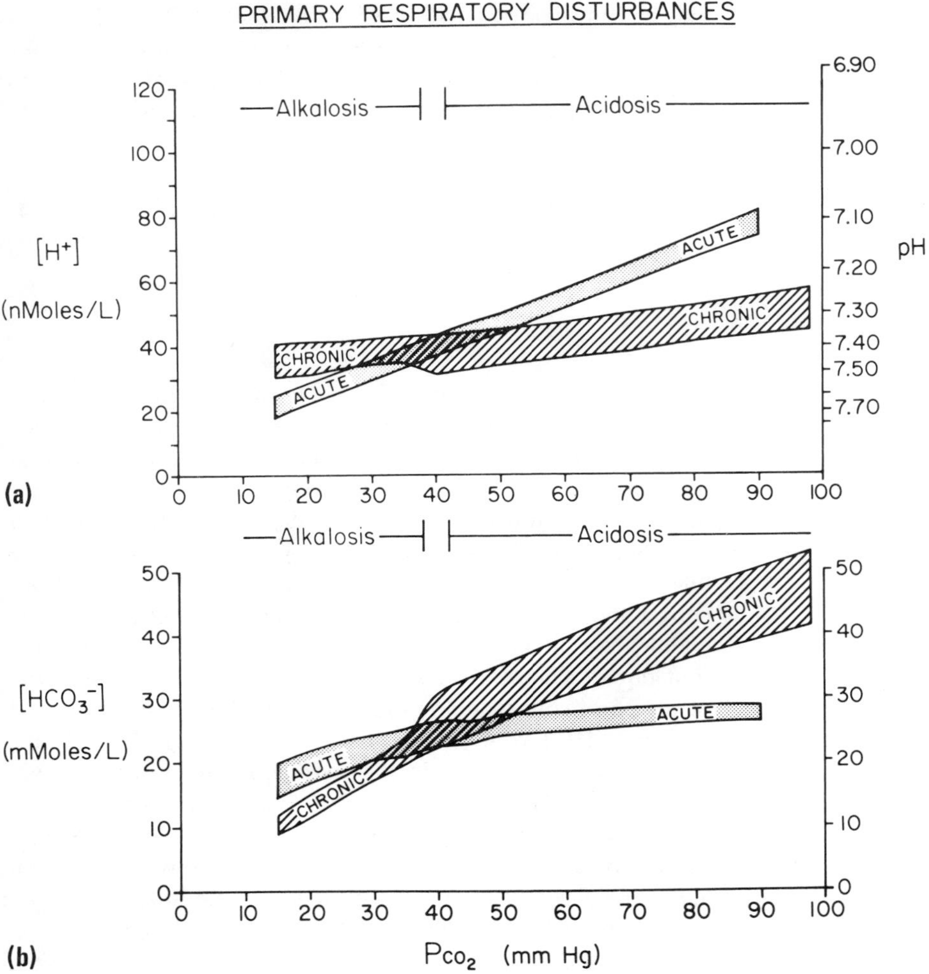

Figure 5-1
The 95% confidence bands for acute and chronic primary respiratory alkalosis and acidosis. *Alkalosis* is here defined as any primary respiratory disturbance in which the arterial P_{CO_2} is less than 38 mm Hg, even though the range of the confidence band may extend to a pH that is usually considered acidotic. Similarly, *acidosis* is here defined as any primary respiratory disturbance in which the arterial P_{CO_2} is greater than 42 mm Hg. Data for acute disturbances were taken from N. C. Brackett, Jr., et al., *N. Engl. J. Med.* 272:6, 1965, and G. S. Arbus et al., *N. Engl. J. Med.* 280:117, 1969; those for chronic disturbances from N. C. Brackett, Jr., et al., *N. Engl. J. Med.* 280:124, 1969, and F. J. Gennari et al., *J. Clin. Invest.* 51:1722, 1972 (slightly adapted from dog to man).

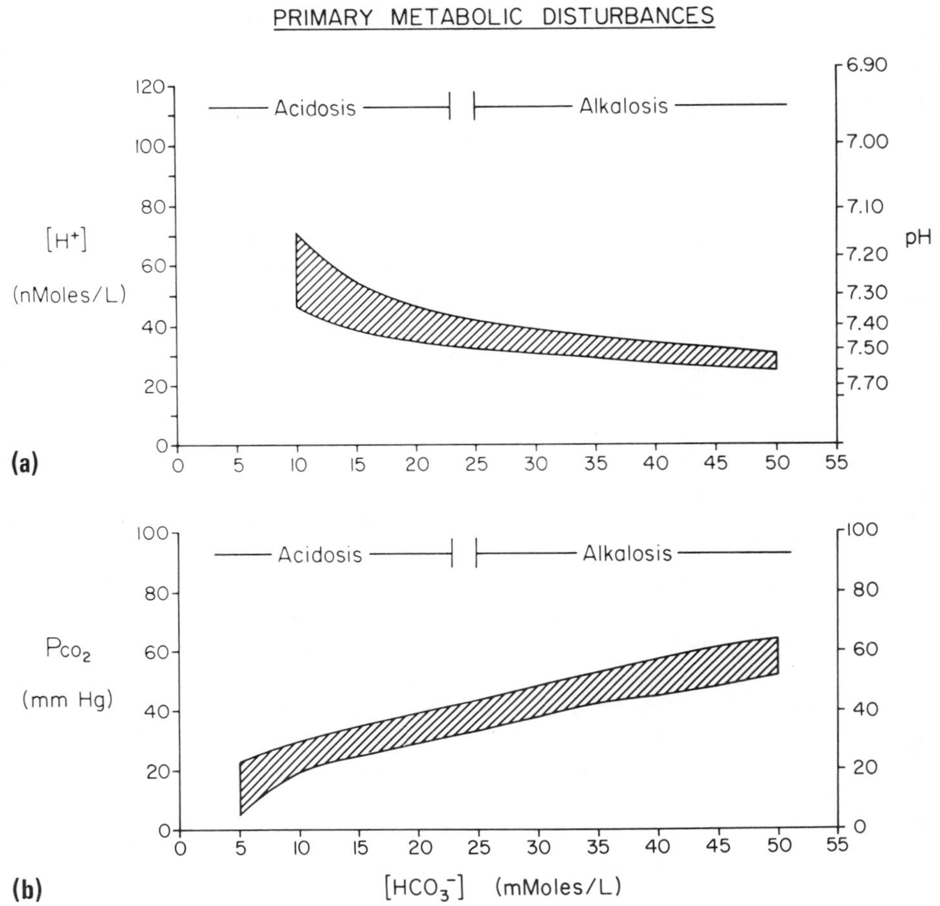

PRIMARY METABOLIC DISTURBANCES

Figure 5-2

The 95% confidence bands for chronic metabolic acidosis and alkalosis. *Acidosis* is here defined as any primary metabolic disturbance in which the arterial $[HCO_3^-]$ is less than 23 mMoles per liter, even though the range of the confidence band may extend to a pH that is usually considered alkalotic. Similarly, *alkalosis* is here defined as any primary metabolic disturbance in which the arterial $[HCO_3^-]$ is greater than 25 mMoles per liter. Data from R. W. Winters (ed.), *The Body Fluids in Pediatrics.* Boston: Little, Brown, 1973; C. van Ypersele de Strihou and A. Frans, *Clin. Sci. Mol. Med.* 45:439, 1973; J. M. Bone et al., *Clin. Sci. Mol. Med.* 46:113, 1974.

admitted to the hospital not because of the chronic emphysema, but because she had a peptic ulcer that had caused her to vomit for three days. Because the predominant change in H^+ balance during vomiting is due to the loss of HCl (Table 1-4), the physician knew that he might be dealing with a mixed disturbance of metabolic alkalosis and respiratory acidosis. The latter disturbance tends to elevate the $[HCO_3^-]$ by the two mechanisms listed in example (1) above; vomiting elevates the $[HCO_3^-]$ by mechanisms described in Chapter 6 (see under Metabolic Alkalosis). The prediction in this patient is therefore that the $[HCO_3^-]$ should be elevated out of proportion to the P_{CO_2} of 68 mm Hg. This prediction is indeed fulfilled, as is reflected by the fact that the point corresponding to the arterial blood values falls outside of the confidence band for chronic respiratory acidosis. Reasoning another way, the physician knew before the arterial sample was drawn that he was probably dealing with a mixed disturbance of alkalosis and acidosis. Whether the arterial pH would be more alkaline than normal or more acid would depend on which of the primary disturbances predominated; in any case, however, it could be predicted that the pH would be more alkaline than that which is seen in 95 percent of patients with uncomplicated chronic emphysema and a P_{CO_2} of 68 mm Hg. This prediction is also fulfilled, as is shown by inspection of Figure 5-1a (and as indeed it must be, since the confidence bands in Figure 5-1a and those in Figure 5-1b portray the same data and are based on the Henderson-Hasselbalch equation; see also Problem 5-2).

3. In the case of a mixed disturbance that has a metabolic component, the confidence bands of Figure 5-2 can be used to answer analogous questions. (In contrast to Figure 5-1, $[HCO_3^-]$ is plotted on the abscissa in Figure 5-2 instead of P_{CO_2}, because in primary metabolic disturbances, $[HCO_3^-]$ is the independent variable.) Again consider the patient cited in example (2) above, who demonstrated emphysema, peptic ulceration, and vomiting and had arterial blood-sample values of pH = 7.44, P_{CO_2} = 68 mm Hg, and $[HCO_3^-]$ = 47 mMoles per liter. This patient was admitted to the hospital because of the ulcer and vomiting, not because of her emphysema. It might be expected, therefore, that attention would be focused on the metabolic alkalosis, in which there is a primary elevation of the $[HCO_3^-]$. This primary event often elicits a secondary, compensatory response of alveolar hypoventilation, and the question that the confidence bands help to answer is whether the elevation of P_{CO_2} is in the range *ordinarily* to be expected in uncomplicated, primary metabolic alkalosis. For the patient being considered, the P_{CO_2} of 68 mm Hg is higher than what occurs in 95 percent of patients or normal subjects in whom a primary metabolic alkalosis has caused the

$[HCO_3^-]$ to rise to 47 mMoles per liter. That is, the patient evidently has hypoventilated more than would be expected as a compensatory response to this degree of primary metabolic alkalosis, and the reason is that the patient has, in addition, a primary cause for alveolar hypoventilation, namely, chronic emphysema.

Note: The use and interpretation of the confidence bands is not always as straightforward as in the preceding three examples. W. B. Schwartz and his associates have rightly emphasized that while values that fall outside of the bands denote a mixed disturbance, *points falling within the bands do not necessarily reflect a single, uncomplicated, primary disturbance of H^+ balance.* The following, not uncommon clinical example will illustrate this point.

4. A middle-aged woman with chronic, obstructive pulmonary disease was admitted to the hospital with a high arterial Pco_2 of 67 mm Hg. It was decided to treat her with mechanical hyperventilation, a maneuver that can suddenly lower the Pco_2 without much altering the $[HCO_3^-]$, thereby producing acute alkalosis (Eq. 5-2); the latter effect often precipitates tetany and convulsions. In order to prevent this well-recognized complication, the patient was first given NH_4Cl, which adds HCl ($2NH_4Cl + CO_2 \rightarrow 2HCl + H_2O + CO(NH_2)_2$). She was then hyperventilated, and some hours later, an analysis of her arterial plasma revealed a pH of 7.42, $[H^+]$ of 38 nMoles per liter, Pco_2 of 30 mm Hg, and $[HCO_3^-]$ of 19 mMoles per liter. These values lie within the confidence bands for chronic disturbances in Figures 5-1 and 5-2. In this case, therefore, the "automatic" usage of the confidence bands might lead the physician to conclude that he is dealing *either* with uncomplicated chronic respiratory alkalosis *or* with uncomplicated chronic metabolic acidosis, when in fact the patient has a mixed disturbance of acute respiratory alkalosis and acute metabolic acidosis. This example emphasizes the point made earlier, namely, that automatic usage of aids or graphs can lead to erroneous conclusions and that *laboratory data should always be interpreted in light of the patient's history.*

Construction of Confidence Bands. The procedure will be described using primary respiratory acidosis as an example. In this disorder, the purpose of the confidence bands is to ascertain the range of pH, $[H^+]$, and $[HCO_3^-]$ that is seen in 95 percent of patients in whom the sole abnormality is an elevation of the Pco_2 to a given level. For example, the question asked may be: When the Pco_2 in a group of patients is raised to 60 mm Hg — and if these patients have no other disturbance of H^+ balance — what will be the range of pH, $[H^+]$, and $[HCO_3^-]$ in 95 percent of these patients? Most readers will recognize this range as being two standard deviations (S.D.) higher or lower than the mean pH, $[H^+]$, or $[HCO_3^-]$ at a Pco_2 of 60 mm Hg; or, stated differently, that any value falling outside of this range will have a *p* value of < 0.05.

The compensatory response to a primary respiratory acidosis is an increased excretion of H^+ and increased reabsorption of HCO_3^- by the kidneys. Some two to five days are required for this mechanism to restore the pH to the near-normal range. That is, although the denominator of the Henderson-Hasselbalch equation increases immediately with the onset of a respiratory acidosis and thus lowers the pH (Eq. 5-2), the compensatory increase of the numerator, $[HCO_3^-]$, takes days to materialize. It is for this reason that the confidence band for *acute* respiratory acidosis has a different slope from the one for the corresponding *chronic* disturbance. If the respiratory center is depressed for a few hours or for a day or two (e.g., as in a suicidal attempt with a barbiturate), then the pH at a Pco_2 of, say, 70 mm Hg will be lower than if the Pco_2 has been raised to this level by chronic obstructive lung disease, because in the first instance renal retention of HCO_3^- has barely set in, whereas in the chronic condition it has been maximized.

The confidence band for acute respiratory acidosis shown in Figure 5-1 was obtained by having normal human subjects breathe a gas mixture containing 7% and then 10% CO_2; oxygen was maintained at 21%, and the remainder of the mixture was made up of nitrogen. A new steady state (i.e., with stable values for the variables given on the ordinates of Figure 5-1) was reached within 10 minutes or less after exposure to the high CO_2 concentration. The data were obtained in normal subjects rather than patients, because one can then be certain that the only abnormality is respiratory acidosis, and because in patients it is often difficult to be sure that they are truly in the acute state. The bands for chronic respiratory acidosis were obtained on patients with alveolar hypoventilation due to various chronic disease processes, such as emphysema, bronchitis, and kyphoscoliosis. These patients were free of other diseases that could lead to primary disturbances in H^+ balance, and they were in the steady state as judged by a Pco_2 that varied by no more than ±4 mm Hg over a period of three days.

The reasoning is analogous for the construction of the confidence bands in respiratory alkalosis (Fig. 5-1). The data for the acute disturbance were obtained on anesthetized patients who for therapeutic reasons had to be mechanically hyperventilated during the course of the operation. As in acute hypercapnia, a new steady state of hypocapnia was attained in these patients within a few minutes after starting the hyperventilation. The data for the confidence bands in chronic respiratory alkalosis were obtained on dogs exposed to an atmosphere of 9% O_2 for one to two weeks. Dogs were used because they tolerate hypoxic breathing much better than humans. The data plotted in Figure 5-1 for chronic respiratory alkalosis were slightly modified, utilizing the small difference in normal acid-base values between dogs and humans.

The construction of confidence bands for primary metabolic disturbances is somewhat simpler in that a distinction need not be made between acute and chronic disturbances. This is because the compensatory response — the "second line of defense," or fast respiratory component — begins within minutes of the primary perturbation and is probably maximized within 6 to 8 hours. Consequently, the compensatory adjustment of the Pco_2 (Eq. 5-2), and hence the restoration of pH, is very rapid and does not require days, as does the compensatory adjustment of the $[HCO_3^-]$ in primary respiratory disturbances. One therefore rarely encounters a patient in whom the compensatory respiratory response is not yet fully developed, and the distinction in confidence bands between acute and chronic metabolic disturbances is seldom, if ever, of clinical importance.

The bands in Figure 5-2 are based on data from patients of all age groups who had primary metabolic disturbances due to various disease processes: renal failure, renal failure treated with alkali added to dialysis fluid, prolonged vomiting, excess intake of alkali, diarrhea, uncontrolled diabetes mellitus, and NH_4Cl ingestion.

Anion Gap

Definition. Figure 5-3 shows that most of the electrical charges on the major cation of plasma — namely, Na^+ — are neutralized by Cl^- and HCO_3^-. The remaining charges *on* Na^+, which amount to 10 to 16 mEq per liter, are covered by some of the negative charges on the other anions in plasma, namely, phosphate, sulfate, organic acids, and proteins. The sum of these charges is called the anion "gap" because they cover the gap of positive charges on Na^+ left, so to speak, by Cl^- and HCO_3^-. The *anion gap* is thus defined as the difference between $[Na^+]$ and the sum of $[Cl^-]$ and $[HCO_3^-]$, all expressed in mEq per liter; or,

$$\text{Anion gap} = [Na^+] - ([Cl^-] + [HCO_3^-]) \qquad (5\text{-}5)$$

If one considers the range of normal concentrations for Na^+, Cl^-, and HCO_3^- listed in Table 1-1, one can derive a *normal range for the anion gap of 10 to 16 mEq per liter.*

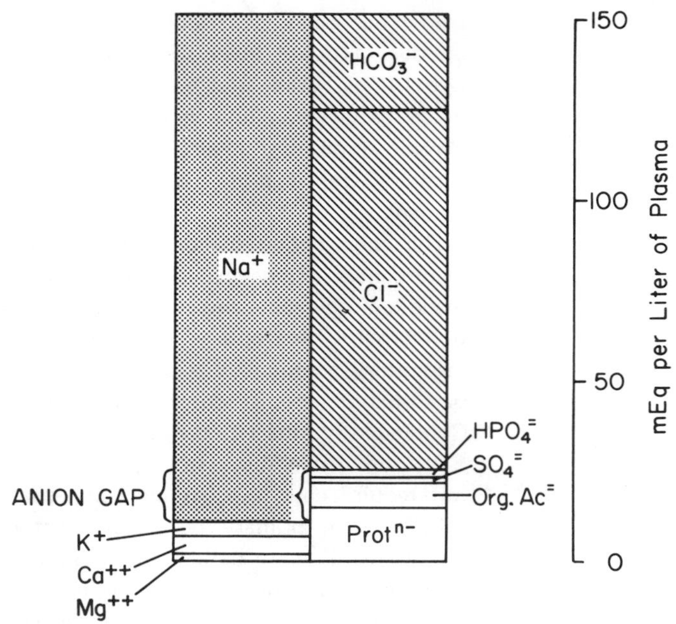

Figure 5-3
Anion gap for normal plasma.

The gap is sometimes referred to as the "sum of unmeasured anions" because phosphate, sulfate, organic acids, and proteins are not as *routinely* measured as are Cl^- and HCO_3^-. In fact, in modern clinical jargon, when a physician refers to "serum electrolytes," he means Na^+, K^+, Cl^-, and HCO_3^-, leaving out the other electrolytes in plasma (Fig. 5-3). Thus, although "sum of unmeasured anions" is a correct description insofar as these anions are often not measured, it is a misnomer because the anion gap does not refer to the total charges on these anions, but only to the equivalents that are required to neutralize the remaining charges on Na^+. Because K^+ is routinely measured as one of the four so-called serum electrolytes, some physicians calculate the anion gap as the difference between the sum of Na^+ and K^+ minus the sum of Cl^- and HCO_3^-. The distinction is arbitrary, and it causes a difference in the average value for the gap of only 3 to 4 mEq per liter. In this text, however, we shall use the definition that is given in equation 5-5.

Meaning of Anion Gap. Examples of the value of the anion gap in various diseases are listed in Table 5-3. *The major clinical usefulness of the anion gap lies in the differential diagnosis of metabolic acidosis;* this fact is reflected in Table 6-2.

An increased anion gap is seen in some forms of metabolic acidosis that are due, at least in part, to an accumulation of organic acids. Perhaps the prototype is uncontrolled diabetes mellitus, in which the plasma concentrations mainly of β-hydroxybutyric acid and acetoacetic acid are greatly increased. In the extracellular fluid, the H^+ from these organic acids is buffered mainly by HCO_3^-, the concentration of which is therefore markedly decreased (Table 5-3); Na^+, however, often remains at a normal concentration, as does Cl^-. It follows from Equation 5-5 that the anion gap must be increased, a point that can also be understood from Figure 5-3 if one visualizes that the major change in the plasma profile is an increase in organic acids at the expense of HCO_3^-.

Another example is spontaneous lactic acidosis, a condition in which the concentration of this organic acid, which is the main end product of anaerobic metabolism, may rise from its normal value of about 1 mEq per liter to 10 or 20 mEq per liter or higher. The extra H^+ is buffered by extracellular HCO_3^- as well as by intracellular buffers, and the result is often a severe acidosis. The cause of spontaneous lactic acidosis is not known; it is suspected that it involves tissue hypoxia, which causes cells to shift from aerobic to anaerobic metabolism. The concentration of lactic acid in plasma may also rise in a number of other conditions in which it may abet an acidosis while not necessarily being the major cause of it; such conditions include uncontrolled diabetes mellitus, treatment of diabetes mellitus with the oral hypoglycemic agent phenformin, renal failure, hepatic failure, septicemia, ethanol intoxication, leukemia, shock, severe exercise, some types of neonatal acidosis, and others. It may also be elevated in some forms of primary respiratory alkalosis (see below). Thus, an increased anion gap is rather frequently caused by a rise in lactate levels.

A more common, single cause of an elevated anion gap, however, is renal failure. In this condition, a number of anions, principally sulfate and phosphate, accumulate by the dynamics outlined in Figure 1-A (see Answers to Problems at the end of this text). The plasma concentration of some organic acids (e.g., uric acid) also rises. The H^+ that is associated with these anions is largely buffered by HCO_3^-, and renal failure is therefore usually accompanied by metabolic acidosis.

It should be emphasized that an increase in the anion gap is not necessarily attended by acidosis. For example, if a patient vomits for several days so that his food intake is nearly nil, then much of the daily supply of energy will be obtained from fat catabolism. This metabolic cycle is accompanied by the production of keto acids, which exist as anions that are not routinely measured. In uncontrolled diabetes mellitus, the accumulation of keto acids results in acidosis, but in prolonged vomiting, this effect is usually overshadowed by the alkalosis resulting from the large loss of

Table 5-3
Values for the anion gap in several disease states. Normal anion gap = 10 to 16 mEq/L

State	Arterial pH	Venous Plasma Concentration (mEq/L)			Anion Gap (mEq/L)	Comments
		Na^+	Cl^-	HCO_3^-		
Uncontrolled diabetes mellitus	7.10	140	100	5	35	Unmeasured anions are mainly β-hydroxybutyric acid and acetoacetic acid
Spontaneous lactic acidosis	7.10	137	87	10	40	Unmeasured anion is lactic acid, which in this patient was 26 mEq/L
Chronic renal failure	7.32	138	95	18	25	Unmeasured anions include organic acids, sulfate, and phosphate. (See Figure 1-A for the dynamics of phosphate retention in renal failure.)
Prolonged vomiting	7.58	146	75	40	31	Unmeasured anions are mainly keto acids produced during increased fat metabolism when the patient is not eating. (*Note:* An increased anion gap does not necessarily mean that the patient is acidotic.)
Psychogenic hyperventilation	7.58	142	102	21	19	The small increase in unmeasured anions represents phosphate and some lactate and pyruvate coming out of cells
Chronic hypoxic hyperventilation	7.38	139	107	16	16	This condition is accompanied by very slight accumulation of organic acids (e.g., lactic acid), which accounts for the anion gap being at the upper limit of normal
Ingestion of NH_4Cl	7.12	143	122	7	14	*Note:* Metabolic acidosis can occur without an increase in anion gap (for reaction, see text)

Diarrhea and other HCO_3^--losing states	7.32	148	116	20	12	(Same comment as above)
Chronic obstructive lung disease	7.38	142	90	38	14	Lactic acid is often — but not invariably — elevated in primary respiratory disturbances
Syndrome of inappropriate ADH secretion (SIADH)	7.41	125	89	22	14	All plasma solutes are diluted by H_2O retention; hence, there is no selective change in concentration of unmeasured anions
SIADH plus laboratory error	7.41	113	89	22	2	The concentration of unmeasured anions could not be reduced so drastically. Therefore, either the reported $[Na^+]$ is too low, or $[Cl^-]$ or $[HCO_3^-]$ too high

gastric HCl and other mechanisms (Table 1-4 and Chap. 6). Another alkalotic state that is often (but not invariably) associated with a slight rise in the anion gap is primary respiratory alkalosis, as occurs in psychogenic hyperventilation or chronic hypoxic hyperventilation (Table 5-3).

Conversely, acidosis is not necessarily accompanied by a rise in the anion gap. Ingestion of NH_4Cl causes a metabolic acidosis through the net addition of HCl. Most of the H^+ produced in this reaction is buffered by extracellular HCO_3^-, thereby reducing the $[HCO_3^-]$. But for every equivalent of HCO_3^- thus taken out of solution, an equivalent of Cl^- is added; hence, the anion gap does not change (Eq. 5-5 and Fig. 5-3). Further examples include diarrhea or loss of other gastrointestinal fluids with high concentrations of HCO_3^-, where again Cl^- "replaces" HCO_3^-. An analogous chain of events keeps the anion gap normal in uncomplicated respiratory acidosis, as in chronic obstructive lung disease when it is not accompanied by a rise in lactic acid levels. The CO_2 that is retained in this condition is hydrated as shown in Equation 5-4. The H^+ from carbonic acid has to be buffered almost exclusively within cells (i.e., by Buf^-), because the main extracellular buffer, HCO_3^-, cannot be used to neutralize this H^+. (This fact is apparent from Equation 5-4; the reaction would have to shift to the left if HCO_3^- were to buffer the H^+, but it is already being shifted to the right by the primary addition of CO_2.) The HCO_3^- that is produced in this reaction stays mainly within the extracellular space. According to Equation 5-5, this addition might be expected to reduce the anion gap; the reduction does not occur, however, because the rise in $[HCO_3^-]$ is accompanied by a reciprocal decrease in $[Cl^-]$ (Table 5-3). The reason for the reciprocity probably involves the prime importance of Na^+ balance; that is, Na^+ balance is usually maintained in uncomplicated chronic obstructive lung disease, the $[HCO_3^-]$ is perforce elevated, and the $[Cl^-]$ "adjusts" to balance the normal plasma concentration of Na^+.

Finally, calculation of the anion gap can be useful in analyzing problems of hyponatremia. In the syndrome of inappropriate ADH secretion (SIADH), for example, hyponatremia is due partly to excessive urinary loss of NaCl but mainly to a positive balance of H_2O (Fig. 2-5). In either case, the anion gap should remain unchanged, in the first instance because Cl^- is lost in roughly equal proportion with Na^+, and in the second instance because the retained H_2O will dilute Na^+, Cl^-, and HCO_3^- equally. Hence, the finding of a normal anion gap will confirm the genuine nature of the hyponatremia, whether it be due to SIADH or some other cause (see Table 3-3). Such confirmation is important because a laboratory error in a single determination is not that rare;

calculation of the anion gap can often detect such error (Table 5-3).

In summary, the anion gap is a useful adjunct in confirming diagnostic suspicions. To repeat a few examples: diabetic acidosis, lactic acidosis, and the acidosis of renal failure must be associated with an increased anion gap; the acidosis of NH_4Cl poisoning and of diarrhea and other bicarbonate-losing states will be accompanied by little if any change in the gap; and the true presence of hyponatremia should be confirmed by a quick calculation of the anion gap before treatment for this condition is begun.

Summary

The analysis of clinical problems of H^+ imbalance is based on the Henderson-Hasselbalch equation (Eq. 5-2). This fact often constitutes a serious stumbling block to the understanding and quantitative management of acid-base disorders, because many physicians are not conversant with the use of logarithms, and such use usually requires log tables or slide rules. In this chapter we first present two useful tools that permit utilization of the Henderson-Hasselbalch equation by means of arithmetic estimates: the conversion of pH to $[H^+]$ and vice versa and the estimation of the $[HCO_3^-]$ or P_{CO_2} (see Problem 5-1).

Two additional helpful tools were presented. One is the use of confidence bands, which help to distinguish chronic from acute respiratory disorders and which predict how much compensatory change in $[HCO_3^-]$ may be expected in pure respiratory disturbances (Fig. 5-1b) or how much compensatory change in P_{CO_2} should be anticipated in pure metabolic derangements (Fig. 5-2b). If a patient's laboratory values fall outside of the confidence bands, a mixed disturbance of H^+ imbalance is indicated; if, however, the values fall within the bands, this fact will not *necessarily* reflect an uncomplicated primary disturbance. The final tool that is discussed is the anion gap, which is calculated as the difference between the plasma $[Na^+]$ and the sum of the plasma $[Cl^-]$ and $[HCO_3^-]$. Because this gap is typically increased or unchanged in certain acid-base disturbances, its quick calculation at the bedside is often of tremendous help in analyzing such disturbances, especially different types of metabolic acidosis (Table 6-2).

In the next chapter it will be illustrated how these tools can be utilized in the management of patients with acid-base disturbances. It has been repeatedly emphasized that the correct analysis of such disturbances, and hence the logical management of such patients, requires an understanding of the dynamics of the disorder. For this reason — and for the reason that a clinical diagnosis should be based on a history and physical examination *supported* by laboratory studies, seldom on laboratory values alone — "automatic" diagrams of H^+ imbalances have not been presented.

Appendix: Nomogram of the Henderson-Hasselbalch Equation

The Henderson-Hasselbalch equation has three variables: pH, $[HCO_3^-]$, and Pco_2; that is,

$$pH = 6.1 + \log \frac{[HCO_3^-]}{0.03Pco_2}$$

When any two of these variables are known, the third can be derived from the nomogram of Figure 5-4 by laying a straightedge to intersect the two known variables. For example, if the laboratory reports that a patient's arterial blood, taken anaerobically, has a pH of 7.32 and a Pco_2 of 32 mm Hg, then the nomogram tells us that the $[HCO_3^-]$ in that same arterial sample must have been 16 mMoles per liter. This conclusion can be verified in a somewhat more cumbersome manner by solving the equation given above.

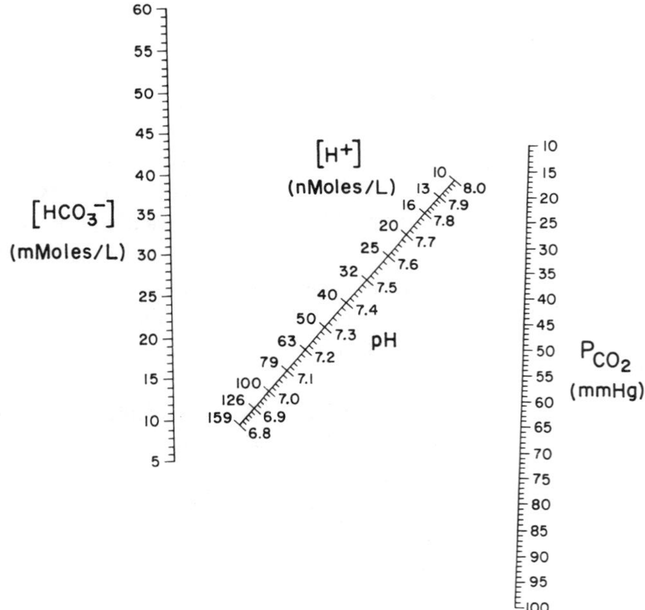

Figure 5-4
Nomogram of the Henderson-Hasselbalch equation. Each variable extends over the ranges shown in Figures 5-1 and 5-2, or slightly beyond. For convenience, H^+ concentrations are also shown. Adapted from F. C. McLean, *Physiol. Rev.* 18:495, 1938; H. W. Davenport, *The ABC of Acid-Base Chemistry* (5th ed.). Chicago: University of Chicago Press, 1969.

Problem 5-1

Under the following columns are listed variables of the Henderson-Hasselbalch equation or the Henderson equation for components of arterial plasma. In each instance, fill in the blank spaces (not occupied by dashes) by supplying both the calculated (Calc.) and the estimated (Est.) values. Also give the units in the parentheses.

	pH		$[H^+]$ ( )		P_{CO_2} ( )		$[HCO_3^-]$ ( )	
	Calc.	Est.	Calc.	Est.	Calc.	Est.	Calc.	Est.
(1)	7.40	—			40	—	24	—
(2)	7.32	—	—	—			15	—
(3)	7.55	—	—	—	44	—		
(4)			65	—	75	—	28	—

Problem 5-2

A 61-year-old woman was transferred from another hospital because she was agitated and hallucinating. She had been admitted to the other hospital 10 days earlier because of nausea and vomiting, and while there, she had become increasingly confused. Her most striking laboratory finding at the other hospital had been a plasma $[HCO_3^-]$ of 50 mMoles per liter.

Some 3½ years before the present admission, she had consulted a physician because of an infection of the urinary tract. At that time, x-rays revealed that both of her kidneys were small, her serum creatinine concentration had been 3.8 mg/100 ml, and the concentration of urea nitrogen in her blood (BUN) was 90 mg/100 ml. These findings were interpreted to reflect chronic renal failure (Chaps. 8 and 10). Several determinations of her plasma

Table 5-4
Results of laboratory tests on a 61-year-old woman on admission to the hospital

Test	On Admission
Arterial blood:	
pH	7.51
P_{CO_2} (mm Hg)	34
Venous plasma:	
$[HCO_3^-]$ (mMoles/L)	45
$[Cl^-]$ (mEq/L)	98
$[Na^+]$ (mEq/L)	152
BUN (mg/100 ml)	82
Creatinine (mg/100 ml)	3.1

$[Ca^{2+}]$ had been borderline high, but this finding was not satisfactorily explained or pursued.

Physical examination on admission revealed a small, thin woman with dry skin and mucous membranes. She was hallucinating, and frequently broke into tears.

Because of her mental status (for which there was no immediate explanation) and because the main laboratory abnormality reported from the other hospital was a very high plasma $[HCO_3^-]$, the studies listed in Table 5-4 were obtained shortly after the patient was admitted.

Analyze the patient's acid-base status. What would you have done next?

Selected References

General

Bates, R. G. *Determination of pH. Theory and Practice.* New York: Wiley & Sons, 1964.

Bittar, E. E. *Cell pH.* Washington, D.C.: Butterworth, 1964.

Davenport, H. W. *The ABC of Acid-Base Chemistry* (5th ed.). Chicago: University of Chicago Press, 1969.
The fifth edition of this inexpensive and useful book gives brief and lucid explanations of many of the other methods currently in use for analyzing clinical problems.

Davis, R. P. Logland: A Gibbsian view of acid-base balance. *Am. J. Med.* 42:159, 1967.

Hills, A. G. *Acid-Base Balance: Chemistry, Physiology, Pathophysiology.* Baltimore: Williams & Wilkins, 1973.

Huckabee, W. E. Henderson vs. Hasselbalch. *Clin. Res.* 9:116, 1961.

Lennon, E. J. Body Buffering Mechanisms. In E. D. Frohlich (ed.), *Pathophysiology: Altered Regulatory Mechanisms in Disease.* Philadelphia: Lippincott, 1972.

Makoff, D. L. Acid-Base Metabolism. In M. H. Maxwell and C. R. Kleeman (eds.), *Clinical Disorders of Fluid and Electrolyte Metabolism* (2nd ed.). New York: McGraw-Hill, 1972.

Masoro, E. M., and Siegel, P. D. *Acid-Base Regulation: Its Physiology and Pathophysiology.* Philadelphia: Saunders, 1971.

Muntwyler, E. *Water and Electrolyte Metabolism and Acid-Base Balance.* St. Louis: Mosby, 1968.

Nahas, G. G. (ed.). Current concepts of acid-base measurement. *Ann. N.Y. Acad. Sci.* 133:1, 1966.
Two of the papers in this symposium, "Terminology of acid-base disorders" and "Statement on acid-base terminology," have also been reproduced in *Ann. Intern. Med.* 63:873, 1965.

Rector, F. C., Jr. (ed.). Symposium on acid-base homeostasis. *Kidney Int.* 1:273, 1972.
This volume contains articles on physiological as well as clinical topics. Among the latter are metabolic alkalosis; acidosis due to renal defects or insufficiency; metabolic, cardiovascular, and pulmonary consequences of acid-base disorders; and pH of cerebrospinal fluid in acidosis and alkalosis.

Schwartz, W. B., and Relman, A. S. Critique of the parameters used in evaluation of acid-base disorders. "Whole-blood buffer base" and "standard bicarbonate" compared with blood pH and plasma bicarbonate concentration. *N. Engl. J. Med.* 268:1382, 1963.

Valtin, H. *Renal Function: Mechanisms Preserving Fluid and Solute Balance in Health.* Boston: Little, Brown, 1973. Chaps. 9 and 10.

Waddell, W. J., and Bates, R. G. Intracellular pH. *Physiol. Rev.* 49:285, 1969.

Weisberg, H. F. Water, Electrolytes, Acid-Base, and Oxygen. In I. Davidson and J. B. Henry (eds.), *Todd-Sanford Clinical Diagnosis by Laboratory Methods* (15th ed.). Philadelphia: Saunders, 1974.

Winters, R. W. (ed.). *The Body Fluids in Pediatrics.* Boston: Little, Brown, 1973.

Arithmetic Approximations

Fagan, T. J. Estimation of hydrogen ion concentration. *N. Engl. J. Med.* 288:915, 1973.

Flenley, D. C. Another non-logarithmic acid-base diagram? *Lancet* 1:961, 1971.

Kassirer, J. P., and Bleich, H. L. Rapid estimation of plasma carbon dioxide tension from pH and total carbon dioxide content. *N. Engl. J. Med.* 272:1067, 1965.

Confidence Bands

Albert, M. S., Dell, R. B., and Winters, R. W. Quantitative displacement of acid-base equilibrium in metabolic acidosis. *Ann. Intern. Med.* 66:312, 1967.

Arbus, G. S., Herbert, L. A., Levesque, P. R., Etsten, B. E., and Schwartz, W. B. Characterization and clinical application of the "significance band" for acute respiratory alkalosis. *N. Engl. J. Med.* 280:117, 1969.

Bone, J. M., Cowie, J., Lambie, A. T., and Robson, J. S. The relationship between arterial PCO_2 and hydrogen ion concentration in chronic metabolic acidosis and alkalosis. *Clin. Sci. Mol. Med.* 46:113, 1974.

Brackett, N. C., Jr., Cohen, J. J., and Schwartz, W. B. Carbon dioxide titration curve of normal man: Effect of increasing degrees of acute hypercapnia on acid-base equilibrium. *N. Engl. J. Med.* 272:6, 1965.

Brackett, N. C., Jr., Wingo, C. F., Muren, O., and Solano, J. T. Acid-base response to chronic hypercapnia in man. *N. Engl. J. Med.* 280:124, 1969.

Cohen, J. J., and Schwartz, W. B. Evaluation of acid-base equilibrium in pulmonary insufficiency. *Am. J. Med.* 41:163, 1966.

Lennon, E. J., and Lemann, J., Jr. Defense of hydrogen ion concentration in chronic metabolic acidosis. A new evaluation of an old approach. *Ann. Intern. Med.* 65:265, 1966.

Schwartz, W. B., Brackett, N. C., Jr., and Cohen, J. J. The response of extracellular hydrogen ion concentration to graded degrees of chronic hypercapnia: The physiologic limits of the defense of pH. *J. Clin. Invest.* 44:291, 1965.

van Ypersele de Strihou, C., and Frans, A. The respiratory response to chronic metabolic alkalosis and acidosis in disease. *Clin. Sci. Mol. Med.* 45:439, 1973.

Anion Gap

Alberti, K. G. M. M., and Nattrass, M. Lactic acidosis. *Lancet* 2:25, 1977.

Alpert, N. R. Lactate production and removal and the regulation of metabolism. *Ann. N.Y. Acad. Sci.* 119:995, 1965.

DeTroyer, A., Stolarczyk, A., Zegers DeBeyl, D., and Stryckmans, P. Value of anion-gap determination in multiple myeloma. *N. Engl. J. Med.* 296:858, 1977.

Eichenholz, A., Mulhausen, R. O., Anderson, W. E., and MacDonald, F. M. Primary hypocapnia: A cause of metabolic acidosis. *J. Appl. Physiol.* 17:283, 1962.

Emmett, M. E., and Narins, R. G. Clinical use of the anion gap. *Medicine* (Baltimore) 56:38, 1977.

Huckabee, W. E. Abnormal resting blood lactate. *Am. J. Med.* 30:840, 1961.

Lancet Editorial. The anion gap. *Lancet* 1:785, 1977.

Lancet Editorial. Lactic acidosis. *Lancet* 2:27, 1973.

Oh, M. S., and Carroll, H. J. The anion gap. *N. Engl. J. Med.* 297:814, 1977.

Seligson, D. The Role of the Laboratory. In M. H. Maxwell and C. R. Kleeman (eds.), *Clinical Disorders of Fluid and Electrolyte Metabolism* (2nd ed.). New York: McGraw-Hill, 1972.

Zborowska-Sluis, D. T., and Dossetor, J. B. Hyperlactatemia of hyperventilation. *J. Appl. Physiol.* 22:746, 1967.

Zilva, J. F. The anion gap. *Lancet* 1:948, 1977.

6 : Disorders of H^+ Balance: Clinical Examples

In this chapter, the analysis of clinical problems of H^+ imbalance is illustrated by means of patient presentations. One or more examples of each of the primary disturbances will be considered, and these are accompanied by tables listing the major disease processes that can lead to that particular acid-base disorder. Further examples, including one involving H^+ balance in the cerebrospinal fluid (CSF), are described in the problems at the end of this chapter.

Metabolic Acidosis

Chronic Renal Failure

The patient is a 32-year-old man who for seven years had been followed by his physician because of chronic renal failure. At age 20, the patient had had a sore throat due to β-hemolytic *Streptococcus* group A; within 2½ weeks after the onset of the sore throat, he suddenly began to pass bright red (bloody) urine. At this time, he was found to be slightly hypertensive, and analysis of his urine revealed a moderate amount of protein and erythrocytes as well as red blood cell casts in the sediment. A diagnosis of acute poststreptococcal glomerulonephritis was made.

Thereafter, the patient was checked by his physician every three to six months. Twelve years after the episode of sore throat, the patient was feeling well except that he seemed to tire somewhat easily. He was working full-time and eating a regular diet. Physical examination was unremarkable except for borderline hypertension (blood pressure 150/90 mm Hg). The following laboratory values were obtained: for venous plasma, Na^+ 142 mEq per liter, K^+ 4.5 mEq per liter, Cl^- 102 mEq per liter, creatinine 6.8 mg/100 ml, and urea nitrogen (BUN) 71 mg/100 ml; for arterial plasma, pH 7.33 and P_{CO_2} 32 mm Hg.

Comment. The history suggests chronic renal failure due to chronic glomerulonephritis. This impression is supported by the elevations in serum creatinine and BUN, which reflect a decrease in the glomerular filtration rate (GFR) (see Chap. 8).

In uncomplicated chronic renal failure, we expect to find a primary metabolic acidosis, which is due mainly to decreased excretion of ammonium and titratable acid (see Table 10-3). Such failure is also associated with a rise in the plasma concentrations of sulfate and phosphate according to the dynamics illustrated in Figure 1-A (see Answer to Problem 1-1 in back of book). Thus, if we are dealing with the uncomplicated metabolic acidosis of chronic renal failure, we would expect the arterial plasma values for this patient to fall within the confidence bands given in Figure 5-2, and we would anticipate an elevation of the anion gap.

Both predictions are fulfilled. By estimation, the $[H^+]$ corresponding to a pH of 7.33 is 40 + 7, or 47 nMoles per liter, and the $[HCO_3^-]$ is 25 × 32/47 (Eq. 5-3), or 17 mMoles per liter. The true value calculated by the Henderson-Hasselbalch equation for $[HCO_3^-]$ would be 16.3 mMoles per liter (see Fig. 5-4). In either case, the arterial values fall within the confidence bands in Figure 5-2 for uncomplicated primary metabolic acidosis; that is, the extent to which the P_{CO_2} is lowered reflects the degree of compensatory hyperventilation that would be expected in an otherwise normal subject who had this amount of metabolic acidosis. The anion gap (Eq. 5-5) is usually calculated using the values obtained on venous serum or plasma. For $[HCO_3^-]$, this value is 2 to 4 mMoles per liter higher than the arterial value, partly because there is an arteriovenous difference between HCO_3^- levels and partly because the total CO_2 content, rather than $[HCO_3^-]$, is ordinarily measured on venous plasma. Again, however, this is a trivial distinction, for whether 16.3, 17, or even 19 mMoles per liter is used for the $[HCO_3^-]$ value, the anion gap is clearly elevated in this patient.

The laboratory values thus confirm the diagnostic impression based on the clinical history. It should be noted that a patient in chronic renal failure — even, as this patient, with a reduction in GFR to less than 15 percent of normal — can remain in balance for Na^+, Cl^-, and K^+ while ingesting a normal diet (Chap. 10). There is, however, a positive balance for H^+; these ions are thought to be buffered mainly by bone, so the arterial pH may remain stable despite a positive balance. The subject of H^+ balance in chronic renal failure is covered in much greater detail in Chapter 10.

Uncontrolled Diabetes Mellitus

A 51-year-old woman had been known to have diabetes mellitus for ten years. She was checked by her physician every two months, and the disease remained in good control as a result of moderate dietary measures and the use of an oral hypoglycemic agent.

Three days before admission, the patient developed a rather severe "cold." She had a mild fever, lost her appetite, and urinated more frequently, especially during the night. On the day of admission to the hospital, she had begun to vomit and she felt short of breath.

Physical examination on admission revealed an acutely ill person whose mucous membranes and axillae were dry. She had periods of deep breathing, called Kussmaul respiration. She was alert. Her temperature was 38.2°C, her pulse rate 100 per minute, her respiratory rate about 24 per minute, and her blood pressure 150/110 mm Hg. A urine specimen obtained on admission contained large amounts of sugar and keto acids; the results of some other laboratory tests on admission are shown in Table 6-1.

Comment. The history is typical of uncontrolled diabetes mellitus, which is commonly set off by an intercurrent illness, such as an infection. The increased urination reflects an osmotic diuresis due to glucosuria, which was confirmed by large amounts of this sugar in the urine. Uncontrolled diabetes mellitus often leads to primary metabolic acidosis, called *ketoacidosis* because it is due to an overproduction of keto acids, mainly β-hydroxybutyric and acetoacetic acids (Table 5-3). This impression is supported by the arterial pH value, which is in the acidotic range. If the hyperventilation that the patient manifested were the primary cause of the acid-base disturbance, the arterial pH should have indicated an alkalosis. Since it did not, the hyperventilation was probably a compensatory response to the rather severe

Table 6-1
Results of laboratory tests on a 51-year-old woman before and during treatment for diabetic ketoacidosis. For $[H^+]$ and $[HCO_3^-]$, the first figure is the calculated value, the one in parentheses the estimated value

Test	On Admission	12 Hours After Admission
Arterial blood:		
pH	7.15	7.40
P_{CO_2} (mm Hg)	13	21
$[H^+]$ (nMoles/L)	71 (65)	40 (40)
$[HCO_3^-]$ (mMoles/L)	4 (5)	13 (13)
Venous plasma:		
$[Na^+]$ (mEq/L)	126	142
$[Cl^-]$ (mEq/L)	90	101
$[K^+]$ (mEq/L)	3.7	3.5
Venous blood:		
Glucose (mg/100 ml)	762	156

metabolic acidosis. If that is correct, the patient's arterial values should fall within the confidence bands in Figure 5-2, whereas if the labored breathing reflected an added, primary respiratory disturbance, the points should fall outside the bands. The arterial $[H^+]$ and $[HCO_3^-]$ can be estimated from the pH and P_{CO_2} that the laboratory reported. With this additional information, the patient's arterial values can be employed in Figure 5-2, and it may be concluded that we are dealing with an uncomplicated metabolic acidosis with appropriate respiratory compensation. The increased anion gap, which was due to the accumulation of keto acids in the plasma, further supports the diagnosis.

The low plasma concentrations of Na^+ and Cl^- are often, but not invariably, seen in uncontrolled diabetes mellitus; they result partly from a shift of H_2O from the intracellular into the extracellular space (see Problem 3-1) and partly from the increased urinary excretion of NaCl that accompanies an osmotic diuresis.

Severe diabetic ketoacidosis often leads to coma; so does severe hypoglycemia, which diabetic patients can develop from relatively too much insulin or other hypoglycemic agents. Therefore, when a diabetic patient is comatose, it is very important to ascertain the blood glucose concentration before giving the patient insulin. In the present case, insulin could be given immediately because the patient was alert; intravenous infusion was therefore started at once through the same needle from which the venous blood had been obtained. During the 12 hours after admission, a total of 3 liters of isotonic saline (Fig. 1-6) was given to correct the volume contraction, and to these infusions were added a total of 250 units of crystalline insulin and a total of about 250 mEq of $NaHCO_3$ (five 50-ml ampules of the concentrated solution; Fig. 1-6). In addition, the patient was urged to drink liquids that are high in K^+, such as bouillon, tea, orange juice, and skim milk. This measure is important because as the hyperglycemia and acidosis are corrected, a shift of K^+ into the cells can lead to dangerous hypokalemia (Fig. 4-2).

The laboratory values after the first 12 hours of treatment are shown in Table 6-1. HCO_3^- is distributed throughout the extracellular space (ECF). Nevertheless, the volume of distribution for HCO_3^- exceeds the ECF, because much H^+ exists within cells; when HCO_3^- is given, intracellular as well as extracellular acidosis is corrected. The former correction occurs by movement of H^+ out of the cells; during this process, a portion of the administered HCO_3^- is consumed, which has the same net effect as a movement of HCO_3^- into the cells. Consequently, one calculates the amount of HCO_3^- to be given *as if* it were distributed into a volume greater than the ECF; in practice, this is done by deciding how many milliequivalents per liter the

$[HCO_3^-]$ is to be raised and multiplying this value by a volume equal to 50 percent of the body weight *in kilograms.* In the present patient, the $[HCO_3^-]$ was deliberately only partially corrected, because as a general rule, it is safer not to correct imbalances abruptly and completely. This patient exemplified this point: *Partial* correction of the $[HCO_3^-]$ *fully* restored the arterial pH to normal because the P_{CO_2} remained low. This phenomenon, which is discussed further in the Answer to Problem 6-1, probably occurs because the HCO_3^- in plasma does not very quickly equilibrate with the HCO_3^- in the cerebrospinal fluid (CSF). Consequently, the pH of CSF remains lower than the arterial pH, and compensatory hyperventilation continues. Therefore, had more HCO_3^- been given to this patient, it is likely that an iatrogenic alkalosis might have complicated the picture.

Because of the lag in reducing compensatory hyperventilation, the acid-base status 12 hours after admission indicated a mixed disturbance of metabolic acidosis and respiratory alkalosis. Accordingly, the arterial values now fell outside the confidence bands in Figure 5-2 as well as outside the bands for *acute* respiratory alkalosis (Fig. 5-1). The anion gap remained high, because much of the β-hydroxybutyrate and acetoacetate that had accumulated had not yet been excreted or metabolized.

Once the acute imbalances of H_2O and electrolytes have been reversed, it is usually safer to curtail or discontinue vigorous intravenous therapy and to allow several days for the patient's renal and respiratory mechanisms to restore values fully to normal. During this period, however, careful observation of the patient, including frequent monitoring of the laboratory values, must be continued.

Causes of Metabolic Acidosis

The causes of metabolic acidosis are listed in Table 6-2. Details about each disorder can be found in a number of standard references (e.g., in the chapter by D. L. Makoff in the book edited by Maxwell and Kleeman). Note that the conditions are divided on the basis of whether they are characterized by an increased anion gap.

Metabolic Alkalosis

Prolonged Vomiting: K^+ Deficiency and Contraction Alkalosis

A 44-year-old man had had a duodenal ulcer for at least eight years. Once previously he had bled from this ulcer, but he had refused an operation. For two weeks before being admitted now, he had been unable to keep down any food; he had lost at least 3 kg, and on admission he was vomiting and very weak. On physical examination, his mucous membranes and axillae were

Table 6-2
Causes of metabolic acidosis. The disorders have been divided into those that are usually accompanied by an increased anion gap and those in which the gap is usually normal. This division reflects the major clinical usefulness of the anion gap

Increased anion gap:
- Uncontrolled diabetes mellitus
- Renal failure (acute and chronic)
- Lactic acidosis
- Administration, ingestion, or intoxication
  - Ethyl alcohol, with "starvation" and production of keto acids
  - Salicylate
  - Methyl alcohol
  - Paraldehyde
  - Ethylene glycol

Normal anion gap:
- Diarrhea or loss of other gastrointestinal fluids with high [HCO_3^-] through fistulas or surgical drainage (see Table 1-4)
- Renal tubular acidosis (see Chap. 12)
- Ureterosigmoidoscopy
- "Expansion acidosis"
- Administration, ingestion, or intoxication
  - NH_4Cl
  - Carbonic anhydrase inhibitors

dry and the skin turgor poor. Blood pressure was 105/70 mm Hg, pulse rate 92 per minute, and respiratory rate 18 per minute. The abdomen was distended, and the deep tendon reflexes were hypoactive.

An electrocardiogram showed flattening of the T waves and prolonged Q-T interval; it was interpreted to be typical of K^+ deficiency (Fig. 4-4). Selected laboratory values, both on admission and 48 hours later, are given in Table 6-3.

Comment. The genesis and maintenance of metabolic alkalosis in prolonged vomiting are shown in Figure 6-1. The primary event during vomiting is the loss of gastric acid as HCl (Table 1-4). In the extracellular fluid, this loss leads to a release of H^+ from carbonic acid and other buffers, loss of Cl^- in relative excess of Na^+, and buildup of $NaHCO_3$, as schematized by the following reaction:

$$H_2CO_3 + Na^+ + Cl^- \rightleftharpoons Na^+ + HCO_3^- + \downarrow H^+ + \downarrow Cl^- \quad (6\text{-}1)$$

The downward arrows in front of the symbols H^+ and Cl^- indicate that the initial event is loss of these ions; thus, the reaction is driven to the right. These events are manifested in the patient by a proportionately greater decrease in the plasma

Table 6-3
Results of laboratory tests on a 44-year-old man before and after treatment for metabolic alkalosis due to prolonged vomiting. For $[H^+]$ and $[HCO_3^-]$, the first figure is the calculated value, the one in parentheses the estimated value

Test	On Admission	48 Hours After Admission
Arterial blood:		
pH	7.53	7.41
P_{CO_2} (mm Hg)	56	51
$[H^+]$ (nMoles/L)	30 (27)	39 (39)
$[HCO_3^-]$ (mMoles/L)	45 (52)	31 (33)
Venous plasma:		
$[Na^+]$ (mEq/L)	132	141
$[Cl^-]$ (mEq/L)	65	97
$[K^+]$ (mEq/L)	2.2	3.4

concentration of Cl^- than of Na^+ and an increase in the concentration of HCO_3^-. The result, according to this analysis, is an uncomplicated metabolic alkalosis, and the arterial points do fall within the confidence bands in Figure 5-2, whether the estimated or calculated values for $[H^+]$ and $[HCO_3^-]$ are used. The anion gap is high, largely for reasons that are unclear, but partly because, in the absence of eating, fat catabolism becomes the source of energy for the patient, and this metabolic process produces keto acids.

As is shown in Figure 6-1, however, the generation of metabolic alkalosis in prolonged vomiting is much more complicated than is set forth above. There are concomitant losses of K^+ and Na^+, partly as a consequence of the composition of gastric juice (Table 1-4), but mainly because of excessive urinary excretion of these two ions. Sodium levels are further reduced in the extracellular space because there is a shift of this ion out of the extracellular and into the intracellular compartment. The loss of NaCl leads to contraction of the extracellular volume, with resulting activation of the renin-angiotensin-aldosterone system (Chap. 14, under Renin-Angiotensin-Aldosterone System). Thus, prolonged vomiting leads to K^+ deficiency and volume contraction, two changes that are known to aggravate metabolic alkalosis. The patient demonstrated evidence of these two further changes. His plasma concentration of K^+ was low, the electrocardiogram showed the typical alterations of K^+ depletion, and his weakness and diminished deep tendon reflexes probably reflected this deficiency (Chap. 4). Decreased extracellular fluid volume was manifested in the loss of body weight (which, however, was due

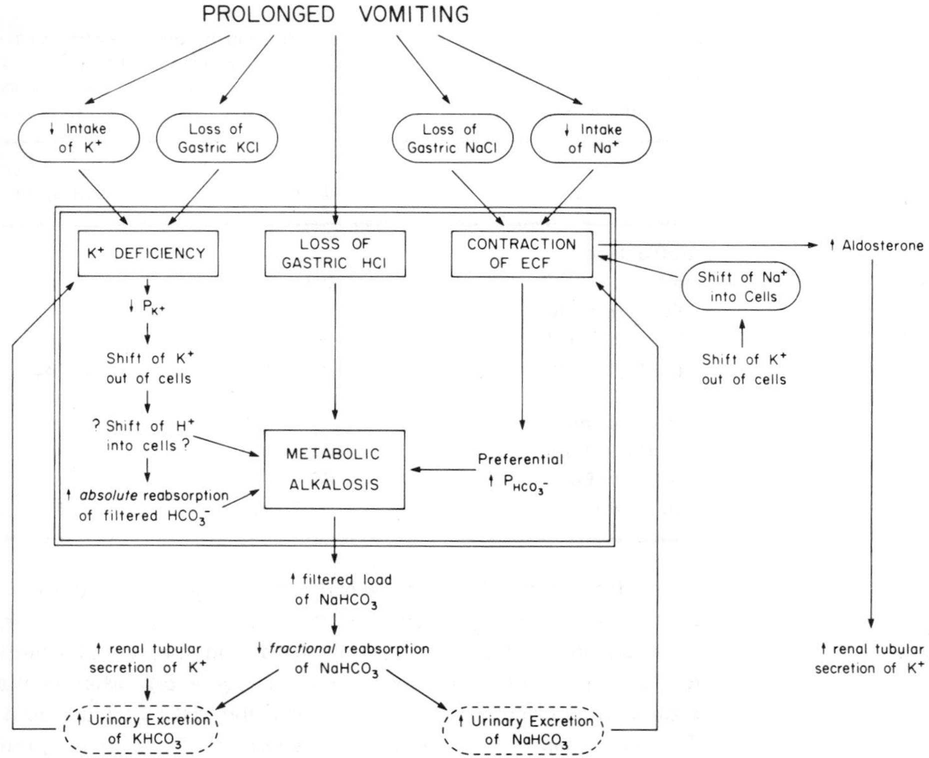

Figure 6-1

The generation of metabolic alkalosis in prolonged vomiting. The three major causes of the alkalosis are shown in the upper boxes. The causes of K^+ deficiency and of contraction of the extracellular fluid volume (ECF) are depicted in the oval rings. The ovals for increased urinary excretion of $KHCO_3$ and $NaHCO_3$ are drawn with dashed lines to indicate that these events are not necessarily seen. When vomiting is prolonged and severe, the rise in plasma HCO_3^- concentration ($P_{HCO_3^-}$) may cause an increase in the filtered load of HCO_3^- that exceeds the tubular capacity to reabsorb HCO_3^-. Under these circumstances, the excretion of HCO_3^- obligates the excretion of K^+ and Na^+; this can lead to rates of urinary excretion for these two ions of 40 to 100 mEq per day, even when the plasma concentrations for K^+ and Na^+ are abnormally low. The concomitant high urinary excretion of HCO_3^- results in alkaline urine with a pH of 7.60 to 8.25. However, when vomiting is less severe or stops, the kidneys can often reabsorb all the increased filtered HCO_3^-; urinary excretion of $KHCO_3$ and $NaHCO_3$ is then normal or curtailed, and the urinary pH is again acid. Based partly on the work of W. B. Schwartz and his associates (*J. Clin. Invest.* 43:1836, 1964; *Am. J. Med.* 40:10, 1966) and adapted from D. W. Seldin and F. C. Rector, Jr., *Kidney Int.* 1:306, 1972.

partly to loss of lean body mass), the dry skin and mucous membranes, the relatively low blood pressure, and the hyponatremia.

Depletion of K^+ during prolonged vomiting has the following origins, the first two of which are relatively minor: (1) The concentration of K^+ in gastric juice is ordinarily higher than in plasma (Table 1-4), and the K^+ is lost as the Cl^- salt. (2) At the same time, the patient does not eat or is unable to retain ingested food; thus his intake of K^+ is curtailed. (3) Most important, there is increased urinary excretion of K^+, which may have at least two causes. One involves the contraction of the extracellular fluid volume and a consequent rise in the plasma concentration of aldosterone, which augments K^+ secretion in the distal renal tubules. The second involves increased urinary excretion of HCO_3^-. As the plasma concentration of HCO_3^- rises (Eq. 6-1), so does the filtered load of HCO_3^- (GFR $\cdot$ $P_{HCO_3^-}$). Although the increased filtered load is accompanied by a rise in the tubular reabsorption of HCO_3^-, the latter adjustment may lag behind the former so that less than the usual 99.9+ percent of the filtered HCO_3^- is reabsorbed; this occurs especially in prolonged and severe vomiting. Consequently, HCO_3^- is excreted in the urine, and one of the cations accompanying it is K^+, whose distal secretion was stimulated by aldosterone. If the vomiting stops or is less severe, tubular reabsorption of HCO_3^- keeps pace with the increased filtered load, and the excessive urinary excretion of HCO_3^- and K^+ stops. If, however, K^+ supplements are given as other than the chloride salt, excessive excretion of K^+ may continue, even though HCO_3^- excretion is no longer increased.

Contraction of the extracellular fluid compartment results from NaCl deficiency, which also has several causes in prolonged, severe vomiting: (1) Gastric juice contains Na^+ and Cl^- (Table 1-4), and the losses are not replaced, because both the intake and retention of food are poor or nonexistent. (2) Hypokalemia causes K^+ to shift out of the cells, and reciprocally, Na^+ ions (and possibly H^+) shift into cells (Fig. 4-2). (3) When the increase in the tubular reabsorption of HCO_3^- does not keep pace with the increase in its filtered load (as described above), there is excessive urinary excretion of Na^+ as well as of K^+. The greater amount of HCO_3^- in the glomerular filtrate exists mainly as the Na^+ salt (Eq. 6-1), and when the urinary excretion of HCO_3^- is increased, that which is not balanced by K^+ is excreted as $NaHCO_3$. In this way, the metabolic alkalosis of prolonged vomiting can lead to increased urinary excretion of Na^+, even in the face of a contracted extracellular fluid volume, which in most other circumstances is associated with avid renal retention of Na^+. It should be emphasized that the Na^+ is excreted as the

HCO_3^- salt, not as the Cl^- salt; NaCl *is* avidly reabsorbed, and it is the obligatory excretion of HCO_3^- that secondarily raises the excretion of Na^+. If the vomiting stops or is curtailed so that virtually all of the filtered HCO_3^- is reabsorbed, then the renal "wasting" of Na^+ stops. As with K^+, however, renal wasting of Na^+ will continue if Na^+ supplements are given as other than the chloride salt.

Once K^+ deficiency and contraction of the extracellular fluid volume have been established, they may cause further alkalosis by the following mechanisms. As K^+ shifts out of the cells, H^+ may enter the cells in exchange. This effect has not been conclusively demonstrated, but to the extent that it occurs, the reciprocal shift leads to extracellular alkalosis and intracellular acidosis (Fig. 4-2). The shift of H^+ into renal tubular cells may explain the phenomenon of increased absolute reabsorption of filtered HCO_3^- as the plasma concentration of K^+ is reduced; that is, an increased concentration of H^+ within renal tubular cells would lead to increased secretion of H^+ and, reciprocally, to increased reabsorption of HCO_3^-. It may seem self-contradictory to invoke increased reabsorption of filtered HCO_3^- as abetting the alkalosis when we have cited evidence above that the urinary excretion of HCO_3^- is increased. The solution to this apparent contradiction is that the increased urinary excretion of HCO_3^- is itself due to the elevated plasma $[HCO_3^-]$, and to the extent that the resulting K^+ depletion causes the reabsorption of more HCO_3^-, it further increases its plasma concentration and the alkalosis.

Contraction of the extracellular compartment can lead to alkalosis not only via increased aldosterone levels and K^+ deficiency, but even when present by itself. It results from a negative balance of Na^+, Cl^-, and H_2O without a loss of HCO_3^-, or at least with a lesser loss than of Na^+, Cl^-, and H_2O. The result is a rise in the extracellular concentration of HCO_3^- and alkalosis. For obvious reasons, this is known as *contraction alkalosis* (Chap. 7 and Problem 7-1).

Returning now to our patient, his treatment during the first 48 hours of hospitalization followed logically from the pathogenesis of his fluid and solute imbalances. The vomiting had led to large deficits of Cl^-, K^+, Na^+, H_2O, and calories, and these losses were replaced by intravenous infusions. During the first 24 hours, he received 3 liters of 5% dextrose in normal saline and 2 liters of normal saline, with 60 mMoles of KCl added to each of the 5 liters (Fig. 1-6). During the subsequent 24 hours, he received 2 liters of 5% dextrose in normal saline and 1 liter of normal saline, with 40 mMoles of KCl added to each liter. This combination replaced the predominant loss of Cl^-, largely corrected the deficit of K^+, and replenished the volume of the extracellular compartment. It is not essential to replace the losses exactly, because with correction of the major derangements, the patient's kidneys will accomplish the fine regulations required for rectifying the imbalances. By 48 hours, the metabolic alkalosis was therefore corrected (Table 6-3). It should be noted, however, that the arterial values now fell slightly above the confidence bands in Figure 5-2. The probable reason is a lag in the correction of the pH of the cerebrospinal fluid (CSF). On admission, the $[HCO_3^-]$ of the CSF, like that of the plasma, was abnormally high. Probably as a result of an alkalotic CSF, there was compensatory hypoventilation and a rise in the Pco_2. With treatment, the plasma $[HCO_3^-]$ dropped considerably, but that of the CSF declined more slowly; consequently, some alkalosis of the CSF persisted even after the plasma pH had returned to normal, and continued alveolar hypoventilation led to a higher Pco_2 than is seen in uncomplicated metabolic alkalosis with a plasma $[HCO_3^-]$ of 31 mMoles per liter.

Over the next week, the patient's condition stabilized so that he could undergo surgery. At operation, it was found that scar tissue, presumably from an old and recurrent peptic ulcer, was almost totally obstructing the pylorus.

W. B. Schwartz and his associates have clarified the importance of replenishing the extracellular fluid volume (ECF) in correcting this type of metabolic alkalosis. They have shown that *once the vomiting has stopped,* the alkalosis can be reversed by giving NaCl alone, even though deficits of K^+ had been incurred. This observation can be explained through the dynamics illustrated in Figure 6-1. The key is to reverse the increase in the *absolute* reabsorption of filtered HCO_3^-, that is, to allow the kidneys to excrete the extra HCO_3^- that has accumulated as a consequence of K^+ deficiency. Reexpansion of the ECF accomplishes this task by reducing the plasma concentration of aldosterone and thereby stopping the renal wasting of K^+. When the kidneys can again conserve this ion avidly, the plasma concentration of K^+ (P_{K+}) will rise, and the chain of events that led to the increased absolute reabsorption of HCO_3^- will be reversed (Fig. 6-1). Reexpansion further aids the reparative process by the following mechanisms: (1) With a rise in P_{K+}, K^+ will again shift into the cells, and in exchange, H^+ may leave the cells (Fig. 4-2); to the extent that this process takes place, it will correct the alkalosis. (2) As the *preferential* rise in $P_{HCO_3^-}$ (contraction alkalosis) is reversed, the intensity of the alkalosis will be lessened.

There is an alternative way of visualizing the efficacy of Cl^- repletion in correcting this type of alkalosis. This view states that contraction of the ECF obligates the avid reabsorption of Na^+.

During selective and severe Cl^- depletion, not enough Cl^- is available to "accompany" all the Na^+ that needs to be reabsorbed; HCO_3^-, being the only other anion present in sufficient quantities in the glomerular filtrate, is therefore reabsorbed with Na^+ at a greater rate than normally. Once the Cl^- deficiency is replenished, Cl^- can again accompany the reabsorbed Na^+, and HCO_3^- can be excreted. The last will correct the alkalosis; furthermore, with the simultaneous repletion of Na^+ and restoration of the ECF, the HCO_3^- will now be excreted as the Na^+ salt, urinary K^+ wasting will cease, and the K^+ depletion can be corrected without supplementation of this ion.

At first glance, Figure 6-1 may appear paradoxical in at least one respect: The key to the correction of the metabolic alkalosis is a decrease in the absolute reabsorption of HCO_3^- (i.e., an increase in its urinary excretion); yet, according to the figure, reversal of the alkalosis would appear to decrease the urinary excretion of HCO_3^- (indicated by dashed ovals in Fig. 6-1). As is shown in Table 6-4, the apparent paradox can be resolved by very small changes in the *fractional* reabsorption of HCO_3^-. The renal handling of HCO_3^- in a healthy adult is shown in the first column of the table, the possible status of the patient on admission in the second column. We postulate that the contraction of the ECF led to a 20 percent decrease in the GFR and that the rapid rise in the $P_{HCO_3^-}$ led to a decrease in the fractional reabsorption of HCO_3^- to 99 percent; the result is an increase in both the absolute reabsorption of HCO_3^- and in its absolute excretion. A possible status during repair (e.g., at 48 hours after admission) is shown in the third column of the table. Reexpansion of the ECF has restored the GFR to normal and has reduced the $P_{HCO_3^-}$. Although the latter change by itself would tend to increase the fractional reabsorption of HCO_3^-, expansion of the ECF has the opposite effect. It is clear that a further decrease in fractional reabsorption of just 1 percent will lead to a reduction

Table 6-4
Renal handling of HCO_3^- in health, during severe metabolic alkalosis from prolonged vomiting, and during correction of the alkalosis

Variable	In Health	Metabolic Alkalosis	Repair
GFR (liters/day)	180	144	180
$P_{HCO_3^-}$ (mEq/L)	24	45	31
Filtered HCO_3^- (mEq/day)	4,320	6,480	5,580
Fractional reabsorption of HCO_3^- (%)	99.9	99	98
Absolute reabsorption of HCO_3^- (mEq/day)	4,316	6,415	5,468
Excretion of HCO_3^- (mEq/day)	4	65	112

in the absolute reabsorption of HCO_3^- and an increase in its absolute excretion.

Causes of Metabolic Alkalosis

The major causes of this disorder are listed in Table 6-5. Many of the mechanisms involved in each of the conditions can be inferred from Figure 6-1. In some instances, however, additional mechanisms or different pathways may be involved. In hyperaldosteronism, for example, the metabolic alkalosis may not be caused primarily or solely by increased tubular secretion of K^+ and K^+ deficiency. Rather, the major causes *may* involve increased reabsorption of Na^+ in the distal tubule and collecting duct that leads to increased secretion of H^+; or possibly direct stimulation of H^+ secretion by the mineralocorticoid is involved. Suffice it to say that the generation and maintenance of metabolic alkalosis often involve complicated processes that have not been fully unraveled; present concepts for each of the conditions listed in Table 6-5 can be reviewed in the references cited at the end of this chapter.

An example of posthypercapnic alkalosis is presented in Problem 6-2.

Table 6-5
Causes of metabolic alkalosis. In order to emphasize the causative role of deficits in the extracellular fluid volume and of Cl^- in some of the disturbances, the list is divided into those disorders that respond to the administration of NaCl and those that do not

Responsive to NaCl:
- Vomiting or gastric drainage
- Diuretic therapy (contraction alkalosis)
- Sudden relief from chronic hypercapnia (posthypercapnic alkalosis)
- Certain types of diarrhea that lead to predominant loss of Cl^- (congenital chloridorrhea)

Unresponsive to NaCl:
- Administration of alkali, especially in renal failure
  - HCO_3^-
  - Salts of organic acids (e.g., lactate, citrate, or acetate) that are oxidized to yield HCO_3^-
- Excess mineralocorticoids
  - Cushing's syndrome
  - Hyperaldosteronism
  - Bartter's syndrome
  - ACTH-secreting tumors
  - Licorice ingestion (mimics hyperaldosteronism)
- Severe K^+ depletion

Respiratory Acidosis

Pulmonary Edema: Acute Respiratory Acidosis

A 59-year-old woman had had a myocardial infarction ten years prior to the present illness and possibly a second infarction about eight years later. Just before the present admission, she had undergone severe physical exertion, and shortly thereafter she experienced chest pain and dyspnea. On arrival in the emergency room, she was unresponsive and cyanotic. Her blood pressure was 90/60 mm Hg and the pulse rate 132 per minute. Her neck veins were distended, and auscultation of the lungs revealed weak breath sounds, reflecting poor entry of air, and many "wet" rales, signifying pulmonary edema. Results of laboratory tests at this time are shown in Table 6-6.

It was concluded that the patient had had another myocardial infarction (which was later confirmed by electrocardiogram) and that she was in pulmonary edema. She was therefore treated with oxygen, positive-pressure assisted ventilation, and intravenous administration of aminophylline. Although she regained consciousness, her course was further complicated by ventricular fibrillation, which was managed by electrical shock and intravenous infusion of $NaHCO_3$. At 3 hours after admission, the pulmonary edema began to clear, she was conscious, and her blood pressure was 150/90 mm Hg; the results of laboratory tests at this time are also shown in Table 6-6.

Comment. When the left side of the heart fails as a pump (as it often does in acute myocardial infarction), the damming of blood in the pulmonary veins leads to increased hydrostatic pressure in the pulmonary capillaries and the formation of edema fluid, first around and then within the alveoli (Chap. 3). The presence of fluid in the alveoli can be heard as "wet" rales, and

Table 6-6
Results of laboratory tests on a 59-year-old woman on admission with pulmonary edema and three hours later when the edema had cleared

Test	On Admission	Three Hours After Admission
Arterial blood:		
pH	6.92	7.46
P_{CO_2} (mm Hg)	76	34
$[HCO_3^-]$ (mMoles/L)	15	23
[Lactate] (mEq/L)	10.7	7.2
Oxygen saturation (%)	70	94

Modified from N. R. Anthonisen and H. J. Smith, *Ann. Intern. Med.* 62:991, 1965.

when sufficient fluid is present to obstruct the airway passages, the physician detects this disorder as poor breath sounds. The result is alveolar hypoventilation, which, in a patient breathing room air, results not only in an elevation of the P_{CO_2} but also in poor oxygen saturation and cyanosis. The logical treatment is to try to improve the heart as a pump, often with digitalis, to assist the patient's ventilation while giving oxygen and to relieve possible bronchospasm with drugs such as aminophylline and morphine.

The elevation of the P_{CO_2} in this patient led to severe acidosis (Table 6-6). According to the reaction shown in Equation 5-4, retention of CO_2 leads to elevation of the plasma concentration of HCO_3^-; inspection of Figure 5-1b shows that in pure acute respiratory acidosis, a rise of the P_{CO_2} to 76 mm Hg would be expected to increase the HCO_3^- concentration to about 26 to 29 mMoles per liter. The fact that this concentration was considerably lower – namely, 15 mMoles per liter – suggests that this patient had a mixed disturbance that included a metabolic acidosis. This acidosis resulted from a deficient supply of oxygen to the tissues (showing up as cyanosis) and a consequent increase in anaerobic metabolism and production of lactic acid.

With two primary causes for acidosis, one would expect the arterial pH to be lower than in an uncomplicated acute respiratory acidosis with a P_{CO_2} of 76 mm Hg; this was indeed the case (Fig. 5-1a). Because the very severe acidosis may have contributed to the patient's clouded mental state as well as to further impairment of myocardial contractility, and because ventricular fibrillation aggravates lactic acidosis by causing further tissue hypoxia, $NaHCO_3$ was given intravenously. Consequently, the plasma HCO_3^- concentration returned to normal within 3 hours after admission, even though the plasma lactate concentration remained elevated. As is so often the case during assisted respiration, the patient was slightly hyperventilated, so the P_{CO_2} fell somewhat below the normal range.

The H^+ imbalance illustrated in this patient is not invariably seen in pulmonary edema. A mixed disturbance of respiratory and metabolic acidosis occurs in perhaps 50 percent of such patients; the remainder may show only metabolic acidosis or only respiratory acidosis, and a few have respiratory alkalosis.

Chronic Obstructive Lung Disease: Chronic Respiratory Acidosis

A 44-year-old woman had had asthma since childhood, and she had been a heavy cigarette smoker since her teens. Over the past four to five years, she had experienced progressive shortness of breath and somnolence, and she had developed some pretibial and ankle edema. She had been on mild diuretic therapy for about two years.

At the time of a routine checkup, the physical examination revealed a cachectic woman who was short of breath and coughed frequently. Her chest was barrel-shaped with an increase in the anteroposterior diameter, the respiratory excursions were poor, and the breath sounds faint. Laboratory studies obtained at this time are shown in Table 6-7.

During the ensuing two months, the patient became increasingly debilitated and somnolent. At the time of her final admission, she was comatose; results of laboratory tests on that admission are also shown in Table 6-7. She died in her sleep 4 hours later.

Comment. Probably as a result of long-standing asthma, smoking, and chronic infection, this patient had severe pulmonary emphysema. The resulting poor alveolar ventilation led to chronic retention of CO_2, which is reflected in the elevated P_{CO_2}. Two mechanisms account for the high $[HCO_3^-]$ in chronic obstructive lung disease: (1) the chemical reaction shown in equation 5-4 and (2) the increase in the tubular reabsorption of filtered HCO_3^- that accompanies a rise in Pa_{CO_2}. If these were the only mechanisms leading to H^+ imbalance in this patient, we would expect the arterial values to fall within the confidence bands for chronic respiratory acidosis in Figure 5-1. The points fall just within the outer limits of the bands, and the reason is almost certainly that a slight elevation of plasma lactic acid occurred as a consequence of the low Pa_{O_2} and tissue hypoxia. This explanation is strengthened by the fact that there was a minimal rise in the anion gap. (Vigorous diuretic therapy can lead to selective depletion of Cl^- and an increase

Table 6-7
Results of laboratory tests on a 44-year-old woman with chronic obstructive lung disease and pulmonary emphysema at the time of a routine checkup and two months later during her terminal admission

Test	Routine Checkup	Terminal Admission
Arterial blood:		
pH	7.34	7.09
P_{CO_2} (mm Hg)	58	52
$[HCO_3^-]$ (mMoles/L)	30	15
P_{O_2} (mm Hg)	45	30
Venous plasma:		
$[Na^+]$ (mEq/L)	139	137
$[Cl^-]$ (mEq/L)	87	88
$[K^+]$ (mEq/L)	4	4
$[HCO_3^-]$ (mEq/L)	33	17

in $[HCO_3^-]$. This complication, illustrated in Problem 7-1, was not present in this patient.)

Long-standing lung disease often leads to hypertension in the pulmonary arteries and thereby to heart failure. It was probably this chain of events that led to edema in this patient. Her somnolence was probably due to retention of CO_2, and the coma due to this factor plus severe acidosis.

During the final admission, the patient was more acidotic than would be expected from an uncomplicated chronic respiratory acidosis with a Pa_{CO_2} of 52 mm Hg (Fig. 5-1) or from an uncomplicated metabolic acidosis with a $[HCO_3^-]$ of 15 mMoles per liter (Fig. 5-2). At this time, she had a mixed respiratory and metabolic acidosis, the latter resulting from further production of lactic acid as reflected in an anion gap of 32 mMoles per liter.

J. B. West, among others, has emphasized that the retention of CO_2 in chronic lung disease may also result from the inequality between the amount of effective ventilation to a given area of the lung and the amount of blood perfusing that area. This mechanism may contribute as well to the retention of CO_2 in certain acute disorders such as pulmonary edema.

Causes of Respiratory Acidosis

Some of the major causes of respiratory acidosis are listed in Table 6-8.

Respiratory Alkalosis

Psychogenic Hyperventilation: Acute Respiratory Alkalosis

A 24-year-old woman was brought to the emergency room by a fellow worker, who reported that the patient said, "I'm going to die." The day before, the patient had had a fight with her boyfriend. She had been up all night and had gone to work without breakfast. At the office she had been distraught, and shortly after arriving there, she became light-headed and then began to hyperventilate uncontrollably. Soon thereafter, her face felt taut, and she began to experience tingling and numbness of the hands and feet. She remembers thinking that she must have had a stroke and that she was going to die. Upon arrival in the emergency room, she still had the same symptoms. She was conscious, breathing rapidly and deeply, and showed carpopedal spasm. Laboratory values obtained on her arterial blood at this time are shown in Table 6-9. It is of interest that the patient's father had died of a cerebrovascular accident two years earlier.

As soon as a brief history and physical examination were obtained, it was concluded that the patient was undergoing psychogenic hyperventilation. She was reassured that she had

Table 6-8
Causes of respiratory acidosis. The list has been divided into causes of acute and chronic respiratory acidosis. The distinction can be arbitrary; if a cause is present long enough (usually several days) to elicit renal compensation, then it may be considered chronic

Acute:
- Drug administration or usage
  - Drugs that depress the medullary respiratory center, especially sedatives during suicidal attempts
  - Opiates, alcohol, or anesthetics
- Asthma
- Mechanical obstruction of airway
- Pulmonary edema
- Familial periodic paralysis (acute hypokalemia or hyperkalemia)

Chronic:
- Emphysema
- Asthma
- Pulmonary fibrosis
- Abnormality of central nervous system
  - Central alveolar hypoventilation
  - Pickwickian syndrome
  - Poliomyelitis
  - Traumatic, neoplastic, or degenerative changes
- Extreme obesity
- Muscular dystrophy
- Kyphoscoliosis
- Myasthenia gravis
- Severe K^+ deficiency
- Polyneuritis

Table 6-9
H^+ balance as reflected in the arterial blood of a 24-year-old woman with psychogenic hyperventilation

Test	On Arrival in Emergency Room	Seven Minutes After Arrival
pH	7.56	7.41
PCO_2 (mm Hg)	23	41
$[H^+]$ (nMoles/L)	27.5	39
$[HCO_3^-]$ (mMoles/L)	20	25

not had a stroke and was not about to die, and then she was asked to breathe in and out from a paper bag. Within less than a minute, she calmed down, and all her signs and symptoms disappeared. Analysis of arterial blood 7 minutes after arrival at the hospital showed a return to normal H^+ balance. The physician on duty in the emergency room spoke with the patient for another 45 minutes, during which period he explained the dynamics of psychogenic hyperventilation. The patient returned to work later that morning.

Comment. Two factors may have contributed to the patient's light-headedness. She may have had hypoglycemia, since she had had nothing to eat. Once she began to hyperventilate, the decreased P_{CO_2} and resultant alkalosis led to increased resistance in the cerebral circulation and hence to some cerebral hypoxia. When the arterial values obtained on the patient's arrival are located on Figure 5-1, it may be seen that the patient had an uncomplicated, acute respiratory alkalosis; the slight decrease observed in $[HCO_3^-]$ resulted from the reaction shown in Equation 5-4. Her neurological manifestations (e.g., tingling, numbness, and carpopedal spasm) were probably due to the alkalosis, which led to a decrease in the plasma concentration of ionized Ca^{2+}.

Both the onset and offset of acute respiratory disturbances can develop very rapidly. The arterial pH begins to rise within 15 to 20 seconds after the beginning of hyperventilation, and for any degree of hyperventilation, it will be close to a new steady-state value within 10 to 15 minutes. Similarly, within less than a minute after the patient began to inspire air with a high P_{CO_2} (having filled the paper bag with CO_2 from her own expiration), her arterial pH began to drop, as reflected in the disappearance of the neurological symptoms and signs.

Causes of Respiratory Alkalosis

Table 6-10 lists some of the major causes of this condition. The division between acute and chronic disturbances can be somewhat arbitrary in certain instances. During short-term assisted hyperventilation, for example, the H^+ imbalance is likely to be only acute. If, however, a patient is mechanically hyperventilated for days or weeks, then the hypocapnia will be present long enough to elicit renal compensation in the form of decreased reabsorption of filtered HCO_3^-. The onset of this renal compensation, which may start within one or two days after the beginning of hyperventilation, constitutes the point at which an acute respiratory disturbance progresses to a chronic one.

Salicylate intoxication leads to a complicated series of H^+ imbalances. It begins as acute respiratory alkalosis while the drug is stimulating the medullary respiratory center, but later it is a

Table 6-10
Causes of respiratory alkalosis

Acute:
- Psychogenic hyperventilation
- Short-term assisted hyperventilation (e.g., during anesthesia)
- Acute hypoxemia
  - Certain patients with pulmonary edema
  - Pulmonary embolism
  - Certain patients with acute atelectasis or pneumothorax
- Drug administration
  - Salicylates; dinitrophenol
- Fever

Chronic:
- Prolonged hypoxemia
  - Residence at high altitude
  - Congenital heart disease
  - Anemia
- Cirrhosis
- Prolonged mechanical hyperventilation, usually for neurological diseases. (Some disorders of the central nervous system may themselves cause hyperventilation.)

mixed disturbance in which metabolic acidosis caused by salicylates (but through unknown mechanisms) usually predominates.

The means whereby cirrhosis leads to respiratory alkalosis are not known. The mechanisms may involve shunting of blood in the lungs, consequent chronic reduction of the partial pressure of oxygen in arterial blood (Pa_{O_2}), and hence stimulation of the respiratory center.

Summary

Clinical examples of each of the primary disturbances of H^+ balance are presented and discussed. Detailed attention is given to the metabolic alkalosis that is caused by prolonged vomiting, because both the generation and maintenance of this type of alkalosis involve complicated and multiple pathways. In addition to the loss of gastric HCl, the roles of K^+ deficiency and contraction of the extracellular fluid volume are stressed, as is the importance of NaCl repletion in correcting the alkalosis.

Examples are given of both acute and chronic respiratory disturbances. The point of transition from the former to the latter may be defined as the time when the abnormal arterial P_{CO_2} changes the rate at which the kidneys reabsorb filtered HCO_3^-, that is, the point at which the renal compensation for a primary respiratory disturbance becomes manifest.

The major clinical causes for each of the primary acid-base disturbances have been listed in tables. Although several of the causes not taken up in this chapter will be further described in the problems and in other chapters, no attempt will be made to consider all the causes. Rather, the purpose has been to illustrate a principle for approaching the systematic and logical analysis of imbalances of H^+. Armed with this approach, the student will be in a position to understand other specific acid-base disorders, as well as to understand other systems for analyzing such disorders.

Problem 6-1

H^+ Imbalance in the Cerebrospinal Fluid. A 44-year-old man was admitted to the hospital with diabetic ketoacidosis that had been precipitated by a respiratory infection. During the three days preceding the admission, he had eaten little and had taken no insulin. Physical examination on admission revealed a lethargic person who, however, could be easily aroused and was able to give a clear history. The patient showed Kussmaul respiration and had a temperature of 39.2°C; his skin and mucous membranes were dry. His acid-base status on admission, in both arterial blood and cerebrospinal fluid (CSF), is shown in Table 6-11. Why was the pH of the CSF so much higher than the arterial pH? What would the pH of the CSF have been if the $[HCO_3^-]$ of CSF had been the same as in arterial blood? Would it then have been possible to arouse the patient?

The patient was treated with intravenous infusions of NaCl, insulin, KCl, and 135 mMoles of $NaHCO_3$ – much as the patient with diabetic ketoacidosis described earlier in this chapter. Al-

Table 6-11
Acid-base status of arterial blood and cerebrospinal fluid (CSF) in a 44-year-old man before, during, and after treatment for diabetic ketoacidosis

Test	On Admission	After 7 Hours of Treatment	After 22 Hours of Treatment
Arterial blood:			
pH	6.99	7.39	7.42
P_{CO_2} (mm Hg)	11	31	35
$[HCO_3^-]$ (mMoles/L)	3	18	22
CSF*:			
pH	7.25	7.14	7.30
P_{CO_2} (mm Hg)	20	41	43
$[HCO_3^-]$ (mMoles/L)	8	13	19

*Normal values for CSF: pH = 7.29 to 7.32; $[HCO_3^-]$ = 20 to 24 mMoles/L; P_{CO_2} = 45 to 50 mm Hg; pK' for Henderson-Hasselbalch equation in CSF = 6.13.

Modified from J. B. Posner, A. G. Swanson, and F. Plum, *Arch. Neurol.* 12:479, 1965.

though the arterial pH was thereby corrected to the normal range (Table 6-11, After 7 Hours of Treatment), the patient was now stuporous and could not converse coherently. How do you explain the mental deterioration? How might the patient have been aroused?

By the next morning, and without further treatment, the patient was quite alert and coherent. How do you explain the spontaneous improvement in mental status?

Two patients, one with an uncomplicated acute respiratory acidosis and the other with a pure metabolic acidosis of 5 hours' duration, each have an arterial pH of 7.20. Which of these patients is likely to have the lower pH in the CSF? Which would be more likely to have an abnormal mental status?

Problem 6-2

Posthypercapnic Alkalosis. A 63-year-old man had had chronic bronchitis for about twenty years, and during the past ten years he had developed emphysema and heart failure. The latter had been treated for three years with a low-salt diet, digitalization, and mild diuretic therapy. On the present hospital admission (which was prompted by increasing dyspnea and somnolence), his laboratory values were those shown in Table 6-12. Analyze his acid-base status at this time. Why was the arterial [HCO_3^-] abnormally high? Why was it even higher in venous plasma? Why was the plasma [Cl^-] low?

Because of the severity of his symptoms resulting from respiratory failure, it was decided to ventilate the patient artificially while giving him oxygen. Within 20 minutes after putting the patient on a mechanical respirator, it was noticed that he had

Table 6-12
Results of laboratory tests on a 63-year-old man with chronic bronchitis, emphysema, and heart failure

Test	On Admission	After 20 Minutes of Hyperventilation
Arterial blood:		
pH	7.29	7.64
PCO_2 (mm Hg)	64	28
[HCO_3^-] (mMoles/L)	30	29
PO_2 (mm Hg)	41	89
Venous plasma:		
[Na^+] (mEq/L)	142	–
[Cl^-] (mEq/L)	88	–
[K^+] (mEq/L)	4.5	–
[HCO_3^-] (mEq/L)	33	–

tetany. Arterial blood values at this time are also shown in Table 6-12. Explain what had happened. How would you correct the situation?

Selected References

General

J.A.M.A. Editorial. Acid-base imbalance in pulmonary edema. *J.A.M.A.* 216:1337, 1971.

Kassirer, J. P. Serious acid-base disorders. *N. Engl. J. Med.* 291:773, 1974.

Kildeberg, P. *Clinical Acid-Base Physiology.* Copenhagen: Munksgaard, 1968.

Lennon, E.J. Body Buffering Mechanisms. In E. D. Frohlich (ed.), *Pathophysiology: Altered Regulatory Mechanisms in Disease.* Philadelphia: Lippincott, 1972.

Makoff, D. L. Acid-Base Metabolism. In M. H. Maxwell and C. R. Kleeman (eds.), *Clinical Disorders of Fluid and Electrolyte Metabolism* (2nd ed.). New York: McGraw-Hill, 1972.

Masoro, E. J., and Siegel, P. D. *Acid-Base Regulation: Its Physiology and Pathophysiology.* Philadelphia: Saunders, 1971.

Welt, L. G. *Clinical Disorders of Hydration and Acid-Base Equilibrium* (3rd ed.). Boston: Little, Brown, 1970.

Winters, R. W. (ed.). *The Body Fluids in Pediatrics.* Boston: Little, Brown, 1973.

Winters, R. W., Engel, K., and Dell, R. B. *Acid-Base Physiology in Medicine: A Self-Instruction Program.* Cleveland: The London Co., 1967.

Metabolic Acidosis

Alberti, K. G. M. M., and Nattrass, M. Lactic acidosis. *Lancet* 2:25, 1977.

Chazan, J. A., Stenson, R., and Kurland, G. S. The acidosis of cardiac arrest. *N. Engl. J. Med.* 278:360, 1968.

Cohen, R. D., and Woods, H. F. *Clinical and Biochemical Aspects of Lactic Acidosis.* Oxford, Eng.: Blackwell, 1976.

Davidson, M. B., Bozarth, W. R., Challoner, D. R., and Goodner, C. J. Phenformin, hypoglycemia and lactic acidosis. Report of attempted suicide. *N. Engl. J. Med.* 275:886, 1966.

Felig, P. Diabetic ketoacidosis. *N. Engl. J. Med.* 290:1360, 1974.

Garella, S., Chang, B. S., and Kahn, S. I. Dilution acidosis and contraction alkalosis: Review of a concept. *Kidney Int.* 8:279, 1975.

Garella, S., Dana, C. L., and Chazan, J. A. Severity of metabolic acidosis as a determinant of bicarbonate requirements. *N. Engl. J. Med.* 289:121, 1973.

Gerich, J. E., Lorenzi, M., Bier, D. M., Schneider, V., Tsalikian, E., Karam, J. H., and Forsham, P. H. Prevention of human diabetic ketoacidosis by somatostatin: Evidence for an essential role of glucagon. *N. Engl. J. Med.* 292:985, 1975.

Goodman, A. D., Lemann, J., Jr., Lennon, E. J., and Relman, A. S. Production, excretion, and net balance of fixed acid in patients with renal acidosis. *J. Clin. Invest.* 44:495, 1965.

Heird, W. C., Dell, R. B., Driscoll, J. M., Grebin, B., and Winters, R. W. Metabolic acidosis resulting from intravenous alimentation mixtures containing synthetic amino acids. *N. Engl. J. Med.* 287:943, 1972.

King, A. J., Cooke, N. H., McCuish, A., Clarke, B. F., and Kirby, B. J. Acid-base changes during treatment of diabetic ketoacidosis. *Lancet* 1:478, 1974.

Lancet Editorial. Lactic acidosis. *Lancet* 2:27, 1973.

Lancet Editorial. Sodium bicarbonate in cardiac arrest. *Lancet* 1:946, 1976.

Lathem, W. Hyperchloremic acidosis in chronic pyelonephritis. *N. Engl. J. Med.* 258:1031, 1958.

Lemann, J., Jr., Litzow, J. R., and Lennon, E. J. The effects of chronic acid loads in normal man: Further evidence for the participation of bone mineral in the defense against chronic metabolic acidosis. *J. Clin. Invest.* 45:1608, 1966.

Medalle, R., Webb, R., and Waterhouse, C. Lactic acidosis and associated hypoglycemia. *Arch. Intern. Med.* 128:273, 1971.

Oliva, P. B. Lactic acidosis. *Am. J. Med.* 48:209, 1970.

Pierce, N. F., Fedson, D. S., Brigham, K. L., Mitra, R. C., Sack, R. B., and Mondal, A. The ventilatory response to acute base deficit in humans. Time course during development and correction of metabolic acidosis. *Ann. Intern. Med.* 72:633, 1970.

Relman, A. S. Lactic acidosis and a possible new treatment. *N. Engl. J. Med.* 298:564, 1978.

Simpson, D. P. Control of hydrogen ion homeostasis and renal acidosis. *Medicine* (Baltimore) 50:503, 1971.

Soler, N. G., Bennett, M. A., Dixon, K., FitzGerald, M. G., and Malins, J. M. Potassium balance during treatment of diabetic ketoacidosis, with special reference to the use of bicarbonate. *Lancet* 2:665, 1972.

Waters, W. C., Hall, J. D., and Schwartz, W. B. Spontaneous lactic acidosis. The nature of the acid-base disturbance and considerations in diagnosis and management. *Am. J. Med.* 35:781, 1963.

Metabolic Alkalosis

Aber, G. M., Sampson, P. A., Whitehead, T. P., and Brooke, B. N. The role of chloride in the correction of alkalosis associated with potassium depletion. *Lancet* 2:1028, 1962.

Cannon, P. J., Heinemann, H. O., Albert, M. S., Laragh, J. H., and Winters R. W. "Contraction" alkalosis after diuresis of edematous patient with ethacrynic acid. *Ann. Intern. Med.* 62:979, 1965.

DeRubertis, F. R., Michelis, M. F., Beck, N., and Davis, B. B. Complications of diuretic therapy: Severe alkalosis and syndrome resembling inappropriate secretion of antidiuretic hormone. *Metabolism* 19:709, 1970.

Eckel, R. E., Norris, J. E. C., and Pope, C. E., II. Basic amino acids as intracellular cations in K deficiency. *Am. J. Physiol.* 193:644, 1958.

Fenn, W. O., and Cobb, D. M. The potassium equilibrium in muscle. *J. Gen. Physiol.* 17:629, 1934.

Fernandez, P. C., and Kovant, P. J. Metabolic acidosis reversed by the combination of magnesium hydroxide and a cation-exchange resin. *N. Engl. J. Med.* 286:23, 1972.

Garella, S., Chang, B. S., and Kahn, S. I. Dilution acidosis and contraction alkalosis: Review of a concept. *Kidney Int.* 8:279, 1975.

Kassirer, J. P., Berkman, P. M., Lawrenz, D. R., and Schwartz, W. B. The critical role of chloride in the correction of hypokalemic alkalosis in man. *Am. J. Med.* 38:172, 1965.

Kassirer, J. P., and Schwartz, W. B. The response of normal man to selective depletion of hydrochloric acid. Factors in the genesis of persistent gastric alkalosis. *Am. J. Med.* 40:10, 1966.

Kassirer, J. P., and Schwartz, W. B. Correction of metabolic alkalosis in man without repair of potassium deficiency. A re-evaluation of the role of potassium. *Am. J. Med.* 40:19, 1966.

Kilburn, K. H. Shock, seizures, and coma with alkalosis during mechanical ventilation. *Ann. Intern. Med.* 65:977, 1966.

Lemann, J., Jr., Lennon, E. J., Goodman, A. D., Litzow, J. R., and Relman, A. S. The net balance of acid in subjects given large loads of acid or alkali. *J. Clin. Invest.* 44:507, 1965.

Nattie, E. E., and Tenney, S. M. Effect of potassium depletion on cerebrospinal fluid bicarbonate homeostasis. *Am. J. Physiol.* 231:579, 1976.

Needle, M. A., Kaloyanides, G. J., and Schwartz, W. B. The effects of selective depletion of hydrochloric acid on acid-base and electrolyte equilibrium. *J. Clin. Invest.* 43:1836, 1964.

Orloff, J. Kennedy, T. J., Jr., and Berliner, R. W. The effect of potassium in nephrectomized rats with hypokalemic alkalosis. *J. Clin. Invest.* 32:538, 1953.

Refsum, H. E. Hypokalemic alkalosis with paradoxical aciduria during artificial ventilation of patients with pulmonary insufficiency and high plasma bicarbonate concentration. *Scand. J. Clin. Lab. Invest.* 13:481, 1961.

Robin, E. D. Abnormalities of acid-base regulation in chronic pulmonary disease, with special reference to hypercapnia and extracellular alkalosis. *N. Engl. J. Med.* 268:917, 1963.

Schwartz, W. B., Hays, R. M., Polak, A., and Haynie, G. D. Effects of chronic hypercapnia on electrolyte and acid-base equilibrium. II. Recovery, with special reference to the influence of chloride intake. *J. Clin. Invest.* 40:1238, 1961.

Schwartz, W. B., van Ypersele de Strihou, C., and Kassirer, J. P. Role of anions in metabolic alkalosis and potassium deficiency. *N. Engl. J. Med.* 279:630, 1968.

Seldin, D. W., and Rector, F. C., Jr. The generation and maintenance of metabolic alkalosis. *Kidney Int.* 1:306, 1972.

Tannen, R. L., Bleich, H. L., and Schwartz, W. B. The renal response to acid loads in metabolic alkalosis; an assessment of the mechanisms regulating acid excretion. *J. Clin. Invest.* 45:562, 1966.

Taradash, M. R., and Jacobson, L. B. Vasodilator therapy of idiopathic lactic acidosis. *N. Engl. J. Med.* 293:468, 1975.

Tuller, M. A., and Mehdi, F. Compensatory hypoventilation and hypercapnia in primary metabolic alkalosis. *Am. J. Med.* 50:281, 1971.

Wallace, M., Richards, P., Chesser, E., and Wrong, O. Persistent alkalosis and hypokalaemia caused by surreptitious vomiting. *Q. J. Med.* 37: 577, 1968.

Respiratory Acidosis

Anthonisen, N. R., and Smith, H. J. Respiratory acidosis as a consequence of pulmonary edema. *Ann. Intern. Med.* 62:991, 1965.

Chazan, J. A., Stenson, R., and Kurland, G. S. The acidosis of cardiac arrest. *N. Engl. J. Med.* 278:360, 1968.

Goldring, R. M., Turino, G. M., and Heinemann, H. O. Respiratory-renal adjustments in chronic hypercapnia in man. Extracellular bicarbonate concentration and the regulation of ventilation. *Am. J. Med.* 51:772, 1971.

Kassirer, J. P. Serious acid-base disorders. *N. Engl. J. Med.* 291:773, 1974.

Makoff, D. L. Acid-Base Metabolism. In M. H. Maxwell and C. R. Kleeman (eds.), *Clinical Disorders of Fluid and Electrolyte Metabolism* (2nd ed.). New York: McGraw-Hill, 1972.

Miller, A., Chusid, E. L., and Samortin, T. G. Acute, reversible respiratory acidosis in cardiogenic pulmonary edema. *J.A.M.A.* 216:1315, 1971.

Polak, A., Haynie, G. D., Hays, R. M., and Schwartz, W. B. Effects of chronic hypercapnia on electrolyte and acid-base equilibrium. I. Adaptation. *J. Clin. Invest.* 40:1223, 1961.

Remmers, J. E., DeGroot, W. J., Sauerland, E. K., and Anch, A. M. Pathogenesis of upper airway occlusion during sleep. *J. Appl. Physiol.* 44:931, 1978.

Robin, E. D. Abnormalities of acid-base regulation in chronic pulmonary disease, with special reference to hypercapnia and extracellular alkalosis. *N. Engl. J. Med.* 268:917, 1963.

Schwartz, W. B., Hays, R. M., Polak, A., and Haynie, G. D. Effects of chronic hypercapnia on electrolyte and acid-base equilibrium. II. Recovery, with special reference to the influence of chloride intake. *J. Clin. Invest.* 40:1238, 1961.

West, J. B. Causes of carbon dioxide retention in lung disease. *N. Engl. J. Med.* 284:1232, 1971.

Respiratory Alkalosis

Brown, E. B., Jr. Physiological effects of hyperventilation. *Physiol. Rev.* 33:445, 1953.

Cohen, J. J., Madias, N. E., Wolf, C. J., and Schwartz, W. B. Regulation of acid-base equilibrium in chronic hypocapnia. Evidence that the response of the kidney is not geared to the defense of extracellular [H^+]. *J. Clin. Invest.* 57:1483, 1976.

Eichenholz, A., Mulhausen, R. O., Anderson, W. E., and MacDonald, F. M. Primary hypocapnia: A cause of metabolic acidosis. *J. Appl. Physiol.* 17:283, 1962.

Eldridge, F., and Salzer, J. Effect of respiratory alkalosis on blood lactate and pyruvate in humans. *J. Appl. Physiol.* 22:461, 1967.

Engel, K., Kildeberg, P., and Winters, R. W. Quantitative displacement of blood acid-base status in acute hypocapnia. *Scand. J. Clin. Lab. Invest.* 23:5, 1969.

Hansen, J. E., Stelter, G. P., and Vogel, J. A. Arterial pyruvate, lactate, pH, and P_{CO_2} during work at sea level and high altitude. *J. Appl. Physiol.* 23:523, 1967.

Hurtado, A., and Aste-Salazar, H. Arterial blood gases and acid-base balance at sea level and at high altitudes. *J. Appl. Physiol.* 1:304, 1948.

J.A.M.A. Editorial. Acid-base imbalance in pulmonary edema. *J.A.M.A.* 216:1337, 1971.

Kassirer, J. P. Serious acid-base disorders. *N. Engl. J. Med.* 291:773, 1974.

Kety, S. S., and Schmidt, C. F. The effect of active and passive hyperventilation on cerebral blood flow, cerebral oxygen consumption, cardiac output, and blood pressure of normal young men. *J. Clin. Invest.* 25:107, 1946.

Kilburn, K. H. Shock, seizures, and coma with alkalosis during mechanical ventilation. *Ann. Intern. Med.* 65:977, 1966.

Makoff, D. L. Acid-Base Metabolism. In M. H. Maxwell and C. R. Kleeman (eds.), *Clinical Disorders of Fluid and Electrolyte Metabolism* (2nd ed.). New York: McGraw-Hill, 1972.

Saltzman, H. A., Heyman, A., and Sieker, H. O. Correlation of clinical and physiologic manifestations of sustained hyperventilation. *N. Engl. J. Med.* 268:1431, 1963.

Stead, E. A., Jr. Hyperventilation. *D.M.* February 1960, pp. 1–32.

Tenney, S. M., and Lamb, T. W. Physiological Consequences of Hypoventilation and Hyperventilation. In W. O. Fenn and H. Rahn (eds.), *Handbook of Physiology,* Section 3, Respiration, vol. 2. Washington, D.C.: American Physiological Society, 1965.

Tyor, M. P., and Sieker, H. O. Biochemical blood gas and peripheral circulatory alterations in hepatic coma. *Am. J. Med.* 27:50, 1959.

Cerebrospinal Fluid

Fencl, V. Distribution of H^+ and HCO_3^- in Cerebral Fluids. In B. K. Siesjö and S. C. Sørensen (eds.), *Ion Homeostasis of the Brain. The Regulation of Hydrogen and Potassium Ion Concentrations in Cerebral Intra- and Extracellular Fluids.* New York: Academic, 1971.

Kalin, E. M., Tweed, W. A., Lee, J., and MacKeen, W. L. Cerebrospinal-fluid acid-base and electrolyte changes resulting from cerebral anoxia in man. *N. Engl. J. Med.* 293:1013, 1975.

Katzman, R., and Pappius, H. M. *Brain Electrolytes and Fluid Metabolism.* Baltimore: Williams & Wilkins, 1973. Chap. 10.

Leusen, I. Regulation of cerebrospinal fluid composition with reference to breathing. *Physiol. Rev.* 52:1, 1972.

Mitchell, R. A., Herbert, D. A., and Carman, C. T. Acid-base constants and temperature coefficients for cerebrospinal fluid. *J. Appl. Physiol.* 20:27, 1965.

Nattie, E. E., and Romer, L. CSF HCO_3^- regulation in isosmotic conditions: The role of brain P_{CO_2} and plasma HCO_3^-. *Respir. Physiol.* 33:17, 1978.

Pappenheimer, J. R. *The Ionic Composition of Cerebral Extracellular Fluid and its Relation to Control of Breathing.* The Harvey Lectures, Series 61, 1965-66. New York: Academic, 1967, pp. 71-94.

Plum, F., and Price, R. W. Acid-base balance of cisternal and lumbar cerebrospinal fluid in hospital patients. *N. Engl. J. Med.* 289:1346, 1973.

Posner, J. B., Swanson, A. G., and Plum, F. Acid-base balance in cerebrospinal fluid. *Arch. Neurol.* 12:479, 1965.

Severinghaus, J. W., and Carcelén, B. A. Cerebrospinal fluid in man native to high altitude. *J. Appl. Physiol.* 19:319, 1964.

Siesjö, B. H. The regulation of cerebrospinal fluid pH. *Kidney Int.* 1:360, 1972.

Winters, R. W., Lowder, J. A., and Ordway, N. K. Observations on carbon dioxide tension during recovery from metabolic acidosis. *J. Clin. Invest.* 37:640, 1953.

7 : Diuretics

Clinical Definition

Diuresis is defined as urine flow that is greater than normal, that is, in excess of 1 ml per minute in an adult human. Strictly speaking, therefore, a diuretic is any agent that increases the flow of urine; the clinical definition, however, is much narrower. Physicians limit the term to drugs that achieve one of two major effects: (1) the mobilization of edema fluid and (2) an osmotic diuresis to increase the renal excretion of toxins. Of these, the first is by far the more common application. In Chapter 3 we emphasized that generalized edema, being an expansion of the interstitial fluid compartment, reflects a positive external balance of Na^+. An acceptable clinical definition of a *diuretic* is therefore a drug that furthers a negative balance of Na^+ by increasing the renal excretion of Na^+ and its attendant anions, mainly Cl^-. Most of the diuretics in current vogue accomplish this purpose by inhibiting the tubular reabsorption of Cl^- (in the ascending thick limb of Henle) or of Na^+ (in the remainder of the nephron).

Some so-called diuretics are actually applied more widely to the treatment of nonedematous states, such as hypertension (Chap. 14), nephrogenic diabetes insipidus (Chap. 13), renal tubular acidosis (Chap. 12), hypercalciuria, hypercalcemia, and intoxications. Such other uses, though important, are merely mentioned here; further details can be found in many of the references cited at the end of this chapter. The present discussion will be limited to the diuretic action of the agents currently used for this purpose.

Classification

Diuretic drugs have been classified according to their chemical structure, mode of action, renal site of action, or their effect on various renal functions. In this chapter, however, we have categorized them according to their current clinical usage and effectiveness (Table 7-1). The last term is used advisedly; it takes into account not only the potency of diuretic action following a single, maximally effective dose, but even more importantly, the efficacy during prolonged use. Thus, mannitol may be the most potent diuretic in the pharmacological sense (Table 7-1), but for reasons detailed below, it is not the most effective agent.

Table 7-1
Classification and properties of diuretics used in clinical practice
The values for urinary excretion indicate rates in adults during normal acid-base balance and maximally effective therapy. They thus serve as a comparison of efficacy, although these peak rates are not necessarily seen during routine treatment

Diuretic	Representative Chemical Structure	Proportion of Filtered Na^+ Excreted (%)	Peak Urinary Excretion $\dot{V}$ (ml/min)	Na^+ (μEq/min)	K^+ (μEq/min)	Cl^- (μEq/min)	HCO_3^- (μEq/min)	Major Site(s) of Action in the Kidney (key in Fig. 7-1)
Healthy state; no diuretic		0.6	1	100	70	100	2	
Moderately effective:								
Chlorothiazide	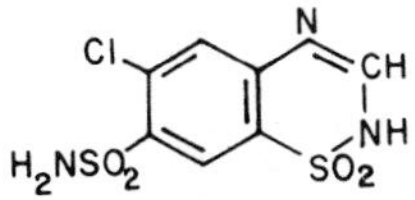 Cl, N, CH, NH, H_2NSO_2, SO_2	8	3	400	150	450	70	3
Very effective:								
Ethacrynic acid	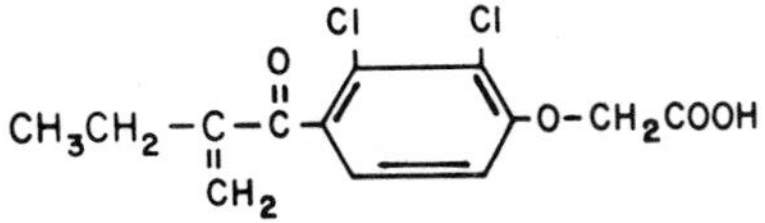 Cl, Cl, O, CH_3CH_2-C-C, CH_2, $O-CH_2COOH$	25	8	1,000	100	1,250	5	2, 3
Furosemide	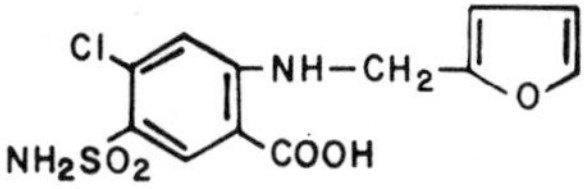 Cl, $NH-CH_2$, O, NH_2SO_2, COOH	25	8	1,000	100	1,250	5	2, 3
Adjuvants:								
Aldosterone antagonists, e.g., spironolactone*	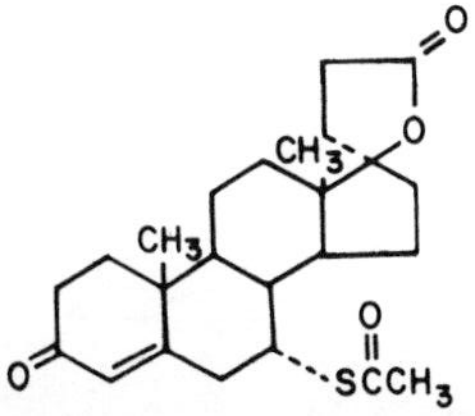 O, O, CH_3, CH_3, O, O, $SCCH_3$	2	1.5	150	50	150	3	4

K^+-sparing, e.g., triamterene		2	3	275	15	250	40	4
Osmotic: Mannitol	$HOH_2C-C(H)(OH)-C(H)(OH)-C(OH)(H)-C(OH)(H)-CH_2OH$	5	10	700	150	1,000	35	2, 3

*Aldosterone antagonists work only in edematous states that are associated with hyperaldosteronism; in these conditions, spironolactone reverses the abnormal pattern of Na^+ and K^+ excretion toward the normal state or slightly beyond.

Adapted from G. H. Mudge, in L. S. Goodman and A. Gilman (eds.), *The Pharmacological Basis of Therapeutics* (5th ed.). New York: Macmillan, 1975; and M. Goldberg, in J. Orloff and R. W. Berliner (eds.), *Handbook of Physiology,* Section 8, Renal Physiology. Washington, D.C.: American Physiological Society, 1973.

The organomercurials are not included in Table 7-1, because they are seldom prescribed today. For many years, these compounds were the most effective diuretics available; they can, in fact, be almost as potent in raising NaCl excretion as ethacrynic acid and furosemide. The discovery of the organomercurials as diuretic drugs, which occurred in the course of treating patients for syphilis, is a fascinating story, and the elucidation of their mode of action was a model of logical pharmacological research. Moreover, one of the most potent oral diuretics in use today — ethacrynic acid — was developed as an outgrowth of understanding the action of organomercurials. Because the mercury compounds must be given parenterally, however, they fell out of use when oral diuretic agents were introduced. Today, organomercurials are rarely employed.

For somewhat analogous reasons, inhibitors of carbonic anhydrase (e.g., acetazolamide) have been omitted from Table 7-1. These drugs reduce the secretion of H^+ and hence the reabsorption of HCO_3^- in the proximal tubules (see Identifying Sites of Renal Action, below), thereby enhancing the excretion of $NaHCO_3$ and especially that of $KHCO_3$. Although they are still used by some physicians to enhance the effect of the "very effective" diuretics that act on the loop of Henle, this application of the carbonic anhydrase inhibitors is relatively rare; they are employed more commonly in nondiuretic applications, such as the treatment of glaucoma, petit mal epilepsy, and conditions where alkalinization of the urine is desired.

The thiazides, ethacrynic acid, and furosemide are currently the most commonly used drugs for mobilizing generalized edema fluid. When one considers that the thiazides can increase the urinary excretion of NaCl threefold or fourfold (Table 7-1), it is clear that their potency should suffice for most clinical problems. Yet, furosemide and ethacrynic acid are used more frequently than the thiazides in the routine treatment of edema. This fact probably reflects the tendency to think that "if a little is good, much is better." In clinical practice, such thinking is usually a mistake; the better rule in handling patients is to give the least amount and number of medications that will do the job and to induce a change in balance slowly rather than rapidly. In this vein, we should introduce here a point that will be emphasized later in this chapter: *A diuretic is far less likely to cause serious imbalance of electrolytes if it is given every other day than if it is given daily.*

The adjuvant diuretics in current use consist of two classes: aldosterone antagonists and those that reduce the renal excretion of K^+. Spironolactone is quite costly, and it is not a very potent natriuretic (Table 7-1). It is therefore most commonly given (often in conjunction with another diuretic) to patients with refractory edema, especially when it is thought to involve hyperaldosteronism. At optimal dosage, triamterene is a fairly effective natriuretic by itself (Table 7-1), even in the absence of aldosterone. Nevertheless, it is used most extensively in conjunction with other diuretics to take advantage of its property of reducing renal K^+ excretion. It has been observed, for example, that when chlorothiazide is used alone and without K^+ supplements, there is a rather high incidence of hypokalemia; on the other hand, when triamterene is given by itself, hyperkalemia may occur. The incidence of both extremes of K^+ balance is reduced when the drugs are used together; furthermore, natriuresis is enhanced by the combination.

At peak effect, the osmotic diuretic mannitol causes the largest increase in urine flow of any of the diuretics in common use; it also quite effectively increases the excretion of NaCl (Table 7-1). One might well ask, therefore, why mannitol is not used in the treatment of edema. There are at least three reasons: (1) it is effective as a diuretic only when given parenterally; (2) when administered as a bolus (Fig. 1-6), it causes an acute rise in plasma osmolality; and therefore (3) a large portion of the water that is lost will come from the intracellular rather than the extracellular space. The first reason obviously makes mannitol less practical and desirable than oral agents in chronic diseases, where diuretics may have to be used for years. The second and third reasons render the use of mannitol less effective in mobilizing edema fluid, as well as possibly being dangerous. Patients with generalized edema have an expanded extracellular fluid volume (Chap. 3). Raising their plasma osmolality will cause water to shift from their intracellular into their extracellular space, and this increment added to an already enlarged ECF may precipitate heart failure and pulmonary edema. This danger lurks especially in congestive heart failure, which is the commonest cause of generalized edema. Even though osmotic diuretics are used primarily to increase the excretion of water rather than Na^+, they are included in Table 7-1 because they are used to induce diuresis and because they satisfy the above definition in that they increase Na^+ excretion.

Identifying Sites of Renal Action

Later in this chapter we shall discuss each diuretic listed in Table 7-1 from the following points of view: (1) its chemical structure; (2) its mode of action, both at the gross and molecular levels; (3) its site(s) of action, especially within the kidney; and (4) its untoward effects. Understanding of item (3) will be aided by first reviewing the rationale for some of the experimental techniques applied to investigating the action of diuretics on the kidney.

Although important facts about the action of diuretics have been gained through various micropuncture techniques, some of the most useful information has been obtained from clearance studies. Such studies have the advantage that they can be conducted not only on kidneys in situ, but also on unanesthetized humans and on human patients. In addition to revealing the magnitude of urine flow and of the excretion of NaCl and other ions (Table 7-1), clearance techniques can often tell us something about the nephron segments where diuretics act. The bases for such deductions are diagrammed in Figure 7-1; they follow from our knowledge of certain aspects of renal physiology.

We know from micropuncture experiments that 80 to 90 percent of the HCO_3^- that is filtered is reabsorbed in the proximal tubule, about 2 percent in the loops of Henle, and perhaps 8 percent in the distal tubule (Fig. 7-2). Hence, any diuretic that causes a moderate increase in the urinary excretion of HCO_3^- might act at any one of these three sites. If, however, a drug induces an increase in HCO_3^- excretion that equals or exceeds 20 percent of the filtered load of HCO_3^- (GFR $\cdot\ P_{HCO_3^-} \approx 3{,}000\ \mu$Eq per minute in an adult human), then it may be concluded that this drug must act at least partly on the proximal tubule (site 1 in Fig. 7-1). Inasmuch as 20 percent of a normal filtered load amounts to about 600 μEq per minute,

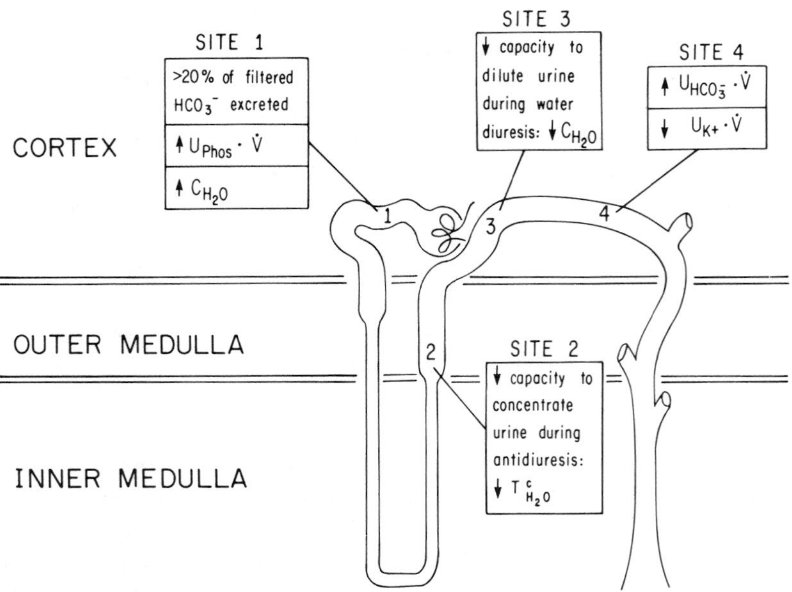

Figure 7-1
Criteria for localizing the sites of action of diuretics in the nephron.

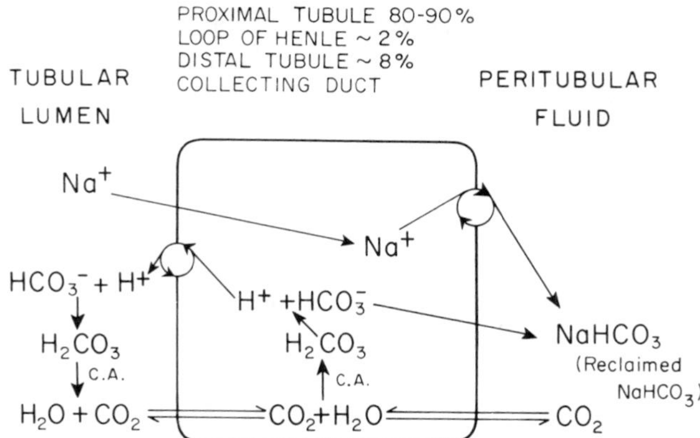

Figure 7-2
Mechanism for the reabsorption of *filtered* HCO_3^-. In the proximal tubular lumen, but not in the distal, tubular fluid is exposed to carbonic anhydrase (*C.A.*). The percentages indicate the proportion of the filtered HCO_3^- that is reabsorbed in each of the nephron segments. From H. Valtin, *Renal Function: Mechanisms Preserving Fluid and Solute Balance in Health.* Boston: Little, Brown, 1973.

it is clear that a major proximal site cannot be invoked to explain the action of any of the diuretics listed in Table 7-1. This effect is seen with carbonic anhydrase inhibitors, such as acetazolamide. It is of interest, however, that the mild increase in HCO_3^- excretion observed with chlorothiazide (Table 7-1) may be due to inhibition of carbonic anhydrase in both the proximal tubule and more distal segments. Although chlorothiazide was developed in the search for potent carbonic anhydrase inhibitors, its major diuretic action does not depend on this property.

Again from micropuncture studies, we know that virtually all the phosphate that is filtered is normally reabsorbed in the proximal tubule. Therefore, a diuretic that consistently increases the urinary excretion of phosphate is thought to act partly on the proximal tubule. Acetazolamide is an example; it can raise the urinary excretion of phosphate to as much as 30 percent of the filtered load. The effect need not be, and probably is not, a direct one on the tubular transport of phosphate, but it may be exerted indirectly by reducing the reabsorption of Na^+.

Clearance experiments can also yield information on whether a diuretic acts on the ascending limb of Henle's loop (ALH; site 2, Fig. 7-1), on the early distal tubule (site 3), or on both. This purpose is accomplished by testing the effect of a given drug *both* in the presence of antidiuretic hormone (ADH) and in its absence. In the first instance, one assesses the influence of the drug on the capacity to concentrate urine, expressed as $T^c_{H_2O}$; in the second, on the capacity to dilute the urine, expressed as C_{H_2O}.

Free water (i.e., water that is free of solutes) is generated by the kidney when solute, mainly NaCl, is reabsorbed to the virtual exclusion of water. This occurs mainly at two sites within the nephron: site 2 in Figure 7-1 (the ascending limb of Henle) and site 3 (the early distal tubule), which like the ALH, is relatively impermeable to water and remains so even in the presence of ADH. Because the generation of free water is a prerequisite to rendering urine more dilute than plasma, site 2, which lies in the medullary region, is known as the *medullary diluting segment,* and site 3 is known as the *cortical diluting segment.*

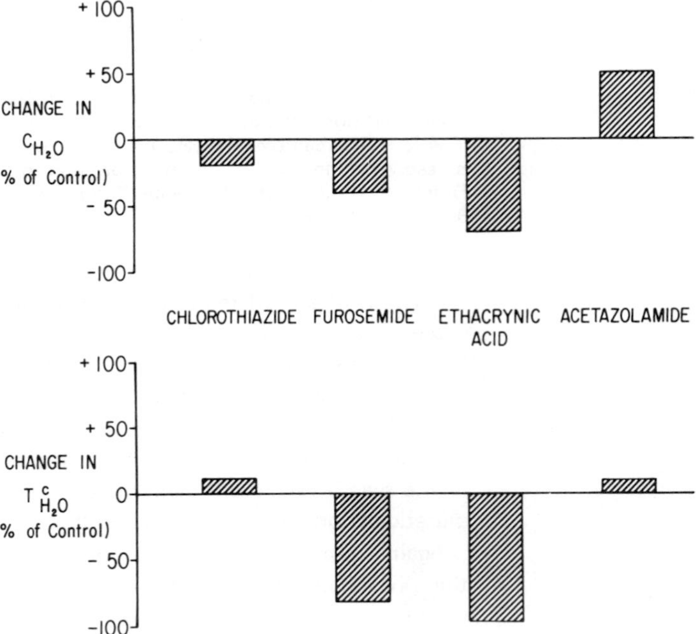

Figure 7-3
Changes in C_{H_2O} (free water clearance) when a diuretic is given in the absence of antidiuretic hormone (ADH) and changes in $T^c_{H_2O}$ (free water reabsorption in the collecting ducts) when the same diuretic is given in the presence of ADH. Modified from M. Goldberg, in J. Orloff and R. W. Berliner (eds.), *Handbook of Physiology,* Section 8, Renal Physiology. Washington, D.C.: American Physiological Society, 1973.

The reasoning for deducing the site of action of a diuretic from its effect on $T^c_{H_2O}$ and C_{H_2O} goes as follows. If a diuretic (e.g., chlorothiazide; Fig. 7-3) inhibits the reabsorption of NaCl in the cortical diluting segment but not in the medullary diluting segment, we would expect a decrease in the capacity of the kidney to dilute the urine, which is gauged as a reduction in the net removal of water from plasma during a water diuresis, or a decreased C_{H_2O}. The capacity to concentrate the urine during antidiuresis, however, should not be compromised, since the reabsorption of NaCl from the ascending limbs of Henle continues unabated. It is this reabsorptive process that initiates the countercurrent multiplier system and creates the corticopapillary interstitial osmotic gradient, which is ultimately responsible for reabsorption of free water from the collecting ducts, increasing $T^c_{H_2O}$ (Fig. 7-3). (The slight increase in $T^c_{H_2O}$ with chlorothiazide may reflect inhibition of carbonic anhydrase and hence increased delivery of Na^+ to site 2; see discussion of acetazolamide, below.) On the other hand, diuretics such as furosemide and ethacrynic acid decrease both C_{H_2O} during water diuresis and $T^c_{H_2O}$ during antidiuresis (Fig. 7-3). This fact is interpreted to reflect inhibition of NaCl transport at both sites 2 and 3 in Figure 7-1. Inhibition at site 2 reduces or abolishes the corticopapillary interstitial osmotic gradient and therefore decreases $T^c_{H_2O}$; inhibition at both sites lessens the generation of free water and therefore reduces C_{H_2O}. If the reasoning is correct, especially in regard to inhibition at site 2, then one should be able to demonstrate a diminution in the corticopapillary gradient as an animal in antidiuresis is given furosemide or ethacrynic acid. The experiment has been done by measuring the interstitial osmolality at various levels in the medulla; these two powerful diuretics do, in fact, obliterate the gradient.

The effect of acetazolamide is also shown in Figure 7-3, even though it is rarely used as a diuretic. As mentioned above, this compound inhibits carbonic anhydrase, including that present in the proximal tubule. Consequently, the amount of Na^+ delivered to the loops of Henle as $NaHCO_3$ (and, for as yet unknown reasons, as NaCl) is increased (Fig. 7-2). If this increment of delivered Na^+ is largely reabsorbed at sites 2 and 3, then C_{H_2O} during water diuresis and $T^c_{H_2O}$ during antidiuresis should be increased. These predictions have been fulfilled experimentally (Fig. 7-3); the fact that $T^c_{H_2O}$ increases proportionately less than C_{H_2O} probably means that most of the increment is reabsorbed at site 3.

If a diuretic decreases the urinary excretion of K^+ — but not if it increases it (see below) — then that drug probably acts on the distal tubule (site 4 in Fig. 7-1). This deduction follows from the fact that K^+ excretion is regulated mainly by modulating the rate of K^+ secretion in the distal tubule (Chap. 4). The modulation may be effected by aldosterone, or it can occur independently of the hormone. Both actions can be influenced by diuretics (Table 7-1): (1) by spironolactone, which inhibits the action of aldosterone and therefore is effective only in its presence, and (2) by triamterene, which can reduce the distal tubular secretion of K^+ even in the absence of aldosterone.

Increases in K^+ excretion, however, cannot be interpreted to reflect a primary action of the diuretic at site 4. Rather, in the case of chlorothiazide, ethacrynic acid, furosemide, and mannitol (Table 7-1), the kaliuresis results indirectly from the inhibition of Na^+ reabsorption at earlier sites in the nephron, mainly the loops of Henle and early distal tubules. The resulting increased delivery of water and NaCl to the distal tubule augments the secretion of K^+, partly because the greater flow rate of tubular fluid provides a greater "sink" for K^+ diffusion and partly because it might increase the electrical potential difference (P.D.) between the distal tubular cell and the lumen.

The conclusions cited above, which are based on clearance studies and patterns of urinary excretion, have been strengthened by evidence obtained through more direct approaches, mainly microtechniques. By obtaining microsamples from the late proximal tubules, as well as the early and late distal tubules at the surface of the kidney, one can calculate the percentages of the filtered loads of water and of NaCl that are reabsorbed in various parts of the nephron, both before and after giving diuretics (Fig. 7-6). Such studies, of course, yield information only about superficial cortical nephrons. Much useful knowledge about nephrons and nephron segments that are not accessible to micropuncture has been obtained through the technique of perfusing isolated renal tubules (Fig. 7-4). This type of work, for example, has established that Cl^-, not Na^+, is actively transported out of the thick ascending limbs of Henle and that this transport is inhibited by potent diuretics such as furosemide and ethacrynic acid.

Many other techniques have been applied to the study of diuretics, such as renal stop-flow analysis, electrolyte transport in various nonrenal systems (e.g., erythrocytes, anuran membranes, and salivary glands), metabolic studies on renal slices, and changes in the intrarenal distribution of blood flow. Results from such studies will be described in the following sections when appropriate.

Moderately Effective Diuretics

We will now describe the different classes of diuretics as they are listed in Table 7-1. The discussion will be limited to the generic compounds given in that table.

Chlorothiazide

Following the discovery that certain sulfonamides could produce a diuresis by inhibiting carbonic anhydrase, a systematic effort was made to synthesize more potent inhibitors of the enzyme. Acetazolamide was one result of this effort. Another outgrowth, chlorothiazide, turned out to be a surprise, for while it had marked diuretic properties, these did not seem to depend on the inhibition of carbonic anhydrase. Thus, by chance (although as part of a systematic search), chlorothiazide was the first of the

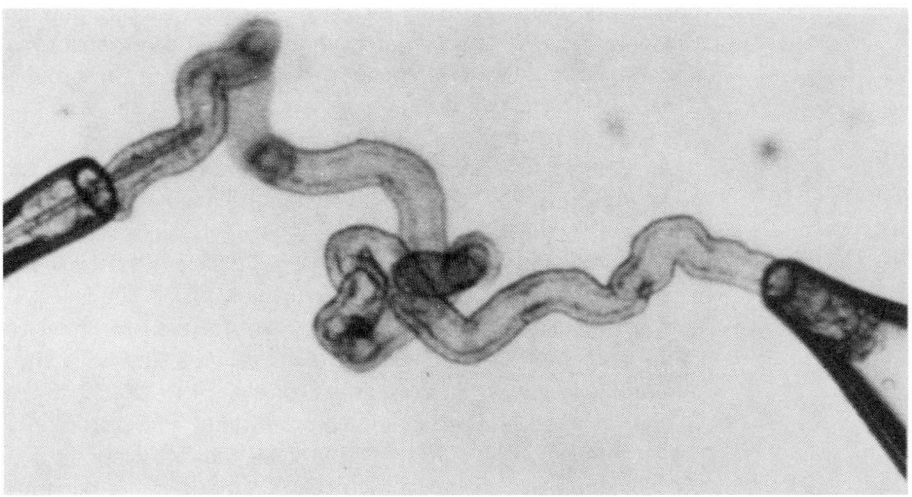

(a)

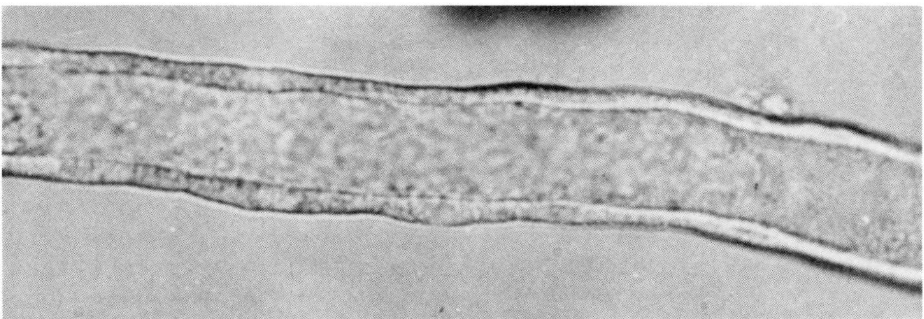

(b)

Figure 7-4
Preparations of isolated, perfused renal tubules.

(a) A segment of proximal convoluted tubule from a rabbit is held between two micropipets and is suspended in a medium of varying composition. Fluid is perfused through the pipet on the left, and it is collected through the pipet on the right. Diameter of the lumen is approximately 20 μm. From M. B. Burg et al., *Am. J. Physiol.* 215:788, 1968.

(b) An isolated, perfused thick ascending limb of Henle from the outer medulla of a rabbit. Diameter of the lumen is approximately 20 μm. From A. S. Rocha and J. P. Kokko, *J. Clin. Invest.* 52:612, 1973.

potent *oral* diuretics to be discovered. It soon became popular, not only because it does not have to be given parenterally, but also because, unlike the organomercurials, its ability to produce a natriuresis and chloruresis does not depend on the acid-base status of the patient.

Chlorothiazide enhances the urinary excretion of Na^+ and Cl^- and, with them, of water (Table 7-1). Its major site of action is the cortical diluting segment (site 3, Fig. 7-1), since it decreases C_{H_2O} without markedly influencing $T^c_{H_2O}$ (Fig. 7-3). Its primary effect may be to inhibit the reabsorption of Cl^- or Na^+. Although this action is independent of an effect on carbonic anhydrase, chlorothiazide does inhibit the enzyme, at least in vitro, and probably thereby increases the excretion of HCO_3^-.

The main adverse effect of chlorothiazide administration is the accompanying kaliuresis (Table 7-1); the latter can lead to K^+ depletion, which may be especially serious if the patient is also receiving digitalis (Chap. 4, under Causes of K^+ Deficiency). Chlorothiazide increases K^+ secretion in the distal tubules mainly by increasing the tubular flow rate and increasing the potential difference between the distal tubular cell and the lumen. The latter effect may be due to inhibition of carbonic anhydrase proximally and the consequent presence of nonreabsorbed HCO_3^- in the distal tubules; this effect of chlorothiazide, which is absent with ethacrynic acid and weak with furosemide, may explain why chlorothiazide is more kaliuretic than the very effective diuretics (Table 7-1). Dangerous K^+ deficiency can be prevented by following the patient carefully; often, an oral K^+ supplement or the concurrent use of triamterene or spironolactone is indicated.

Chlorothiazide may reduce the GFR, possibly through direct action on the renal vessels as well as through contraction of the ECF. It should therefore be used with caution in patients who have edema of renal origin. The drug may also inhibit the renal excretion of uric acid, possibly by competing for the active secretory system for weak acids. This effect can lead to hyperuricemia and gout. A rather common complication is the development of hyponatremia (Fig. 2-6 and Table 3-3).

Other Uses. Despite their potency as diuretics, the thiazides are actually used more widely as *antihypertensive agents.* This action of the thiazides may be due to a direct vasodilator action in addition to their ability to mobilize edema.

The thiazides are thus far unique among diuretics in that they are capable of causing a natriuresis while simultaneously decreasing the excretion of Ca^{2+}. This property makes them useful agents in some patients with *hypercalciuric stone disease.*

Finally, thiazide diuretics are sometimes used in the treatment of *nephrogenic diabetes insipidus.* This seemingly paradoxical application was mentioned in Chapter 2 (see Causes and Treatment of Diabetes Insipidus); it may involve decreased generation of free water in the cortical diluting segment.

Very Effective Diuretics

The two drugs in this category that are most extensively used in the United States — furosemide and ethacrynic acid — were developed simultaneously and independently in the early 1960s. Ethacrynic acid was synthesized as part of a search for compounds that bind renal sulfhydryl groups, the rationale being that such binding may be the mechanism underlying the potent saluretic action of the organomercurials. Although furosemide and ethacrynic acid are different in some respects — for example, in regard to mild inhibition of carbonic anhydrase, their phosphaturic action, their dose-response curves, and their effectiveness in experimental animals — their major characteristics are so similar (Table 7-1) that they will be considered here together.

Ethacrynic Acid and Furosemide

These drugs are often also called high-ceiling diuretics, because they cause the most profound increase in the urinary excretion of water and NaCl of any known agents (Table 7-1). This powerful action depends on their ability to inhibit the active transport of Cl^- out of the thick ascending limb of Henle and hence the reabsorption of NaCl from this portion of the nephron; for this reason, they are also called loop diuretics. This capability is reflected in the decreased C_{H_2O} in the absence of ADH and the decreased $T^c_{H_2O}$ in its presence (Fig. 7-3), as well as in the elimination of the corticopapillary interstitial osmotic gradient, signifying temporary abolition of the countercurrent multiplier system. The urine is consequently isosmotic during peak diuresis with these drugs. The molecular mode of action of these two compounds is not yet known, but both have been shown to inhibit active Cl^- reabsorption from the isolated, perfused thick ascending limb of Henle (Fig. 7-4).

In view of the handling of Na^+ by the various segments of the nephron (Fig. 7-5), it is not surprising that the ability to inhibit NaCl transport in the ascending limb of Henle should be essential to marked saluresis. Nearly 70 percent of the filtered Na^+ is ordinarily reabsorbed in the proximal tubules, about 25 percent in the loops of Henle, 5 percent in the distal tubules, and approximately 3 percent in the collecting ducts. According to these values, one might expect the greatest natriuresis from a drug that inhibits Na^+ reabsorption from the proximal tubules. The loops of Henle, however, have a large capacity for conserving Na^+, and they characteristically reabsorb most of the increment of NaCl that might be delivered to them from the proximal

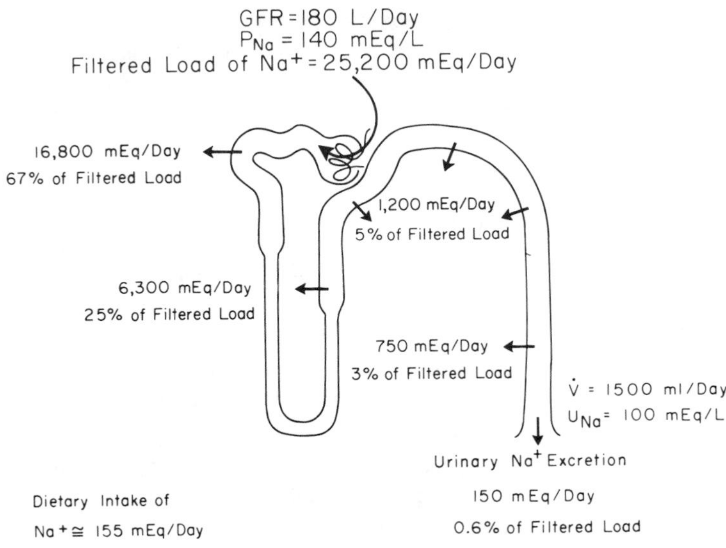

Figure 7-5
Renal handling of Na^+ in a healthy adult human. The diagram of the nephron represents the composite of the roughly two million nephrons of both kidneys. From H. Valtin, *Renal Function: Mechanisms Preserving Fluid and Solute Balance in Health.* Boston: Little, Brown, 1973.

tubules. Although normally about 25 percent of the filtered Na^+ is reabsorbed in the loops (specifically in the ascending limbs and perhaps principally in the thick ascending limbs), this figure can rise to about 50 percent when Na^+ reabsorption in the proximal tubules is reduced. The distal tubules and collecting ducts, however, have a limited capacity to increase Na^+ reabsorption. Hence, when the reabsorption of NaCl is inhibited in the loops, most of this moiety is excreted; 25 percent or more of the filtered NaCl can therefore be excreted at peak diuresis with ethacrynic acid and furosemide (Table 7-1). (Under some circumstances, up to 45 percent of the filtered load may be excreted with these agents; this fact may reflect some effect on the proximal tubules as well.)

The main untoward effects of the high-ceiling diuretics result from their potency. Both the magnitude and the rapidity of the diuretic and saluretic effect (Table 7-1) can lead to deleterious reduction of the extracellular fluid volume, hepatic coma in patients with liver disease, and hyponatremia as well as other electrolyte imbalances. Among the last, potentially the most serious are K^+ deficiency (see Problem 4-1) and contraction alkalosis (see Problem 7-1). The K^+ deficiency accompanying the use of these drugs probably arises mainly from the high flow rate of tubular fluid in the distal tubules and collecting ducts, which provides a large sink for K^+ secretion; it is often aggravated by the reduction of the extracellular fluid volume, which leads to hyperaldosteronism. Contraction alkalosis with these agents results from the fact that relative to the composition of plasma, the loss of water exceeds that of HCO_3^- and the loss of Cl^- exceeds that of Na^+ (this effect is further explained in the Answer to Problem 7-1). Both of the adverse effects are prevented most easily by treating patients relatively slowly, which can be accomplished not only through cautious dosage, but often through prescribing these powerful drugs to be taken on alternate days rather than daily.

Both ethacrynic acid and furosemide are actively secreted by the organic-acid transport system in the proximal tubules. Probably for this reason, both can block the secretion of uric acid and precipitate attacks of gout in susceptible patients, and they may potentiate the nephrotoxicity of aminoglycoside antibiotics. Other toxic effects are rare; their discussion can be found in standard texts.

Other Uses. These diuretics are often used in *acute renal failure;* their efficacy and mode of action in this application are uncertain (see Chap. 9). Inasmuch as these drugs — in contrast to the thiazides — increase the urinary excretion of calcium, they may also be used to treat *hypercalcemia.* In this application, however, the concomitant urinary losses of water, Na^+, Cl^-, and Mg^{2+} must be replaced.

Adjuvants

The drugs in this category are seldom used alone, because they have a relatively weak diuretic and saluretic action. They are employed mainly for two auxiliary purposes: (1) for treating patients with edema who are relatively refractory to the diuretics discussed above, especially when hyperaldosteronism is involved (e.g., patients with cirrhosis and ascites; Fig. 3-3c) and (2) to prevent K^+ deficiency during the prolonged use of chlorothiazide, furosemide, or ethacrynic acid.

Spironolactone

The observation that progesterone could block the renal effects of the adrenal mineralocorticoid, deoxycorticosterone, prompted the development of antagonists to aldosterone, the most potent natural mineralocorticoid. Spironolactone, a steroid that is similar in chemical structure to aldosterone, appears to act through competitive binding to the nuclear receptor for aldosterone in the kidney and other tissues. In a patient with adrenal insufficiency (Addison's disease) who lacks endogenous aldosterone, for example, it can be shown that (1) exogenous aldosterone reduces the urinary excretion of Na^+ and raises that of K^+, (2) spironolactone can reverse these effects of exogenous aldosterone, (3) the antagonistic actions of spironolactone can be nullified by large doses of aldosterone, but (4) when given by itself, spironolactone has no effect. Analogous results can be observed in other systems, such as the toad bladder in vitro.

The kaliuretic effect of aldosterone is thought to occur at site 4 in the distal tubule (Fig. 7-1), and this therefore seems to be the main place within the kidney where spironolactone acts. Inasmuch as normally only about 5 percent of the filtered Na^+ is reabsorbed in the entire distal convolution (Fig. 7-5), it is not surprising that spironolactone does not have a strong natriuretic effect; at peak diuresis it may increase the excretion of Na^+ to about 2 percent of the filtered load.

Although untoward effects are rare, spironolactone is a dangerous drug to employ in patients with renal failure. In such patients, this diuretic can cause fatal hyperkalemia, even when used in conjunction with a kaliuretic drug, such as chlorothiazide.

Other Uses. These are limited to distinguishing primary aldosteronism from a rare hereditary disorder called pseudoaldosteronism. The latter mimics some of the effects of hyperaldosteronism, but it does so in the presence of subnormal production of the hormone. Predictably, spironolactone will reverse some of the abnormalities of primary aldosteronism but not those of pseudoaldosteronism.

Triamterene

This drug is a pteridine derivative. Like spironolactone, it reduces the urinary excretion of K^+, especially when used in conjunction with chlorothiazide, ethacrynic acid, or furosemide, which increase K^+ excretion. The mode of action of triamterene differs, however, from that of spironolactone, for unlike the latter, triamterene can act in the absence (as well as the presence) of aldosterone. Furthermore, the diuretic and natriuretic effects resulting from maximal doses of triamterene and spironolactone are additive, which would not be expected if they utilized the same mechanism.

The pattern of urinary excretion with triamterene — namely, mild diuresis and saluresis combined with decreased excretion of K^+ and a small increase in HCO_3^- excretion (Table 7-1) — strongly suggests that the drug acts on the distal tubule (Fig. 7-1). The fact that it does not change C_{H_2O} during water diuresis localizes its action to the late distal tubule, or site 4 in Figure 7-1. Although the gross location of its site of action is therefore the same as that of spironolactone, the cellular, subcellular, or, at the very least, molecular sites of action must be different for the two drugs, since one agent depends on the presence of aldosterone and the other does not.

Triamterene inhibits Na^+ transport in the toad bladder and reduces the electrical potential (P.D.) across this membrane in vitro. Because the toad bladder is analogous in many functional respects to the mammalian distal tubule, these results suggest that triamterene may decrease the tubular secretion of K^+ by reducing the P.D. between the distal tubular cell and the lumen.

Untoward effects of triamterene are usually negligible. When used in large doses, it can reduce the GFR and hence raise the BUN and serum creatinine concentration (Chap. 8). Supplements of K^+ should not be given when triamterene is used, because the combination can lead to dangerous hyperkalemia. It is important to be reminded of this fact, since triamterene is often prescribed when the use of chlorothiazide, furosemide, or ethacrynic acid has led to K^+ depletion, and, in such a case, K^+ supplementation may have been started as a first step.

Other Uses. Triamterene is uniquely suited for the treatment of pseudoaldosteronism (see Spironolactone, above), since the drug can exert its effects in the absence of aldosterone.

Osmotic Diuretics

The rate of urine flow is ultimately a function of the rate at which filtered water is reabsorbed from the renal tubules, and this reabsorptive rate is governed largely by differences between the osmolality of tubular fluid and that within the intercellular spaces or of the surrounding interstitium. The increase in urine flow that is seen with the diuretics considered thus far involves this phenomenon; that is, it results from the osmotic retention of water inside the tubules because the NaCl that is normally reabsorbed stays within the tubules. In this sense, all saluretic agents might be considered osmotic diuretics, but the pharmacological definition of these agents is much more restricted. We define an *osmotic diuretic* as an exogenous substance, usually a nonelectrolyte, that increases urine flow when its filtered load is increased. Effective osmotic diuretics therefore have the following properties: (1) they are relatively small molecules that are not bound to plasma proteins, so they are freely filterable at the glomerulus; (2) they are poorly or not at all reabsorbed by the renal tubules; and (3) they are pharmacologically inert, so their only primary effect is to raise the osmolality of tubular fluid.

There is an irony in the above definition. The most common clinical example of an osmotic *diuresis* is probably that which occurs in uncontrolled diabetes mellitus. In that instance, the filtered load of glucose (GFR $\cdot$ P_G) is increased because the plasma concentration of the sugar (P_G) has risen, and the glucose stays within the tubules because the maximal capacity of the tubular epithelium to reabsorb glucose (Tm_G) has been exceeded. Glucose, however, does not fall within the definition of an osmotic diuretic given above, because it is not usually employed as an exogenous compound to induce diuresis.

Osmotic diuretics are not given for mobilizing edema fluid, even though they are effective in raising the excretion of NaCl (Table 7-1). The reasons for this fact – namely, that this type of diuretic must be administered parenterally and that it mobilizes mainly intracellular, not extracellular, fluid – were discussed earlier in this chapter (see Classification).

Mannitol

Mannitol is a six-carbon sugar, it has a molecular weight of 182, and it is not bound to plasma proteins; it is therefore freely filtered through the glomerular capillary membrane. Under most circumstances, it is not at all reabsorbed by the renal tubules or reabsorbed very little. Furthermore, it is neither metabolized by the body nor excreted by any organ other than the kidney. Mannitol is thus very similar to inulin, and once it has been injected (usually intravenously), it is all filtered and remains within the tubular system until it is excreted in the urine.

The first impulse might be to think that mannitol acts by raising the osmolality of fluid in the collecting ducts and retarding the reabsorption of water from them, thereby causing an increase in urine flow. Clearance and micropuncture studies have shown, however, that the inhibition of water reabsorption occurs in the proximal tubules, loops of Henle, and early distal tubules. Figure 7-6a, which portrays the results of studies in dogs, shows that whereas in antidiuresis at least 98 percent of the filtered water was reabsorbed, the amount was reduced to 72 percent when mannitol was infused intravenously. The illustration shows further that 10 percent less water was reabsorbed from the proximal tubules during mannitol diuresis than during antidiuresis and that 21 percent less of the filtered load was reabsorbed in the loops of Henle and early distal tubules. It may be concluded that inhibition of water reabsorption in the proximal tubules, the loops of Henle, and the early distal tubules can account for the extra water that appeared in the urine. (Although this interpretation must be qualified to the extent that micropunctures at the surface of the kidney yield information only about superficial cortical nephrons, the conclusion is probably valid.)

A similar picture emerges for the fraction of filtered Na^+ that is reabsorbed in the various nephron segments (Fig. 7-6b). The fraction of filtered Na^+ in the urine rose from about 1 percent during antidiuresis to 13 percent during mannitol diuresis. This increment was due partly to the inhibition of Na^+ reabsorption in the proximal tubules, but mainly to inhibition in the loops of Henle and early distal tubules.

The inhibition of Na^+ reabsorption by mannitol is thought to

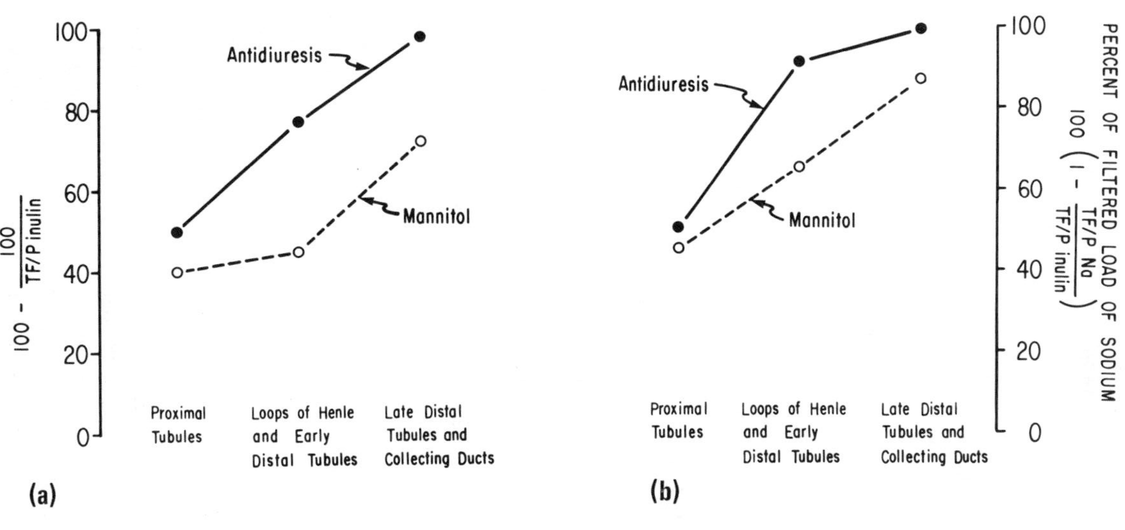

Figure 7-6
Results of micropuncture experiments in dogs showing inhibition of (a) water reabsorption and (b) Na^+ reabsorption during mannitol diuresis. In both cases, the inhibition occurs partly in proximal tubules, but mainly in loops of Henle and early distal tubules. Note that *cumulative* values for reabsorption have been plotted. From J. F. Seely and J. H. Dirks, *J. Clin. Invest.* 48:2330, 1969.

be secondary to the inhibition of water reabsorption. Water is necessarily retained within the proximal tubules, because mannitol decreases the osmotic difference between fluid in the tubular lumen and that in the surrounding interstitium. The retention of water in turn dilutes the Na^+ within the proximal tubules, and this effect slightly retards the rate at which Na^+ is reabsorbed from them. Essentially the same phenomenon, only more pronounced, occurs in the loops of Henle and early distal tubules. (Inasmuch as active reabsorption of Cl^- is the primary event in the thick ascending limb of Henle, one should really refer to the inhibition of the reabsorption of NaCl.) Much less water is reabsorbed from the descending limbs of Henle during mannitol infusion than during antidiuresis, because mannitol reduces the difference between the osmolality of tubular fluid and that of the interstitium. This difference is further reduced as a result of the decrease in interstitial osmolality during mannitol diuresis, both because less NaCl is reabsorbed from the ascending limb (see next sentence) and because less urea is reabsorbed from the collecting ducts. The retention of water in the descending limb dilutes the NaCl within that limb and the ascending limb, and thereby retards NaCl movement out of the latter segment. The diluting effect retards NaCl reabsorption more in the ascending limbs than in the proximal tubules (Fig. 7-6); this phenomenon is thought to reflect the fact that the ascending limb normally operates near the limiting concentration difference for NaCl, beyond which this solute cannot be transported out of the tubular lumen.

In parts of the above description, the terms "loops of Henle" and "ascending limbs" have been used somewhat loosely to refer to both sites 2 and 3 in Figure 7-1. The interpretations of clearance experiments in which C_{H_2O} and $T^c_{H_2O}$ are measured are not as clear-cut in the case of mannitol as in the other diuretics. Hence, it is not yet known whether mannitol inhibits Na^+ reabsorption at site 2 or 3, but it may be predominantly at site 3.

Aside from the possibility of exacerbating heart failure, the main untoward effect of mannitol is related to the increases in Na^+ and K^+ excretion that it secondarily induces (Table 7-1). Excretion of K^+ is increased because of both decreased reabsorption in the proximal tubules and loops of Henle and increased secretion in the distal tubules. In most instances, mannitol is used over brief periods of time, so serious depletion of Na^+ and K^+ does not occur. The probability of increasing the excretion of these ions is such, however, that the danger of their depletion must be kept in mind.

Uses. An intravenous infusion of mannitol is the most reliable means of increasing urine flow. This property is utilized in many cases of intoxication when a high tubular flow rate can increase the urinary excretion of the toxicant by either retarding its reabsorption or increasing its tubular secretion. Mannitol is also used in the prophylaxis, diagnosis, and treatment of acute renal failure (Chap. 9).

The nondiuretic uses of mannitol relate to its distribution within the extracellular space. This property selectively raises the osmolality of the extracellular fluid and can therefore be utilized to draw water out of the cells. Mannitol is commonly used for this purpose in neurosurgery to relieve cerebral edema.

Guidelines

Some useful admonitions can be voiced for the wise management of edematous patients. Although such guidelines are particularly apt for the clinical use of diuretics, many are equally applicable to other problems.

Adequate Treatment of Primary Disease

Not all generalized edema requires treatment with diuretics. Often, the adequate management of the primary disease that has given rise to edema will result in the reduction or disappearance of the edema.

Sometimes, a patient will seem to be refractory to diuretic therapy. The tendency in such instances is to increase the dosage of the diuretic, to work with a combination of diuretic agents, or to turn to more potent diuretics. Not infrequently, however, the problem can be solved through more vigorous management of the primary disease or by starting treatment of the primary disease in the first place. Insidious congestive heart failure is a prime example, especially when it occurs in association with a noncardiac disease such as the nephrotic syndrome; often edema that seems to be refractory to treatment can be reduced or eliminated by digitalizing the patient or adjusting the patient's intake of salt. Suffice it to say that whenever the edema does not seem to be responding to the diuretic regimen, one should re-examine the adequacy of treatment of the primary disease or search for an associated disorder (e.g., congestive heart failure).

Slow Change Is Better than Rapid Change

The serious complications of diuretic therapy — namely, drastic reduction in the volume of extracellular fluid, hyponatremia, contraction alkalosis, and K^+ depletion — usually result from the injudicious use of diuretics. Although they are seen most commonly when the "very effective" diuretics are used, such adverse consequences occur not only because of the magnitude of the change, but also (and often more so) because of the *rapidity* of change. Except in true emergencies (e.g., pulmonary edema), it is a good rule to restore fluid and solute balance slowly. If therapy is instituted when the patient is desperately ill and if after a few hours or a day of treatment, one can see that the patient is improving, then it is usually safer to allow a number of days to pass for the imbalance to be corrected. In general, the aim of a prescription should be to progress *toward* the normal state, not to reach that state in a single step. In that way, advantage can also be taken of the patient's regulatory functions to help in the restoration of balance. Currently in the United States, nearly 15 percent of hospital admissions are precipitated by something the physician did to or for the patient, and frequently that "something" – be it a medication or some other therapeutic or diagnostic procedure – was not essential to the patient's recovery.

Specifically in the case of diuretics, it would probably be wise in most patients to try the moderately effective thiazides before resorting to ethacrynic acid or furosemide. Furthermore, many complications, especially K^+ depletion, could probably be prevented if the drugs were given every other day rather than daily. This fact brings to mind another deplorable *tendency:* the inclination to add a drug when a complication arises, rather than to reduce or eliminate the drug that is causing the complication. Although the adjuvant diuretics can be very useful, their application would often be obviated if the primary diuretic agent had been given more prudently.

Simple Measures Are Better than Complicated Ones

The utility of determining *body weight* in the management of fluid balance has been mentioned in previous chapters. Probably no single measure is as inexpensive, accurate, and useful for gauging the adequacy of diuretic therapy as weighing the patient once a day, preferably first thing in the morning, nude, and immediately after he has urinated. It is a far more reliable guide than a continuous recording of the patient's intake and output ("I. and O."). Too few physicians stop to think that an order for I. and O., which takes but seconds to write, will demand considerable time from attending personnel, yet seldom yields information that is accurate enough to be useful. Even when an assessment of the patient's salt intake is required, simply talking to the patient is likely to be more productive than requesting that the intake be recorded. It is not unheard of that the written account shows the patient's salt intake to be very low (e.g., because a low-salt diet had been ordered), while conversation with the patient reveals that he has used the saltshaker that was inadvertently left on his tray.

These principles apply as well when diuretic therapy is given to a patient who continues to work and live at home. Much useful information regarding the efficacy of treatment can be obtained by having the patient record his weight daily and having him urinate into a discarded milk bottle to estimate his daily urine output to the nearest half-liter, as well as by obtaining a history about nocturia and diet at frequent follow-up visits.

Summary

Although many therapeutic agents have a diuretic effect, this chapter has been limited to drugs that are used in clinical practice for inducing diuresis. They fall into two categories: (1) drugs that mobilize edema fluid and (2) osmotic diuretics. Because drugs falling in the first category are used much more commonly than those in the second, most clinicians would define a "diuretic" as a drug that increases the renal excretion of Na^+ and its accompanying anions, mainly Cl^-.

Diuretics that mobilize edema fluid can be subclassified into moderately effective agents, which are mainly the thiazides, and the very effective or "high-ceiling" diuretics, furosemide and ethacrynic acid. These drugs are often given in conjunction with adjuvants in order to achieve a greater diuresis or to prevent K^+ deficiency; the adjuvants may be subclassified into those that counteract aldosterone (i.e., the spironolactones) and those that reduce the urinary excretion of K^+ through a mechanism that is independent of aldosterone (namely, triamterene).

Chlorothiazide, the first of the potent oral diuretics to be developed, can cause the excretion of as much as 8 percent of the filtered load of Na^+ (Table 7-1). It decreases C_{H_2O} in the absence of ADH, but causes little change in $T^c_{H_2O}$ when ADH is present; it therefore acts mainly by inhibiting the reabsorption of NaCl from the cortical diluting segment of the nephron. It may also mildly inhibit carbonic anhydrase and thereby slightly increase the excretion of HCO_3^-. Because it may reduce the GFR (possibly through a direct action on renal vessels), chlorothiazide should be used cautiously in patients with renal failure.

At peak diuresis, the very effective diuretics furosemide and ethacrynic acid can cause the excretion of as much as 25 percent of the filtered load of Na^+; it is because of this massive effect that they are often called high-ceiling diuretics. They are also known as loop diuretics, because it is their inhibition of NaCl transport out of the ascending limbs of Henle that makes them such powerful diuretic agents. Their major and primary effect may be to block active reabsorption of Cl^- from the thick ascending limbs of Henle.

When used alone, the adjuvants have a relatively weak saluretic effect. They are therefore used mainly (1) to augment the effect of another diuretic, especially in patients with hyperaldosteronism, and (2) to reduce the distal tubular secretion of K^+. The spironolactones accomplish both purposes through competitive inhibition of aldosterone; triamterene serves the second purpose through a mechanism in the distal tubule that is independent of aldosterone.

Mannitol is the agent most commonly used to induce osmotic diuresis. It is freely filtered, and once in the tubules, it is reabsorbed from them very little if at all. Consequently, it causes osmotic retention of H_2O within the tubules and ultimately diuresis. Mannitol causes a negative balance primarily of intracellular H_2O, not of extracellular NaCl, and it is therefore used to increase urine flow rather than to mobilize edema fluid. The saluresis results secondarily because the H_2O that is retained within the tubules reduces the concentration of NaCl therein and thereby retards the reabsorption of NaCl. Mannitol acts mainly in the loops of Henle and early distal tubules, but also in the proximal tubules.

The major complications of diuretic therapy are K^+ deficiency, contraction alkalosis, and hyponatremia (these adverse effects are illustrated in Problems 4-1, 7-1, and 7-2, respectively). The complications might often be prevented if a mild diuresis were effected slowly by (1) using an agent of moderate potency when a very powerful one is not needed and (2) prescribing diuretics to be taken every second or third day rather than daily.

Problem 7-1

This problem and the next describe two complications of diuretic therapy. They have been chosen to illustrate further how important questions of fluid and electrolyte balance should be diagnosed and handled. It should be emphasized that the adverse effects here mentioned are not unique to the particular diuretics that were used, and that millions of patients who take diuretics do not experience these complications.

Contraction Alkalosis. The following report has been adapted from a balance study performed by P. J. Cannon, H. O. Heinemann, M. S. Albert, J. H. Laragh, and R. W. Winters (*Ann. Intern. Med.* 62:979, 1965).

The patient was a 62-year-old man who had had arteriosclerotic cardiovascular disease for many years. He had been adequately digitalized and had been on chlorothiazide for several years. During the two months prior to admission, he had become increasingly breathless, especially on exertion, and he had gained weight. On a follow-up visit, he was in obvious congestive heart failure, and he showed moderately severe, pitting presacral and pretibial edema (Fig. 3-3a). The patient agreed to enter the metabolic research ward, where his response to more vigorous diuretic therapy could be studied.

During the entire period of study, including the control period, he received the same diet, which was adequate in calories but contained only 5 mEq of Na^+ and of Cl^- per day. The average values obtained for two control days are shown in Table 7-2.

Table 7-2
Results of balance studies on a 62-year-old man with arteriosclerotic cardiovascular disease maintained on a diet containing 5 mEq of Na^+ and of Cl^- per day

		Urinary Excretion					Plasma Concentrations					
							Venous			Arterial		
Period	Body Weight (kg)	$\dot{V}$ (ml/day)	Na^+ (mEq/day)	K^+ (mEq/day)	Cl^- (mEq/day)	HCO_3^- (mEq/day)	Na^+ (mEq/L)	K^+ (mEq/L)	Cl^- (mEq/L)	HCO_3^- (mEq/L)	pH	PCO_2 (mm Hg)
Control	94.0	410	2	42	2	0.1	137	4.6	98	23	7.42	38
Therapy (with ethacrynic acid, 50 mg 4 times daily for 3 days)	89.5	3,108	233	64	266	1.1	135	3.9	87	29	7.50	39

Modified from P. J. Cannon, H. O. Heinemann, M. S. Albert, J. H. Laragh, and R. W. Winters, *Ann. Intern. Med.* 62:979, 1965.

The patient was then given ethacrynic acid, 50 mg by mouth four times daily for three days. The average values for urinary excretion during this period, as well as plasma concentrations and the body weight at the end of the period, are also presented in Table 7-2.

Analyze the patient's H^+ balance after three days of diuretic therapy. To what extent can the rise in plasma [HCO_3^-] be accounted for by contraction of the ECF?

Problem 7-2

Hyponatremia Induced by Diuretics. A 47-year-old woman was brought to the emergency room because she had had a generalized seizure at home, following which she remained confused. She had been on a low-salt diet since age 27, when hypertension was diagnosed. At age 31, she had undergone bilateral lumbar sympathectomy for high blood pressure, and she had experienced postural hypotension since then. Somehow she had also gained the impression that a high fluid intake was beneficial, and it was estimated that she drank 5 to 10 liters per day.

The patient had taken furosemide (20 to 40 mg per day) for hypertension and what she perceived to be facial swelling. She had taken this medication intermittently during the previous two years and again for three weeks before the present episode. During the last period, she had become increasingly weak, lethargic, anorectic, and nauseated; during the three days before the seizure, she had become disoriented, agitated, and combative. She had vomited several times.

Physical examination revealed a body weight of 53 kg, a blood pressure of 130/85 mm Hg, pulse of 100 per minute, respiration of 18 per minute, and a normal temperature. She was semicomatose, thrashing about in bed, and responsive only to painful stimuli. Her mucous membranes and axillae were not conspicuously dry, skin turgor was good, and she had no edema. The results of neurological examination were entirely normal.

Pertinent laboratory data on admission to the emergency room are shown in Table 7-3. In addition, the result of a lumbar puncture was normal, as were x-rays of the skull and chest. It was also learned that three times during the past 3½ years, she had been admitted to other hospitals, and the history and physical and laboratory findings had been virtually identical to those of the present episode; each time she had been on diuretics, twice on furosemide and once on an unknown diuretic.

What is the probable diagnosis in this patient? How would you have treated her?

(This report has been abstracted from F. R. de Rubertis, M. F. Michelis, N. Beck, and B. B. Davis, *Metabolism* 19:709, 1970.)

Table 7-3
Laboratory data obtained on a 47-year-old woman at the time of her admission to the emergency ward. The patient had just had a generalized seizure.

Test	On Admission
Venous blood or plasma:	
Na^+ (mEq/L)	112
K^+ (mEq/L)	3.1
Cl^- (mEq/L)	69
HCO_3^- (mMoles/L)	29
BUN (mg/100 ml)	10
Creatinine (mg/100 ml)	0.7
Sugar (mg/100 ml)	147
Osmolality (mOsm/kg H_2O)	232
Urine:	
$\dot{V}$ (ml/min)	0.7
Osmolality (mOsm/kg H_2O)	600
Glucose	0

Selected References

General

Baer, J. E., and Beyer, K. H. Renal pharmacology. *Annu. Rev. Pharmacol.* 6:261, 1966.

Baer, J. E., and Beyer, K. H. Subcellular Pharmacology of Natriuretic and Potassium-sparing Drugs. In K. D. G. Edwards (ed.), *Drugs Affecting Kidney Function and Metabolism.* New York: Karger, 1972.

Burg, M. B. Mechanisms of Action of Diuretic Drugs. In B. M. Brenner and F. C. Rector, Jr. (eds.), *The Kidney.* Philadelphia: Saunders, 1976.

Cannon, P. J. Diuretic Therapy in Patients with Renal Disease. In R. W. Winters (ed.), *The Body Fluids in Pediatrics.* Boston: Little, Brown, 1973.

Dirks, J. H. Use of Micropuncture in Localizing Diuretic Action. In A. F. Lant and G. M. Wilson (eds.), *Modern Diuretic Therapy in the Treatment of Cardiovascular and Renal Disease.* Amsterdam: Excerpta Medica Foundation, 1973.

Frazier, H. S., and Yager, H. The clinical use of diuretics. *N. Engl. J. Med.* 288:246 and 455, 1973.
This interesting summary includes a comparison of the cost of various diuretic regimens.

Goldberg, M. The Renal Physiology of Diuretics. In J. Orloff and R. W. Berliner (eds.), *Handbook of Physiology,* Section 8, Renal Physiology. Washington, D.C.: American Physiological Society, 1973.

Grossman, R. A., and Goldberg, M. The use of diuretics in renal disease. *Kidney* 7:1, 1974.

Kassirer, J. P., and Harrington, J. T. Diuretics and potassium metabolism: A reassessment of the need, effectiveness and safety of potassium therapy. *Kidney Int.* 11:505, 1977.

Lant, A. F., and Wilson, G. M. (eds.). *Modern Diuretic Therapy in the Treatment of Cardiovascular and Renal Disease.* Amsterdam: Excerpta Medica Foundation, 1973.

Loggie, J. M. H., Kleinman, L. I., and Van Maanen, E. F. Renal function and diuretic therapy in infants and children. Part I. *J. Pediatr.* 86:485, 1975; Part II, *ibid.* 86:657, 1975; and Part III, *ibid.* 86:825, 1975.

Martinez-Maldonado, M., Eknoyan, G., and Suki, W. N. Diuretics in nonedematous states. Physiological basis for the clinical use. *Arch. Intern. Med.* 131:797, 1973.

Mudge, G. H. Diuretics and Other Agents Employed in the Mobilization of Edema Fluid. In L. S. Goodman and A. Gilman (eds.), *The Pharmacological Basis of Therapeutics* (5th ed.). New York: Macmillan, 1975.

Pitts, R. F. *The Physiological Basis of Diuretic Therapy.* Springfield, Ill.: Thomas, 1959.

Puschett, J. B. Physiologic basis for the use of new and older diuretics in congestive heart failure. *Cardiovasc. Med.* 2:119, 1977.

Schrier, R. W. Disorders of Sodium Metabolism and Use of Diuretics. In R. W. Schrier (ed.), *Renal and Electrolyte Disorders.* Boston: Little, Brown, 1976.

Seely, J. F., and Dirks, J. H. Site of action of diuretic drugs. *Kidney Int.* 11:1, 1977.

Seldin, D. W. (ed.). The Physiology of Diuretic Agents. *Ann. N.Y. Acad. Sci.* 139:273, 1966.

Seldin, D. W., Eknoyan, G., Suki, W. N., and Rector, F. C., Jr. Localization of diuretic action from the pattern of water and electrolyte excretion. *Ann. N.Y. Acad. Sci.* 139:328, 1966.

Seldin, D. W., and Rector, F. C., Jr. Evaluation of Clearance Methods for Localization of Site of Action of Diuretics. In A. F. Lant and G. M. Wilson (eds.), *Modern Diuretic Therapy in the Treatment of Cardiovascular and Renal Disease.* Amsterdam: Excerpta Medica Foundation, 1973.

Suki, W. N., Eknoyan, G., and Martinez-Maldonado, M. Tubular sites and mechanisms of diuretic action. *Annu. Rev. Pharmacol.* 13:91, 1973.

Thurau, K., and Jahrmärker, H. (eds.). *Renal Transport and Diuretics.* New York: Springer, 1969.

Weston, R. E. Pathogenesis and Treatment of Edema with Special Reference to Use of Diuretics. In M. H. Maxwell and C. R. Kleeman (eds.), *Clinical Disorders of Fluid and Electrolyte Metabolism* (2nd ed.). New York: McGraw-Hill, 1972.

Moderately Effective Diuretics and Organomercurials

Burg, M. B. The Mechanism of Action of Diuretics in Renal Tubules. In L. G. Wesson and G. M. Fanelli, Jr. (eds.), *Recent Advances in Renal Physiology and Pharmacology.* Baltimore: University Park Press, 1974.

Cafruny, E. J. The site and mechanism of action of mercurial diuretics. *Pharmacol. Rev.* 20:89, 1968.

Clapp, J. R., and Robinson, R. R. Distal sites of action of diuretic drugs in the dog nephron. *Am. J. Physiol.* 215:228, 1968.

Clapp, J. R., Watson, J. F., and Berliner, R. W. Effect of carbonic anhydrase inhibition on proximal tubular bicarbonate reabsorption. *Am. J. Physiol.* 205:693, 1963.

Earley, L. E., and Orloff, J. Thiazide diuretics. *Annu. Rev. Med.* 15:149, 1964.

Edmonds, C. J., and Jasani, B. Total-body potassium in hypertensive patients during prolonged diuretic therapy. *Lancet* 2:8, 1972.

Edwards, B. R., Baer, P. G., Sutton, R. A. L., and Dirks, J. H. Micropuncture study of diuretic effects on sodium and calcium reabsorption in the dog nephron. *J. Clin. Invest.* 52:2418, 1973.

Eknoyan, G., Suki, W. N., and Martinez-Maldonado, M. Effect of diuretics on urinary excretion of phosphate, calcium, and magnesium in thyroparathyroidectomized dogs. *J. Lab. Clin. Med.* 76:257, 1970.

Kunau, R. T., Jr. The influences of the carbonic anhydrase inhibitor, benzolamide (CL-11,366), on the reabsorption of chloride, sodium, and bicarbonate in the proximal tubule of the rat. *J. Clin. Invest.* 51:294, 1972.

Lancet Editorial. Big doses of frusemide in renal failure. *Lancet* 2:803, 1971.

Lancet Editorial. Slow-K, quick quick, slow. *Lancet* 2:1123, 1974.

Maren, T. H. Carbonic anhydrase: Chemistry, physiology, and inhibition. *Physiol. Rev.* 47:595, 1967.

Maren, T. H., and Wiley, C. E. Renal activity and pharmacology of n-acyl and related sulfonamides. *J. Pharmacol. Exp. Ther.* 143:230, 1964.

Meng, K. Mikropunktionsuntersuchungen über die saluretische Wirkung von Hydrochlorothiazid, Acetazolamid, und Furosemid. *Arch. Pharmakol. Exp. Pathol.* 257:355, 1967.

Mudge, G. H., and Hardin, B. Response to mercurial diuretics during alkalosis: A comparison of acute metabolic and chronic hypokalemic alkalosis in the dog. *J. Clin. Invest.* 35:155, 1956.

Taggart, J. V. (ed.). Chlorothiazide and other diuretic agents. *Ann. N.Y. Acad. Sci.* 71:323, 1958.

Vogl, A. The discovery of the organic mercurial diuretics. *Am. Heart. J.* 39:881, 1950.

Weiner, I. M., Levy, R. I., and Mudge, G. H. Studies on mercurial diuresis: Renal excretion, acid stability and structure-activity relationships of organic mercurials. *J. Pharmacol. Exp. Ther.* 138:96, 1962.

Very Effective Diuretics

Beyer, K. H., Baer, J. E., Michaelson, J. K., and Russo, H. F. Renotropic characteristics of ethacrynic acid: A phenoxyacetic saluretic-diuretic agent. *J. Pharmacol. Exp. Ther.* 147:1, 1965.

Birtch, A. G., Zakheim, R. M., Jones, L. G., and Barger, A. C. Redistribution of renal blood flow produced by furosemide and ethacrynic acid. *Circ. Res.* 21:869, 1967.

Burg, M. B. The Mechanism of Action of Diuretics in Renal Tubules. In L. G. Wesson and G. M. Fanelli, Jr. (eds.), *Recent Advances in Renal Physiology and Pharmacology*. Baltimore: University Park Press, 1974.

Burg, M., and Green, N. Effect of ethacrynic acid on the thick ascending limb of Henle's loop. *Kidney Int.* 4:301, 1973.

Burg, M., and Stoner, L. Renal tubular chloride transport and the mode of action of some diuretics. *Annu. Rev. Physiol.* 38:37, 1976.

Burg, M., Stoner, L., Cardinal, J., and Green, N. Furosemide effect on isolated perfused tubules. *Am. J. Physiol.* 225:119, 1973.

Burke, T. J., Robinson, R. R., and Clapp, J. R. Determinants of the effect of furosemide on the proximal tubule. *Kidney Int.* 1:12, 1972.

Clapp, J. R., Nottebohm, G. A., and Robinson, R. R. Proximal site of action of ethacrynic acid: Importance of filtration rate. *Am. J. Physiol.* 220:1355, 1971.

Down, P. F., Polak, A., Rao, R., and Mead, J. A. Fate of potassium supplements in six outpatients receiving long-term diuretics for oedematous disease. *Lancet* 2:721, 1972.

Duarte, C. G., Chomety, F., and Giebisch, G. Effect of amiloride, ouabain, and furosemide on distal tubular function in the rat. *Am. J. Physiol.* 221:632, 1971.

Epstein, M., Hollenberg, N. K., Guttmann, R. D., Conroy, M., Basch, R. I., and Merrill, J. P. Effect of ethacrynic acid and chlorothiazide on intrarenal homodynamics in normal man. *Am. J. Physiol.* 220:482, 1971.

Fichman, M. P., Vorherr, H., Kleeman, C. R., and Telfer, N. Diuretic-induced hyponatremia. *Ann. Intern. Med.* 75:853, 1971.

Goldberg, M. Ethacrynic acid: Site and mode of action. *Ann. N.Y. Acad. Sci.* 139:443, 1966.

Goldberg, M., McCurdy, D. K., Foltz, E. L., and Bluemle, L. W., Jr. Effects of ethacrynic acid (a new saluretic agent) on renal diluting and concentrating mechanisms: Evidence for site of action in the loop of Henle. *J. Clin. Invest.* 43:201, 1964.

Hagedorn, C. W., Kaplan, A. A., and Hulet, W. H. Prolonged administration of ethacrynic acid in patients with chronic renal disease. *N. Engl. J. Med.* 272:1152, 1965.

Klahr, S., Yates, J., and Bourgoignie, J. Inhibition of glycolysis by ethacrynic acid and furosemide. *Am. J. Physiol.* 221:1038, 1971.

Kleeman, C. R., Okun, R., and Heller, R. J. The renal excretion of sodium and potassium in patients with chronic renal failure (CRF) and the effect of diuretics on the excretion of these ions. *Ann. N.Y. Acad. Sci.* 139:520, 1966.

Knauf, H., Schollmeyer, P., and Steinhardt, H. J. The separate modes and sites of action of furosemide and amiloride. *Clin. Nephrol.* 3:148, 1975.

Puschett, J. B., and Goldberg, M. The acute effects of furosemide on acid and electrolyte excretion in man. *J. Lab. Clin. Med.* 71:666, 1968.

de Rubertis, F. R., Michelis, M. F., Beck, N., and Davis, B. B. Complications of diuretic therapy: Severe alkalosis and syndrome resembling inappropriate secretion of antidiuretic hormone. *Metabolism* 19:709, 1970.

Schrier, R. W., Lehman, D., Zacherle, B., and Earley, L. E. Effect of furosemide on free water excretion in edematous patients with hyponatremia. *Kidney Int.* 3:30, 1973.

Sullivan, L. P., Tucker, J. M., and Scherbenske, M. J. Effect of furosemide on sodium transport and metabolism in toad bladder. *Am. J. Physiol.* 220:1316, 1971.

Adjuvants

Baba, W. I., Lant, A. F., Smith, A. J., Townshend, M. M., and Wilson, G. M. Pharmacological effects in animals and normal human subjects of the diuretic amiloride hydrochloride (MK-870). *Clin. Pharmacol. Ther.* 9:318, 1968.

Baba, W. I., Tudhope, G. R., and Wilson, G. M. Triamterene, a new diuretic drug. I. Studies in normal man and in adrenalectomized rats. *Br. Med. J.* 2:756, 1962.

Baba, W. I., Tudhope, G. R., and Wilson, G. M. Site and mechanism of action of the diuretic, triamterene. *Clin. Sci.* 27:181, 1964.

Ball, G. M., and Greene, J. A., Jr. Localization of the site of action of triamterene diuretic. *Proc. Soc. Exp. Biol. Med.* 113:326, 1963.

Crabbé, J. Decreased effectiveness of aldosterone on active sodium transport by the isolated toad bladder in the presence of other steroids. *Acta Endocrinol. (Kbh.)* 47:419, 1964.

Duarte, C. G., Chomety, F., and Giebisch, G. Effect of amiloride, ouabain, and furosemide on distal tubular function in the rat. *Am. J. Physiol.* 221:632, 1971.

Gatzy, J. The effect of K^+-sparing diuretics on ion transport across the excised toad bladder. *J. Pharmacol. Exp. Ther.* 176:580, 1971.

Guignard, J. -P., and Peters, G. Effects of triamterene and amiloride on urinary acidification and potassium excretion in the rat. *Eur. J. Pharmacol.* 10:255, 1970.

Liddle, G. W. Aldosterone antagonists. *Arch. Intern. Med.* 102:998, 1958.

McKenna, T. J., Donohoe, J. F., Brien, T. G., Healy, J. J., Canning, B. St. J., and Muldowney, F. P. Potassium-sparing agents during diuretic therapy in hypertension. *Br. Med. J.* 2:739, 1971.

Nielsen, O. E., and Lassen, J. B. Triamterene activity investigated by the stop flow technique and in vitro studies on carbonic anhydrase. *Acta Pharmacol. Toxicol. (Kbh.)* 20:351, 1963.

Vander, A. J., Wilde, W. S., and Malvin, R. L. Stop-flow analysis of aldosterone and steroidal antagonist SC-8109 on renal tubular sodium transport kinetics. *Proc. Soc. Exp. Biol. Med.* 103:525, 1960.

Osmotic Diuretics

Gennari, F. J., and Kassirer, J. P. Osmotic diuresis. *N. Engl. J. Med.* 291:714, 1974.

Goldberg, M., McCurdy, D. K., and Ramirez, M. A. Differences between saline and mannitol diuresis in hydropenic man. *J. Clin. Invest.* 44:182, 1965.

Goldberg, M., and Ramirez, M. A. Effects of saline and mannitol diuresis on the renal concentrating mechanism in dogs: Alterations in renal tissue solutes and water. *Clin. Sci.* 32:475, 1967.

Kauker, M. L., Lassiter, W. E., and Gottschalk, C. W. Micropuncture study of effects of urea infusion on tubular reabsorption in the rat. *Am. J. Physiol.* 219:45, 1970.

Rapoport, S., Brodsky, W. A., West, C. D., and Mackler, B. Urinary flow and excretion of solutes during osmotic diuresis in hydropenic man. *Am. J. Physiol.* 156:433, 1949.

Seely, J. F., and Dirks, J. H. Micropuncture study of hypertonic mannitol diuresis in the proximal and distal tubule of the dog kidney. *J. Clin. Invest.* 48:2330, 1969.

Wesson, L. G., Jr., and Anslow, W. P., Jr. Excretion of sodium and water during osmotic diuresis in the dog. *Am. J. Physiol.* 153:465, 1948.

8 : Clinical Assessment of Renal Function

When managing a patient who *may* have renal disease, a physician seeks answers to the following questions: (1) Does the patient have renal disease? If yes, (2) What is the cause of the renal disease? (3) What is the extent of renal impairment? (4) What is the rate of progression of the disease? These questions can usually be answered by a relatively small number of procedures, some of which will be described in detail in this chapter.

Important Questions

Does the Patient Have Renal Disease?

The biggest help to answering this question is the patient's history. Again, it should be emphasized that when seeing a patient for the first time, the physician should allot the bulk of the time to obtaining an accurate history and most of the remainder to the physical examination. When there is a question of renal disease, a careful analysis of freshly voided urine and microscopic examination of the urinary sediment should be part of the initial visit. Other tests should be ordered judiciously, and in the vast majority of clinical problems, they should serve to confirm, refine, and quantify the diagnosis that has been reached on the basis of the history, physical examination, and urinalysis.

A useful source of historical information is the patient's record, either at hospitals or doctors' offices. It is often invaluable, for example, to learn that the patient's blood pressure or routine urinalysis was normal in the recent — or even not too recent — past. The particular historical points that should be ascertained can be found in any standard textbook of medicine. Likewise, details about the urinalysis can be looked up in a number of texts that are listed at the end of this chapter, and they will not be described here. Suffice it to say that a finding of proteinuria or of erythrocytes, leukocytes, or casts can constitute important supporting evidence, not only for determining the presence of renal disease but also for identifying the cause of that disease.

Two simple laboratory tests – the blood urea nitrogen concentration (BUN) and the serum concentration of creatinine – can be of tremendous help in establishing the presence of renal disease. These two tests are discussed extensively below.

What Is the Cause of the Renal Disease?

Once more, the patient's history is the most helpful aid to answering this question. Was there a preceding sore throat, an abrupt or gradual onset, recurrent infection of the urinary system, fever and chills, hypertension, edema, hematuria, instrumentation of the urinary tract or other surgical procedures, a familial incidence of renal disease, or other systemic disease, and so on? Once a likely diagnosis has been made on the basis of the history, valuable supportive information can be gained from a careful urinalysis, especially from the microscopic examination of the urinary sediment. Relatively heavy proteinuria, for example, is more compatible with disorders of the glomeruli (e.g., some form of glomerulonephritis) than with diseases such as pyelonephritis, which affect primarily the tubules and the interstitium. Similarly, a preponderance of erythrocytes over leukocytes speaks more for glomerular than for tubular disorders; proteinaceous casts of tubules in which erythrocytes have been entrapped – called *red cell casts* – establish that the bleeding comes from the kidneys, rather than from extrarenal tissue; and so on. Additional procedures – for example, ultrasonography, intravenous pyelography (I.V.P.) and other radiological examinations, cystoscopy, and certain serological tests – are often very helpful. Perhaps surprisingly, renal biopsy is frequently not the final arbiter, although it is invaluable in some instances, especially when combined with immunochemical and ultrastructural techniques.

What Is the Extent of Renal Impairment?

Although the findings of the history and physical examination (e.g., the presence or absence of nausea and anorexia, hypertension, impairment of neurological function, and so on) will answer this question in a general way, we rely on laboratory tests for a quantitative assessment. One simple measure, too often overlooked, is to determine the size of the kidneys by means of roentgenographic or ultrasonic techniques (Fig. 8-1). If a kidney is smaller than normal – shorter than about 12.5 cm in an adult woman and about 13 cm in an adult man – then chances are that the amount of renal parenchyma in that kidney is reduced; if both kidneys appear smaller, a reduction in total functioning renal tissue is likely. On the other hand, kidneys of normal size do not necessarily exclude renal impairment; in amyloidosis, for example, the kidneys may be normal in size or enlarged, even though the amount of functioning tissue has been greatly decreased.

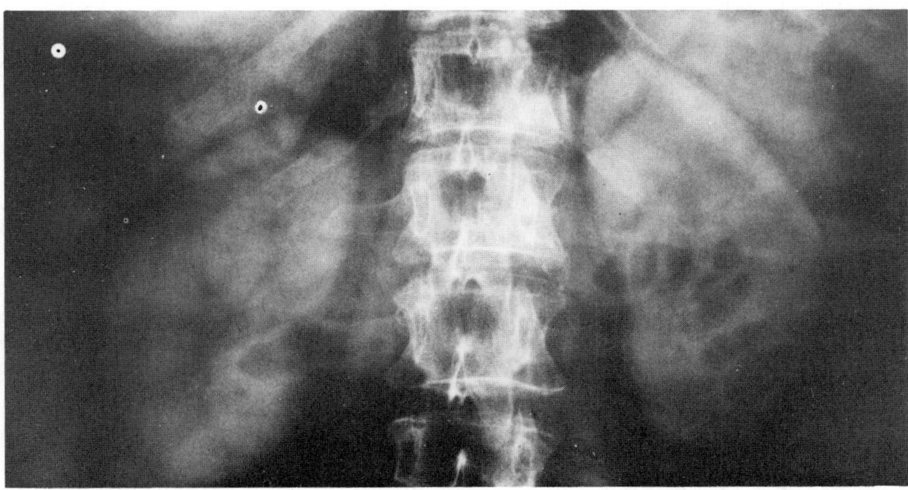

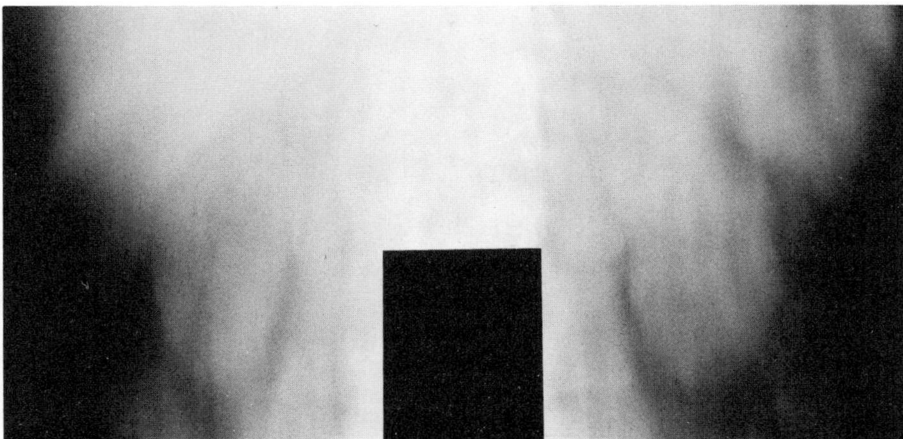

Figure 8-1
X-rays showing the size of the kidneys of two patients. At the top are the normal kidneys of a 52-year-old woman as revealed by a flat plate of the abdomen; at the bottom, the small kidneys of a 50-year-old man with chronic glomerulonephritis as visualized by tomography. Courtesy of Harte C. Crow.

Ideally, one would like to know which parts of the kidney (i.e., the glomeruli or the tubules, and if the latter, which tubular segments) are primarily affected by disease and to what extent. Some major renal functions are listed in the first column of Table 8-1, and specific tests by which these functions *could* be measured in patients are given in the second column. In routine clinical tests, however, some accuracy and specificity are often sacrificed for the sake of safety, convenience, and economy (see Chap. 1, under Clinical Tests Are Estimates). The actual tests used in patients that yield approximate assessments of the func-

Table 8-1
Tests to assess renal function

Function	Specific Test	Clinical Approximation
Rate of glomerular filtration (GFR)	Clearance of inulin (C_{In})	Blood urea nitrogen (BUN) Serum creatinine concentration Clearance of endogenous creatinine
Permeability of glomerular capillaries	Clearance of neutral or charged polysaccharides of varying molecular dimensions (e.g., dextrans or polyvinylpyrrolidones)	Protein excretion (24-hour)
Effective renal plasma flow (ERPF)	Clearance of PAH at low plasma concentration of PAH[a]	Rapid-sequence I.V.P. (Chap. 14)
Renal plasma flow (RPF)	C_{PAH}/E_{PAH}[b]	Renal scan with radioisotopes
Renal blood flow (RBF)	$C_{PAH}/E_{PAH}(1 - Hct)$	Renal angiography (Problem 14-1)
Transport in proximal tubules	Tm_G (reabsorptive)[c] Tm_{PAH} (secretory)	Urinary excretion of amino acids, glucose, phosphate, or uric acid (Chap. 12)
Transport in loops of Henle and early distal tubules	Generation of free water: C_{H_2O} during water diuresis $T^c_{H_2O}$ during antidiuresis (Fig. 7-3)	Maximal and minimal urine specific gravity and osmolality (Chaps. 2 and 13)
Concentration and dilution of urine	Maximal and minimal U/P osmolality[d] $T^c_{H_2O}$ during antidiuresis C_{H_2O} during water diuresis	Maximal and minimal urine specific gravity and osmolality Hickey-Hare test (Chaps. 2 and 13)
Acidification of urine	Renal threshold for HCO_3^- $Tm_{HCO_3^-}$ (Fig. 12-7) Urinary pH	Urinary excretion of HCO_3^- and urinary pH during NH_4Cl-induced metabolic acidosis (Chap. 12; RTA)

[a]PAH = *p*-aminohippurate.
[b]C_{PAH} = clearance of PAH; E_{PAH} = extraction ratio for PAH = $(Pa_{PAH} - Pv_{PAH})/Pa_{PAH}$, where Pa_{PAH} and Pv_{PAH} are arterial and venous plasma PAH concentrations, respectively.
[c]Tm = transport maximum; Tm_G = transport maximum for glucose.
[d]U/P osmolality = ratio of urine osmolality to plasma osmolality.

tion in question are shown in the third column of Table 8-1. The frequent referrals in this column to other chapters indicate that many of the clinical tests are used primarily for diagnosing and quantifying specific (and mostly rare) diseases of the kidneys, not to gauge a decrease in general renal function. For example, although an impairment in the dilution and concentration of urine occurs in renal failure, most nephrologists limit the use of urine specific gravity and osmolality determinations to diagnosing disorders of water balance (Chaps. 2 and 13). Furthermore, although renal failure from whatever cause usually is accompanied by decreased renal plasma flow (RPF), decreased proximal tubular transport, and decreased excretion of acid, the clinical tests that measure these functions are customarily limited to the diagnosis of specific renal vascular disorders and hypertension (Chap. 14) or discrete tubular dysfunctions (Chap. 12).

Thus, the extent of renal impairment is mainly determined by the BUN, the serum creatinine concentration, and the clearance of endogenous creatinine. These are all tests of glomerular function (Table 8-1); this limitation for measuring renal reserve can be justified by the structural and functional interdependence of the vascular and tubular components of the kidney. The glomerulonephritides, for example, affect first the glomerular capillaries and therefore will decrease the GFR. Because the renal circulation runs in series, however, the renal blood flow is likely to decline simultaneously, and the consequent diminution of blood flow in the peritubular capillaries may thus quickly lead to disturbances of tubular function as well. Conversely, pyelonephritis afflicts primarily the tubular and interstitial structures in the renal medulla; it therefore initially and predominantly compromises the ability to concentrate urine. However, because of the intertwining and continuity of tubular and vascular structures, pyelonephritis will quickly involve cortical functions as well, so the GFR will also decrease. Some diseases (e.g., the nephrotic syndrome) will alter the permeability of glomerular capillaries without influencing the GFR; in these instances, the amount of protein excreted during a 24-hour period can be correlated with the degree of damage. In most cases, though, the degree of functional impairment from any generalized renal disease, whether its initial impact is on the tubular or the vascular system, will be reflected in the amount of decrease of the GFR.

What Is the Rate of Progression of Renal Disease?

For the reasons just outlined, this question is also most readily answered by the first four simple tests listed in the third column of Table 8-1. The utility of these measures in a patient with one form of chronic glomerulonephritis is shown in Figure 8-2. This man was known to have glomerulonephritis, and he was

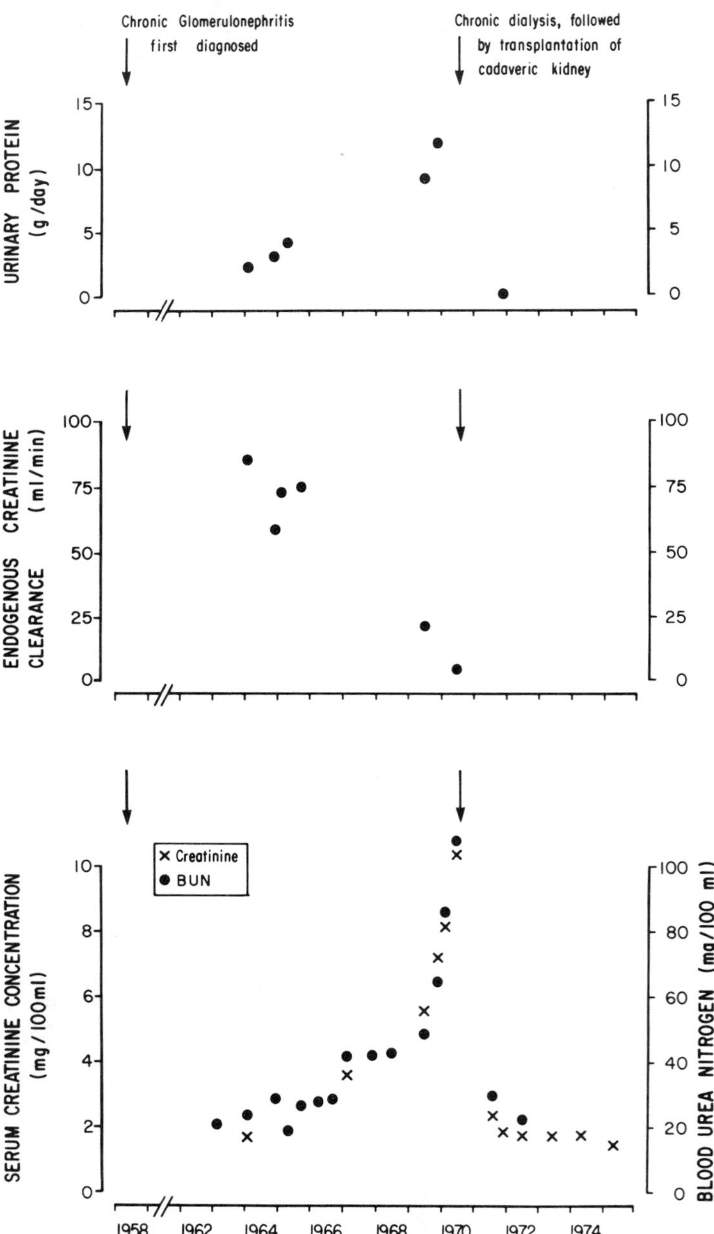

Figure 8-2
Serial determinations of the four tests most commonly used to follow the progression of renal disease. The clinical history for the patient is given in the text, and each of the tests is described in subsequent sections.

seen by his physician every three months or more often as required. The progression of his disease was reflected by the gradual rise of the BUN, serum creatinine concentration, and 24-hour protein excretion, and the fall in the endogenous creatinine clearance. The changes were correlated with increasing symptoms of renal failure: anorexia, nausea, weakness, lethargy, and malaise. These symptoms, signs, and a few laboratory values were used to determine the time when the patient should be managed through chronic dialysis and ultimately through transplantation. In 1978, this patient was feeling well and leading a full professional and personal life.

Although the tests shown in Figure 8-2 are those most commonly used to follow the progression of renal disease, it should be stressed that they are not the only tests. The routine urinalysis, especially insofar as it gives a semiquantitative assessment of the degree of proteinuria and abnormal elements (e.g., casts) in the urinary sediment, is an inexpensive and valuable aid; so, too, is the HCO_3^- concentration in venous plasma (Chap. 10) and the calculation of the anion gap (Table 5-3 and Fig. 1-A). And all tests must always be evaluated in light of how the patient is faring.

Rate of Glomerular Filtration (GFR)

The remainder of this chapter will be devoted to discussing clinical tests of glomerular function. The other tests listed in Table 8-1 have been or will be taken up in other chapters.

Serum Creatinine

The relationship between the GFR and the concentration of creatinine in serum is shown in Figure 8-3 (the blood urea nitrogen concentration, or BUN, is also graphed in this figure and will be discussed in the subsequent section). Although individual points have not been plotted in Figure 8-3, the curve represents an empirical relationship based on data obtained from healthy subjects and patients. The graph describes a rectangular hyperbola, which means that in the steady state and at any value of the GFR, the product of the serum creatinine concentration times the GFR equals a constant value. The dynamics of this relationship are summarized in Figure 8-4.

Creatinine is derived from creatine, which as creatine phosphate, is found mainly in muscle cells, especially in those of skeletal muscles. The dietary intake of meat is so small compared to the total muscle mass of an individual that far and away the principal source of creatinine is the metabolism of muscle. Since *in any one individual* this metabolism proceeds at a fairly stable rate, the daily production of creatinine is also quite constant. It varies with age, sex, and size (Table 1-3), but for the purpose of illustration, we shall use a value of 1.8 g per day. Creatinine is excreted solely by the kidneys, and in humans this

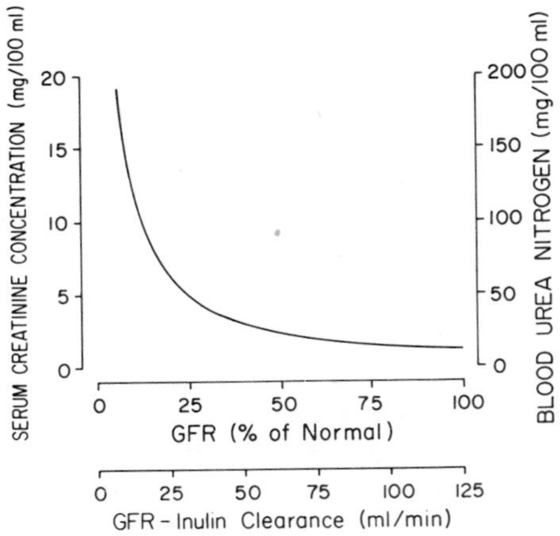

Figure 8-3
Relationship between the rate of glomerular filtration (GFR) and the serum creatinine concentration on the one hand, and the blood urea nitrogen concentration (BUN) on the other. Absolute values for the GFR, as determined by inulin clearance, refer to measurements in adults. The graph is based on values obtained from healthy subjects and from patients who are in nitrogen balance on a normal protein intake. Although there is considerable scatter of these values among individuals, a single average curve has been drawn; however, for a particular person whose GFR has been reduced by, say, 50 percent, the serum creatinine concentration could lie anywhere between about 1.4 and 3.0 mg/100 ml.

process is accomplished overwhelmingly by filtration, with a small fraction undergoing tubular secretion. For practical purposes, then, we can say that creatinine is handled like inulin, so the filtered load (GFR · P_{Creat}) represents the amount of creatinine that is excreted. For a normal GFR of 180 liters per day and a normal plasma creatinine concentration of 1 mg/100 ml (or 10 mg per liter), the filtered load, and hence the rate of excretion, would be about 1,800 mg per day. Since this value also represents the daily production of creatinine, the normal individual is thus in balance for creatinine.

If this individual now sustains damage to the kidneys so that the GFR is decreased, he will temporarily go into positive balance for creatinine. This consequence is inevitable, because the filtered load of creatinine decreases while the daily production of creatinine, being dependent mainly on the total muscle mass, remains at the normal value. As a result of the positive balance, the serum creatinine level rises, and as it does so, the filtered load increases so that the daily increments of positive balance become less. The serum creatinine concentration will level off at a value where the product of the decreased GFR and the increased serum creatinine concentration will again equal the normal rate of production of creatinine. Thus, if the degree of renal damage is such that the

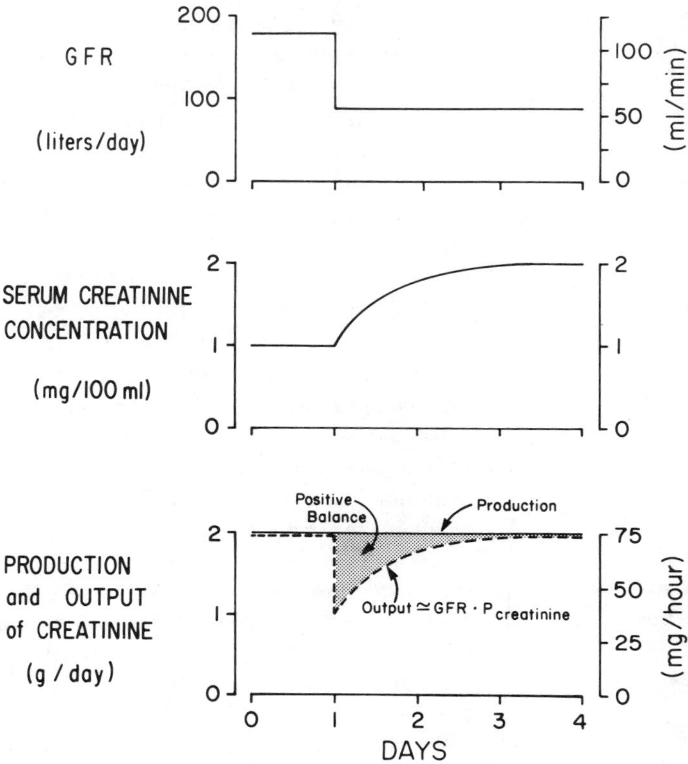

Figure 8-4
Dynamics for the restoration of creatinine balance when the glomerular filtration rate (GFR) is reduced to 50 percent of its normal value. Alternative units for the GFR and for the production and output of creatinine are given for the ordinates on the right; the fact that the ordinates on the left and right do not precisely match quantitatively serves to emphasize that the values shown are approximate. Modified from J. P. Kassirer, *N. Engl. J. Med.* 285:385, 1971.

GFR is reduced by 50 percent (Figs. 8-3 and 8-4), the new steady-state value for serum creatinine will, in this instance, be 2.0 mg/100 ml, for it is at this value that the filtered load — namely, 90 liters per day times 20 mg per liter — will again equal the normal rate of production of creatinine, or 1.8 g per day. Alternatively, if the extent of renal damage is relatively mild so that the GFR is reduced by only 25 percent, the serum creatinine concentration will rise to 1.3 mg/100 ml (135 liters per day $\times$ 13 mg per liter $\approx$ 1.8 g per day).

The normal range for the serum creatinine concentration is 0.7 to 1.5 mg/100 ml (Table 1-1); this seemingly wide range results mainly from variation in the age, sex, and size of individuals (see Comments, Table 1-3) and partly from errors in measurement. In many patients, therefore, the serum creatinine concentration does not rise out of the normal range until the GFR has been reduced by at least 40 percent (Fig. 8-3). This fact has led to the *erroneous* statement that the serum creatinine does not rise until a rather large degree of renal impairment has occurred. In fact, it must rise as soon as the GFR begins to decrease, but because the relationship follows that of a rectangular hyperbola, the initial rise is gradual (Fig. 8-3) and, given the possibility of variation in measurement, may be imperceptible. Although a serum creatinine concentration of 1.5 mg/100 ml or even a little higher may be seen in healthy individuals, such values are very likely to reflect reduction in renal function *when observed in a patient with a history suggesting renal disease.* It is probably in this kind of situation — that is, when the serum creatinine concentration is at the upper limits of normal — that determination of the 24-hour endogenous creatinine clearance can be of the greatest help in deciding whether the GFR is decreased (see below).

Blood Urea Nitrogen (BUN)

The determinants of the BUN (Table 8-2) are analogous to those for creatinine, but they are slightly more complicated. The normal value for the BUN concentration is 9 to 18 mg/100 ml; the range is wide mainly because of variation in protein intake (see below; also Comments, Table 1-1).

Normal Protein Intake. Urea is the major end product of nitrogen metabolism, and ordinarily its daily production depends mainly on the dietary intake of protein. Urea is excreted almost solely by the kidneys through a combination of filtration and tubular reabsorption; roughly 40 to 50 percent of the filtered load of urea is excreted. A normal adult weighs about 70 kg, and he eats about 70 g of protein per day. With an average nitrogen content for protein of 16 percent (see Lean Tissue Balance, Table 1-5), his daily nitrogen production is about 11 g per day, or approximately 7.5 mg per minute. If his GFR and BUN are normal — that is, 125 ml per minute and 12 mg/100 ml, respectively — the filtered load of urea nitrogen will equal 15 mg per minute (Table 8-2). At a normal urine flow, roughly 50 percent of the filtered urea nitrogen is reabsorbed, and 50 percent, or 7.5 mg per minute, is excreted. Since under these conditions, the amount of urea nitrogen excreted equals its production, the individual is in urea balance.

Increased Protein Intake in Health. Unlike the serum creatinine concentration, which varies minimally with changes in dietary protein, the BUN depends critically upon the protein intake. If the healthy man described above doubles his protein intake and hence the production of urea nitrogen (Table 8-2), then, so long as he excretes only 7.5 mg of urea nitrogen per

Table 8-2
Determinants of the blood urea nitrogen (BUN)[a]

Condition	GFR (ml/min)	BUN (mg/100 ml)	Urea Nitrogen[b] (mg/min) Filtered	Reabsorbed	Excreted	Produced	Remarks
Normal protein intake in health	125	12	15	7.5	7.5	7.5	Balance; i.e., urea excretion = urea production
Double protein intake in health	125	12	15	7.5	7.5	15	BUN, but not creatinine, will double without impairment of renal function
	125	18[c]	22.5	11.3	11.3	15	
	125	24	30	15	15	15	
Renal disease	75	12	9	4.5	4.5	7.5	BUN may be at upper limit of normal despite 40% decrease in renal function
	75	16[c]	12	6	6	7.5	
	75	20	15	7.5	7.5	7.5	
Further deterioration of renal function	25	20	5	2.5	2.5	7.5	Absolute increase in BUN (and creatinine) is greater the more advanced the renal failure (Fig. 8-3)
	25	40[c]	10	5	5	7.5	
	25	60	15	7.5	7.5	7.5	
Double protein intake in renal disease	25	60	15	7.5	7.5	15	In renal disease, an increase in dietary protein can cause a dramatic rise in BUN, but not in serum creatinine (see Fig. 8-6)
	25	90[c]	22.5	11.3	11.3	15	
	25	120	30	15	15	15	

[a]The schema is based on the assumption that 50% of the filtered urea is reabsorbed and 50% excreted. To the extent that these proportions vary (especially in renal disease), the absolute values will be slightly different (e.g., those of the BUN/creatinine ratio and the effect of dehydration and overhydration).
[b]Concentrations of urea are usually determined by measuring the amount of nitrogen in urea; hence, the expression "urea nitrogen." The two nitrogen atoms constitute 28/60 of the urea molecule: $CO(NH_2)_2$. One can therefore estimate the blood urea concentration by multiplying the BUN by two.
[c]Intermediate values represent partial attainment of a new steady state.

minute, he will be in positive urea balance and his BUN will rise. When it has risen by 50 percent to 18 mg/100 ml, the filtered load (and hence the excretion of urea nitrogen) will have increased, but not sufficiently to eliminate positive urea balance. Only when the BUN has doubled, thereby doubling the filtered load and the excretion of urea nitrogen, will he again be in balance.

Note that doubling a normal BUN raises its value into the abnormal range. This fact may lead to an erroneous diagnosis of renal failure if it is based solely on the BUN. An example of where this error was committed is shown in Figure 8-5. The values graphed in this figure are from a boy who was born April 22, 1970. At five weeks of age, he developed hemolytic anemia (possibly as part of the hemolytic-uremic syndrome), which was associated with a very high BUN and a serum creatinine concentration that was somewhat elevated. The high BUN probably resulted from increased protein catabolism following the destruction of erythrocytes as well as possibly from mild contraction of the extracellular fluid volume (Table 8-3) and some decrease in the GFR; the elevation in creatinine probably reflected only the last event. An intravenous pyelogram (I.V.P.) was done in June 1970, and even though gas-filled bowel overlying the kidneys made a reliable interpretation impossible, the radiologist mentioned the possibility of "renal dysplasia." Ever

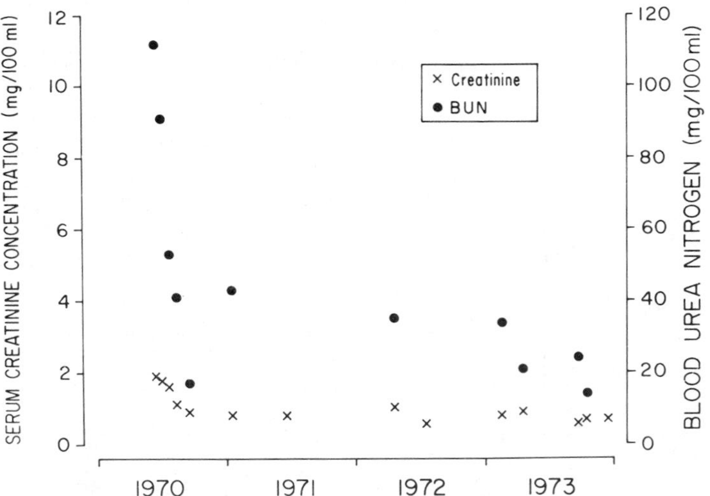

Figure 8-5
High BUN-to-creatinine ratios in a young boy. Even though there was some renal failure in early 1970 as reflected by the increased serum creatinine concentration (the normal value at 1 month of age is approximately 0.5 mg/100 ml), the elevated *ratio* at that time was due mainly to increased protein catabolism from hemolytic anemia. The high ratios subsequently were caused by a high dietary intake of milk. For details, see text.

since then, and because of recurrent, high BUN values, the child has been considered to be in chronic renal failure. When the problem was reassessed in 1973, a consulting nephrologist pointed out not only that the BUN/creatinine ratio was far in excess of the normal value of 10 (Fig. 8-5; also below), but also that the serum creatinine concentration did not fluctuate like the BUN but had been consistently in the normal range since late 1970. These findings suggested that the high BUN values reflected elevated production of urea, not a decreased GFR. It was then discovered that the patient's mother considered milk to be healthy and was giving the child so much milk to drink that his calculated protein intake was four to five times the normal daily allowance. The child's high BUN was "cured" just by reducing his milk intake. Although the possibility that he sustained a renal injury right after birth should be kept in mind, the history does not justify labeling this patient with the stigma of chronic renal failure.

Renal Disease. It is not uncommon for renal disease to result in a permanent reduction of the GFR to 60 percent of the normal value, that is, to about 75 ml per minute, as in the example cited in Table 8-2. This degree of renal impairment can occur without the patient even being aware of having been ill, and such patients can lead an active life on a normal diet. Their production of urea nitrogen will therefore remain at the normal rate, and according to the dynamics previously discussed (also Fig. 8-4), such patients will regain urea balance at a new and elevated BUN. Even with a 40 percent reduction in GFR, however, the BUN will barely rise out of the normal range (Fig. 8-3). As was the case with the serum creatinine concentration, this fact sometimes lulls physicians into the false impression that the patient's kidneys have not been damaged. As pointed out above, it is probably in this situation that measurement of the 24-hour endogenous creatinine clearance has its greatest value.

Further Deterioration of Renal Function. Once slight reduction of renal function has raised the BUN (and serum creatinine) to the upper limits of normal, however, further renal damage leads to a precipitous rise in these variables. This fact is reflected in the steep slope of the curve in Figure 8-3 when the GFR is decreased to less than 50 percent of normal (also Table 8-2). When the hypothetical patient with renal disease showed further deterioration of renal function so that his GFR declined by a factor of three (i.e., from 75 ml per minute to 25 ml per minute), the BUN had to rise threefold so long as the patient ate the normal amount of protein. Although the precipitous rise has the same mathematical meaning as the more gradual increase seen during early renal damage, it does have a more ominous functional connotation, for it shows that the patient is beginning to run out of renal reserve.

Increased Protein Intake in Renal Disease. The final example in Table 8-2 shows that even a very alarming rise in the BUN does not necessarily signify a further decrease in renal reserve. Doubling the intake of protein must double the BUN, whether it occurs in health or renal disease. Thus, when a patient with a GFR of 25 ml per minute and a BUN of 60 mg/100 ml eats twice as much protein as before, the BUN increases to 120 mg/100 ml. A clinical example of this phenomenon is shown in Figure 8-6.

The patient for whom the data are depicted (Fig. 8-6) was a 54-year-old man who had several subdural hematomas after he fell off a truck. He had a long and complicated hospitalization, involving a number of neurosurgical procedures, protracted coma, and pneumonia. The cause of his renal failure was never determined. On the 46th day of illness, a nephrologist was called in because it was feared that the rapidly rising BUN reflected a sudden deterioration of renal function. A review of the record at this time revealed that on about the 41st hospital day, the patient, who had eaten poorly, was force-fed a high-protein diet through a stomach tube. The impression that this procedure — and not progressing renal failure — was the cause of the rising BUN was confirmed by the failure of the serum creatinine level to increase simultaneously and by the prompt decrease of the BUN when the protein intake was reduced. Seven years after the

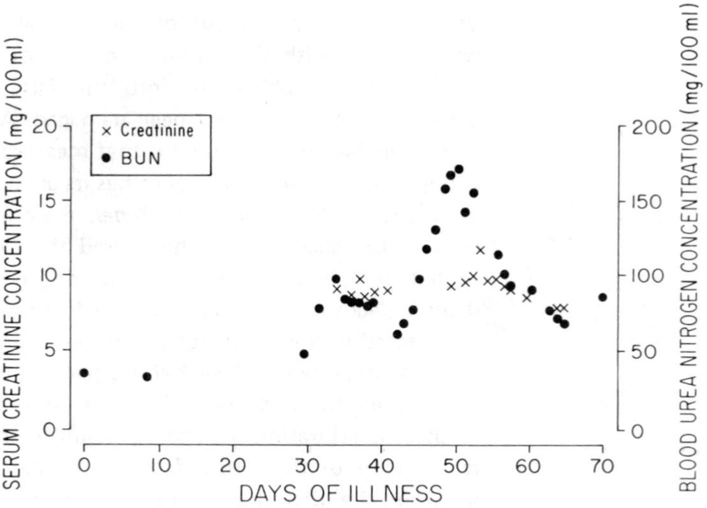

Figure 8-6
Dramatic and selective rise of the BUN in a patient with renal failure who was suddenly started on a high-protein intake on day 41. Details are given in the text.

accident, the patient was living in a county home, showing signs of residual brain damage. His serum creatinine concentration and BUN had stabilized at about 2 mg/100 ml and 20 mg/100 ml, respectively. (*Note:* It seems easy to analyze the situation correctly in retrospect, especially when given the graph of Figure 8-6. Sometimes it is difficult to discern a pattern when looking at isolated laboratory data; graphing values is therefore often very helpful.)

Creatinine Versus BUN

Considering the vagaries of the BUN, especially when contrasted with the reliability of the serum creatinine concentration as a measure of the GFR, why is the BUN still used so extensively? There are at least two good reasons. (1) The BUN determination is a simple, inexpensive, and reproducible test that gives a semi-quantitative assessment of renal function in the vast majority of patients. (2) When the BUN and the serum creatinine concentrations are determined simultaneously in the same patient, the combination frequently yields a more complete evaluation than either test alone. Ordinarily, the BUN/creatinine ratio is about 10, as is evident from several of the preceding figures. Therefore, if the BUN is roughly 10 times greater than the serum creatinine, one may not only conclude that the measurements are correct, but one can also gauge the extent of renal damage without further tests. For example, if the BUN is about 50 mg/100 ml and the serum creatinine about 5 mg/100 ml, one can conclude with considerable assurance that the patient's GFR has been reduced to approximately 25 percent of normal and that an endogenous creatinine clearance test, if done (Fig. 8-2), would yield a result of about 25 to 35 ml per minute. Conversely, a ratio that consistently and markedly deviates from 10 should arouse suspicions of associated, nonrenal factors (Figs. 8-5 and 8-6).

BUN/Creatinine Ratio. Conditions that can cause deviations of the BUN/creatinine ratio from its normal value of about 10 are shown in Table 8-3. Any increase in the amount of protein that is metabolized to urea – be it exogenous from diet or endogenous from internal bleeding, destruction of blood (Fig. 8-5), increased catabolism, or decreased anabolism – will lead to a selective rise of the BUN. Dehydration tends to increase the ratio, not because it may lower the GFR (which would have the same proportional effect on the BUN and serum creatinine levels), but because a slowing of the rate of tubular flow increases the percentage of the filtered load of urea that is reabsorbed. The consequent decrease in the amount of urea excreted will cause a positive balance of urea until a rise in the BUN reestablishes balance. A low rate of creatinine production, as in asthenic individuals, is a rare cause of an increased ratio.

Table 8-3
Causes of alterations in the BUN/creatinine ratio

Increased ratio:
- Increased urea production, as in
  - Increased dietary protein
  - Gastrointestinal bleeding (digestion of erythrocytes and plasma proteins)
  - Hemolytic anemia
  - Fever
  - Inhibition of protein anabolism by adrenal steroids or tetracyclines
  - Gluconeogenesis
- Dehydration (through increased fractional reabsorption of urea)
- Decreased creatinine production, as in prolonged starvation

Decreased ratio:
- Decreased urea production, as in
  - Low dietary protein
  - Severe liver damage
- Overhydration (through decreased fractional reabsorption of urea)
- Increased creatinine production, as in rhabdomyolysis

Decreases in the ratio are usually not as striking or as common as increases. Severe damage to the liver may impair the urea cycle sufficiently to result in decreased urea production. Overhydration as a result of events opposite to those described above for dehydration may lead to an increase in the fraction of the filtered load of urea that is excreted and hence to a temporary, negative urea balance.

Clearance of Endogenous Creatinine

The BUN and serum creatinine concentrations provide an estimate of the GFR. The GFR can be measured accurately by means of the inulin clearance test (Table 8-1), but this procedure is not practicable for patients, since it would involve a continuous intravenous infusion of inulin and an accuracy of urine collection that can be achieved in most patients only through urethral catheterization. What is required for quantification of the GFR in patients is an *endogenous* substance that has a stable plasma concentration and that, like inulin, is freely filtered at the glomerulus, is neither reabsorbed nor secreted by renal tubules, and can be readily measured in urine and plasma. No such endogenous compound has yet been found. Creatinine approaches – but by no means meets – these ideal criteria; its plasma concentration in any one person probably fluctuates by no more than 10 percent during a 24-hour period, but it is partly secreted by the renal tubules of man, and most methods used to quantify it in plasma measure some substance in addition to creatinine, the so-called noncreatinine chromogen. Nevertheless, the value for the endogenous creatinine clearance is, on the average, equal to the simultaneously determined inulin clearance under many circumstances. The agreement, however, probably results from the cancellation of equal and opposite errors in the creatinine clearance test, rather than from creatinine being handled just like inulin. Furthermore, the agreement breaks down in renal disease, just when an accurate measure of the GFR might be most wanted; the discrepancy occurs because both the renal handling and the metabolism of creatinine change as renal function declines. An additional drawback of the creatinine clearance determination is that it requires an accurate measure of urine flow without catheterizing the patient. In order to circumvent this difficulty, the clearance of endogenous creatinine can be determined during a 24-hour period.

The opinion of nephrologists is divided regarding the usefulness of creatinine clearance as a clinical test. In view of the possible sources of error cited above and the wide range of normal values among individuals (85 to 125 ml per minute per 1.73 m^2 body surface area in women; 97 to 140 ml per minute per 1.73 m^2 in men), it is difficult to see what advantages the creatinine clearance test offers over the simpler determinations of BUN and serum creatinine levels. There is one situation, however, in which the clearance test can help, and that is in patients with *possible* renal disease whose BUN and serum creatinine concentrations are at the upper limits of normal. Such values are compatible with normal renal function, or they could reflect as much as a 50 percent reduction in renal reserve. If the latter is the case, the 24-hour endogenous creatinine clearance is likely to fall below the normal range, and if this finding proves consistent on a repeated clearance test, the likelihood of the patient's having suffered renal damage would be great.

In closing this section it should be stated that a precise measurement of the GFR is not critical to the optimal management of patients with renal disease. If a patient has a BUN of 36 mg/100 ml and a serum creatinine concentration of 3.2 mg/100 ml, it is not important to know whether the GFR is 30 ml per minute or 45 ml per minute; what is important is the recognition that the patient has moderately severe renal failure, because he has lost approximately two-thirds of normal renal function. Similarly, in another patient, if the BUN is 108 mg/100 ml and the serum creatinine is 10.4 mg/100 ml (Fig. 8-2), it is not essential to know whether the GFR is 5 ml per minute or 10 ml per minute; in either case, it will be known that the patient has very advanced renal disease and that he may soon need dialysis or transplantation. Furthermore, the right time for beginning such measures will be determined, not on the basis of the endogenous creatinine clearance test nor even on the basis of the BUN and serum creatinine concentrations, but rather on the patient's symptoms and signs.

Permeability of Glomerular Capillaries

One important feature of normal renal function is the selective permeability of the glomerular capillaries, which permits free filtration of plasma water and its nonprotein constituents (often called crystalloids) while largely preventing blood cells and protein macromolecules (the colloids) from entering Bowman's space. This characteristic is decreased in many disorders of the kidneys, and it is not surprising, therefore, that proteinuria is one of the commonest and earliest signs of renal disease. If the degree of proteinuria is to be accepted as a semiquantitative measure of glomerular permeability, however, it must be shown that the protein that appears in the urine entered the tubular system by way of glomerular filtration and not by some other route.

Mechanisms of Proteinuria

There are four possible ways by which abnormal quantities of protein can enter the urinary system: (1) by increased filtration of normal plasma proteins because of a defect in the filtration barrier of the glomerular capillaries, (2) through filtration of small proteins that are produced systemically in abnormal amounts, (3) as a result of decreased tubular reabsorption of the relatively small amount of protein that is normally filtered, or (4) through secretion of protein into the tubular lumina or into the ureters or bladder. There is now considerable experimental evidence that the first is by far the most common mechanism. In the majority of *renal* diseases that are associated with heavy proteinuria (Table 8-4), the major urinary proteins are identical with those in normal plasma. Although such a pattern does not exclude some of the other routes of entry mentioned above, the evidence shown in Figure 8-7 points convincingly to increased glomerular permeability as the principal mechanism. Dextrans are polysaccharides that, like inulin, can be infused intravenously; they are filtered but neither reabsorbed nor secreted by the renal tubules. They are available in varying molecular weights (M.W.), ranging from less than 4,000 (i.e., less than that of inulin, which has a molecular weight of about 5,000) to more than 100,000, which exceeds the molecular weight of serum albumin (69,000). Normally, dextran of M.W. 4,000 is filtered as readily as inulin, and the renal clearance of that dextran is equal to the clearance of inulin. As dextrans of increasing molecular weight are infused, they are filtered less readily, and at a molecular weight of around 50,000, they are just barely filtered and therefore just detectable in normal urine (Fig. 8-7). This finding is consistent with inde-

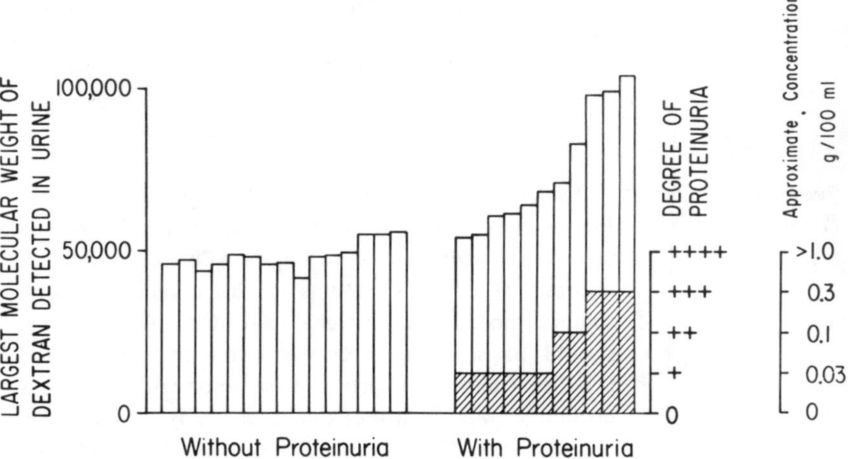

Figure 8-7
Correlation between the largest size of dextran that can pass through the glomerular filter (and therefore be detected in urine) and the appearance and degree of proteinuria in human patients. Each bar represents the results in a single patient. The open columns refer to the size of dextran molecules; the shaded columns to the degree of proteinuria. Similar results have been obtained with another polysaccharide, polyvinylpyrrolidone. The approximate concentrations of protein (g/100 ml) that correspond to the clinical designations of one-plus, two-plus, three-plus, and four-plus proteinuria are indicated on the second ordinate. Modified from G. Wallenius, *Acta Soc. Med. Upsal.* 59 (Suppl. 4):1, 1954.

pendent evidence that small amounts of serum albumin can pass through the filtration barrier of normal glomerular capillaries. When dextrans of M.W. 55,000 or greater appear in the urine, this finding is not only associated with proteinuria, but the degree of proteinuria can be roughly correlated with the size of the dextran that must have passed through the glomerular filter in order to be excreted. The association and correlation strongly suggest that the proteins entered the urinary system through a more "leaky" filter. In addition, it has been shown that normally, fixed negative charges on the glomerular capillary wall influence the filtration of solute particles. It is possible that the number of these charges – and hence the filtration barrier to polyanions (e.g., albumin) – may be reduced in some forms of glomerular disease.

Sometimes, however, proteinuria is caused predominantly by another mechanism. An example of the second mechanism listed above is the urinary excretion of Bence Jones proteins in multiple myeloma (Fig. 8-8). The third and fourth possible causes listed may be more theoretical than real. It is possible, however, that decreased reabsorption of proteins that are normally filtered occurs in certain discrete tubular dysfunctions, for example, in some patients with the Fanconi syndrome (Chap. 12). The fourth mechanism may be the cause of proteinuria in some instances, such as pyelonephritis, where tubular damage predominates, or when the damage is mainly to the lower urinary tract (e.g., in ureteral obstruction or cystitis).

Twenty-four Hour Protein Excretion

Qualitative and Quantitative Electrophoretic Pattern in Health. Figure 8-8a has been included to permit comparison of the abnormal pattern shown in Figure 8-8b and to stress that electrophoresis of urinary proteins is now a valuable diagnostic tool, though mostly for nonrenal disorders. A couple of cautions should be sounded in connection with Figure 8-8a, however. (1) The figure may give a false impression of the amount of protein in normal urine; this quantity is so minimal (up to 150 mg per day) that normal urine must be concentrated 50- to 100-fold by dialysis in order to discern the profile shown in Figure 8-8a. In fact, tor clinical purposes the protein concentration of normal urine is considered to be zero, because routine tests have a sensitivity of only about 100 mg per liter, and ordinarily the urinary protein concentration is below this value (Table 1-3). Thus, the important diagnostic information to be

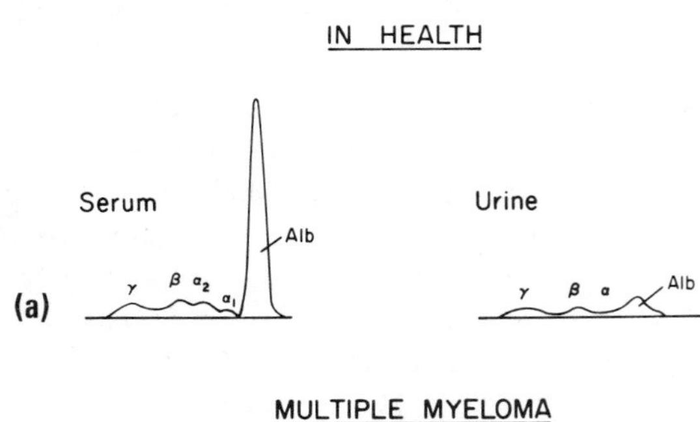

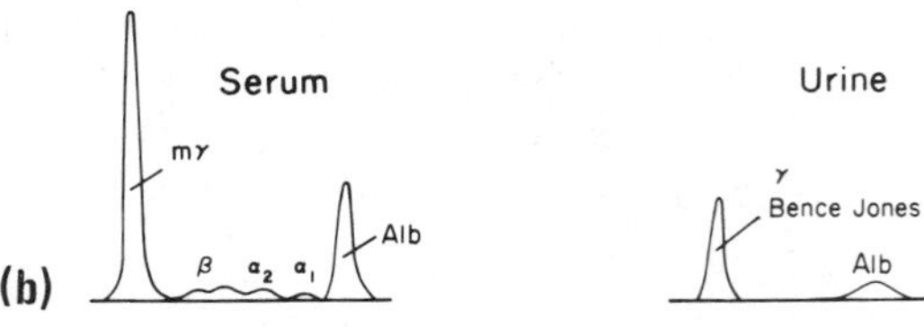

Figure 8-8
Electrophoretic patterns for proteins in serum and urine of (a) a healthy individual and (b) a patient with multiple myeloma. Urine samples were concentrated by dialysis prior to electrophoresis. *Alb* = albumin; α, β, γ = α-, β-, and γ-globulins; $m\gamma$ = myeloma globulin in γ region; *Bence Jones* = Bence Jones protein. Adapted from E. F. Osserman, in P. B. Beeson and W. McDermott, *Textbook of Medicine* (14th ed.). Philadelphia: Saunders, 1975.

derived from urinary protein electrophoresis concerns the pattern, not the quantity, of the proteins. (2) Viewed roughly, the figure may also give the false impression that the proteins that normally appear in the urine are simply those that have been filtered from normal plasma. Actually, 20 to 30 percent of normal urinary protein is the Tamm-Horsfall protein, a mucoprotein of high molecular weight (7×10^6), which is not present in plasma but is thought to be derived from cells lining the loops of Henle, distal tubules, and collecting ducts. Furthermore, some of the globulins in serum are so large that they can barely, if at all, pass through the filtering membrane of glomerular capillaries. Urinary albumin, however, is probably derived from filtered plasma and constitutes about 25 percent of normal protein.

Nevertheless, much of the protein that normally appears in urine is thought to be the result of selective glomerular filtration and of nonselective tubular reabsorption, chiefly in the proximal tubules. Micropuncture samples from the proximal tubules of rats and dogs have shown concentrations for albumin and γ-globulin in the range of perhaps 1 to 10 mg/100 ml of tubular fluid. Since a normal plasma protein concentration is at least a thousand times greater than this value (Table 1-1), the finding shows that the normal glomerular capillary is a very effective filter. If the results can be extrapolated to man (as seems likely), they would show, moreover, that a large amount of filtered protein must normally undergo tubular reabsorption. Assuming the concentration of total protein in the fluid of Bowman's space to be 5 mg/100 ml (or 50 mg per liter), the filtered load of protein at a normal GFR of 180 liters per day would be 9,000 mg per day. Since no more than 150 mg per day is excreted, the difference must be reabsorbed.

Quantitation in Renal Disease

Urine flow can normally vary over such a wide range from one moment to the next that a protein concentration on a random specimen can give only a semiquantitative appraisal of the degree of proteinuria. Although this estimate, which is recorded on a scale of "pluses" or as approximate concentrations (Fig. 8-7), is valuable, a more accurate quantitation is often desirable. For example, a patient with questionable renal disease may show intermittent or minimal proteinuria on random samples. Or, in the patient for whom results are shown in Figure 8-2, every urine specimen since 1965 was reported as "4+ " or "> 1.0 g/100 ml"; however, a more accurate measure was needed to evaluate the rate of progression of his disease. Similarly, a patient with the nephrotic syndrome may continue to show "4+ proteinuria" as he is being treated, even though more precise quantitation will indicate a large and meaningful decrease in the amount of protein being excreted. In such instances, determination of the 24-hour protein excretion is a relatively simple and inexpensive test that usually gives the needed information.

A 24-hour urine sample is collected as follows. On first arising in the morning, the patient empties his bladder into the toilet and he notes the time of this voiding. He then saves all urine during the ensuing 24 hours, up to and *including* the voiding at the same hour the next morning.

In addition to having prognostic value (Fig. 8-2), the quantitation of proteinuria can also help in diagnosis. Some conditions (Table 8-4) are characterized by heavy proteinuria, by which we mean more than 4.0 g per day or consistently three-plus to four-plus (Fig. 8-7) on random specimens. In other conditions, mild or intermittent proteinuria – that is, <0.5 g per day, or zero to one-plus – is typical. Details about these conditions can be found in standard textbooks.

Summary

A partial list of the numerous tests used to evaluate renal function is given in Table 8-1. In addition, the patient's history, the physical examination, and the routine urinalysis (including an expert assessment of the urinary sediment) are of paramount importance. Many of the tests are described in the preceding and succeeding chapters. Here, we have restricted detailed discussion to the four tests that are used most commonly to establish the presence, extent, and rate of progression of renal impairment: the BUN, serum creatinine, 24-hour endogenous creatinine clearance, and 24-hour protein excretion tests. Although all four tests reflect glomerular function, their use to evaluate general renal function is justified by the structural and functional interdependence of the tubular and vascular elements of the kidney.

Endogenous creatinine is excreted almost solely by glomerular filtration, and its rate of production depends almost entirely on the lean muscle mass, which is quite constant in any one individual. As the GFR and hence the urinary excretion of creatinine decrease, the individual goes into positive balance for creatinine, because the production of creatinine continues at the normal rate. Consequently, the creatinine concentration in plasma rises, and it will level off at that point where the filtered load of creatinine – that is, the product of the lower GFR and the higher plasma creatinine concentration – will again equal the filtered load in the normal state (Fig. 8-4). In other words, at any given rate of production of creatinine, the serum creatinine concentration will rise in proportion to the decrease in GFR; it is for this reason that the serum creatinine concentration rather accurately gauges the GFR, and this is also why the curve in Figure 8-3 describes a rectangular hyperbola.

Table 8-4
Conditions typically associated with heavy or light proteinuria

Common causes of heavy proteinuria:
- Nephrotic syndrome
- Subacute and chronic glomerulonephritides
- Renal disease of diabetes mellitus (so-called intercapillary glomerulosclerosis)
- Renal disease of severe hypertension (so-called malignant nephrosclerosis)
- Amyloidosis
- Systemic lupus erythematosus
- Vasculitis (e.g., periarteritis nodosa)
- Multiple myeloma
- Renal venous congestion
  - Severe congestive heart failure
  - Constrictive pericarditis
  - Renal vein thrombosis(?)

Conditions in which proteinuria is usually mild, intermittent, or absent:
- Chronic pyelonephritis
- Renal disease of mild hypertension (so-called benign nephrosclerosis)
- Obstruction
- Stones
- Latent glomerulonephritis
- Polycystic disease
- Hypokalemic or hypercalcemic nephropathy
- Discrete tubular dysfunctions [e.g., Fanconi's syndrome or renal tubular acidosis (RTA)]
- Congestive heart failure
- Neoplasms
- Malformations
- Nonspecific
  - Postural proteinuria(?)
  - Exercise, fever, or exposure to cold

Adapted from N. G. Levinsky, *D.M.* March 1967.

The dynamics that determine the blood urea nitrogen concentration (BUN) are analogous but somewhat more complicated. Unlike creatinine, urea is not only filtered but also reabsorbed; normally, about 50 to 60 percent of the filtered load undergoes tubular reabsorption, and this proportion increases during dehydration and decreases during high rates of urine flow. Furthermore, in contrast to the production of creatinine, that of urea depends principally on the daily intake of protein; hence, at any given GFR, the BUN rises or falls in direct relation to the protein intake or to other events (e.g., gastrointestinal bleeding) that change the rate of urea production (Tables 8-2 and 8-3). Despite such factors that may complicate the interpretation of the BUN values, this test is a simple and reliable indicator of the GFR in the vast majority of patients. When determined simultaneously on the same sample of plasma, the BUN and creatinine levels can serve as instantaneous checks on the accuracy of the laboratory determination, and any marked deviation of the BUN/creatinine ratio from its normal value of about 10 may provide a clue to certain complicating conditions (Table 8-3).

The 24-hour endogenous creatinine clearance determination is most useful in patients whose history suggests that they may have suffered renal damage and in whom the BUN and serum creatinine concentrations are at the upper limits of normal. In these instances, a carefully executed creatinine clearance determination that is verified by consistent results on repeated testing can usually settle the question of whether the "high normal" BUN and serum creatinine values reflect merely the wide range of normality or a roughly 40 to 50 percent decrease in renal reserve. In other situations, the creatinine clearance test adds little useful information to the BUN and serum creatinine values, especially in advanced renal disease when it is no longer an accurate measure of the GFR.

Proteinuria is one of the earliest signs of renal impairment, and in most diseases of the kidney, it reflects increased permeability of the glomerular capillaries. The quantitation of proteinuria can aid in differential diagnosis (Table 8-4) as well as in prognosis (Fig. 8-2). Although a quick and useful estimate of the degree of urinary protein excretion can be gained from the routine urinalysis where results are expressed in "plus" ratings or as approximate concentrations (Fig. 8-7), the extent of proteinuria is best quantified by measuring the 24-hour protein excretion. The pattern of urinary proteins as determined by electrophoresis is useful in the diagnosis of certain nonrenal disorders (e.g., multiple myeloma) or discrete tubular disorders (Chap. 12); this technique is not ordinarily employed in the diagnosis or management of the common diseases of the kidney.

Problem 8-1

A 47-year-old man was referred to a nephrologist because his physician had found the patient's BUN and serum creatinine concentrations to be 38 mg/100 ml and 3.5 mg/100 ml, respectively. He had twice repeated these tests over a ten-day period, and they had remained in the same range. Abnormal findings that the physician noted on routine urinalysis included a protein concentration of 0.1 g/100 ml and a urinary sediment that contained about three hyaline and granular casts per high-power field and approximately 20 white blood cells and 40 erythrocytes per ten high-power fields. The patient reported having had frequent sore throats, including two episodes during the previous three months; he had had no signs or symptoms of acute or chronic renal disease. He had been in the Navy during World War II and had always considered himself to be in good health. He had sought out a doctor now because for about the past six months, he had just not felt "right"; his appetite, however, had remained good and his weight stable.

When the nephrologist took the patient's history, he obtained no additional facts. The findings on physical examination were entirely normal, including the blood pressure.

1. What do you estimate the patient's GFR to be?
2. What tests of renal function did the nephrologist probably order?
3. Is the patient's daily excretion of urea probably in the normal range, greater than normal, or less than normal?

Problem 8-2

From age 19 onward, a woman, now aged 43, had been on a dietary fad in order to stay thin. For the three years beginning at age 40, she had eaten only one meal a day, which she had at night, and this consisted of about 3 pounds of cod together with a milk-protein powder and some cauliflower and cabbage. On Mondays, when she could not obtain fresh fish, she substituted meat and cottage cheese for cod. During the day, her intake was limited to large amounts of coffee. It was estimated that this diet provided her with an average daily intake of 366 g of protein, 11 g of fat, 6 g of carbohydrate, 18 mEq of Na^+, and 84 mEq of K^+. She weighed 45 kg, had a blood pressure of 115/65 mm Hg and a pulse rate of 72 per minute, and appeared to be in good health.

While on this diet, her BUN was 70 mg/100 ml and her serum creatinine concentration 0.6 mg/100 ml. The results of the urinalysis were entirely normal, and she was not anemic.

Explain these findings, with particular emphasis on whether this woman is in renal failure and what you would estimate her GFR to be.

(This problem has been adapted from P. Richards and C. L. Brown, *Lancet* 2:207, 1975.)

Problem 8-3

On a routine preschool checkup, a 15-year-old boy was found to have borderline high blood pressure (140/80 mm Hg) and minimal proteinuria (0.01 g/100 ml) on two random urine specimens; these samples showed no other abnormality. Except for the possible high blood pressure, the findings on physical examination were normal.

The patient reported having sustained a "ruptured kidney" from a football injury 4½ years earlier. There was some gross hematuria for three days; the injury was allowed to heal spontaneously without medications or surgical intervention. Two years prior to the present checkup, the results of a urinalysis performed as part of a precamp physical examination were entirely normal. The blood pressure at that time was 120/80 mm Hg.

How should the physician handle this patient?

Selected References

General

Chapman, W. H., Bulger, R. E., Cutler, R. E., and Striker, G. E. *The Urinary System. An Integrated Approach.* Philadelphia: Saunders, 1973.

de Wardener, H. E. *The Kidney. An Outline of Normal and Abnormal Structure and Function* (4th ed.). Edinburgh: Churchill/Livingstone, 1973.

Edelmann, C. M., Jr. (ed.). *Pediatric Kidney Disease.* Boston: Little, Brown, 1978.

Kassirer, J. P. Clinical evaluation of kidney function — glomerular function. *N. Engl. J. Med.* 285:385, 1971.

Kassirer, J. P. Clinical evaluation of kidney function — tubular function. *N. Engl. J. Med.* 285:499, 1971.

Mitch, W. E., Walser, M., Buffington, G. A., and Lemann, J., Jr. A simple method of estimating progression of chronic renal failure. *Lancet* 2:1326, 1976.

Papper, S. *Clinical Nephrology* (2nd ed.). Boston: Little, Brown, 1978.

Peters, J. P., and Van Slyke, D. D. *Quantitative Clinical Chemistry,* vol. 1, Interpretations. Baltimore: Williams & Wilkins, 1946.

Relman, A. S., and Levinsky, N. G. Clinical Examination of Renal Function. In M. B. Strauss and L. G. Welt (eds.), *Diseases of the Kidney* (2nd ed.). Boston: Little, Brown, 1971.

Rutherford, W. E., Blondin, J., Miller, J. P., Greenwalt, A. S., and Vavra, J. D. Chronic progressive renal disease: Rate of change of serum creatinine concentration. *Kidney Int.* 11:62, 1977.

Schreiner, G. E., and Maher, J. F. *Uremia: Biochemistry, Pathogenesis, and Treatment.* Springfield, Ill.: Thomas, 1961.

Shaw, S. T., Jr., and Benson, E. S. Renal Function and Its Evaluation. In I. Davidsohn and J. B. Henry (eds.), *Todd-Sanford Clinical Diagnosis by Laboratory Methods* (15th ed.). Philadelphia: Saunders, 1974.

Smith, H. W. *The Kidney. Structure and Function in Health and Disease.* New York: Oxford University Press, 1951.

Wallach, J. B. *Interpretation of Diagnostic Tests: A Handbook Synopsis of Laboratory Medicine* (3rd ed.). Boston: Little, Brown, 1978.

Glomerular Filtration Rate (GFR)

Berlyne, G. M., Varley, H., Nilwarangkur, S., and Hoerni, M. Endogenous-creatinine clearance and glomerular-filtration rate. *Lancet* 2:874, 1964.

Bleiler, R. E., and Schedl, H. P. Creatinine excretion: Variability and relationships to diet and body size. *J. Lab. Clin. Med.* 59:945, 1962.

Borsook, H., and Dubnoff, J. W. The hydrolysis of phosphocreatine and the origin of urinary creatinine. *J. Biol. Chem.* 168:493, 1947.

Cole, B. R., Giangiacomo, J., Ingelfinger, J. R., and Robson, A. M. Measurement of renal function without urine collection. A critical evaluation of the constant-infusion technic for determination of inulin and para-aminohippurate. *N. Engl. J. Med.* 287:1109, 1972.

Dodge, W. F., Travis, L. B., and Daeschner, C. W. Comparison of endogenous creatinine clearance with inulin clearance. *Am. J. Dis. Child.* 113:683, 1967.

Dosseter, J. B. Creatininemia versus uremia. The relative significance of blood urea nitrogen and serum creatinine concentrations in azotemia. *Ann. Intern. Med.* 65:1287, 1966.

Gault, M. H., Dixon, M. E., Doyle, M., and Cohen, W. M. Hypernatremia, azotemia, and dehydration due to high-protein tube feeding. *Ann. Intern. Med.* 68:778, 1968.

Hsu, C. H., Kurtz, T. W., Massari, P. U., Ponze, S. A., and Chang, B. S. Familial azotemia. Impaired urea excretion despite normal renal function. *N. Engl. J. Med.* 298:117, 1978.

Israelit, A. H., Long, D. L., White, M. G., and Hull, A. R. Measurement of glomerular filtration rate utilizing a single subcutaneous injection of ^{125}I-iothalamate. *Kidney Int.* 4:346, 1973.

Katz, M. A. Ablutional azotemia – the bathtub principle. *N. Engl. J. Med.* 282:572, 1970.
This letter to the editor stirred up a dialogue between Dr. Katz and Dr. J.-P. Habicht. The subsequent letters were also published (*N. Engl. J. Med.* 282:1376, 1970; 283:436, 1970; 283:437, 1970).

Kumar, R., Steen, P., and McGeown, M. G. Chronic renal failure or simple starvation? A case report. *Lancet* 2:1005, 1972.

Lancet Editorial. Urea metabolism in man. *Lancet* 2:1407, 1971.

Miller, B. F., Leaf, A., Mamby, A. R., and Miller, Z. Validity of the endogenous creatinine clearance as a measure of glomerular filtration rate in the diseased human kidney. *J. Clin. Invest.* 31:309, 1952.

Oester, A., Wolf, H., and Madsen, P. O. Double isotope technique in renal function testing in dogs. *Invest. Urol.* 6:387, 1969.

Richards, P., and Brown, C. L. Urea metabolism in an azotaemic woman with normal renal function. *Lancet* 2:207, 1975.

Schirmeister, J., Willmann, H., Kiefer, H., and Hallauer, W. Für und wider die Brauchbarkeit der endogenen Kreatininclearance in der funktionellen Nierendiagnostik. *Dtsch. Med. Wochenschr.* 89:1640, 1964.

Schmidt-Nielsen, B. (ed.). *Urea and the Kidney.* Amsterdam: Excerpta Medica Foundation, 1970.

Sirota, J. H., Baldwin, D. S., and Villarreal, H. Diurnal variations of renal function in man. *J. Clin. Invest.* 29:187, 1950.

Wolpert, E., Phillips, S. F., and Summerskill, W. H. J. Transport of urea and ammonia production in the human colon. *Lancet* 2:1387, 1971.

Proteinuria

Bohrer, M. P., Baylis, C., Humes, H. D., Glassock, R. J., Robertson, C. R., and Brenner, B. M. Permselectivity of the glomerular capillary wall. Facilitated filtration of circulating polycations. *J. Clin. Invest.* 61:72, 1978.

Cortney, M. A., Sawin, L. L., and Weiss, D. D. Renal tubular protein absorption in the rat. *J. Clin. Invest.* 49:1, 1970.

Dirks, J. H., Clapp, J. R., and Berliner, R. W. The protein concentration in the proximal tubule of the dog. *J. Clin. Invest.* 43:916, 1964.

Kark, R. M. Proteinuria II: Diagnosis and management. *Hosp. Pract.* 6(6): 59, 1971.

Leber, P. D., and Marsh, D. J. Micropuncture study of concentration and fate of albumin in rat nephron. *Am. J. Physiol.* 219:358, 1970.

Levinsky, N. G. The interpretation of proteinuria and the urinary sediment. *D.M.* March 1967.

Manuel, Y., Revillard, J. P., and Betuel, H. (eds.). *Proteins in Normal and Pathological Urine.* Baltimore: University Park Press, 1970.

Morgensen, C. E., Vittinghus, E., and Sølling, K. Increased urinary excretion of albumin, light chains, and β_2-microglobulin after intravenous arginine administration in normal man. *Lancet* 2:581, 1975.

Pollak, V. E. Proteinuria I: Mechanisms. *Hosp. Pract.* 6(6):49, 1971.

Robinson, R. R. Proteinuria. In C. M. Edelmann, Jr. (ed.), *Pediatric Kidney Disease.* Boston: Little, Brown, 1978.

Thompson, A. L., Durrett, R. R., and Robinson, R. R. Fixed and reproducible orthostatic proteinuria. VI. Results of a 10-year follow-up evaluation. *Ann. Intern. Med.* 73:235, 1970.

Wallenius, G. Renal clearance of dextran as a measure of glomerular permeability. *Acta Soc. Med. Upsal.* 59 (Suppl. 4):1, 1954.

Urinalysis

Bradley, G. M., and Benson, E. S. Examination of the Urine. In I. Davidsohn and J. B. Henry (eds.), *Todd-Sanford Clinical Diagnosis by Laboratory Methods* (15th ed.). Philadelphia: Saunders, 1974.

Hendler, E. D., Kashgarian, M., and Hayslett, J. P. Clinicopathological correlations of primary haematuria. *Lancet* 1:458, 1972.

Levinsky, N. G. The interpretation of proteinuria and the urinary sediment. *D.M.* March 1967.

Lippman, R. W. *Urine and the Urinary Sediment. A Practical Manual and Atlas* (2nd ed.). Springfield, Ill.: Thomas, 1957.
This book contains many useful photomicrographs of the urinary sediment.

Weller, J. M., and Green, J. A., Jr. *Examination of the Urine. A Programmed Text.* New York: Appleton-Century-Crofts, 1966.

Other Tests

Harrington, J. T., and Cohen, J. J. Measurement of urinary electrolytes — indications and limitations. *N. Engl. J. Med.* 293:1241, 1975.

Heptinstall, R. H. *Pathology of the Kidney* (2nd ed.). Boston: Little, Brown, 1974.

Isaacson, L. C. Urinary osmolality and specific gravity. *Lancet* 1:72, 1959.

Lindeman, R. D. Percutaneous renal biopsy. *Kidney* 7:1, 1974.

Miles, B. E., Paton, A., and de Wardener, H. E. Maximum urine concentration. *Br. Med. J.* 2:901, 1954.

Muehrke, R. C., and Pirani, C. L. Renal Biopsy: An Adjunct in the Study of Kidney Disease. In D. A. K. Black (ed.), *Renal Disease* (3rd ed.). Oxford, Eng.: Blackwell, 1972.

Olsson, O. Renal Radiography. In M. B. Strauss and L. G. Welt (eds.), *Diseases of the Kidney* (2nd ed.). Boston: Little, Brown, 1971.

Schoen, E. J., Young, G., and Weissman, A. Urinary specific gravity versus total solute concentration: A critical comparison. I. Studies in normal adults. *J. Lab. Clin. Med.* 54:277, 1959.

Schreiner, G. E. Renal Biopsy. In M. B. Strauss and L. G. Welt (eds.), *Diseases of the Kidney* (2nd ed.). Boston: Little, Brown, 1971.

Sunderman, F. W., and Sunderman, F. W., Jr. (eds.). *Laboratory Diagnosis of Kidney Diseases.* St. Louis: Green, 1970.

Wolf, A. V., and Pillay, V. K. G. Renal concentration tests; osmotic pressure, specific gravity, refraction and electrical conductivity compared. *Am. J. Med.* 46:837, 1969.

9 : Acute Renal Failure: The Abrupt Cessation of Multiple Balances

Up to now we have discussed balances and imbalances of major substances such as H_2O, Na^+, K^+, and H^+. In most disturbances involving these substances, be they extrarenal or renal in origin, temporary imbalance is followed by a new steady state in which balance is restored, albeit usually at some abnormal value, as of plasma concentration or body fluid volume. Thus, in a disturbance leading to chronic generalized edema, there is a period of positive balance of NaCl and H_2O, which is often followed by a new steady state in which the balance for NaCl and H_2O is restored, but at an expanded extracellular fluid volume. Or, in most diseases of the kidneys, there is a positive balance of inorganic phosphate, which is succeeded by a restoration of phosphate balance, either at a normal plasma phosphate concentration in mild disease or at an elevated plasma phosphate concentration in advanced renal impairment (see Answer to Problem 1-1).

During acute renal failure – but not in chronic – one sees an exception to this pattern. The kidneys, having failed abruptly, are unable to maintain or restore solute and water balance unless and until they recover; in the meantime, the physician must assume this role by regulating the intake and output of water and major solutes.

Definitions

In the context of the above discussion, *acute renal failure* may be defined as the sudden inability of the kidneys to regulate water and solute balance, be that in the face of a reduced, normal, or high urine flow. In the majority of instances, however, there is *oliguria* (a decrease in the urine flow to the range of 50 to 400 ml per day) or *anuria* (an absence of urine or less than 50 ml per day); we shall limit the present discussion to this condition, that is, *to acute oliguric renal failure.* Thus, for the purposes of this chapter, as well as to conform to the meaning intended by most clinicians when they speak of acute renal failure, we shall apply the definition used by S. S. Franklin and M. H. Maxwell: "an abrupt, frequently reversible impairment or cessation of renal function, which is usually manifested by oliguria or anuria."

Table 9-1
Representative causes of acute renal failure

I. Prerenal
   Hypotension (e.g., trauma, myocardial infarction, septicemia)
   Hemorrhage, external or internal (e.g., obstetric, traumatic, surgical)
   Contraction of body fluid volumes, especially extracellular volume (e.g., severe gastroenteritis, "third space" effect)
   Major surgical procedures (e.g., operations on the heart, biliary tract, and major vessels)

II. Postrenal
   Lower urinary tract obstruction (e.g., benign or malignant hypertrophy of the prostate)
   Upper urinary tract obstruction (e.g., uterine tumor pressing on both ureters, renal stone in the ureter of a single kidney)

III. Renal
   A. Initial damage to tubular epithelium
      1. Ischemia
         Prerenal causes if sufficiently severe and prolonged
         Trauma ("crush syndrome")
         Burns
         Obstetric disorders
         Transfusion reactions
         Sepsis
         Thrombosis or embolization of major renal vessels
      2. Toxins
         Heavy metals (e.g., mercuric chloride)
         Organic solvents (e.g., carbon tetrachloride, methanol)
         Glycols (e.g., ethylene glycol or antifreeze)
         Drugs (e.g., methoxyflurane, cytolytic agents, diphenylhydantoin, gentamicin, amphotericin)
         Pesticides (e.g., chlorinated hydrocarbons)
         Others (e.g., uric acid, mushrooms, snake bites, radiographic contrast agents, nontraumatic rhabdomyolysis)
   B. Initial damage to glomeruli and small renal vessels
      Acute glomerulonephritides
      Polyarteritis nodosa
      Lupus erythematosus
      Hemolytic-uremic syndrome
      Goodpasture's syndrome
      Serum sickness
      Malignant hypertension

Causes of Acute Renal Failure

As a guide to therapy, it is useful to classify the causes of acute renal failure into three general categories: prerenal, postrenal, and renal. Some representative examples for each category are set forth in Table 9-1. The list is by no means exhaustive, and for a more complete description of causes, students should consult standard textbooks or the appendix to this chapter.

Prerenal Causes

This type of acute renal failure describes an oliguric state that is due to inadequate blood perfusion of the kidneys and which can be reversed if the systemic cause of the ischemia is corrected before renal cell damage occurs. The renal circulation is exquisitely sensitive to disturbances of body homeostasis. Any of the insults listed in section I of Table 9-1 are likely to be accompanied by an abrupt and drastic reduction in renal perfusion, even in the absence of overt shock; the ischemia is thus probably due to intense constriction of certain renal vessels. Furthermore, there may be a redistribution of what little blood perfuses the kidneys, so a selective reduction in perfusion of the superficial cortex results.

The probable dynamics of prerenal acute renal failure are shown in Figure 9-1. As the renal blood flow decreases, so does the GFR, and these events are usually accompanied by an increase in the *fraction* of the glomerular filtrate that is reabsorbed, at least in the proximal tubules. Consequently, oliguria sets in. Ordinarily, most renal oxidative energy is utilized in the reabsorption of the filtered Na^+. This fact probably explains the observation that the renal blood flow (RBF) has to be decreased to about 5 percent of the normal value before ischemic damage occurs. Initially, as the RBF and GFR are reduced, so is the filtered load of Na^+ (GFR · P_{Na^+}), and hence the tubular reabsorption of Na^+ and the renal O_2 consumption are also reduced. As GFR approaches zero, the oxygen consumption approximates the basal rate that is required to keep renal cells alive even when

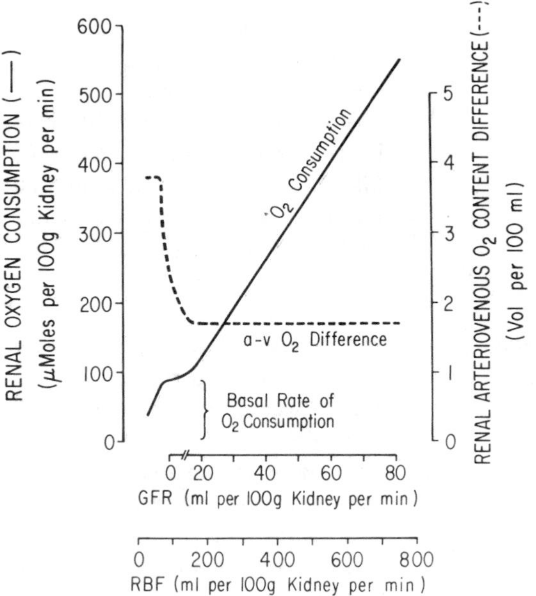

Figure 9-1
Relationship between changes in renal blood flow (RBF) or glomerular filtration rate (GFR), and renal oxygen consumption in dogs. The graph shows that the *basal* rate of oxygen consumption is compromised only when renal perfusion is reduced drastically; it is probably for this reason that prerenal acute renal failure can be corrected abruptly and completely even though it might have been preceded by a severe reduction in the GFR and oliguria. Adapted from H. Valtin, *Renal Function: Mechanisms Preserving Fluid and Solute Balance in Health.* Boston: Little, Brown, 1973.

they are not reabsorbing Na^+; in the face of a further reduction in RBF, this basal requirement is met by the extraction of more oxygen from each unit of blood flowing through the kidneys. It is only at very low RBF, when the extraction of oxygen and hence the arteriovenous oxygen content difference are maximal, that a further decrease in RBF leads to damaging ischemia of renal cells. Therefore, if the cause of a given prerenal ischemia can be corrected before this critical point is reached, the kidney can immediately resume normal function as the rates of perfusion and filtration are restored to normal. It also follows that prerenal acute renal failure can evolve into the "renal" category if deleterious ischemia has been present for a critical period of time. In fact, renal ischemia is perhaps the commonest cause of the *renal* form of acute renal failure (see below).

Postrenal Causes

Postrenal acute renal failure refers to an *abrupt* diminution or cessation of urine flow that is caused by the obstruction of the urinary passages distal to the kidneys (Table 9-1). The importance of recognizing this entity, like that of recognizing prerenal failure, is that normal renal function can be quickly restored if the cause is removed. Chronic obstruction can lead to irreversible renal damage (Chap. 11), but obstruction lasting only a few hours or days may not.

Although simultaneous blockage of both ureters is quite rare, it occurs with sufficient frequency that it must be borne in mind. Likewise, the physician should always be alert to the possibility that the patient may have only one kidney and that it has become obstructed; about one person in 800 is born with only a single kidney.

Renal Causes

These causes of acute renal failure are so called because they result in damage to the renal parenchyma, which either may take days or weeks to be repaired or may be irreversible. It is therefore of obvious therapeutic importance to distinguish this category from those of prerenal and postrenal causes, since prompt correction of the latter types may prevent a prolonged illness. Once *renal* acute renal failure has been diagnosed, the physician must regulate the patient's solute and water balance during the period that the patient's kidneys are unable to do so (see below).

The renal-disorder category of acute renal failure can be divided roughly into those conditions that cause initial damage to the tubular epithelium and those that injure the glomerular capillaries and other small renal vessels. Such classification refers to the primary site of injury; because both the renal vasculature and the tubular system run in series and are intertwined both anatomically and functionally, initial damage to the tubules will quickly involve the vessels, and vice versa.

Initial Damage to Tubular Epithelium. When tubular damage is involved — a far more common cause of acute renal failure than initial injury to the small vessels — the condition is often referred to as *acute tubular necrosis* (ATN). Such damage is produced most commonly by renal ischemia and by toxins. Cellular damage resulting from *ischemia* is frequently an outgrowth of prerenal acute renal failure if the causes listed under that category (Table 9-1) lead to a critical degree of renal tissue hypoxia. There are other causes, however, that commonly lead to renal parenchymal damage and acute renal failure by the ischemic route. Among others, these include (1) trauma, as in battle casualties or vehicular accidents, which is also called *crush syndrome,* because during World War II it was first recognized as a cause of acute renal failure in London air-raid victims whose limbs had been compressed by falling debris; (2) extensive burns, leading to contraction of the body fluid volumes; (3) obstetric disorders, such as septic abortion, premature separation of the placenta, or severe hemorrhage; (4) adverse reactions to blood transfusions; (5) overwhelming sepsis; and (6) blockage of major renal vessels. Although hypotension and fluid volume contraction may contribute to the renal ischemia in any of the above disorders, disseminated intravascular coagulation with blockage of the microcirculation of the kidneys may be the more critical change in many or most instances.

There is a long list of *toxins* that have been shown to damage the tubular epithelium and lead to acute renal failure; some examples are listed in Table 9-1. For the following reasons, the kidneys may be especially susceptible to toxins: (1) The inordinately high rate of renal blood flow causes the kidneys to be exposed to a great amount of the offending compound. (2) Extensive tubular reabsorption of water may expose the tubular epithelium to high concentrations of the toxin. This process may be aggravated because with the slow flow of tubular fluid that occurs during oliguria, the "sink" for secretion of the toxin is curtailed so that the poison accumulates within the cell. (3) Certain toxins may be transported by specific carriers of the tubular epithelium, and that epithelium may therefore be selectively exposed to the poison. (4) Depending on how the compounds are handled by the kidneys, they may become concentrated by participating in the countercurrent system.

Initial Damage to Glomeruli and Small Vessels. This classification is based on the site of primary damage; to the extent that injury to small vessels will lead to renal ischemia, however, there is overlap with the previous category. The causes are diverse (Table 9-1), encompassing immune-complex disorders, connective-tissue diseases, and possibly disseminated intravascular coagulation (e.g., in the hemolytic-uremic syndrome). Acute renal failure occurs commonly in the hemolytic-uremic syndrome and in Goodpasture's syndrome, whereas it is a much less frequent concomitant of the other disorders that have been listed.

The mechanisms whereby damage to the glomerular capillaries cause decreased filtration are just being defined. They probably vary among the different conditions, and they may involve mainly a decrease in glomerular plasma flow or predominantly a decrease in the filtration coefficient, K_f (Eq. 3-2), depending on the nature of the initial insult.

Mechanisms of Oliguria

One of the areas of greatest controversy in acute renal failure concerns the pathogenesis of oliguria. The causes are obvious in the prerenal and postrenal forms, namely, the lack of glomerular filtration and the obstruction of the outflow channel, respectively. The controversy is limited to the mechanism of oliguria in the renal-disorder category of acute renal failure. The causes proposed by the three main theories are (1) back-leakage of the glomerular filtrate through the injured tubular epithelium; (2) obstruction of the tubules by cellular debris, which may secondarily decrease the GFR; and (3) a primary decrease in the GFR due to vasoconstriction. Experimental evidence has been obtained that both favors and opposes each theory, and each therefore has its proponents and opponents.

Back-Leakage

It is proposed that plasma continues to be filtered into Bowman's space, but that virtually all of it back-diffuses through the damaged tubular epithelium. Several lines of evidence favor this theory: (1) In 1929, A. N. Richards reported direct observations on the kidneys of frogs that had been poisoned with mercuric chloride. During the time when he could see a greater than normal blood flow through the glomeruli at the surface of the kidney, he could collect abundant, apparently normal filtrate from Bowman's space; yet at the same time, the kidney was producing no urine. (2) Careful microdissection studies, begun by J. Oliver and his colleagues, often reveal the kind of damaged tubular epithelium that might permit back-leakage. In subsequent experiments in which microdissection has been combined with prior functional studies, tubular fluid could be obtained from severely damaged tubules. (3) In the hands of some investigators (but not of others) the dye, lissamine green — which ordinarily becomes more concentrated in the more distal tubular segments because, like inulin, it is not reabsorbed — becomes less concentrated in rats with experimental toxic acute renal failure, suggesting that the dye has leaked out of the tubules.

If inulin were also to leak out of the tubules, then the determination of its clearance would give falsely low values for the

GFR. It is possible that this experimental error has contributed to the notion that the GFR is decreased in all instances of acute renal failure.

Tubular Obstruction

Another theory states that the renal tubules (not the large collecting conduits, as in postrenal acute renal failure) become occluded by debris that is sloughed from damaged tubular epithelium. This obstruction, in turn, would raise the intratubular hydrostatic pressure, including that within Bowman's space, and thereby lead to a secondary decrease in the GFR. Cited in favor of this hypothesis are the following findings: (1) frequent casts within the tubular lumina, (2) increased intraluminal hydrostatic pressure as measured by micropuncture, (3) dilation of some tubular lumina, and (4) edema of the kidney, which, given the relatively inexpansible renal capsule, might be expected to raise the intratubular hydrostatic pressure. These findings are not conclusive, however, because they are not seen in all models of acute renal failure, nor even in all tubules of the same model. In a single experimental animal, for example, there may be some collapsed rather than dilated tubules, some with low rather than high hydrostatic pressure, some without casts, and so on. It seems more likely, therefore, that intratubular obstruction may be a contributing factor rather than the sole factor, at least in some models or in some tubules.

It is also possible that tubular obstruction could be an initial event that leads to vasomotor changes in the glomerular vessels and thereby secondarily causes a decrease in the GFR. For example, if a single tubule is obstructed temporarily by the microinjection of an oil droplet, an initial phase of elevated intratubular hydrostatic pressure is followed about 24 hours later by the constriction of the afferent arteriole, a consequent decrease in the sGFR (i.e., in the glomerular filtration rate of the single, affected nephron), and a decrease in the intratubular pressure within that nephron.

Vasomotion

In human patients as well as in various experimental animal models, the renal type of acute renal failure is associated with a selective and marked reduction of the blood supply to most of the cortex, while that to the medullary regions appears to be better preserved (Fig. 9-2). This finding has given rise to the hypothesis that a change in the resistance of the glomerular arterioles leads to a *primary* decrease in the GFR and hence to oliguria. This theory is supported by micropuncture studies, which show a decrease in the filtration rate of a single nephron (sGFR) at the same time the hydrostatic pressure in the proximal tubule of that nephron is lower than normal (not higher than

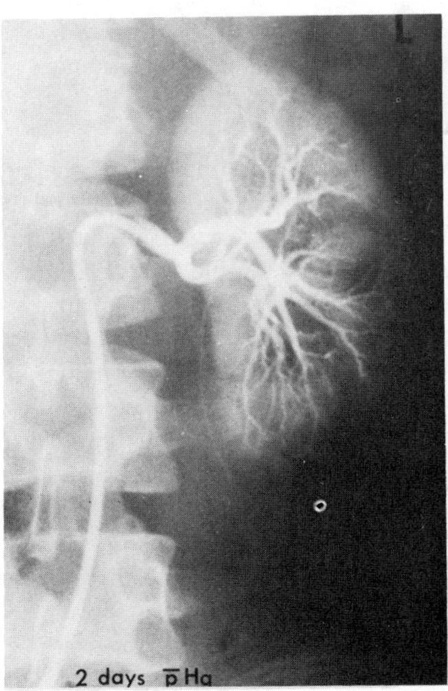

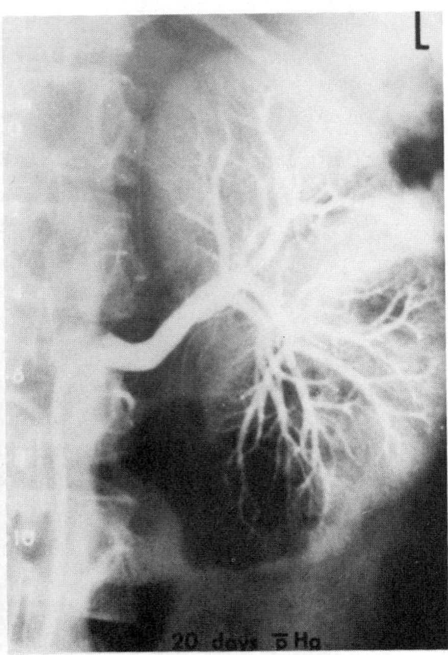

Figure 9-2
Selective renal arteriograms on a 19-year-old college student who ingested an unknown amount of mercuric chloride. The arteriogram taken on the second day of severe acute oliguric renal failure (*left*) shows attenuation of the renal vasculature and decreased opacification (nephrogram) of the cortex, especially along the right lower border. The arteriogram obtained one week after return of normal urine flow (*right*), or three weeks after the onset of oliguria, shows reappearance of opacification in the cortex. From N. K. Hollenberg et al., *Medicine* (Baltimore) 47:455, 1968.

normal, which would be required if tubular obstruction had caused a *secondary* decrease in the sGFR). The further finding in the same experiments that the hydrostatic pressure in the efferent arteriole is decreased shows that constriction of the afferent arteriole, rather than dilation of the efferent arteriole, is likely to be the cause of the decreased sGFR.

Juxtaglomerular Apparatus and the Renin-Angiotensin System. The "vasomotor" hypothesis has been extended by an additional theory, which is currently under intensive debate. This theory, first proposed in its essence by N. Goormaghtigh and then refined and championed most vigorously by K. Thurau and his colleagues, is illustrated in Figure 9-3. It is proposed that when the tubular epithelium is damaged (e.g., by ischemia or toxins), the capacity of the proximal tubule and the loop of Henle to reabsorb NaCl is diminished. Consequently, more NaCl than normally is delivered to the beginning of the distal tubule, where the juxtaglomerular apparatus (JGA) is located. It is further postulated that the increased delivery of NaCl is somehow

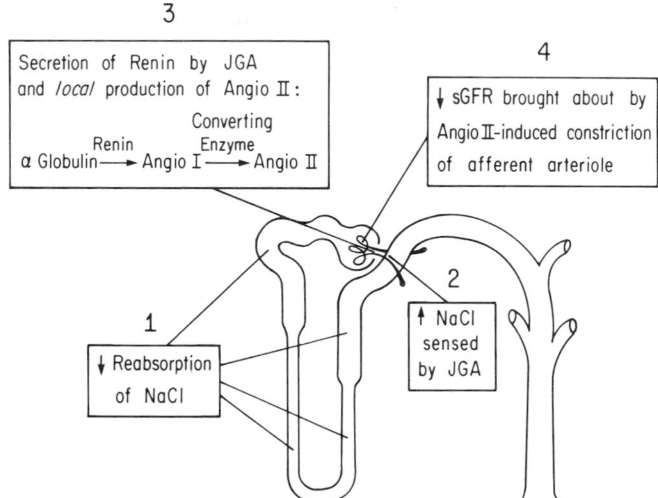

Figure 9-3
One theory of the pathogenesis of oliguric acute renal failure. The numbered, sequential steps are described in the text. *JGA* = juxtaglomerular apparatus; *Angio* = angiotensin; *sGFR* = filtration rate of a single glomerulus.

sensed by the JGA — be that through an increased concentration of Cl^- or Na^+ or through some other consequence of increased delivery — which then secretes renin and thereby stimulates the conversion of a plasma α_2-globulin to angiotensin I and then to angiotensin II *at that particular JGA.* (For a more detailed description of this reaction, see Fig. 14-1.) The locally produced angiotensin II, it is proposed, then causes constriction of the afferent arteriole belonging to the JGA-glomerular complex in question and thereby reduces or abolishes the sGFR in that nephron. To the extent that most or all of the tubules are damaged in a given instance of acute renal failure, this mechanism would lead to the reduction or cessation of filtration in virtually all glomeruli and hence to oliguria.

Evidence favoring this hypothesis includes the following findings: (1) hypertrophy and increased granularity of the JGA in many instances of acute renal failure (which is the finding that first prompted Goormaghtigh to propose the theory); (2) frequent elevation of the plasma renin concentration; (3) micropuncture evidence for a feedback system that reduces the sGFR when the delivery of NaCl to the area of the JGA is increased; (4) demonstration within single JGAs of all the elements — for example, substrate, renin, and converting enzyme (Fig. 14-1) — that are required for the local production of angiotensin II and appropriate changes in this production when the feedback mechanism is manipulated; and (5) prevention of the experimental production of acute renal failure by the prior administration of salt loads, a maneuver that is known to deplete the kidney of its renin content. There is also, however, evidence against the hypothesis, such as the failure (thus far) to prevent experimental acute renal failure through the inhibition of renin, angiotensin, or converting enzyme.

Thus, the available experimental evidence does not rule conclusively for or against this theory. One interesting consequence of the theory (should it ultimately turn out to be correct) is that by shutting off glomerular filtration and thereby preventing dangerous wastage of NaCl, the kidney, far from having failed, would be effectively carrying out one of its most vital functions.

There is as yet no conclusive evidence that unequivocally favors any one of the above theories for the causation of the renal type of acute renal failure, that is, whether it be back-leakage, tubular obstruction, or vasomotion. Most workers view the last as the major mechanism leading to oliguria in most instances of the renal form of acute renal failure. It is possible, however, that the other mechanisms predominate in some cases, and it may well be that two or even all three processes may be interrelated and contribute simultaneously to the oliguria (Fig. 9-4).

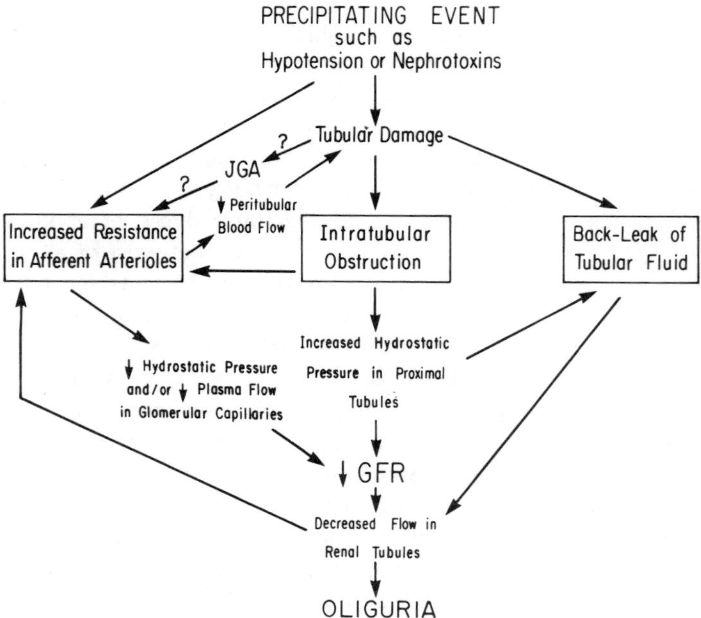

Figure 9-4
Possible schema for the causation of oliguria in acute renal failure in which the three major theories of its etiology may be reconciled. The theories are stated in the boxes, and the arrows indicate the possible interrelations among them. Adapted from W. F. Finn et al., *Circ. Res.* 36:675, 1975.

Treatment

It is of the utmost importance to establish the cause of the acute renal failure (Table 9-1), especially since the correction of a prerenal or postrenal cause may quickly reestablish urine flow and thus prevent a prolonged illness. When the renal form of acute renal failure is involved, the precipitating cause should also be treated whenever possible in order to forestall further damage to the kidneys.

Restoration of Urine Flow

Even when the renal form is present, most physicians consider it worthwhile to try to increase the urine flow by administering hypertonic mannitol, giving one of the very powerful diuretics (i.e., furosemide or ethacrynic acid), or both. The means by which these agents sometimes restore urine flow is not known. With mannitol, the mechanism may involve "flushing out" debris that might be obstructing the tubules. In the case of diuretic administration, this effect may also occur. Of possibly greater importance, however, is the fact that the diuretics are known to increase blood flow to the superficial cortex, and they *may* interfere with the signal at the JGA that would shut off glomerular filtration. It is not settled, though, whether any of these effects of mannitol or the diuretics are instrumental in reestablishing urine flow even when they do take place. Furthermore, insofar as the presence of oliguria might signal not so much renal failure but rather a compensatory response in order to preserve NaCl (see Juxtaglomerular Apparatus and the Renin-Angiotensin System, above), restoring normal urine flow might be illogical. Nevertheless, most physicians find it easier to regulate fluid and solute balance in a patient with acute renal failure who is producing ample urine than in one who is in failure and oliguric.

It should be emphasized that usually only a single dose of the agents should be tried: a 50-ml bolus of 25% mannitol or 200 mg of furosemide or ethacrynic acid intravenously. If the attempt fails to restore urine flow, then the patient may be oliguric or anuric for anywhere from a few hours to three or four weeks. During this period, which may be required for the kidneys to heal, it is the physician's task to regulate fluid and solute balance for the patient, because the patient's kidneys cannot do it themselves. Such imposed regulation of water and of a number of important solutes is described next.

H_2O Balance

A patient who is oliguric will quickly and dangerously expand his body-fluid volumes unless he curtails his water intake. By just how much he needs to reduce the fluid intake may be determined from Figure 9-5. Suppose a given oliguric patient is excreting only 100 ml of urine per day. Adding this amount to

INTAKE PLUS ENDOGENOUS PRODUCTION ml/day			OUTPUT ml/day		
Water as fluid	1,200		Urine		1,500
Water in food	1,000		Insensible		900
Water of oxidation	300		Respiratory	400	
			Skin	500	

Internal Cycling of Gastrointestinal Fluid	Secreted		Reabsorbed			
Saliva	1,500					
Gastric juice	2,500					
Bile	500					
Pancreatic juice	700					
Intestinal juice	3,000					
	8,200	−	8,100	=	Water in stool	100

FLUID BALANCE	2,500		2,500

Figure 9-5
Average turnover of water in a healthy adult. This figure is the same as Figure 1-5, in the appendix to Chapter 1; it is repeated here to supplement the text and to emphasize the importance of water balance in oliguric acute renal failure.

a daily insensible water loss of 900 ml (and possibly another 100 ml if he has bowel movements) makes his total output of water equal to 1,100 ml per day. An oliguric patient is usually so sick that he is not eating; hence, the 1,000 ml of water that is ordinarily contained in food is omitted from the "Intake" column (Fig. 9-5). If the patient therefore restricts his intake of fluid to 800 ml per day, he will be in balance for water (800 + 300). Under these conditions, however, he would go into a form of hyposmotic expansion (Table 2-4). This would happen because, with the patient not eating, the daily water of oxidation comes mainly from the breakdown of endogenous fats and proteins rather than of food. In the process, therefore, the patient will replace solid cellular tissue with water. Even though the patient will be in external balance, he will be in internal imbalance, and there will be a net shift of water from the intracellular into the extracellular compartment. The potentially serious consequences of heart failure and pulmonary edema can be avoided by reducing the water intake by an amount approximately equal to the daily water of oxidation. Hence, the total water intake of a severely oliguric adult patient should not exceed 500 ml per day, and usually it is less than that.

Body Weight

The above values and those shown in Figure 9-5 are rough estimates that can vary considerably. If a patient is febrile, for example, his water loss from the skin, both insensible and through sweat, may double or triple. Further, if he is in the postoperative state and has drainage tubes in the gastrointestinal tract (a rather common occurrence), then his fluid loss by that route could amount to a liter or more per day. On the other hand, fever and other catabolic states will increase the water of oxidation and hence the total fluid input. Measuring these variables may be impossible or is at best cumbersome and inaccurate, especially in a very sick patient. The easiest and probably the most accurate means of preventing dangerous expansion of the body-fluid compartments is therefore to weigh the patient at least once a day and to strive for a weight loss of about 250 g (about 0.5 pound) each day. This is best accomplished by projecting a line of desired weight loss on a flow chart and seeing how closely the daily weights approximate the ideal line (Fig. 9-6).

Na^+ Balance

The great threat produced by water imbalance is the expansion of the extracellular compartment and the precipitation of heart failure. This outcome could be seriously aggravated if there is also a positive balance for Na^+. Most patients with severe oliguria should therefore receive no Na^+ whatsoever, either as NaCl or as $NaHCO_3$. Exceptions include patients who have large losses of gastrointestinal secretions, especially from the small bowel (Table 1-4), who are sweating profusely, who are losing serum through burns, or who have other, obvious extrarenal losses of Na^+.

K^+ Balance

Besides H_2O and Na^+ overload, the other major threat of fluid and solute imbalance in acute renal failure is hyperkalemia. Although a positive Na^+ balance can usually be prevented merely by not giving the patient any Na^+, this simple measure does not suffice to prevent dangerous hyperkalemia. The reason for this difficulty is analogous to that discussed above for H_2O balance; that is, internal imbalance for K^+ is a threat to life even if external K^+ balance is achieved. If an individual is starved, he will break down endogenous tissue (i.e., cells) to provide the minimum amount of energy required to sustain life. Cells have a high content of K^+, and their obligatory breakdown therefore shifts K^+ from the intracellular into the extracellular pool. Inasmuch as this K^+ load cannot be excreted by the kidneys of an oliguric patient, the plasma K^+ concentration tends to rise. The problem is aggravated by the fact that the extracellular pool of K^+ is small (Fig. 4-1) and that even a moderate rise in its plasma concentration — for example, to no more than 8 mEq per liter — can be fatal (see Chap. 4, under Effects of Hyperkalemia). Fatal hyperkalemia is also a special threat when acute renal failure has resulted from trauma or other conditions that are associated with increased breakdown of tissue.

In order to guard against dangerous hyperkalemia, the serum K^+ concentration is measured daily, and the electrocardiogram (ECG) is monitored at least once a day (Fig. 4-4). Several measures are also immediately instituted with the onset of oliguria to try to prevent hyperkalemia. Chief among these is regulation of the diet, which should be free of protein and high in carbohydrate (and possibly in essential amino acids). Protein is omitted not to minimize the rise of urea in the blood but to eliminate any exogenous source of K^+. The diet is high in carbohydrate in order to supply enough calories to reduce endogenous protein catabolism and hence to hold the internal release of K^+ to a minimum. An intake of 100 to 200 g of sugar achieves this goal; although some nephrologists prefer to give the sugar intravenously as a 5% or 10% solution of dextrose in water, a very simple and effective means is to dissolve 200 g of sugar in the daily allowance of water and let the patient sip this solution throughout the 24 hours. Lactose is often preferred to glucose because patients find it less nauseating. To vary the diet (!) the calories can also be supplied by a mixture of equal portions of corn (Karo) syrup and ginger ale, and the potion is usually more palatable if it is well cooled. Sourballs or other hard, clear candy can further supplement the caloric intake. There is recent evidence that an even greater protein-sparing effect can be achieved by adding essential amino acids. The administration of anabolic steroids (e.g., testosterone) may also help to decrease the breakdown of endogenous protein, although the effectiveness of such agents in very ill, uremic patients has not been proved.

If, despite these dietary measures, the serum K^+ concentration rises or the ECG suggests hyperkalemia, then an ion-exchange resin, sodium polystyrene sulfonate (Kayexalate), can be given by mouth or by retention enemas. Inasmuch as this resin exchanges mainly K^+ for Na^+, it will add some Na^+ to the patient; this drawback, however, is seldom a major problem.

Not infrequently, a patient with acute renal failure will be in the postoperative state and he may well have surgical tubes draining gastrointestinal secretions. Since some of these secretions are rather rich in K^+ (Table 1-4), such drainage often alleviates the problem of hyperkalemia. Alternatively, the induction of diarrhea — for example, with an osmotic agent like sorbitol (a polyhydric alcohol) — can serve as an extrarenal route for the excretion of K^+.

In some patients, however, especially those who are in a catabolic state or have sustained trauma, the serum K^+ concentration continues to rise despite the above measures. In such patients, dialysis, either of the peritoneal type or through use of an artificial kidney, is instituted (see below). If the situation is critical, even faster measures for combating hyperkalemia are used, such as intravenous administration of calcium or of glucose plus insulin (Table 4-3).

H^+ Balance

With the affected kidneys virtually unable to excrete the H^+ of fixed acids, the patient develops a metabolic acidosis. Even though this imbalance tends to aggravate the hyperkalemia (Figs. 4-2 and 4-3), the acidosis is usually of a mild degree and need not be treated. In fact, the treatment, which usually consists of giving $NaHCO_3$ or sodium lactate, can itself be so dangerous that it is better to avoid it. The infusion of alkalinizing sodium salts can precipitate heart failure and pulmonary edema. Many patients in acute renal failure also have an elevation of the serum inorganic phosphate concentration and with it a reciprocal lowering of the serum calcium concentration. Inasmuch as the portion of the total serum calcium that exists in the free, unbound state is lower at an alkaline than an acid pH, sudden alkalinization in a patient with renal failure can precipitate hypocalcemic tetany, convulsions, or both (see Chap. 6, under Respiratory Alkalosis). The diet described above, which supplies enough calories to minimize the breakdown of endogenous tissues, not only slows down the development of hyperkalemia but also that of the acidosis, since the production of keto acids will be kept to a minimum. Acidosis also tends to be no problem in patients whose gastric juice is being removed through surgical drainage tubes.

Conservative Management

Many patients with oliguric acute renal failure can be treated very adequately by the simple, so-called conservative regimen outlined above. This fact is illustrated in Figure 9-6, which shows the course of a 23-year-old woman who had an obstetrical hemorrhage and became oliguric after an incompatible blood transfusion. These events occurred at a small community hospital without house staff. The simplicity and efficacy of the conservative management is emphasized by the fact that the patient remained at this hospital throughout her illness and was treated by her own physician, who was helped by a daily telephone consultation with a nephrologist at a major medical center some 70 miles away. Each day, the two doctors discussed the following points: how the patient was feeling, her body weight, her urine output during the previous 24 hours, her serum K^+ concentration, and her ECG. She was given 200 g of lactose dissolved in the daily allowance of water and she sipped this mixture over the

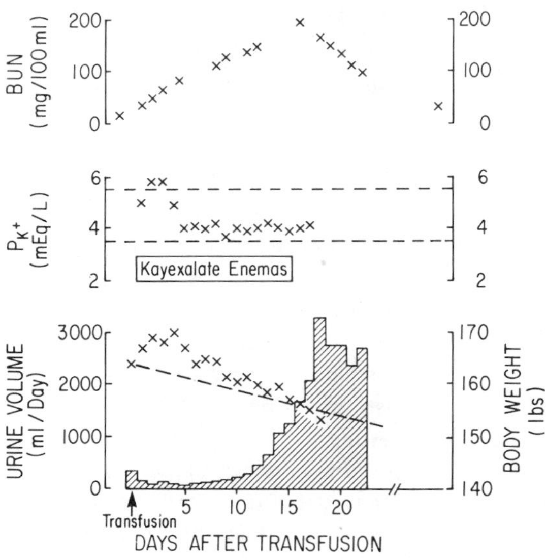

Figure 9-6
Course of oliguric acute renal failure due to obstetrical hemorrhage in a 23-year-old woman. The area between the dashed lines in the middle graph delimits the normal range for plasma potassium concentration. The sloping dashed line in the lower graph corresponds to a weight loss of 1/2 pound (250 g) per day. BUN = blood urea nitrogen; P_{K^+} = plasma potassium concentration.

24-hour period. On the basis of her known normal weight, it was determined that during the first four days of oliguria, the patient's fluid volumes became expanded from the administration of intravenous fluids. Initially, therefore, the daily fluid intake was limited to 200 ml per day until about day 9, when her body weight approached the ideal slope described by a weight loss of 250 g (0.5 pound) per day. Thereafter, and with increasing urine output, the daily intake of water was increased, and the question of whether the right amount was being given was settled by watching the body weight. The patient was given the ion-exchange resin, Kayexalate, 40 g in 200 ml of 25% sorbitol every 6 hours, by retention enemas in order to forestall hyperkalemia. Except for the values on days 2 and 3, this measure, combined with the elimination of K^+ from the diet, kept the serum K^+ concentration within the normal range and prevented abnormalities of the ECG. By the tenth day, it was clear that the urine flow was increasing, and by day 13, the flow exceeded the range that is usually considered oliguric. Several months after the illness, the patient's BUN was 14 mg/100 ml, which signaled complete recovery and healing of the injured renal tissue; such full recovery is typical of patients who survive the acute episode.

Two further features about this course should be noted. Immediately after the oliguric phase, the urine flow rose to slightly diuretic levels. This phenomenon — known as the *diuretic phase* of acute renal failure — is often, though not invariably, seen. The diuresis is frequently much more severe than shown in Figure 9-6, in which case it may reflect excretion of the NaCl and water that was excessively retained while the patient was oliguric. Judging by the weight loss, however, this was not likely to be the explanation in the present patient. It is therefore possible that the diuresis resulted partly from incomplete recovery of tubular cells and hence from some decrease in the tubular reabsorption of NaCl and water. Occasionally, the diuresis is so marked that suddenly the patient requires vigorous replacement of water and NaCl; more commonly, however, the patient's own thirst and appetite, combined with reestablished renal function, will suffice to restore solute and water balance.

The BUN continued to rise for at least three days after normal urine flow resumed; the same observation would have held for the serum creatinine concentration, had it been measured. The explanation for this common finding lies in the relationship between the filtration and the reabsorption of water. To take the present patient as an example, let us suppose that in health, she had a GFR of 100 ml per minute, which would keep her BUN and serum creatinine concentrations at normal levels. Let us suppose, further, that on day 15, her GFR was 20 ml per minute. If at this time she reabsorbed 19.3 ml per minute, she would have excreted 0.7 ml per minute, which would be in accordance with her urine output of about 1,000 ml on that day. The GFR of 20 ml per minute, however, falls far short of the rates of filtration for urea and creatinine that are required to keep her in balance for these two solutes (see Chap. 8, under Rate of Glomerular Filtration). Consequently, the concentrations of these solutes in the blood will continue to rise, and they will not begin to fall until the GFR has been restored to a value where the filtered load for urea and creatinine will be so large that their rates of urinary excretion will exceed their rates of production.

Dialysis

Although many and perhaps most patients with acute renal failure can be managed by the conservative method, this is not possible for all. The problem of maintaining solute and water balance becomes particularly difficult in oliguric patients who are in a catabolic state (e.g., after surgical operations or severe trauma). In such patients, the release of water and K^+ from the cells and the production of keto acids may be so great that conservative measures do not suffice to prevent dangerously positive balances for these substances. In that event, one resorts to either peritoneal or machine dialysis. Moreover, some nephrologists advocate early, prophylactic dialysis in virtually all patients with acute renal failure because it might curtail the course or improve the prognosis. In the case of the patient illustrated in Figure 9-6, they would have instituted dialysis around day 8 or earlier. Although there is some evidence that this method of treatment may reduce the mortality from acute renal failure — which is still at a disturbingly high rate of 50 percent — the statistics probably apply mainly to patients with high risk, such as those with increased catabolism.

Principles of Dialysis. The two methods of dialysis that are used in patients are shown in Figure 9-7. In *peritoneal dialysis,* the patient's plasma is dialyzed against a solution that is put into the abdominal cavity; the semipermeable barrier is some membrane(s) that lies between the interior of the splanchnic vessels and the abdominal cavity, possibly mainly the vessels of the omentum. In adult patients, 2 liters of the dialysis solution are usually instilled, kept within the abdominal cavity for 20 to 40 minutes to allow for passive transport of diffusible compounds into or out of the solution, and then removed by gravity drainage. The process is repeated until the therapeutic goal is accomplished, usually for at least 24 hours.

The composition of a common dialysis solution is shown in Figure 1-6. The solution is devoid of those substances that one wishes to remove from the patient; substances that one wishes to add to the patient are present in high concentrations within the dialysis solution; and those for which one wishes to maintain normal plasma concentrations in the patient occur in the same concentrations within the solution as within the plasma. The osmolality of the solution is adjusted by the addition of glucose; usually the solution is slightly hyperosmotic to the patient's plasma, so expansion of the patient's fluid volumes can be prevented. The first category — namely, the substances to be removed — includes K^+, urea, creatinine, and the so-called middle molecules such as guanidine, which may be responsible for some of the symptoms of the uremic syndrome. Many of these molecules have not been identified; they are called "middle molecules" because they have intermediate molecular weights, and it is possible that they constitute some of the uremic toxins that cause the distressing symptoms of nausea, vomiting, twitching, somnolence, and coma, among others. This topic is discussed further in the next chapter; suffice it to say here that urea and creatinine are in themselves relatively harmless and that their elimination by dialysis may simply reflect the degree to which as yet unidentified toxic compounds are removed simultaneously. The second category — namely, the substances to be added —

involves mainly buffers for H^+; they are added in the form of lactate or acetate, which, when metabolized, raise the plasma HCO_3^- concentration in the patient. The third category — solutes that are to be kept normal — applies mainly to Na^+, Cl^-, Ca^{2+}, and Mg^{2+}.

The principles are the same when dialysis is carried out with an *artificial kidney,* but in that case the patient's arterial blood is passed through very fine channels or tubing made up of an artificial semipermeable membrane (Fig. 9-7). The tubing is contained in a small "kidney" that is continuously rinsed by dialysis solution; this solution is supplied by a delivery system that monitors composition, temperature, and pressure. It takes about 6 hours to achieve a given therapeutic goal with machine dialysis, and about four times longer to reach the same goal by the peritoneal route. This fact, it should be emphasized, does not necessarily make the artificial kidney "better," since it is often to the patient's advantage to correct imbalances slowly (see Chap. 7, under Guidelines).

Indications for Dialysis. There are no absolute rules governing when dialysis should be used in acute renal failure. Some nephrologists immediately turn to this mode of therapy on the conviction that prophylactic dialysis reduces morbidity and mortality, especially in hypercatabolic patients. Others, however, prefer to start with the conservative management and will intervene with dialysis when one or more of the following circumstances becomes manifest: (1) severe uremia (serum creatinine concentration of 10 to 13 mg/100 ml), with symptoms such as nausea, vomiting, neuromuscular irritability, somnolence, or distressing malaise; (2) uncontrollable hyperkalemia; (3) uncontrollable expansion of the extracellular fluid volume; and (4) severe metabolic acidosis that may be contributing to the drowsiness and disorientation.

Of course, dialysis is used in a number of other conditions, notably in chronic renal failure (Chap. 10) and in poisonings. The present description has been limited to the application of dialysis in acute renal failure.

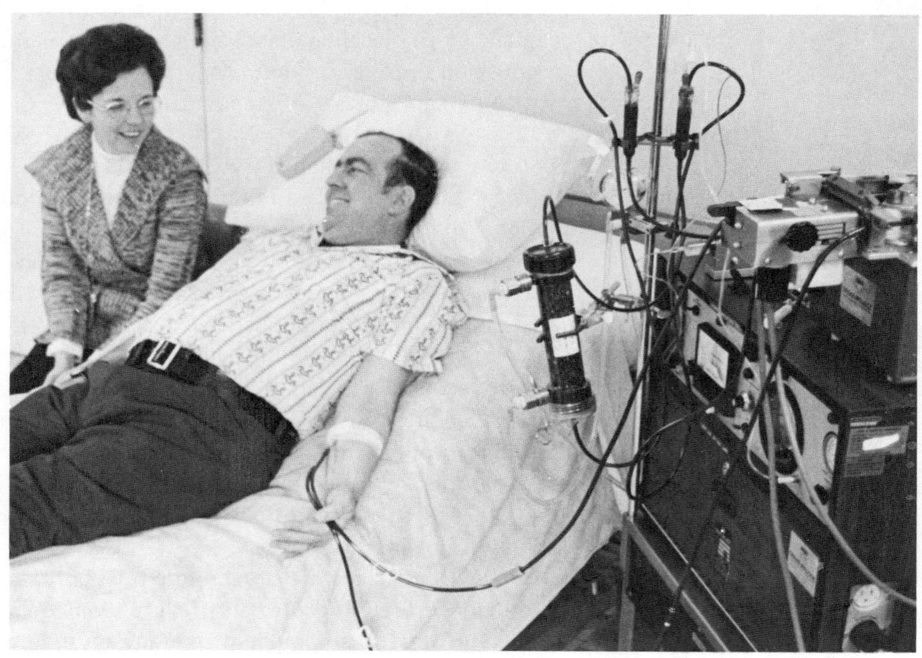

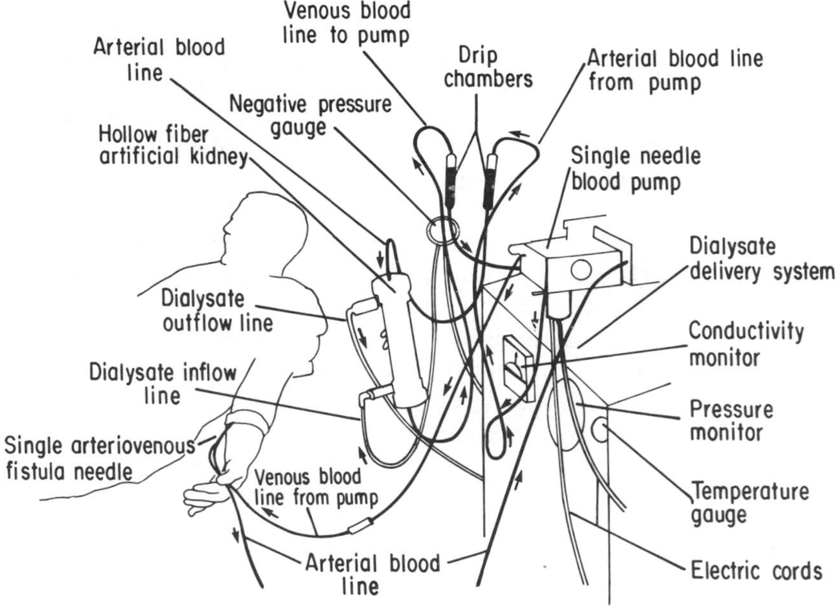

Figure 9-7
Dialysis by means of an artificial kidney in an adult patient with chronic renal failure (*above*) and peritoneal dialysis being carried out on an infant with acute renal failure from the hemolytic-uremic syndrome (*right*). Photograph above courtesy of C. F. Runge.

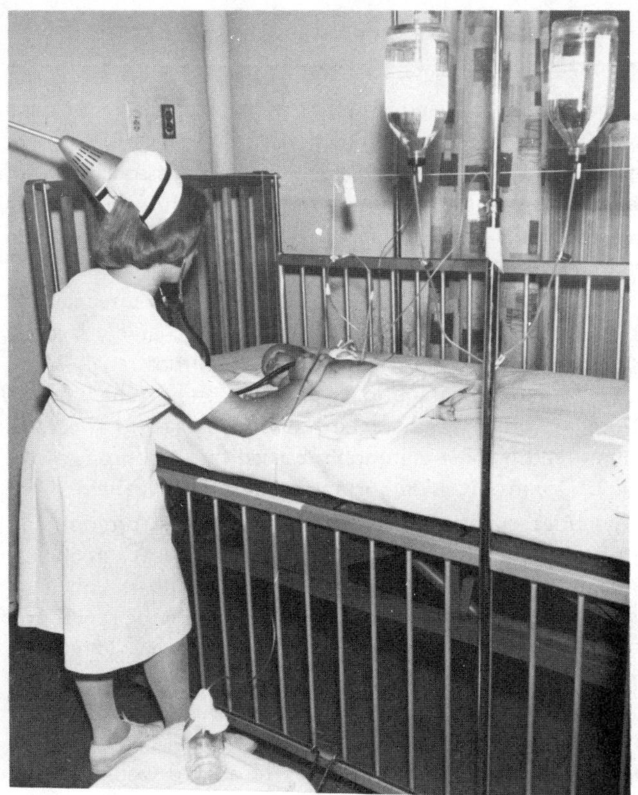

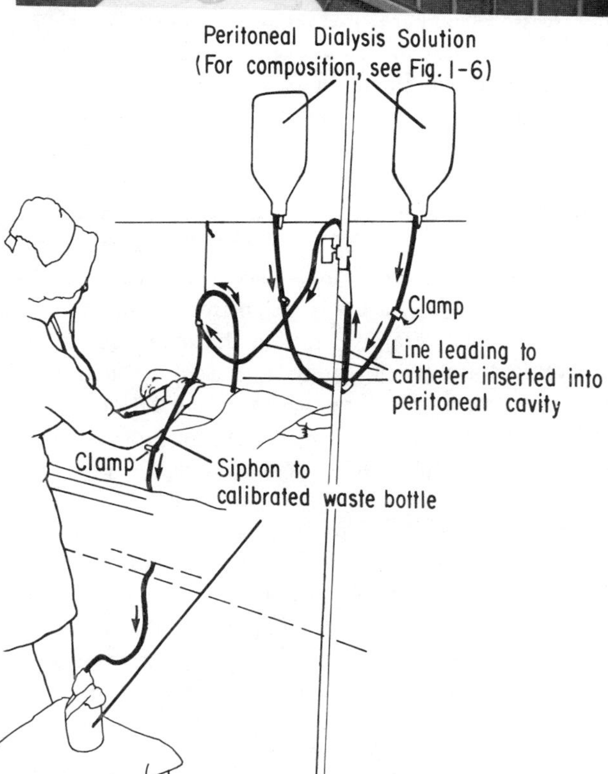
Peritoneal Dialysis Solution
(For composition, see Fig. 1-6)
Clamp
Line leading to
catheter inserted into
peritoneal cavity
Clamp
Siphon to
calibrated waste bottle

Summary

Acute renal failure is a sudden deficiency or cessation of renal function. In the vast majority of patients (perhaps 90 percent of those in acute renal failure), the condition is associated with oliguria (defined as the production of 50 to 400 ml of urine per day) or anuria (<50 ml per day); it can, however, occur in the face of a normal or high urine output.

Causes of acute renal failure may be classified into three general categories (Table 9-1): (1) prerenal, which is characterized by inadequate blood perfusion of the kidneys; (2) postrenal, which is due to obstruction of the urinary passages distal to the kidneys; and (3) renal, which is characterized by damage to the renal parenchyma and is most commonly caused by prolonged, severe ischemia or toxins. It is important to determine which of the three categories a patient falls into, because the prompt correction of either the prerenal or the postrenal causes can obviate cellular damage and thereby prevent a prolonged illness.

The mechanisms that bring about oliguria during the renal form of acute renal failure have not been conclusively identified. Three main theories have been proposed: (1) back-leakage of the glomerular filtrate through injured tubular epithelium, (2) intratubular obstruction that may secondarily decrease the GFR, or (3) a primary decrease in the GFR due to altered vasomotion of certain renal vessels, perhaps mainly the afferent arterioles. These mechanisms are not mutually exclusive, and it is possible that one or the other predominates at various times and in various types of the renal form of acute renal failure. The cause(s) for a possible primary decrease in the GFR (the third theoretical cause listed above) is the subject of intense debate. One postulate states that as the renal tubules are injured and hence reabsorb less NaCl, the greater delivery of NaCl out of the loops of Henle is somehow sensed by the specialized macula densa cells at the early distal tubule. A signal is then transmitted to the granular cells of the JGA, which sets into motion the *local* production of renin and angiotensin II and ultimately leads to constriction of the afferent arteriole and a reduction in the filtration rate of the single, affected nephron (sGFR). When this process occurs in a large number of single nephrons, the total GFR will be decreased.

Treatment of acute renal failure begins by identifying and correcting its cause. This first step is especially important, because if the origin is prerenal or postrenal, its elimination can forestall a prolonged illness. Once it is established that the renal form of acute renal failure is involved, an attempt to reestablish normal urine flow with a single trial of mannitol, furosemide, or ethacrynic acid is probably justified. If that effort fails, then the patient may be oliguric for up to three or four weeks, during which period the physician must regulate water and solute balance for the patient.

Water balance is most easily achieved by monitoring the patient's body weight. The patient should be given a daily allowance of fluid that will lead to a weight loss of about 250 g per day. Such loss is essential in order to prevent expansion of the body-fluid compartments with endogenous water of oxidation. Potentially dangerous expansion of the extracellular fluid volume is further prevented by eliminating all Na^+ from the diet. One of the chief threats to life in acute renal failure is hyperkalemia. It can be avoided in most patients by a diet that is free of protein and K^+ but which contains enough calories in the form of carbohydrate to reduce endogenous catabolism to a minimum; the addition of essential amino acids is a new and alternative means of minimizing negative nitrogen balance. The serum K^+ concentration and the electrocardiogram (ECG) are monitored daily, and if hyperkalemia threatens, an ion-exchange resin (e.g., Kayexalate) is added to the regimen. In the majority of patients, water and solute balance can be achieved, even for periods of weeks, by these simple measures and by a "diet" that provides 200 g of sugar dissolved in the daily ration of water. For some patients, however, more vigorous measures – for example, dialysis or those listed in Table 4-3 for hyperkalemia – may be required or deemed desirable.

The period of oliguria may be followed by a diuretic phase. Although the diuresis usually does not pose critical therapeutic problems, especially not if the requisite weight loss was achieved during the period of oliguria, the physician must still be alert to the possibility of negative water and solute balance occurring during the diuretic phase.

Problem 9-1

A 41-year-old woman was transferred to a major medical center because of oliguric acute renal failure. For about six months, she had noticed a lower abdominal mass, which apparently had not increased in size. Her last menstrual period had started 26 days before the present admission. About four weeks prior to admission, she had had a flu-like illness characterized by fever and rhinitis but not by sore throat. She then began to have severe sweats at night and urinary urgency. Two days prior to transfer, the patient had been admitted to another hospital because of shaking chills, fever, nausea, vomiting, abdominal discomfort, and back pain. Physical examination at that time revealed a pale woman in acute distress, with a temperature of 39°C and a blood pressure of 170/100 mm Hg. A lower abdominal mass could be palpated. The most striking findings noted during this short admission were a hematocrit of 27 percent, a white blood cell count of 38,000 per cubic millimeter with a marked shift to the left, and lack of urination. When the urinary bladder was catheterized, 50 ml of urine was obtained; this specimen showed a specific gravity of 1.017, and two to three white cells and more than 100 red cells per high-power field. Notable normal values included that of the serum potassium concentration, and of the BUN (15 mg/100 ml). A cystoscopy was performed, as was a retrograde pyelographic study of the left kidney; neither examination revealed any obstruction of the urinary tract. The patient was then transferred to the larger hospital.

Now, on about the third day of acute renal failure, the previous findings were confirmed and additional abnormalities were noted. The abdominal mass was firm, smooth, and round, and it extended in the midline to a point about 10 cm above the symphysis pubis. The patient still did not urinate spontaneously, but catheterization yielded 15 ml of urine, which showed a specific gravity of 1.020, two-plus protein (for quantitative estimate, see Fig. 8-7), two-plus hemoglobin, and two to three white cells, innumerable red cells, some bacteria, and a few, coarsely granular casts per high-power field. The BUN was 30 mg/100 ml, the serum creatinine concentration 4.9 mg/100 ml, and the serum K^+ concentration 4.9 mEq per liter. There were striking hematological abnormalities as reflected in a hematocrit of 25 percent, a white blood cell count of 45,700 (82 percent of which were neutrophils), and a smear of the peripheral blood that showed very marked microangiopathic changes in the form of burr cells, cellular fragments, anisocytosis, and poikilocytosis.

On the fifth day of illness, the patient underwent a pelvic examination under anesthesia, which disclosed an enlarged uterus with multiple, firm, irregular nodules; scrapings from the uterine cavity revealed menstrual endometrium. Because the patient still had not urinated spontaneously by the sixth day of illness, she was again catheterized, and 15 ml of urine, having the same characteristics as those previously described, was obtained. A percutaneous (often called closed) renal biopsy was done on the same day. The biopsy specimen showed fibrin thrombi in the interlobular arteries, afferent arterioles, and glomerular capillaries; endocapillary swelling of the glomeruli; and necrosis of the proximal and distal tubules; there was hemorrhagic infarction of 80 to 85 percent of the glomeruli. The findings added up to a pathological diagnosis of renal cortical necrosis which, in the light of the microangiopathic hemolytic anemia, was considered to be due to the *hemolytic-uremic syndrome.* On the seventh day of illness, the BUN was 95 mg/100 ml and the serum creatinine concentration 11.2 mg/100 ml.

From the day of transfer to the second hospital, the patient was treated with fluid restriction and a diet that was low in K^+ and protein. Dialysis with an artificial kidney was begun during the first week. After two weeks, the patient began to produce urine, with an increase in output of about 50 ml per day. By the end of one month, the urine flow averaged approximately 750 ml per day, and it then rose to about 1 liter per day. Dialysis was stopped at the beginning of the fifth month; three weeks later, the serum creatinine concentration was 6.0 mg/100 ml, the endogenous creatinine clearance was 13 liters per 24 hours, and the patient looked and felt remarkably well.

This clinical history has been abstracted and simplified from the *New England Journal of Medicine* (293:1247, 1975). It appeared as part of a weekly series of clinicopathological conferences, which are published regularly in that and other journals and which contain learned discussions of differential diagnosis. One reason for selecting this particular history is to point out to students that although this book stops short of discussing specific diseases, it nevertheless should whet the appetite for reading other material, such as the journals and standard textbooks in clinical disciplines.

Even though the beginning student is not expected to have mastered the refined points of differential diagnosis, it is time that he or she deal with some general questions that a physician faces when managing a patient with acute renal failure. (1) Was the patient described above oliguric or anuric? Why is it important to make this distinction? (2) Is it better to pass a urinary catheter several times (as was done in this patient), or should a so-called indwelling catheter have been kept within the urethra during the first few days or weeks? (3) Why was there so much concern about the nature of the abdominal mass in this patient? (4) Should cystoscopy and retrograde pyelography be performed in patients such as this? Why was a retrograde pyelogram not obtained on the right kidney as well as the left? (5) Is it important to know whether a patient has two kidneys? (6) At what rate are the BUN and serum creatinine concentrations expected to rise in an otherwise uncomplicated instance of oliguric acute renal failure? Why is it important to consider this question?

Appendix

For those who want to read more about the gamut of causes and courses of acute renal failure, the following references contain detailed clinical histories. The sources are listed in chronological order.

Bull, G. M., Joekes, A. M., and Lowe, K. G. Renal function studies in acute tubular necrosis. *Clin. Sci.* 9:379, 1950 (Appendix 2, beginning on p. 395).

Swan, R. C., and Merrill, J. P. The clinical course of acute renal failure. *Medicine* (Baltimore) 32:215, 1953 (Appendix, beginning on p. 283).

Munck, O. *Renal Circulation in Acute Renal Failure.* Oxford, Eng.: Blackwell, 1958 (Supplement, beginning on p. 38).

Crandell, W. B., Pappas, S. G., and Macdonald, A. Nephrotoxicity associated with methoxyflurane anesthesia. *Anesthesiology* 27:591, 1966 (mostly examples of nonoliguric acute renal failure).

Hollenberg, N. K., Epstein, M., Rosen, S. M., Basch, R. I., Oken, D. E., and Merrill, J. P. Acute oliguric renal failure in man: Evidence for preferential renal cortical ischemia. *Medicine* (Baltimore) 47:455, 1968 (Appendix, beginning on p. 470).

Baker, G. P., Jr., and Blennerhassett, J. B. Persistent abdominal pain and oliguria. *N. Engl. J. Med.* 283:305, 1970 (another clinicopathological conference, or CPC).

Klahr, S., and Lynch, R. Renal failure after transplantation. *Am. J. Med.* 58:537, 1975 (another CPC).

Grantham, J. J., and Cuppage, F. Rapidly progressive renal failure in a young woman. *N. Engl. J. Med.* 293:922, 1975 (another).

Harrington, J. T., and McCluskey, R. T. Fever, rash and renal failure after upper-respiratory-tract infection. *N. Engl. J. Med.* 293:1308, 1975 (and yet another).

Selected References

General

Anderson, R. J., Linas, S. L., Berns, A. S., Henrich, W. L., Miller, T. R., Gabow, P. A., and Schrier, R. W. Nonoliguric acute renal failure. *N. Engl. J. Med.* 296:1134, 1977.

Bluemle, L. W., Jr., Potter, H. P., and Elkinton, J. R. Changes in body composition in acute renal failure. *J. Clin. Invest.* 35:1094, 1956.

Bluemle, L. W., Jr., Webster, G. D., Jr., and Elkinton, J. R. Acute tubular necrosis. Analysis of one hundred cases with respect to mortality, complications, and treatment with and without dialysis. *Arch. Intern. Med.* 104:180, 1959.

Bywaters, E. G. L., and Beall, D. Crush injuries with impairment of renal function. *Br. Med. J.* 1:427, 1941.

de Wardener, H. E. *The Kidney. An Outline of Normal and Abnormal Structure and Function* (4th ed.). Edinburgh: Churchill/Livingstone, 1973.

Flamenbaum, W., and Kaufman, J. S. Acute renal failure. *Kidney* 9:21, 1976.

Franklin, S. S., and Maxwell, M. H. Acute Renal Failure. In M. H. Maxwell and C. R. Kleeman (eds.), *Clinical Disorders of Fluid and Electrolyte Metabolism* (2nd ed.). New York: McGraw-Hill, 1972.

Friedman, E. A., and Eliahou, H. E. (eds.). *Proceedings of the Acute Renal Failure Conference.* DHEW Publication No. (NIH)74-608. Washington, D.C.: U.S. Government Printing Office, 1974.
This volume contains up-to-date presentations and useful discussions of the pathogenesis, prognosis, and treatment of acute renal failure. The book can be purchased from the Superintendent of Documents, U.S. Government Printing Office, Washington, D.C. 20402.

Harrington, J. T., and Cohen, J. J. Acute oliguria. *N. Engl. J. Med.* 292:89, 1975.

Kirkland, K., Edwards, K. D. G., and Whyte, H. M. Oliguric renal failure: A report of 400 cases including classification, survival, and response to dialysis. *Australas. Ann. Med.* 14:275, 1965.

Lancet Editorial. Acute renal failure. *Lancet* 2:134, 1973.

Lewers, D. T., Mathew, T. H., Maher, J. F., and Schreiner, G. E. Long-term follow-up of renal function and histology after acute tubular necrosis. *Ann. Intern. Med.* 73:523, 1970.

Linton, A. L. Acute renal failure. *Can. Med. Assoc. J.* 110:949, 1974.

Lordon, R. E., and Burton, J. R. Post-traumatic renal failure in military personnel in southeast Asia. *Am. J. Med.* 53:137, 1972.

Merrill, J. P. *The Treatment of Renal Failure* (2nd ed.). New York: Grune & Stratton, 1965.

Merrill, J. P. Acute Renal Failure. In M. B. Strauss and L. G. Welt (eds.), *Diseases of the Kidney* (2nd ed.). Boston: Little, Brown, 1971.

Milne, M. D. (ed.). Management of renal failure. *Br. Med. Bull.* 27:95, 1971.

Papper, S. *Clinical Nephrology* (2nd ed.). Boston: Little, Brown, 1978.

Schreiner, G. E. Acute Renal Failure. In D. A. K. Black (ed.), *Renal Disease* (2nd ed.). Philadelphia: Davis, 1967.

Schrier, R. W., and Conger, J. D. Acute Renal Failure: Pathogenesis, Diagnosis, and Management. In R. W. Schrier (ed.), *Renal and Electrolyte Disorders.* Boston: Little, Brown, 1976.

Stott, R. B., Cameron, J. S., Ogg, C. S., and Bewick, M. Why the persistently high mortality in acute renal failure? *Lancet* 2:75, 1972.

Vertel, R. M., and Knochel, J. P. Nonoliguric acute renal failure. *J. A. M. A.* 200:598, 1967.

Williams, G. S., Klenk, E. L., and Winters, R. W. Acute Renal Failure in Pediatrics. In R. W. Winters (ed.), *The Body Fluids in Pediatrics.* Boston: Little, Brown, 1973.

Pathogenesis

Arendhorst, W. J., Finn, W. F., and Gottschalk, C. W. Nephron stop-flow pressure response to obstruction for 24 hours in the rat kidney. *J. Clin. Invest.* 53:1497, 1974.

Arendhorst, W. J., Finn, W. F., and Gottschalk, C. W. Pathogenesis of acute renal failure following temporary renal ischemia in the rat. *Circ. Res.* 37:558, 1975.

Arieff, A. I., and Massry, S. G. Calcium metabolism of brain in acute renal failure. Effects of uremia, hemodialysis, and parathyroid hormone. *J. Clin. Invest.* 53:387, 1974.

Bank, N., Mutz, B. F., and Aynedjian, H. S. The role of "leakage" of tubular fluid in anuria due to mercury poisoning. *J. Clin. Invest.* 46:695, 1967.

Biber, T. U. L., Mylle, M., Baines, A. D., and Gottschalk, C. W. A study by micropuncture and microdissection of acute renal damage in rats. *Am. J. Med.* 44:664, 1968.

Bohle, A., and Thurau, K. Ein Dialog: Funktion und Morphologie der Niere im akuten Nierenversagen. *Verh. Dtsch. Ges. Inn. Med.* 80:565, 1974.

Brown, J. J., Gleadle, R. I., Lawson, D. H., Lever, A. F., Linton, A. L., Macadam, R. F., Prentice, E., Robertson, J. I. S., and Tree, M. Renin and acute renal failure: Studies in man. *Br. Med. J.* 1:253, 1970.

Chedru, M. -F., Baethke, R., and Oken, D. E. Renal cortical blood flow and glomerular filtration in myohemoglobinuric acute renal failure. *Kidney Int.* 1:232, 1972.

Chonko, A. M., Stein, J. H., and Ferris, T. F. Renin and the kidney. *Nephron* 15:279, 1975.

Cox, J. W., Baehler, R. W., Sharma, H., O'Dorisio, T., Osgood, R. W., Stein, J. H., and Ferris, T. F. Studies on the mechanism of oliguria in a model of unilateral acute renal failure. *J. Clin. Invest.* 53:1546, 1974.

Daugharty, T. M., Ueki, I. F., Mercer, P. F., and Brenner, B. M. Dynamics of glomerular ultrafiltration in the rat. V. Response to ischemic injury. *J. Clin. Invest.* 53:105, 1974.

Dev, B., Drescher, C., and Schnermann, J. Resetting of tubulo-glomerular feedback sensitivity by dietary salt intake. *Pflügers Arch. Eur. J. Physiol.* 346:263, 1974.

Earley, L. E. Pathogenesis of oliguric acute renal failure. *N. Engl. J. Med.* 282:1370, 1970.

Finn, W. F., Arendhorst, W. J., and Gottschalk, C. W. Pathogenesis of oliguria in acute renal failure. *Circ. Res.* 36:675, 1975.

Flamenbaum, W. Pathophysiology of acute renal failure. *Arch. Intern. Med.* 131:911, 1973.

Flamenbaum, W., Kotchen, T. A., and Oken, D. E. Effect of renin immunization on mercuric chloride and glycerol-induced renal failure. *Kidney Int.* 1:406, 1972.

Flanigan, W. J., and Oken, D. E. Renal micropuncture study of the development of anuria in the rat with mercury-induced acute renal failure. *J. Clin. Invest.* 44:449, 1965.

Frega, N. S., DiBona, D. R., Guertler, B., and Leaf, A. Ischemic renal injury. *Kidney Int.* 10 [Suppl. 6] : S-17, 1976.

Goormaghtigh, N. Vascular and circulatory changes in renal cortex in the anuric crush-syndrome. *Proc. Soc. Exp. Biol. Med.* 59:303, 1945.

Granger, P., Dahlheim, H., and Thurau, K. Enzyme activities of the single juxtaglomerular apparatus in the rat kidney. *Kidney Int.* 1:78, 1972.

Grantham, J. J. Pathophysiology of Hyposmolar Conditions: A Cellular Perspective. In T. E. Andreoli, J. J. Grantham, and F. C. Rector, Jr. (eds.), *Disturbances in Body Fluid Osmolality.* Washington, D.C.: American Physiological Society, 1977.

Henry, L. N., Lane, C. E., and Kashgarian, M. Micropuncture studies of the pathophysiology of acute renal failure in the rat. *Lab. Invest.* 19:309, 1968.

Hollenberg, N. K., Adams, D. F., Oken, D. E., Abrams, H. L., and Merrill, J. P. Acute renal failure due to nephrotoxins. Renal hemodynamic and angiographic studies in man. *N. Engl. J. Med.* 282:1329, 1970.

Hollenberg, N. K., Epstein, M., Rosen, S. M., Basch, R. I., Oken, D. E., and Merrill, J. P. Acute oliguric renal failure in man: Evidence for preferential renal cortical ischemia. *Medicine* (Baltimore) 47:455, 1968.

Hollenberg, N. K., Sandor, T., Conroy, M., Adams, D. F., Solomon, H. S., Abrams, H. L., and Merrill, J. P. Xenon transit through the oliguric human kidney: Analysis by maximum likelihood. *Kidney Int.* 3:177, 1973.

Jaenike, J. R. Micropuncture study of methemoglobin-induced acute renal failure in the rat. *J. Lab. Clin. Med.* 73:459, 1969.

Leckie, B., Gavras, H., McGregor, J., and McElwee, G. The conversion of angiotensin I to angiotensin II by rabbit glomeruli. *J. Endocrinol.* 55:229, 1972.

Levinsky, N. G. Pathophysiology of acute renal failure. *N. Engl. J. Med.* 296:1453, 1977.

Macknight, A. D. C., and Leaf, A. Regulation of cellular volume. *Physiol. Rev.* 57:510, 1977.

Mauk, R. H., Patak, R. V., Fadem, S. Z., Lifschitz, M. D., and Stein, J. H. Effect of prostaglandin E administration in a nephrotoxic and a vasoconstrictor model of acute renal failure. *Kidney Int.* 12:122, 1977.

Mitch, W. E., and Walker, W. G. Plasma renin and angiotensin II in acute renal failure. *Lancet* 2:328, 1977.

Morgan, T., and Davis, J. M. Renin secretion at the individual nephron level. *Pflügers Arch. Eur. J. Physiol.* 359:23, 1975.

Navar, L. G., Burke, T. J., Robinson, R. R., and Clapp, J. R. Distal tubular feedback in the autoregulation of single nephron glomerular filtration rate. *J. Clin. Invest.* 53:516, 1974.

Oken, D. E., Arce, M. L., and Wilson, D. R. Glycerol-induced hemoglobinuric acute renal failure in the rat. I. Micropuncture study of the development of oliguria. *J. Clin. Invest.* 45:724, 1966.

Oken, D. E., Cotes, S. C., Flamenbaum, W., Powell-Jackson, J. D., and Lever, A. F. Active and passive immunization to angiotensin in experimental acute renal failure. *Kidney Int.* 7:12, 1975.

Oken, D. E., Mende, C. W., Taraba, I., and Flamenbaum, W. Resistance to acute renal failure afforded by prior renal failure: Examination of the role of renal renin content. *Nephron* 15:131, 1975.

Oliver, J., MacDowell, M., and Tracy, A. The pathogenesis of acute renal failure associated with traumatic and toxic injury. Renal ischemia, nephrotoxic damage and the ischemuric episode. *J. Clin. Invest.* 30:1307, 1951.

Reubi, F. C. The pathogenesis of anuria following shock. *Kidney Int.* 5:106, 1974.

Richards, A. N. Direct observations of change in function of the renal tubule caused by certain poisons. *Trans. Assoc. Am. Physicians* 44:64, 1929.

Richards, C. J., and DiBona, G. F. Acute renal failure: Structural-functional correlation. *Proc. Soc. Exp. Biol. Med.* 146:880, 1974.

Riley, A. L., Alexander, E. A., Migdal, S., and Levinsky, N. G. The effect of ischemia on renal blood flow in the dog. *Kidney Int.* 7:27, 1975.

Ruiz-Guiñazú, A., Coelho, J. B., and Paz, R. A. Methemoglobin-induced acute renal failure in the rat. In vivo observation, histology, and micropuncture measurements of intratubular and postglomerular vascular pressures. *Nephron* 4:257, 1967.

Schnermann, J., Hermle, M., Schmidmeier, E., and Dahlheim, H. Impaired potency for feedback regulation of glomerular filtration rate in DOCA escaped rats. *Pflügers Arch. Eur. J. Physiol.* 358:325, 1975.

Sevitt, S. Pathogenesis of traumatic uraemia. A revised concept. *Lancet* 2:135, 1959.

Summers, W. K., and Jamison, R. L. The no reflow phenomenon in renal ischemia. *Lab. Invest.* 25:635, 1971.

Tanner, G. A., Sloan, K. L., and Sophasan, S. Effects of renal artery occlusion on kidney function in the rat. *Kidney Int.* 4:377, 1973.

Thiel, G., McDonald, F. D., and Oken, D. E. Micropuncture studies of the basis for protection of renin depleted rats from glycerol induced acute renal failure. *Nephron* 7:67, 1970.

Thurau, K. (ed.). Experimental acute renal failure. *Kidney Int.* 10 [Suppl. 6] : S-1, 1976.

Thurau, K., and Boylan, J. W. Acute renal success. The unexpected logic of oliguria in acute renal failure. *Am. J. Med.* 61:308, 1976.

Treatment

Abel, R. M., Beck, C. H., Jr., Abbott, W. M., Ryan, J. A., Jr., Barnett, G. O., and Fischer, J. E. Improved survival from acute renal failure after treatment with intravenous essential L-amino acids and glucose. *N. Engl. J. Med.* 288:695, 1973.

Bailey, R. R., Natale, R., Turnbull, D. I., and Linton, A. L. Protective effect of frusemide in acute tubular necrosis and acute renal failure. *Clin. Sci. Mol. Med.* 45:1, 1973.

Berlyne, G. M., Bazzard, F. J., Booth, E. M., Janabi, K., and Shaw, A. B. The dietary treatment of acute renal failure. *Q. J. Med.* 36:59, 1967.

Birtch, A. G., Zakheim, R. M., Jones, L. G., and Barger, A. C. Redistribution of renal blood flow produced by furosemide and ethacrynic acid. *Circ. Res.* 21:869, 1967.

Borst, J. G. G. Protein katabolism in uraemia. Effects of protein-free diet, infections, and blood-transfusions. *Lancet* 1:824, 1948.

Bull, G. M., Joekes, A. M., and Lowe, K. G. Conservative treatment of anuric uraemia. *Lancet* 2:229, 1949.

Cantarovich, F., Galli, C., Benedetti, L., Chena, C., Castro, L., Correa, C., Perez-Loredo, J., Fernandez, J. C., Locatelli, A., and Tizado, J. High dose frusemide in established acute renal failure. *Br. Med. J.* 4:449, 1973.

Elliott, R. W., Kerr, D. N. S., and Lewis, A. A. G. (eds.). Frusemide in renal failure. *Postgrad. Med. J.* 47 [Suppl.] : 3, 1971 (April).

Gordon, A., DePalma, J. R., and Maxwell, M. H. Water, Electrolyte, and Acid-Base Disorders Associated with Acute and Chronic Dialysis. In M. H. Maxwell and C. R. Kleeman (eds.), *Clinical Disorders of Fluid and Electrolyte Metabolism* (2nd ed.). New York: McGraw-Hill, 1972.

Greenberg, G. R., Marliss, E. B., Anderson, G. H., Langer, B., Spence, W., Tovee, E. B., and Jeejeebhoy, K. Protein-sparing therapy in postoperative patients. Effects of added hypocaloric glucose or lipid. *N. Engl. J. Med.* 294:1411, 1976.

Grossman, R. A., and Goldberg, M. The use of diuretics in renal disease. *Kidney* 7:1, 1974.

Kaufmann, F., and Lunglmayr, G. Effect of mannitol diuresis on enzyme activity of the rat kidney in experimental acute renal failure. *Nephron* 8:463, 1971.

Luke, R. G., Linton, A. L., Briggs, J. D., and Kennedy, A. C. Mannitol therapy in acute renal failure. *Lancet* 1:980, 1965.

Massry, S. G., Arieff, A. I., Coburn, J. W., Palmieri, G., and Kleeman, C. R. Divalent ion metabolism in patients with acute renal failure: Studies on the mechanism of hypocalcemia. *Kidney Int.* 5:437, 1974.

Morris, C. R., Alexander, E. A., Bruns, F. J., and Levinsky, N. G. Restoration and maintenance of glomerular filtration by mannitol during hypoperfusion of the kidney. *J. Clin. Invest.* 51:1555, 1972.

10 : Chronic Renal Failure: Adaptation of Balances

Definitions

Chronic renal failure may be defined as the state that results from a large, irreversible reduction in the number of functioning nephrons; "large" denotes a reduction of somewhere in excess of 60 percent of the nephrons existing in health. In addition to irreversibility, chronic renal failure is distinguished from acute renal failure in a number of other aspects: the chronic form is usually more gradual in its development, it is often progressive, and most importantly, it involves adaptive mechanisms whereby the kidneys can maintain balances for water and solutes with a sufficient degree of precision to allow survival *on a normal dietary intake.* It is in the last respect that chronic renal failure differs so strikingly from acute renal failure (Chap. 9), during which the patient's intake of water and solutes must be meticulously regulated in order to prevent fatal imbalances. In this chapter, we shall first describe the anatomical and functional changes that occur when the kidneys are damaged by diseases that lead to chronic renal failure (Table 10-1); we shall then consider how the handling of water and solutes by the damaged kidneys is altered to prevent or minimize imbalances.

The term *uremia* arose from the concept that urine, or at least one of its major constituents, urea, was retained in the blood when the kidneys failed. Even though the term is often used synonymously with chronic renal failure, it can and should be applied to any clinical state where failure of the kidneys, be it acute or chronic, has led to an elevation of the BUN and serum creatinine concentrations. Although the BUN and creatinine levels reflect glomerular but not necessarily tubular function (Table 8-1), the term "uremia" nevertheless adequately describes renal failure, whether it was initiated by a process such as glomerulonephritis (which injures primarily the glomerular capillaries), a process such as poisoning with heavy metals (which damages primarily the tubules), or, for that matter, a primary process that initially damages the nonglomerular vessels or the interstitium. In all cases, the GFR will be decreased, for as a result of the interdependence of the vascular and tubular components of the kidney, the entire nephron will soon be involved (see Chap. 8, under What Is the Extent of Renal Impairment? Thus, a common feature of all types of chronic renal failure (Table 10-1) is *a reduction of the GFR.*

Two further terms should be explained. *Chronic Bright's disease* is still sometimes used as a generic expression to be applied to any disorder due to any of the causes listed in Table 10-1 when they have led to chronic renal failure. The name is derived from that of Richard Bright, the British physician who first described the association of the uremic syndrome with pathological processes of the kidney. Chronic renal failure, especially when it is far advanced, is sometimes referred to by clinicians as *end-stage kidney disease.*

Causes and Incidence of Chronic Renal Failure

Despite the wide spectrum of diseases that can eventuate in chronic renal failure (Table 10-1), the end result is by and large the same: a reduction occurs in the number of nephrons, that is, in the amount of functioning renal tissue. It is for this reason that chronic renal failure can be considered as a single pathological entity, even though many specific diseases are involved.

Loss of renal function is a major health problem. In the United States alone, 50,000 to 100,000 men, women, and children die annually as a result of some form of renal disease. Further, disorders of the kidneys that may lead to chronic renal failure are a major cause of morbidity and of absenteeism; an estimated 12 million people in the United States are affected by renal disease each year.

Anatomical and Functional Changes

In the chronically diseased kidney as in the normal kidney, there appears to be a close correlation between structure and function. Although the various disorders listed in Table 10-1 usually result in some specific anatomical changes that a pathologist can recognize, there are also certain features that are common to most forms of chronic renal disease. Usually, the kidneys are small, weighing as little as one-third of normal (Fig. 10-1a); the cortical zone is often narrowed, and it may be difficult to identify the glomeruli on gross inspection. The functional counterpart of this appearance is a decreased GFR. The renal plasma flow (RPF), however, may be normal or decreased less than the GFR; therefore, the filtration fraction is often reduced.

Microscopically, the key descriptive word is *heterogeneity* (Fig. 10-1b). Glomeruli, even in a single kidney, can vary from being hypertrophied, to normal in appearance, to being completely hyalinized. Tubules are greatly reduced in number, and those that remain may be atrophic, normal, or hypertrophic, shortened or lengthened, and narrowed or dilated; they may be

Table 10-1
Causes of chronic renal failure[a]

1. Immunological disorders
   - Glomerulonephritides[b]
   - Lupus erythematosus
   - Polyarteritis nodosa
   - Goodpasture's syndrome
2. Infections
   - Pyelonephritis[b]
   - Tuberculosis
3. Urinary obstruction
   - Prostatic hypertrophy
   - Renal calculi (bilateral or in a single kidney)
   - Urethral constriction
   - Neoplasms
4. Metabolic disorders
   - Diabetes mellitus[b]
   - Amyloidosis
   - Gout
5. Vascular disorders
   - Hypertension (benign and malignant)[b]
   - Infarctions
   - Sickle-cell anemia
6. Hereditary and congenital disorders
   - Alport's syndrome
   - Polycystic disease
   - Renal hypoplasia
7. Nephrotoxins
   - Analgesic nephropathy
   - Other drugs
   - Heavy metal poisoning
   - Industrial solvents
8. Others
   - Radiation nephritis
   - Multiple myeloma
   - Leukemia
   - Hypercalcemia

[a]The list is not exhaustive, and the placement of some diseases into one category rather than another is arbitrary.
[b]These are some of the more common causes of chronic renal failure. Although certain other conditions (e.g., prostatic hypertrophy and renal calculi) have a high incidence, they do not frequently lead to chronic renal failure.

totally affected by the pathological process or, more commonly, show spotty involvement. Arcuate and interlobular arteries are narrowed, and the consequent ischemic changes probably contribute to the damage. Much of the interstitium is fibrotic. Glomeruli of normal appearance may be attached to very abnormal tubules, and vice versa.

The function of individual nephrons (as determined by micropuncture) is also much more heterogeneous in the diseased than in the normal kidney. For example, in autologous immune-complex nephritis in rats — an experimental counterpart of the

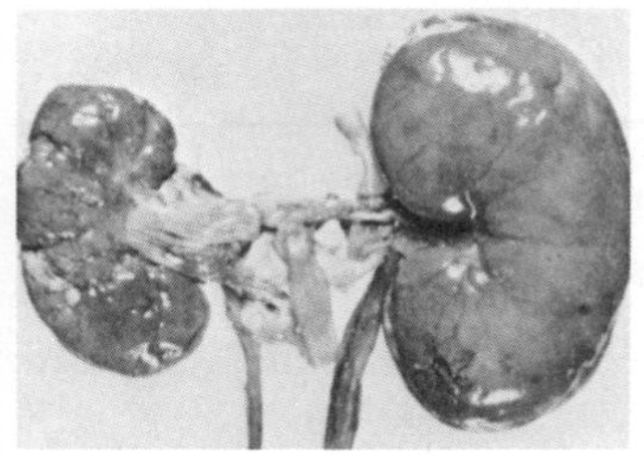

(a)

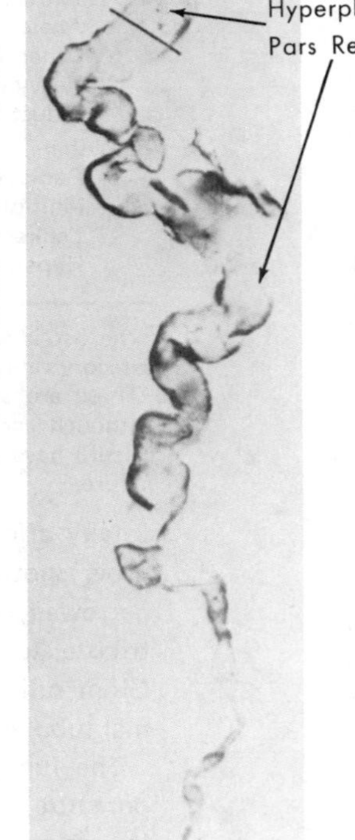

(b)

Figure 10-1
(a) Kidneys of a dog 88 days after the experimental induction of unilateral glomerulonephritis. The characteristic atrophy of the diseased kidney is striking. From N. S. Bricker et al., *Am. J. Med.* 28:77, 1960.

(b) Microdissected glomerulus and proximal tubule of a rat 25 days after exposure to a combination of two nephrotoxins, potassium dichromate and mercuric chloride. The heterogeneous involvement by the pathological process is shown; in other nephrons of the same rat, the distribution would be different and the glomerulus, as well as the tubules, would be affected. Nephrons such as these have been studied by micropuncture; not only do they produce urine, but they also maintain proximal glomerulotubular balance for sodium and water. From R. A. Kramp et al., *Kidney Int.* 5:147, 1974.

most common form of glomerulonephritis in humans — the glomerular filtration rates of single nephrons (sGFR) as well as the proximal intratubular pressures vary over a much wider range than in normal rats (Fig. 10-2a and b). Despite the large

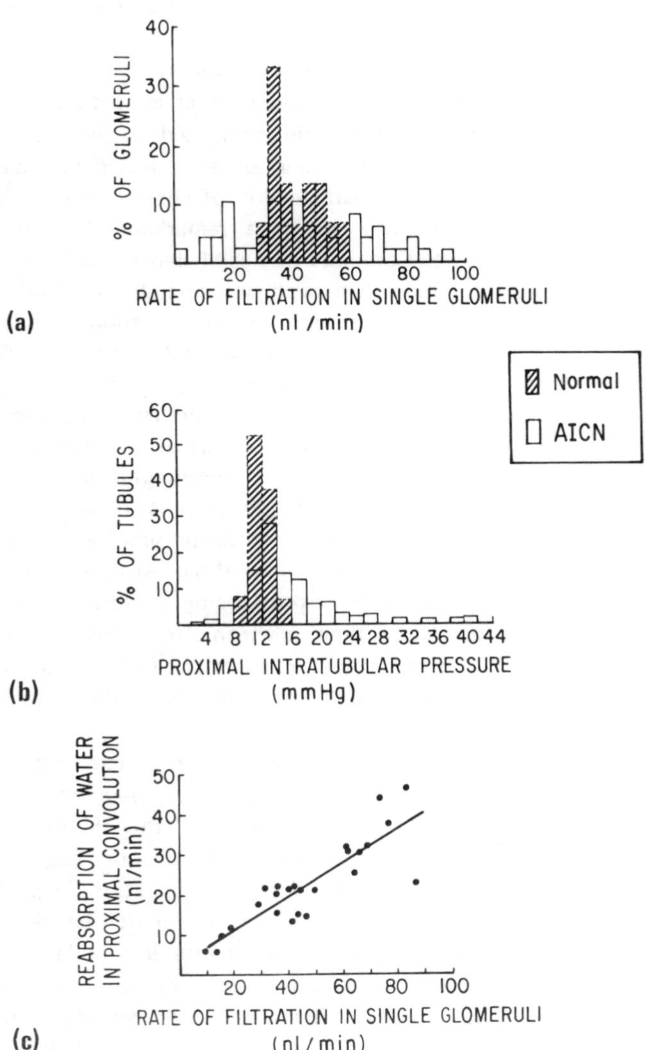

Figure 10-2
Filtration rate in single glomeruli (a) and hydrostatic pressures in single proximal tubules (b) of normal rats (shaded columns) and rats with autologous immune-complex nephritis (AICN). The much wider range of values in the diseased animals reflects the heterogeneity of nephron function that is characteristic of chronic renal failure. Despite the heterogeneity, however, glomerulotubular balance is maintained within the proximal tubule, as shown by the direct correlation between the variables graphed in part (c). Modified from M. E. M. Allison et al., *J. Clin. Invest.* 53:1402, 1974.

differences in the amount of filtrate delivered to a given proximal tubule, however, and despite the great variation in the pathological involvement and consequent anatomy and function of that tubule, the amount of water reabsorbed from it is finely attuned to the amount of filtrate that it receives (Fig. 10-2c). That is, proximal glomerulotubular balance for Na^+ and water is maintained.

The preservation of balance between glomerular and tubular functions by a kidney that is as diseased as the one shown in Figure 10-1a and composed of nephrons as variable in both structure and function as reflected in Figures 10-1b and 10-2a and b is characteristic of chronic renal failure, and this balance is perhaps the most remarkable feature of this pathological state. Complete or near balance can be demonstrated not only for individual nephrons, but also for their aggregate. Thus, the maximal capacity of all the tubules in a diseased kidney to reabsorb glucose (Tm_G) and phosphate (Tm_{Phos}) or to secrete *p*-aminohippuric acid (Tm_{PAH}) is closely correlated with the GFR of that kidney. Inasmuch as diseased nephrons thus adapt to their new state, it has been suggested by C. W. Gottschalk that it may be most meaningful to both think and speak of *adaptive nephrons* in chronic renal failure. In the sense that virtually all nephrons adapt simultaneously, some experts speak of the "homogeneity of glomerulotubular balance"; this phraseology (at the risk of being confusing) stresses the point that at any given time in chronic renal failure, the numerous nephrons of diverse function adapt to a common setting. If we are speaking of proximal glomerulotubular balance for salt and water, this setting is the same as that existing in health; if we use the term to refer to the entire tubular system, the setting will be at a new level, as described in the next paragraph.

In subsequent sections of this chapter, we will describe how the rates of tubular reabsorption (e.g., of water, sodium, or phosphate) or of tubular secretion (e.g., of potassium) are altered in order to preserve external balance for these substances. At first glance, this change in tubular function may seem to conflict with the demonstration of glomerulotubular balance cited above. The solution to the apparent conflict lies in the realization that we are talking about different balances. Above, we considered the balance between the amount of Na^+ and water filtered into a single nephron and the fraction of those filtered loads that was reabsorbed in the *proximal* convolutions of the particular nephron. Alternatively, we described the balance between the maximal capacity of all tubules within a diseased kidney to transport glucose or PAH and the capacity of all glomeruli in that kidney to produce filtrate. In subsequent sections, on the other hand, we shall talk about the maintenance of external balance — namely, intake plus endogenous production equals output (Chap. 1) — which is often achieved by altering tubular transport. It is not self-contradictory to assert that in chronic renal failure, constant fractions of the filtered Na^+ and water are reabsorbed in the proximal convolutions, while external balance for these two substances is achieved by decreasing the fractions of their filtered loads that are reabsorbed by the entire tubular system; the observed decrease would simply have to occur beyond the proximal convolutions. Nor is it self-contradictory to say that the greatest amount of phosphate that can be reabsorbed by a diseased kidney (Tm_{Phos}) is reduced in approximate proportion to the decrease in GFR of that kidney, yet external balance for phosphate is maintained by reducing the fraction of the filtered phosphate that the kidney reabsorbs (see Answer to Problem 1-1 and Fig. 1-A). It is important to keep these distinctions in mind as we proceed. In either context — that is, with respect to either glomerulotubular balance or external balance — the nephrons can be said to have adapted.

Uremia

The development of uremia and some of the influences of this state can be demonstrated in a model of unilateral chronic renal disease that was devised by N. S. Bricker and his colleagues; some aspects pertaining to the GFR and the renal excretion of NH_4^+ during metabolic acidosis in a dog are illustrated in Figure 10-3. As a preliminary procedure, two hemibladders are created surgically so urine can be collected from each kidney separately; stage I represents this state. The GFRs for the control kidney and the experimental (at this stage, still healthy) kidney were 22.4 and 25.6 ml per minute, respectively, and the urinary excretion rates of NH_4^+ during experimentally induced metabolic acidosis were 23.0 and 29.1 μEq per minute, respectively. Pyelonephritis was then induced in the experimental kidney, creating a picture like that shown in Figure 10-1a, and about one month later, both kidneys were again studied during stage II. Although the GFR of the experimental kidney was reduced to 45 percent of its value in stage I, that of the healthy, control kidney had undergone a compensatory increase; consequently, the total GFR was still 82 percent of the value during stage I and uremia was prevented. Similar compensation occurred in regard to the excretion of NH_4^+. Although this rate was reduced in the diseased kidney, it was sufficiently increased in the healthy one so that, for roughly the same degree of acidosis, the total excretion of NH_4^+ was about equal to that in stage I. Note also that a kind of glomerulotubular balance — which, in this instance, was gauged as the rate of maximal tubular secretion of NH_3

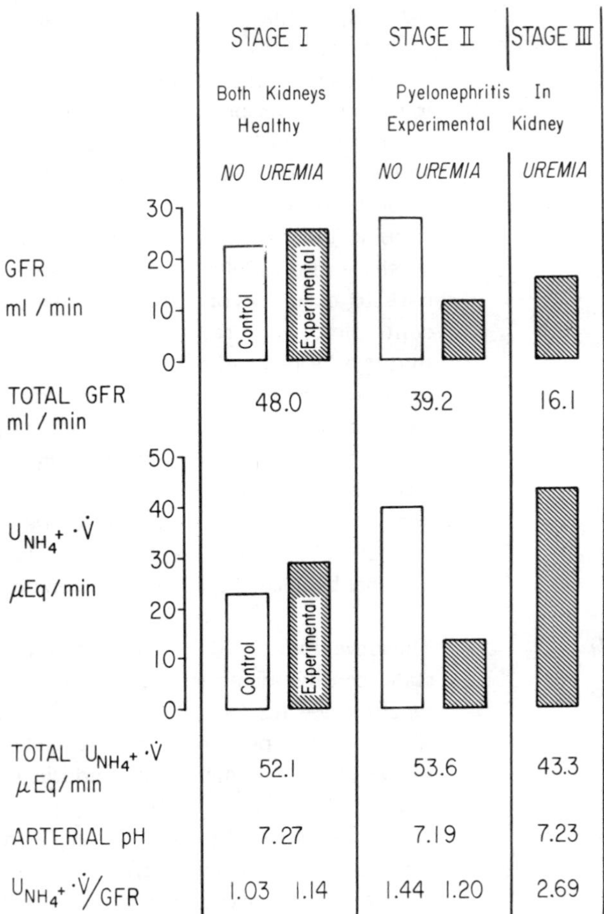

Figure 10-3
Development and influence of uremia during experimental, unilateral, chronic pyelonephritis in a dog (N. S. Bricker et al., *J. Clin. Invest.* 43:1915, 1964). The data for stage II were obtained about one month after the induction of pyelonephritis in the experimental kidney; those for stage III, five days after removal of the control kidney. Results are qualitatively similar after the induction of other types of renal disease (such as glomerulonephritis) or in predominantly unilateral pyelonephritis in man. Data from E. J. Dorhout Mees et al., *J. Clin. Invest.* 45:289, 1966.

per unit of glomerular filtrate, and reflected as $U_{NH_4^+} \cdot \dot{V}$/GFR — was maintained by the diseased kidney; the control kidney showed slight "tubular predominance" in the sense that the compensatory tubular production of NH_3 exceeded the compensatory increase in GFR.

Stage III represents the status five days after removal of the control kidney. Although there was some compensatory increase in the GFR of the diseased kidney, it was not sufficient to prevent uremia, because now the total GFR had been reduced to 34 percent of the value in stage I. Through as yet largely unknown mechanisms, the uremic environment increases the ability of the diseased kidney to produce NH_3, and the excretion of NH_4^+ by this kidney, again for a similar degree of acidosis, approached the normal value, although it was not sufficient to preserve H^+ balance. Tubular predominance, which is characteristic of a number of functions during chronic renal failure, was now prominent.

Figure 10-3 illustrates several important points. (1) Chronic renal disease and chronic renal failure are not necessarily synonymous. During stage II, there was chronic pyelonephritis in the experimental kidney. However, the animal was not in renal failure, not only because the number of functioning nephrons had been reduced by less than 60 percent of the healthy value (see Definitions, at the beginning of this chapter), but also because there had been a compensatory increase in the function of the remaining nephrons. (2) Chronic renal failure arises essentially from a *critical reduction in the number of nephrons,* not from damage to the nephrons. Thus, even diseased nephrons, such as the one shown in Figure 10-1b, increased their glomerular filtration rate and their production of NH_3 (stage III, Fig. 10-3, and Fig. 10-2a), but the uremic state of chronic renal failure did not set in until the number of nephrons was drastically reduced by removing one kidney. (3) The uremic environment somehow induces compensatory changes. It is unlikely that, during the five-day interval between stages II and III, there was much change either in the number of nephrons in the experimental kidney or in the degree of their pathological involvement. Yet, the total GFR for these nephrons and the rate at which they produced NH_3 — as well as most other functions that, although not shown in Figure 10-3, have been measured — were increased when uremia set in.

In most instances, it is not yet known what factors in the uremic environment induce the compensatory changes. As discussed below (see Handling of Water and Major Solutes), they may include increased levels of parathyroid hormone, an as yet hypothetical natriuretic hormone, uremic toxins such as guanidine, guanidinosuccinic acid, and methylguanidine (called "middle molecules" because of their intermediate molecular weight), as well as a number of other compounds that are retained in renal failure but have not yet been identified. Nor are the induced changes necessarily beneficial to the organism; they may work to its detriment, as the term "toxin" implies. For example, one aspect of the uremic environment, hyperparathyroidism, will compensate renal function for the preservation of phosphate balance, but it will simultaneously contribute to the undesirable consequence of renal osteodystrophy (see Trade-Off Hypothesis, under Phosphate, Calcium, and Bone, below).

Function per Nephron

Inasmuch as chronic renal failure results from a reduction in the number of nephrons, it becomes important for understanding the dynamics of this pathological state to be able to estimate the number of remaining nephrons. The best method – short of some statistical count postmortem, which obviously could not be done in vivo – is to equate the reduction in GFR with a proportional decrease in the number of nephrons. Thus, if a healthy individual with roughly 2 million nephrons in both kidneys had a GFR of 125 ml per minute, then we can estimate that in chronic renal failure when his GFR is 25 ml per minute, he has about 400,000 nephrons left. To the extent that the diseased kidney has undergone functional hypertrophy without the addition of nephrons (as in the transition from stage II to stage III in Figure 10-3), this method based on the GFR will slightly overestimate the number of nephrons. For practical purposes, however, the estimate is accurate enough, so when we express a given function per GFR (e.g., $U_{NH_4^+} \cdot \dot{V}$/GFR in Fig. 10-3), we can think of it as reflecting how that function is being carried out *on the average* by each nephron. It is also clear from this example that in chronic renal failure, we often have the situation where a function is reduced in its aggregate (e.g., GFR and $U_{NH_4^+} \cdot \dot{V}$ in stage III) but is increased by each remaining nephron.

Osmotic Diuresis per Nephron

An individual in chronic renal failure can remain in external balance for water and most key solutes of the extracellular fluid on a *normal diet* until the final stages of the disease. This was the case, for example, in the dog for which data are shown in Figure 10-3. Since this animal stayed in balance during stage III, when he had the same dietary intake as during stage I but only about one-third the number of nephrons, it follows that about three times more water and solute must have traversed and been excreted by each nephron during stage III than during stage I. This fact is illustrated more quantitatively in Table 10-2, which illustrates the status for a human patient in chronic renal failure.

In health, the hypothetical patient considered in Table 10-2 presumably had approximately 2 million nephrons, which excreted about 1 ml of water (i.e., of urine) per minute. Theoretically and on the average, therefore, the flow rate in the terminal portion of each nephron was 0.5 nanoliter (nl) per minute. (This value represents an oversimplification in that the terminal portion of the nephron – namely, the collecting duct – results

Table 10-2
Osmotic diuresis per nephron in chronic renal failure

	Healthy State	Diseased State
Number of nephrons	2,000,000	400,000
Water:		
Volume filtered by all nephrons (GFR)	100 ml/min	30 ml/min
Volume filtered per nephron (sGFR)	50 nl/min	75 nl/min
Volume excreted by all nephrons ($\dot{V}$)	1 ml/min	1 ml/min
Volume excreted per nephron	0.5 nl/min	2.5 nl/min
Fraction of filtered water reabsorbed	99%	96.7%
Sodium:		
Plasma concentration	140 mEq/L	140 mEq/L
Filtered load for all nephrons	14 mEq/min	4.2 mEq/min
Filtered load per nephron	7 nEq/min	10.5 nEq/min
Excreted by all nephrons	144 mEq/day	144 mEq/day
Excreted per nephron	72 nEq/day	360 nEq/day
Fraction of filtered load reabsorbed	99.3%	97.6%

from the confluence of several nephrons. The actual flow rate per collecting duct is therefore several times higher. The oversimplification, however, does not invalidate the argument as it applies to the flow rate of a single nephron through its distal tubule, nor as it applies to the flow rates of the collecting ducts in renal disease if these conduits are reduced in proportion to the reduction in the number of nephrons.) Let us say that in the diseased state, the number of functioning nephrons has been diminished to one-fifth of the normal complement, a situation fully compatible with balance on a normal diet. The output of urine is still 1 ml per minute, but it is now five times higher per nephron — that is, 2.5 nl per minute — than it was during health. In other words, in chronic renal failure, the inevitable consequence of maintaining external balance for water on a normal water intake is a diuresis in each functioning nephron.

If there has been a compensatory increase in the filtration rate of single glomeruli (sGFR), this effect will contribute to an increased rate of flow per nephron. This fact is also shown in Table 10-2. In the healthy state, with an assumed GFR of 100 ml per minute, the average filtration rate in each nephron will be 50 nl per minute. (This value may not be unreasonable for humans; it does not, of course, take into account the probability that in humans as in other animals, the superficial cortical nephrons may have a lower sGFR than the juxtamedullary nephrons.) In the hypothetical diseased state illustrated in Table 10-2, the number of nephrons was reduced by a factor of five. If there were no compensatory increase, the GFR *would* be approximately 20 ml per minute; with the increase, however, it might be 30 ml per minute, as shown in the table. The filtration rate per individual nephron (sGFR) in the diseased state might therefore be about 75 nl per minute. (A compensatory increase in the filtration rate of single nephrons can occur in diseases that affect primarily the glomerulus — see Fig. 10-2a — as well as in nonglomerular diseases; it is not yet known, however, whether there can be an increase in the *average* value in primary glomerular disorders.)

Table 10-2 illustrates another important consequence of external balance on a normal diet with a decreased number of nephrons: there is a reduction in the fractional reabsorption. In health, with 100 ml of water filtered per minute and 1 ml per minute excreted, 99 percent of the filtered water was reabsorbed; the same percentage would be calculated on the basis of the filtration and excretion rates of single nephrons. In disease, on the other hand, with 30 ml per minute filtered and 1 ml per minute excreted, the fraction of filtered water reabsorbed is reduced to 96.7 percent.

The same arguments and calculations that have been applied above to water balance also hold for sodium (Table 10-2). A normal intake of Na^+ is about 152 mEq per day (Fig. 7-5), and about 95 percent of this amount, or 144 mEq per day, will be excreted by the kidneys. By employing the oversimplification that was applied to the calculation for water, it can be calculated that each nephron in health excretes approximately 72 nanoequivalents (nEq) of Na^+ per day. In the balanced, diseased state on the same intake, the urinary excretion of Na^+ will be, by definition, 144 mEq per day, and the average excretion of Na^+ by each nephron will therefore be about 360 nEq per day, that is, an amount five times greater than in the healthy state. This increased excretion of solute per nephron is enhanced not only by other dissolved substances in the urine — such as chloride, potassium, phosphate (Fig. 1-A), and ammonium — but also by a maintained normal filtered load of those solutes (e.g., urea) whose plasma concentration increases as the number of nephrons declines (Table 8-2). Thus, in chronic renal failure, the increased flow of water in each nephron is accompanied by an increased flow of solute, and there is therefore an *osmotic diuresis per nephron.* (Despite the generalized increased flow of solutes in each nephron, however, the total excretion of each key solute is regulated with remarkable precision; this fact is discussed in greater detail later.)

As in the case of water, so for sodium it can be calculated that the amount of Na^+ filtered into each nephron rises during chronic renal failure and that balance for Na^+ on a normal diet can be maintained only by decreasing the fraction of the filtered Na^+ that is reabsorbed (Table 10-2).

Consequences of Osmotic Diuresis per Nephron. One of the most striking results of an osmotic diuresis – surprising, a priori, to most people – is a reduction in the ability to both concentrate and dilute the urine. This phenomenon can be demonstrated by infusing mannitol into a healthy individual (Fig. 10-4). The experiment is carried out by giving increasing amounts of mannitol; since this sugar, like inulin, is freely filtered but neither reabsorbed nor secreted (see Chap. 7, under Mannitol), its increased administration is accompanied by greater excretion, and this fact is reflected in the rising rate of solute excretion ($U_{Osm} \cdot \dot{V}$) shown on the abscissa in Figure 10-4. If mannitol is thus infused into an individual who is initially in antidiuresis – which is reflected in Figure 10-4 by a starting urine osmolality of 1,400 mOsm/kg H_2O – this osmolality falls exponentially, even though the plasma concentration of vasopressin remains maximal. (Maximal concentration can be assured not only because mannitol raises the plasma osmolality and hence stimulates the secretion

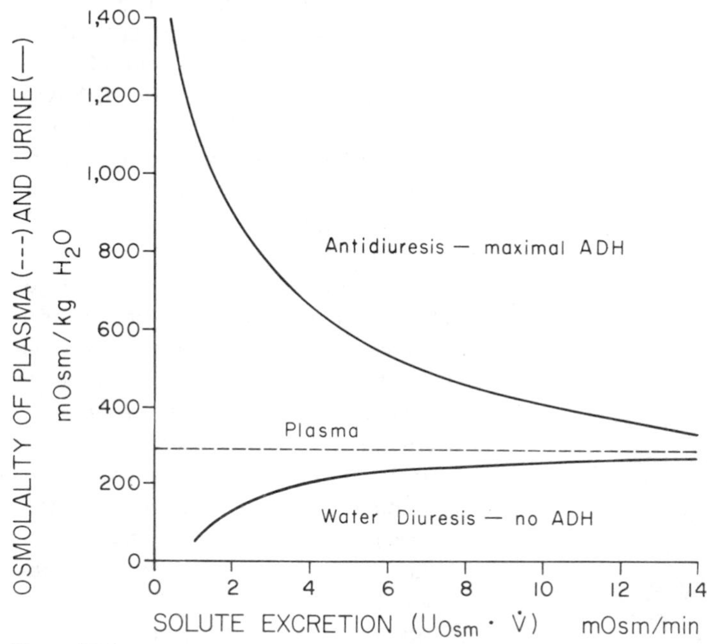

Figure 10-4
Effect of osmotic diuresis on the urine osmolality of a normal subject. These results can be obtained in humans or experimental animals through the intravenous infusion of mannitol or other solutes such as glucose, sucrose, xylose, or urea. *ADH* = antidiuretic hormone (vasopressin). Adapted from D. W. Seldin et al., in M. B. Strauss and L. G. Welt (eds.), *Diseases of the Kidney* (2nd ed.). Boston: Little, Brown, 1971, p. 218.

of endogenous vasopressin – see Figure 2-1b – but also by giving exogenous vasopressin along with the mannitol.) On the other hand, if the infusion of mannitol is begun when the individual is in water diuresis, the urine osmolality will rise as the rate of solute excretion increases, even though the plasma concentration of vasopressin remains nil. (The condition of zero concentration can be assured by running the trial in experimental animals or patients with complete hypothalamic diabetes insipidus.)

Mannitol and other diuretics diminish the ability to concentrate urine through mechanisms that were explained in Chapter 7. The ultimate basis for this effect is the reduction or elimination of the corticopapillary interstitial osmotic gradient, which itself probably has three causes during osmotic diuresis: (1) the inhibition of Na^+ (Cl^-) reabsorption from the ascending limbs of Henle (see Fig. 7-1, site 2), (2) the dilution of urea within the medullary collecting ducts and hence diminished deposition of urea in the inner medullary interstitium, and (3) increased reabsorption of water from the medullary collecting ducts as a result of increased delivery of water from more proximal segments. The diminished ability to dilute the urine in the absence of vasopressin probably results from the inhibition by mannitol of Na^+ (Cl^-) reabsorption from both the medullary and cortical diluting segments (see Fig. 7-1, sites 2 and 3, and Fig. 7-6).

The results shown in Figure 10-4 were obtained in normal subjects. They almost certainly pertain to chronic renal failure as well, although the extrapolation is probably oversimplified (see next paragraph). In both instances, there is an osmotic diuresis per nephron. In the healthy subject, an increased total osmotic load traverses a normal complement of nephrons; in the patient, a normal total osmotic load goes through a reduced number of nephrons. Thus, the results shown in Figure 10-4 explain two of the hallmarks of chronic renal failure: the excretion of a urine of relatively fixed specific gravity or osmolality – known as *isosthenuria* – and an *inflexibility* in handling either a dearth or an excess of water. It is clear from Figure 10-4 that the greater the rate of solute excretion, the more likely the urine osmolality is to be equal to that of plasma. An analogous situation occurs in chronic renal failure, because the greater the reduction in the number of nephrons, the greater the degree of osmotic diuresis per nephron. It is not surprising, therefore, that patients with advanced chronic renal failure excrete urine that tends to be fixed at a specific gravity of about 1.010, corresponding to an osmolality of about 300 mOsm/kg H_2O. (Hence the term *isosthenuria,* meaning a urine having the "same strength" as plasma.) The inflexibility of responding to an excess or lack of water follows from the isosthenuria. If a patient is unable to dilute the urine to a minimal value, he or she will not be able to excrete a water load as quickly as a normal person. Further, if the patient is unable to concentrate the urine maximally, he will take longer to adjust to a deficiency of water than the healthy person, and the patient may develop serious volume contraction during the period of adjustment. Thus, although chronically diseased kidneys can maintain balance, they are not nearly as flexible as normal kidneys in responding to perturbations of intake.

The above explanation, which is based on observations during osmotic diuresis in normal subjects (Fig. 10-4), is probably oversimplified, at least in regard to the deficiency in diluting the urine. Thus, in uremia, this deficiency depends not so much on the inability of each nephron to generate free water (C_{H_2O}/GFR), which value is nearly normal, but more so on the fact that there are not enough nephrons to produce a normal total amount of free water. To phrase the point differently, the inability to reduce urine osmolality to the minimal value in chronic renal failure is a function more of the reduction in number of nephrons than of osmotic diuresis.

Osmotic diuresis has a number of other consequences, among them an increase in the excretion of Na^+ (Table 7-1) that results from decreased tubular reabsorption (Fig. 7-6). Again, this effect, which is demonstrable in healthy kidneys, seems analogous to that of an osmotic diuresis per nephron in diseased kidneys, where Na^+ balance is maintained through decreased fractional reabsorption (Table 10-2). In fact, a number of years ago, R. Platt and his colleagues showed that many of the features of human chronic renal failure could be reproduced in rats merely by excising one kidney and part of the other, thereby causing an osmotic diuresis in the remaining, healthy nephrons. From these experiments, plus those of N. S. Bricker and his co-workers (Fig. 10-3) that showed the remarkable maintenance of balance by diseased kidneys, arose the proposal that in chronic renal failure, urine may be formed mainly by unaffected nephrons that are subjected to an osmotic diuresis as well as to other consequences of the reduction in the number of nephrons. Subsequently, however, it was demonstrated by micropuncture and microdissection techniques that even diseased nephrons not only produce urine but also maintain balance (Fig. 10-2c). The current view is, in a sense, an amalgamation of both theories: Although diseased nephrons continue to function and adapt in order to maintain balance, the key to the development of chronic renal failure is the loss of nephrons.

Handling of Water and Major Solutes

In conjunction with Table 10-2, we developed the concept that if balance for a given substance is to be maintained in the face of a reduction in the number of nephrons but with continued normal acquisition of the substance, then each nephron must excrete more of that substance. This rule would not hold if the substance could be eliminated by extrarenal routes, such as increased excretion by the gastrointestinal tract or increased catabolism by the liver. Although such accommodations do occur in chronic renal failure (e.g., for urea and K^+), the contribution of these mechanisms is never so large as to eliminate the necessity for a renal adjustment. The mechanism for the renal adaptation varies with the way in which a given substance is normally handled, that is, whether by filtration only (a mode that is approached by creatinine), or by filtration plus passive reabsorption (as is urea), or by filtration plus active reabsorption (as is phosphate), or by filtration plus secretion (as is K^+). We shall now consider how the handling of water and some major solutes is altered in chronic renal failure, not only by the kidneys but also by other organs.

Creatinine and Urea

The changes in the handling of these two compounds as the kidneys fail were described in detail in Chapter 8 (see Rate of Glomerular Filtration); this aspect will therefore only be summarized here. Even though small amounts of creatinine are secreted and even though roughly 50 percent of the filtered urea is reabsorbed, the rate of excretion of both compounds — and therefore their balance — depends on the rate at which they are filtered. Hence, as the GFR falls, the filtered loads of creatinine and urea (GFR $\cdot$ P_{Creat} and GFR $\cdot$ P_{Urea}) can be restored to normal only by allowing their plasma concentrations to rise. External balance for creatinine and urea is thus maintained during chronic renal failure, not by an intrinsic renal adaptation, but through a rise in their plasma concentrations. This mechanism for the restoration of balance is modified by several relatively minor factors, which are described next.

Influence of Osmotic Diuresis. Since urea is transported mainly passively in the mammalian nephron, its rate of reabsorption depends in part on its concentration within the tubular lumen. During osmotic diuresis, which exists in each nephron during chronic renal failure, the fraction of filtered water that is reabsorbed is decreased (Table 10-2); inasmuch as proximal glomerulotubular balance is maintained in most nephrons (Fig. 10-2c), the decrease in reabsorption must occur mainly in the more distal segments. With decreased fractional reabsorption of water, the intratubular concentration of urea will be lower than it would be in the nondiuretic state; hence the fraction of filtered urea that is reabsorbed is also decreased, and this effect tends to slightly lower the plasma concentration of urea at which external balance can be attained.

Similarly, an osmotic diuresis per nephron also tends to increase the tubular secretion of creatinine (possibly through a "sink" effect) and thereby also slightly lowers the plasma concentration of creatinine at which balance for this solute can be reached.

Changes in Metabolism. Both in healthy persons and in patients with chronic renal failure, urea – though a breakdown product of protein – can be reutilized for protein synthesis (Fig. 10-5). Through the mediation of bacterial enzymes, urea is hydrolyzed within the gastrointestinal tract. The resulting NH_3 is absorbed and carried via the portal circulation to the liver. There, keto-acid skeletons of amino acids are transaminated to form amino acids, which can then be utilized to form proteins. This process is accelerated in uremia, probably because the production of NH_3 within the gastrointestinal tract is increased. The process is also stimulated by dietary protein restriction, which is instituted in many or most patients with chronic renal failure. Insofar as the recycling of endogenous ammonia reflects an increased breakdown of urea, it also reflects a decrease in the net daily production of urea. This effect, then, may slightly decrease the amount of urea that needs to be excreted by the kidneys and hence decrease the degree to which the plasma concentration of urea must rise in order to restore balance.

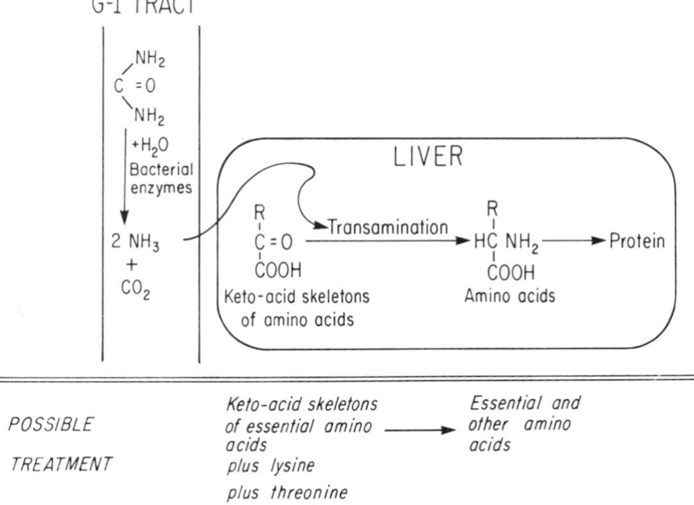

Figure 10-5
Recycling of endogenous ammonia. This process, which is accelerated in uremia and by protein depletion, *might* be utilized in the treatment of chronic renal failure by administering just two essential amino acids but otherwise providing keto-acid skeletons and no protein whatsoever. This possibility is currently under intensive investigation. *G-I* = gastrointestinal tract.

Analogous arguments apply to creatinine, since the daily production of creatinine may be lower in chronic renal failure than in health, possibly because of some muscle wasting.

The mechanism depicted in Figure 10-5 might be utilized for the treatment of chronic renal failure, and such possibilities are being explored. Natural proteins contain a number of substances that may be harmful in renal failure: for example, H^+, K^+, and phosphate (see below). It might be possible to eliminate dietary proteins altogether and to provide patients with just the two essential amino acids that cannot be biosynthesized by transamination, namely, lysine and threonine. The remaining essential amino acids can be produced by providing their keto-acid skeletons. Such a regimen, which was proposed several years ago independently by Giovannetti and Giordano and their respective colleagues, would have the dual benefit of promoting protein anabolism while reducing certain complications of renal failure, such as metabolic acidosis and bone disease (see below). Further trials and the development of palatable, protein-free diets are currently underway.

Water

The characteristics of water excretion in chronic renal failure – isosthenuria and inflexibility – were discussed above in conjunction with Figure 10-4. A few points will be expanded here.

Progressive Decrease in Fractional Reabsorption. In discussing Table 10-2, it was pointed out that on a normal water intake, external balance could be maintained only by decreasing the fraction of filtered water that is reabsorbed. This fraction must decrease progressively as more nephrons are lost. Let us say, for example, that in the diseased state cited in Table 10-2, the nephrons are further reduced to a total complement of 100,000. With one-twentieth of the normal number of nephrons, one would calculate a GFR of about 5 ml per minute, which, if there is a compensatory increase, might approximate 8 ml per minute. With a continued normal fluid intake and hence a continued urine flow of 1 ml per minute, the fraction of filtered water that is excreted would be 12 percent, and thus the fraction that is reabsorbed would be 88 percent. With a further reduction of the GFR to 4 ml per minute (a situation still compatible with life), the fractional reabsorption of water would have to decline to 75 percent.

Decreased Flexibility. The last example can also serve to amplify the concept of inflexibility. After drinking a liter of water, a healthy person can increase his urine flow to about 15 ml per minute. Obviously, a patient with severe chronic renal disease, having a GFR of 4 ml per minute, cannot respond as effectively to a water load. Even if he were to reabsorb none of the filtered water, the urine flow could not exceed 4 ml per minute. It therefore takes such a patient much longer than the healthy subject to excrete a water load, and in the meantime, having retained the water, the patient may develop dangerous hyponatremia. It is by virtue of this mechanism of water retention, as well as through that of urinary "sodium wasting," that renal failure is included as a cause of hyponatremia (Table 3-3).

Nocturia and Polyuria. Another numerical example will show that patients with advanced chronic renal failure must have some polyuria; this effect arises from the limitation on concentrating the urine. In order to stay in solute and water balance, a healthy subject may excrete 600 mOsmoles per day in 1 liter of urine; his average urine osmolality is therefore 600 mOsm/kg H_2O. If a patient in chronic renal failure ingests and produces the same amount of solute (namely, 600 mOsmoles per day) but is unable to concentrate his urine (i.e., has a urine osmolality that is "fixed" at 300 mOsm/kg H_2O), he will then have to increase his urine flow to 2 liters per day. He will therefore also have to increase his fluid intake slightly in order to stay in water balance. The obligatory, higher-than-normal urine flow also points up the importance of not depriving patients in chronic renal failure of water (e.g., before diagnostic tests), at least not in the same routine manner that is used with other patients. Such deprivation can lead to serious contraction of the body-fluid volumes and further reduction in the GFR.

Because the required increase in urine flow is relatively small, patients are often not aware of polyuria during the day. Nocturia, however, is a common symptom of chronic renal failure. It results not only from the mechanism described above, but also perhaps from a reversal in the diurnal rhythm.

Sodium

Progressive Decrease in Fractional Reabsorption. As was true for water, the chief mechanism for maintaining Na^+ balance on a normal intake is to decrease the fraction of the filtered Na^+ that is reabsorbed, which is called the *fractional reabsorption.* It was shown in Table 10-2 that with a decrease in the GFR from 100 ml per minute to 30 ml per minute, the fractional reabsorption of Na^+ had to decline from 99.3 percent of the filtered load to 97.6 percent if balance were to be maintained. As the GFR – and hence the filtered load of Na^+ – declines further, a progressively greater fraction of the filtered load escapes reabsorption. This fact is illustrated in Figure 10-6a, where a progressive decrease in fractional reabsorption in patients at various stages of chronic renal failure is reflected in an exponential rise of the fractional excretion, that is, of the fraction of the filtered load of Na^+ that is excreted.

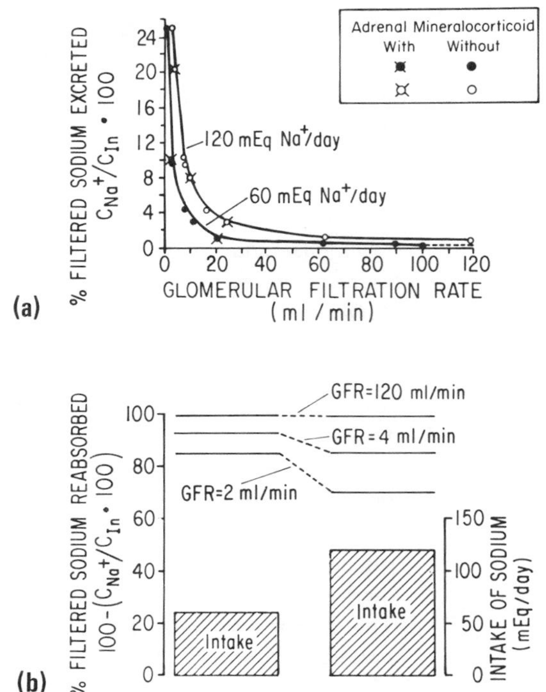

Figure 10-6
(a) Fraction of the filtered sodium that is excreted (called the "fractional sodium excretion") in healthy subjects with a normal GFR and in patients with varying degrees of chronic renal failure. Some patients had one or another form of glomerulonephritis, some pyelonephritis, and some polycystic disease. The subjects were tested in the steady state while on the relatively low sodium intake of 60 mEq per day and while on a normal intake of 120 mEq per day. Administration of high doses of adrenal mineralocorticoid did not alter the adaptive response; hence, a decrease in the plasma concentration of these steroids does not seem to be responsible for the reduced tubular reabsorption of sodium. Note that the fractional excretion required to maintain balance rises sharply as the GFR decreases and that the difference between the fractional excretions at the two rates of intake also rises exponentially. The last point is further illustrated in part (b). Redrawn from E. Slatopolsky et al., *J. Clin. Invest.* 47:521, 1968.

(b) The decrease in fractional reabsorption (slope of the dashed lines) required to maintain balance at the higher intake of sodium is greater the more severe the reduction in renal function. Adapted from N. S. Bricker, *Am. J. Med.* 46:1, 1969.

Figure 10-6 illustrates several other points. (1) A diminution in the plasma concentration of aldosterone is not responsible for the decreased tubular reabsorption of Na^+, for when high doses of mineralocorticoid were given to the patients, the points fell on the same curve as that for patients not given adrenal steroids (Fig. 10-6a). (2) Even in very severe chronic renal failure (i.e., even with a GFR as low as 2 ml per minute), patients can stay in Na^+ balance, whether the intake be normal (e.g., at 120 mEq per day) or moderately reduced (e.g., at 60 mEq per day). (3) The reduction in the fractional reabsorption of Na^+ that is required to stay in balance as the Na^+ intake is increased is greater as the degree of chronic renal failure becomes greater (Fig. 10-6b). Conversely, the augmentation of fractional reabsorption when the Na^+ intake is curtailed is greater, the more severe the renal failure. Thus, in Figure 10-6b, an almost imperceptible change of 0.25 percent in the fractional reabsorption is required for a healthy person with a GFR of 120 ml per minute to stay in balance as the Na^+ intake is changed from 60 mEq per day to 120 mEq per day, or vice versa. The same adjustment, however, requires a 7.5 percent change in the reabsorptive rate by a patient in severe chronic renal failure whose GFR is 4 ml per minute, or a 15 percent change if the GFR is 2 ml per minute. This fact is part of the reason why such patients, though they can stay in Na^+ balance, are less flexible in adjusting to sudden changes in Na^+ intake (see below).

Mechanism(s) for Decreased Reabsorption. These mechanisms are still not fully understood. The factors that normally adjust Na^+ balance – the sGFR, intrarenal shifts in the sGFR, the levels of aldosterone and natriuretic hormone, and Starling forces (Chap. 3) – are unlikely to provide the sole explanation. We have just cited, for example, the apparent lack of influence of aldosterone in modulating the fractional reabsorption of Na^+ (Fig. 10-6a). But even though the mechanism has not been identified, the kind of experimental evidence shown in Figure 10-7 suggests that the mechanism is precise and specific for Na^+.

The experiment was conducted on dogs in whom chronic renal failure was mimicked through inducing an increasing loss of nephrons, first by infarcting about 80 percent of one kidney (stage II, Fig. 10-7) and then by removing the opposite kidney (stage III). The stages are analogous to those shown in Figure 10-3, but in the experiment being described now, the two kidneys were not studied separately. Rather, two groups of animals were studied: in one, the intake of Na^+ remained normal at 120 mEq per day while the number of nephrons was diminished, and in the other, the Na^+ intake was reduced in exact proportion to

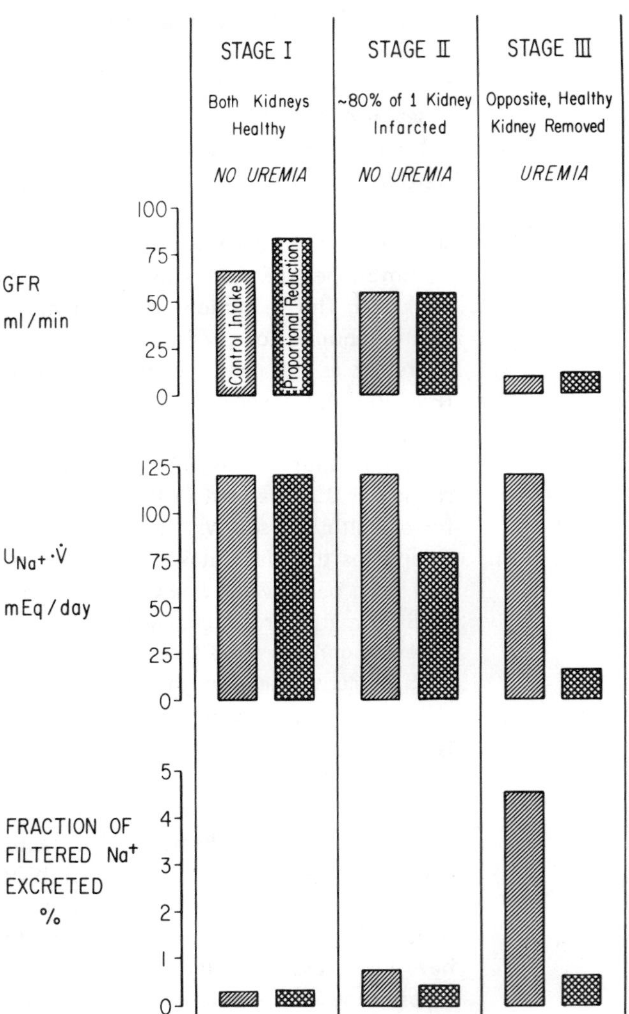

Figure 10-7
Renal handling of Na^+ in dogs in which chronic renal disease was mimicked by reducing the number of nephrons in one kidney through ligation of renal arteries (stage II) and subsequently by removing the other kidney (stage III). In this graph, the columns at each stage do *not* represent separate kidneys from the same animal. Rather, one group of dogs received the same amount of Na^+ through all three stages (shaded columns), while the other group received amounts of Na^+ that were reduced in proportion to the decrease in GFR (cross-hatched columns). All animals remained in external balance for Na^+. Maintenance of a normal Na^+ intake, as reflected by a constant excretion of Na^+ ($U_{Na^+} \cdot \dot{V}$), resulted in adaptive increases in the fractional excretion of Na^+; this adaptive response was obviated through reduction of the Na^+ intake. In these experiments there was evidence for the production of a natriuretic humoral substance in the dogs in which fractional excretion increased. Adapted from R. W. Schmidt et al., *J. Clin. Invest.* 53:1736, 1974.

the decrease in GFR. The main rationale of the study was that if the decreased fractional reabsorption of Na^+ that is seen in chronic renal failure is an adaptive mechanism to maintain balance and is specific for Na^+, then the phenomenon of decreased fractional reabsorption should not be seen in uremic dogs in which the need for an adaptive tubular mechanism has been obviated by maintaining balance through an adjustment of Na^+ intake. As can be seen in Figure 10-7, the prediction was fulfilled. All dogs were in Na^+ balance; hence, the rate of Na^+ excretion ($U_{Na^+} \cdot \dot{V}$) reflects the intake of Na^+. As the number of nephrons was reduced, the dogs who, like human patients, continued to eat a normal amount of Na^+, increased their fractional Na^+ excretion by decreasing its fractional reabsorption. In the animals that had decreased Na^+ intake, however, the fractional excretion — and hence the fractional reabsorption — did not change, even though their degree of renal failure was similar to that of the first group. (It should be cautioned at this point that reducing the Na^+ intake in patients with chronic renal failure is potentially hazardous. If the obligatory Na^+ excretion, which will be discussed below, is not covered by intake, then the patient's extracellular fluid volume will contract and a further decrease in the GFR may ensue. Most patients with advanced chronic renal failure require an intake of at least 20 mEq of Na^+ per day.)

In this experiment, there was also observed an increase in the plasma concentration of a humoral substance that increased fractional Na^+ excretion when injected into rats. Although this kind of evidence suggests that the endogenous production of a natriuretic hormone may be responsible for the fine adjustment of Na^+ reabsorption in chronic renal failure, final judgment on this point must await further experimental evidence.

Decreased Flexibility. Although patients in chronic renal failure (even severe failure) can remain in Na^+ balance on varying intakes of Na^+, the range of intake is much more restricted than in healthy persons, as is the ability to adjust to a sudden change of intake. For example, when Na^+ intake is restricted in a healthy individual, he can reduce the urinary excretion of Na^+ practically to zero; when he receives an excess of Na^+, he can promptly increase the urinary Na^+ excretion to well above 500 mEq per day. In contrast, once the GFR of a patient in chronic renal failure has dropped below 25 to 30 ml per minute, he may have an obligatory urinary Na^+ excretion of about 25 mEq per day, and he may not be able to excrete much more than 150 to 200 mEq of Na^+ per day.

All the reasons for a limit on the amount of Na^+ that can be excreted in chronic renal failure are not yet known. Obviously, the total number of nephrons remaining sets some limit. Thus, a patient with such severe loss of nephrons that his GFR is reduced to 2 ml per minute could *theoretically* excrete all the filtered load of Na^+, or up to about 400 mEq per day, if there were no tubular reabsorption of Na^+ whatsoever. That degree of inhibition does not, however, occur for Na^+ reabsorption. In the example shown in Figure 10-6b, a patient with a GFR of 2 ml per minute was able to stay in balance on an intake of 120 mEq of Na^+ per day by reducing the fractional reabsorption to 70 percent. There is a limit to the reduction, however, which is somewhere around 50 percent of the filtered load when the GFR is 2 ml per minute. The maximum that such a patient could excrete is therefore around 200 mEq per day. Thus, it is probably the reduction in the number of nephrons coupled with a limit to the inhibition of tubular reabsorption that sets the ceiling for Na^+ excretion. Accordingly, most patients in severe chronic renal failure are given about 35 to 70 mEq of Na^+ per day. It is not known why the fractional reabsorption cannot be inhibited beyond about 50 percent.

The reasons for an obligatory minimal excretion of Na^+ in chronic renal failure are better understood. One is the osmotic diuresis per nephron; it is known that a concomitant of osmotic diuresis is an increased excretion of Na^+ (Chap. 7 and Table 7-1). Another reason is that there is, in advanced renal failure, a rise in the plasma concentrations of phosphate and sulfate (see below) and hence a rise in the load of these solutes that is filtered into each nephron. These anions are not completely reabsorbed. Thus, as their filtered load is increased, so is their rate of excretion, and Na^+ is one of the cations that accompanies them. Finally, in chronic renal failure, there are regulatory influences that decrease the fractional reabsorption of Na^+ (Fig. 10-6). Whatever these influences may be — that is, whether they involve the production of a natriuretic hormone or something else — perhaps patients cannot quickly and sufficiently reduce urinary Na^+ excretion because, with the regulatory system "revved up" so to speak, the natriuretic influences continue at a high level even after the Na^+ intake has been curtailed. Because of the obligatory excretion of Na^+, most patients with advanced renal failure require an intake of at least 20 mEq of Na^+ per day.

Potassium

Increased Tubular Secretion. In striking contrast to acute renal failure where fatal hyperkalemia is one of the major problems of management (Chap. 9), the plasma concentration of K^+ stays normal in chronic renal failure despite a continuing normal intake of K^+. This fact and the means whereby the adaptation is accomplished are illustrated in Figure 10-8. The experimental

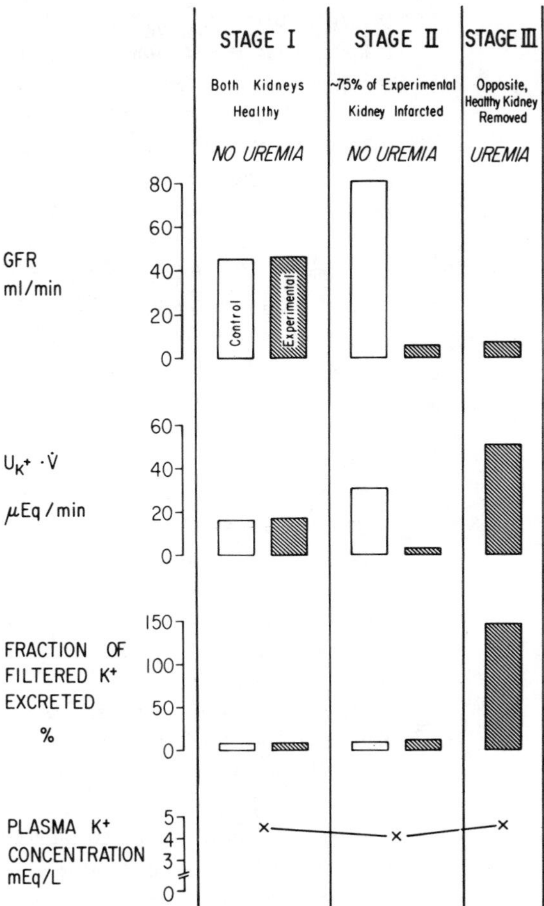

Figure 10-8
Maintenance of external balance for K^+ in a dog before and after experimental induction of chronic renal failure. The model is similar to that described in Figure 10-7, but in the experiment shown here, each kidney of the same animal was studied separately. For K^+, external balance is preserved on a constant intake by increasing the tubular secretion — and hence the urinary excretion — of K^+. The graph also emphasizes that during chronic renal failure (in contrast to acute renal failure), the plasma K^+ concentration remains normal. Adapted from R. G. Schultze et al., *J. Clin. Invest.* 50:1061, 1971.

model is the same as that described previously, that is, one in which chronic renal failure is mimicked by reducing the number of nephrons through the infarction of one kidney and the removal of the other. The stages are those described for Figures 10-3 and 10-7, and in the study under consideration, function was tested separately for the control and experimental kidneys.

In stage I, the two kidneys functioned more or less identically. After the loss of at least 75 percent of the nephrons in the experimental kidney (stage II), there was a compensatory increase in the GFR and the excretion of K^+ by the control kidney;

the total urinary excretion of K^+ was therefore the same as in stage I, balance was maintained, and the plasma K^+ concentration remained normal. At this stage, each kidney excreted approximately 10 percent of its filtered load of K^+.

The biggest challenge to K^+ balance occurred when the number of functioning nephrons was drastically reduced through the removal of the control kidney; the data graphed at stage III were obtained seven days after the nephrectomy. Even though only about 10 percent of the normal complement of nephrons remained during this stage, the urinary excretion of K^+ ($U_{K^+} \cdot \dot{V}$) was even greater than previously, and this adaptation was accomplished by converting net tubular reabsorption of K^+ (with 10 percent of the filtered load being excreted) to net tubular secretion (with more than 100 percent of the filtered load being excreted).

Note that the adaptive response for K^+ is not limited by the degree to which tubular reabsorption can be inhibited, as is the case for Na^+ (discussed above) or phosphate (see below and Fig. 1-A). Unlike these two substances, K^+ can be secreted, and both in a healthy person on a high-K^+ intake and in a patient with chronic renal failure, up to 3½ times more K^+ can be excreted than was filtered.

The factors that accelerate K^+ secretion during chronic renal failure are not known. In health, these factors (Chap. 4) include a high flow rate for Na^+ within the tubules, an increased plasma concentration of adrenal mineralocorticoids, an increased excretion of anions (e.g., sulfate and phosphate) to which the distal parts of the nephron are relatively impermeable, an increased flow rate of fluid within the tubules, and extracellular alkalosis. Although all but the last of these factors are or may be present in chronic renal failure, it can be shown that none is the sole or major stimulator of K^+ secretion in this disease state. For example, the urinary excretion of K^+ remained at a very high value during stage III (Fig. 10-8), even when the tubular flow rate of water and Na^+ was decreased by constricting the renal artery. In fact, as was true for the regulation of Na^+ (Fig. 10-7), the urinary excretion of K^+ is so finely attuned to the needs for balance that it seems unlikely that any general change that accompanies chronic renal failure is the major modulator of K^+ excretion; it is more likely that an as-yet-unidentified factor(s) is responsible.

Increased Fecal Excretion. Very late in chronic renal disease – possibly at the point where adaptive K^+ secretion is at a maximum, that is, at about 350 percent of the filtered load when the GFR is about 4 ml per minute – there is an adaptive increase in the fecal excretion of K^+. Whereas in health about 10 percent of the daily intake of K^+ is excreted in the stool (Fig. 4-1), this value can exceed 50 percent of the daily intake during advanced chronic renal failure. The mechanism(s) for this gastrointestinal adaptation is not known. It occurs in the absence of diarrhea and appears to be specific for renal failure in that the K^+ content of the stool from uremic patients is greater than that of diarrheal stool, and the adaptive changes are reversed by renal transplantation.

Decreased Flexibility. In contrast to the situation in health when a surcharge of 100 to 200 mEq of K^+ can be excreted within hours, in chronic renal disease the plasma K^+ concentration may rise to dangerous levels when a load of K^+ is suddenly imposed. Such loads might arise from K^+ supplements given with diuretics, from an intercurrent illness (e.g., a febrile episode causing increased breakdown of tissue), or from transfusion of old blood in which hemolyzed erythrocytes have released K^+ into the plasma. Studies have not yet been done to ascertain whether the obligatory high rate of K^+ excretion would continue if a patient with chronic renal failure were suddenly deprived of K^+. This possibility seems likely, however, not only because the system for tubular secretion is already "revved up," but also because even in health the renal adjustment to a low K^+ intake is sluggish (Chap. 4).

Phosphate, Calcium, and Bone

Progressive Decrease in Fractional Reabsorption. The adjustments in the renal handling of phosphate during progressive chronic renal disease were described in the Answer to Problem 1-1. The illustration from that answer is reproduced here as Figure 10-9. In summary, during the early stages of chronic renal failure, external balance for phosphate is maintained by decreasing the fraction of the filtered phosphate that is reabsorbed. This adjustment is mediated by the parathyroid hormone (PTH) (see below; also Figs. 10-10 and 10-11). There is disagreement whether the hypothetical state of column (b) in Figure 10-9 occurs; some believe that it is this transient positive balance for phosphate – which causes short periods of hyperphosphatemia and consequent hypocalcemia – that stimulates the secretion of PTH. When renal disease has caused a loss of nephrons to the extent that the GFR has been decreased to about one-fifth of normal, the tubular reabsorption of phosphate cannot be reduced further. At this point (i.e., at a GFR of about 25 ml per minute in adults), the plasma phosphate concentration rises and external balance is maintained through an increase in the filtered load of phosphate.

Parathyroid Hormone (PTH). The role of PTH in modulating the fractional reabsorption of phosphate was neatly demonstrated

	HEALTH	RENAL DISEASE (Early)		RENAL DISEASE (Late)	
	(a) Steady State:	*(b) Hypothetical:*	*(c) Actual:*	*(d) Transient:*	*(e) New Steady State:*
	Balance	*Positive Balance*	*Balance*	*Positive Balance*	*Balance*
INTAKE OF PHOSPHATE (mMoles/Day)	20	20	20	20	20
GFR (L/Day)	180	90	90	10	10
PLASMA PHOSPHATE CONCENTRATION (mMoles/L)	1.2	1.2	1.2	1.2	2.2
FILTERED LOAD OF PHOSPHATE $GFR \cdot P_P$ (mMoles/Day)	216	108	108	12	22
PHOSPHATE REABSORBED (mMoles/Day) [Fractional Reabsorption]	196 [91%]	98 [91%]	88 [82%]	1 [10%]	2 [10%]
PHOSPHATE EXCRETED $\dot{V} \cdot U_P$ (mMoles/Day)	20	10	20	11	20
MECHANISM BY WHICH BALANCE IS ATTAINED			Decreased Fractional Reabsorption		Increased P_P and hence increased Filtered Load

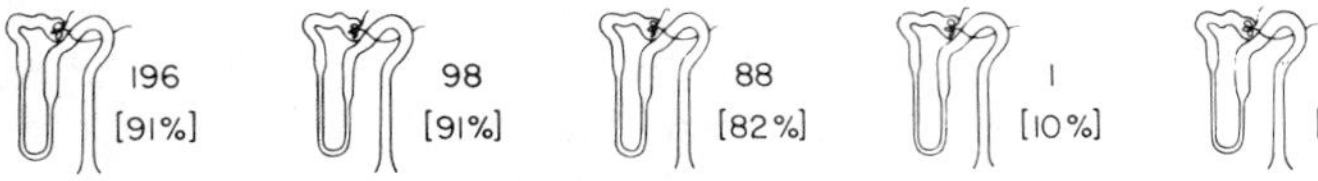

Figure 10-9
Dynamics involved in the maintenance of external balance for phosphate during chronic renal failure.

in the series of experiments shown in Figure 10-10. Although the experimental method for inducing the loss of nephrons was slightly different from those described for the experiments in connection with some of the previous figures, the three stages are analogous in that stage I represents the healthy state, stage II a moderate loss of nephrons without uremia, and stage III chronic renal failure with uremia. Two groups of dogs were tested; in one, the intake of phosphate remained constant throughout, and in the other, the phosphate intake was reduced in exact proportion to the decrease in GFR. In the first group, the adjustment shown in column (c) of Figure 10-9 occurred: There was a progressive decline in the fractional reabsorption of phosphate that was accompanied by a progressive rise in the plasma concentration of PTH. It was reasoned that if the increase in PTH resulted from the need to maintain phosphate balance through a PTH-mediated decrease in tubular reabsorption, then both the increase in the plasma concentration of PTH and the decrease in reabsorption should disappear if external balance is established instead by lowering the

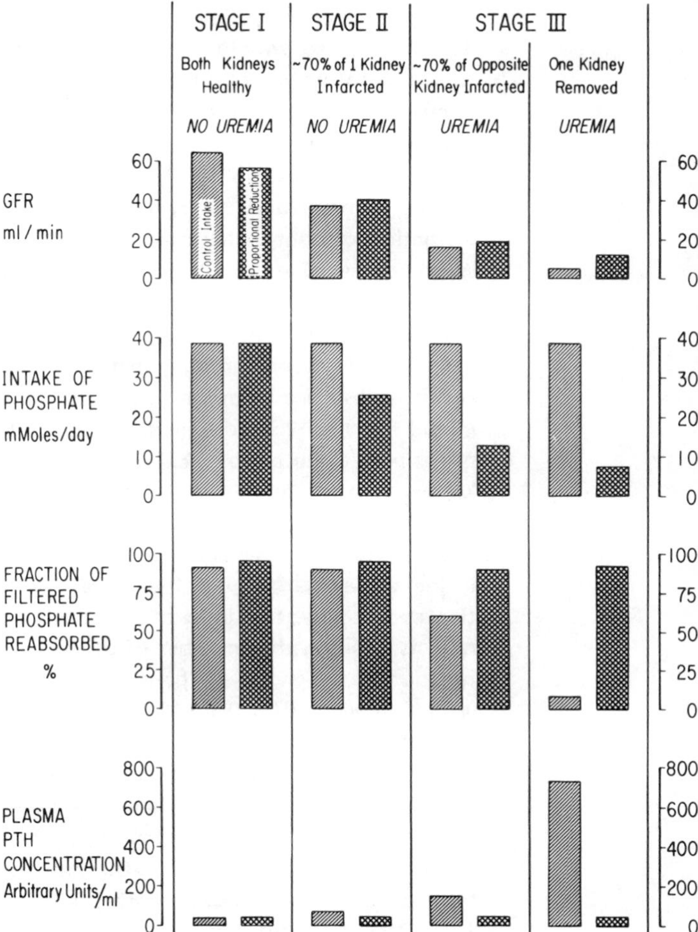

Figure 10-10
Renal handling of phosphate before and after experimental induction of chronic renal failure in dogs. In this graph, each set of columns represents different animals, not different kidneys. When the intake of phosphate was kept constant (shaded columns), a rise in the plasma concentration of parathyroid hormone (PTH) caused a progressive decline in the tubular reabsorption of phosphate. However, when external balance for phosphate was maintained by decreasing dietary phosphate in proportion to the decline in GFR (cross-hatched columns), the hormonal and tubular adjustments did not occur. Data from E. Slatopolsky et al., *J. Clin. Invest.* 50:492, 1971; E. Slatopolsky et al., *Kidney Int.* 2:147, 1972.

intake of phosphate. The fulfillment of these predictions (Fig. 10-10), coupled with the known effect of PTH in reducing the tubular reabsorption of phosphate (Fig. 10-11), leaves little doubt about the role of PTH in the renal handling of phosphate during chronic renal failure.

Renal Osteodystrophy, PTH, and Vitamin D. One of the serious complications of chronic renal failure is the defective formation of bone called osteodystrophy. This complication has several causes (Fig. 10-12), which can be better comprehended if the normal regulation and major actions of PTH and vitamin D_3 are understood (Fig. 10-11). Vitamin D_3 is derived from 7-dehydrocholesterol through ultraviolet irradiation of the skin, and it is absorbed from the gut. The vitamin is converted (mainly in the liver) to 25-hydroxyvitamin D_3 (25-OH-D_3), which does not appear to have biological effects of its own. The most active known form of vitamin D — namely, 1,25-dihydroxyvitamin D_3 or 1,25-$(OH)_2$-D_3) — is formed exclusively in the kidneys by the hydroxylation of 25-OH-D_3. Inasmuch as 1,25-$(OH)_2$-D_3 is made in the kidney but acts on other target tissues — namely, the intestine and bone — this form of vitamin D is truly a hormone and reflects, along with a number of other substances, the endocrine function of the kidneys. The renal production of 1,25-$(OH)_2$-D_3 is stimulated by PTH (Fig. 10-11), and this phenomenon serves as one of the links between the two compounds in regulating calcium balance. In the presence of hypocalcemia, the production of PTH by the parathyroid glands is accelerated. The resulting increase in the plasma concentration of PTH not only stimulates the production of 1,25-$(OH)_2$-D_3 but also the renal reabsorption of Ca^{2+}. An elevation of the plasma concentration of 1,25-$(OH)_2$-D_3 contributes to the pool of extracellular Ca^{2+} by enhancing the intestinal absorption of Ca^{2+} and, together with PTH, by increasing the mobilization of Ca^{2+} from bone.

During chronic renal failure, the rates of these normal mechanisms are altered (Fig. 10-12). The plasma concentration of PTH is chronically elevated (Fig. 10-10), and this change may have several causes. If, as some investigators believe, the hypothetical state of column (b) in Figure 10-9 results in transient periods of hyperphosphatemia and hypocalcemia, the latter will stimulate production of PTH as shown in Figure 10-11. In any case, late in renal failure when the plasma phosphate concentration rises (Fig. 10-9, column e), this mechanism almost certainly contributes to the hyperparathyroidism. The loss of renal tissue in chronic renal failure would be expected to result in decreased production of 1,25-$(OH)_2$-D_3, and this inhibition is abetted by hyperphosphatemia. Furthermore, during chronic renal failure, there is a relative resistance to vitamin D_3 that cannot be explained merely

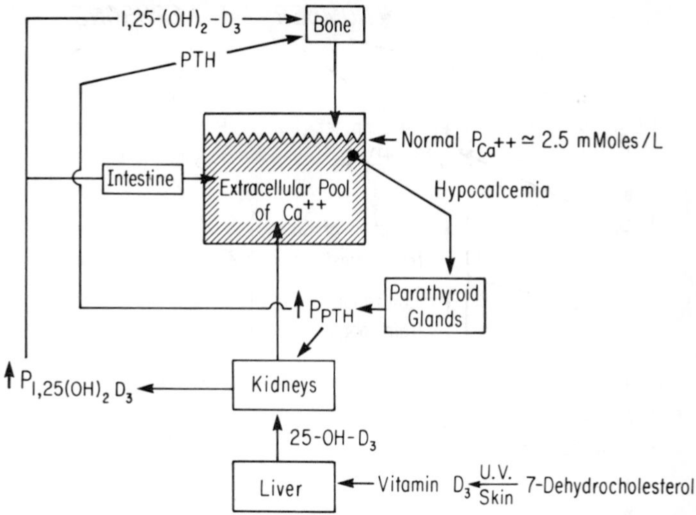

MAJOR ACTIONS

Parathyroid Hormone (PTH):

- ↓ renal reabsorption of phosphate (not shown above)
- ↑ renal reabsorption of Ca^{++}
- ↑ renal production of 1,25-(OH)$_2$-D$_3$
- mobilization of Ca^{++} from bone

1,25-dihydroxyvitamin D$_3$ (1,25-(OH)$_2$-D$_3$):

- ↑ intestinal absorption of Ca^{++} and phosphate
- ↑ mobilization of Ca^{++} and phosphate from bone
- may ↑ renal reabsorption of Ca^{++} and phosphate

Figure 10-11
Mechanisms that raise the pool of extracellular calcium in response to hypocalcemia. The chain of events, which involves most of the known actions of parathyroid hormone and 1,25-dihydroxyvitamin D$_3$, is described in the text. $P_{\ \ ++}$ = plasma calcium concentration; P_{PTH} = plasma concentration of parathyroid hormone; *25-OH-D$_3$* = 25-hydroxyvitamin D$_3$; *U.V.* = ultraviolet light; $P_{1,25(OH)_2D_3}$ = plasma concentration of 1,25-dihydroxyvitamin D$_3$. Modified from H. F. DeLuca, *J. Lab. Clin. Med.* 87:7, 1976.

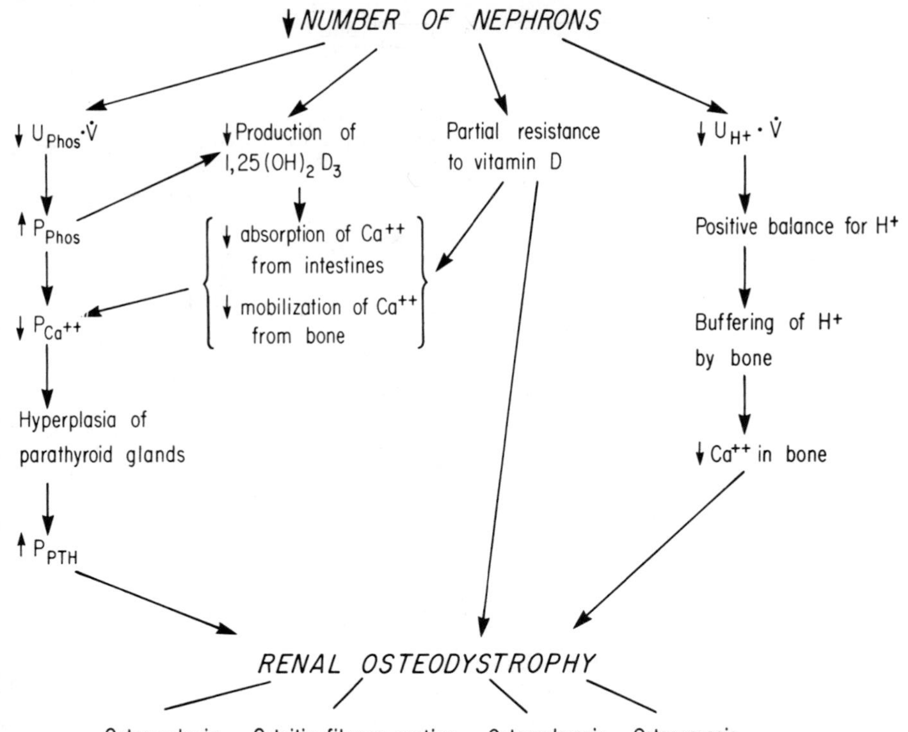

Figure 10-12
Possible pathways by which chronic renal failure leads to hyperparathyroidism and osteodystrophy. The various forms of defective bone formation may coexist in the same patient. $U_{Phos} \cdot \dot{V}$ and $U_{H^+} \cdot \dot{V}$ = urinary excretion of phosphate and hydrogen ions, respectively; P_{Phos}, $P_{Ca^{++}}$, and P_{PTH} = plasma concentrations of phosphate, calcium, and parathyroid hormone, respectively; $1,25(OH)_2D_3$ = 1,25-dihydroxyvitamin D_3. The figure is a composite of several diagrams from H. E. de Wardener, *The Kidney* (4th ed.). Edinburgh: Churchill/Livingstone, 1973, p. 186; C. R. Kleeman and O. S. Better, *Kidney Int.* 4:73, 1973; H. F. DeLuca, *Kidney Int.* 4:80, 1973; C. D. Arnaud, *Kidney Int.* 4:89, 1973.

by the decreased production of 1,25-$(OH)_2$-D_3. Both changes — that is, both the decreased production of 1,25-$(OH)_2$-D_3 and the relative resistance to it — probably contribute to diminished absorption of Ca^{2+} from the gut and to reduced mobilization of Ca^{2+} from bone. Thus, all the mechanisms shown in Figure 10-12 that lead to hyperparathyroidism seem to work through the common pathway of hypocalcemia. In addition to the elevation of plasma PTH, two other mechanisms may contribute to the osteodystrophy of chronic renal failure. One is the positive balance of H^+ (discussed below), which results in buffering by bone tissue and hence the loss of Ca^{2+} from bone. The other is the relative resistance to 1,25-$(OH)_2$-D_3, which, insofar as it applies to bone, may be responsible for some of the bone disease.

In chronic renal failure, several forms of osteodystrophy may be seen simultaneously in the same patient. Osteomalacia results from the defective mineralization of the osteoid matrix, osteitis fibrosa cystica ensues from prolonged decalcification, and osteosclerosis refers to a radiographic denseness in portions of certain bones, which may result from a redistribution of Ca^{2+} within bone. Osteoporosis, which denotes a rarefaction of bone, is seen less frequently than the other forms of bone disorders in chronic renal failure.

Treatment. On the basis of the scheme shown in Figure 10-12, one might infer that renal osteodystrophy would be treatable by preventing hyperphosphatemia or by giving 1,25-$(OH)_2$-D_3. Such measures have been and continue to be tried with some success. Gels that bind phosphate in the gut (and therefore prevent its absorption) may be combined with dietary phosphate restriction. From the results shown in Figure 10-10, one might conclude that merely restricting phosphate intake in proportion to the decrease in GFR might suffice. This possibility is being explored. That measure by itself, however, might not prevent hypocalcemia, since it would not correct the lack of 1,25-$(OH)_2$-D_3 or the partial resistance to it. Various forms of vitamin D — most notably a synthetic analogue, 1-α-hydroxycholecalciferol, that is converted in vivo to 1,25-$(OH)_2$-D_3 — are effective in some patients. Again, however, the problem is not so simple, since some patients (though not others) develop hypercalcemia when the 1-α analogue is given. Sometimes a more direct attack on the hyperparathyroidism is taken by administering Ca^{2+} supplements or excising parathyroid tissue. To date, patients have responded differently to varying regimes, which probably means that several different mechanisms can lead to renal osteodystrophy. It seems certain that more rational therapy, arising from further understanding of the causes of bone disease in chronic renal failure, will soon be available.

Trade-Off Hypothesis. The development of hyperparathyroidism in chronic renal failure, coupled with the kind of results shown in Figure 10-10, has prompted N. S. Bricker to propose the "trade-off hypothesis." The idea is that a price is exacted for the pleasure of eating a fairly normal diet in chronic renal failure. In the case of phosphate, balance *on a normal intake* can be maintained only through decreased renal tubular reabsorption, which entails hyperparathyroidism, and the price is thus osteodystrophy. The fact that the price might not have to be paid or might be much lower if the phosphate intake were curtailed (Fig. 10-10) has interesting therapeutic implications. It has been suggested that analogous trade-offs might apply to other substances: Is it possible, for example, that osteodystrophy is also the price of a normal protein diet, because some of the H^+ produced during the catabolism of protein must be buffered by bone (Fig. 10-12)? Or might the price for the decreased renal tubular reabsorption of Na^+ (Fig. 10-7) be the undesirable consequences of lessened Na^+ transport in other, extrarenal tissues?

Hydrogen Ion

Pattern in Chronic Renal Failure. Some typical features of H^+ balance during chronic renal failure are shown in Table 10-3. The following points should be noted: (1) When the GFR has been reduced to less than about 20 ml per minute, there is a mild metabolic acidosis characterized by a modest decrease in the plasma concentration of HCO_3^-. This acidosis is usually stable and becomes more severe only as further renal failure develops, either because of an acute, intercurrent episode or because of the progression of the basic disease. (2) The ability to acidify the urine (i.e., to reduce the urine pH) is preserved, even though the rate of H^+ excretion is reduced. (The distinction between acidification and H^+ excretion is discussed below.) (3) The total urinary excretion of H^+ is reduced, largely because of the renal disease but partly because patients in chronic renal failure often eat less protein than healthy persons, so their production of nonvolatile acids is decreased. (4) Despite the lesser excretion of H^+ and even though there is a positive external balance for H^+, the acidosis is stable unless deterioration of renal function occurs. (5) The proportional reduction in the excretion of H^+ as NH_4^+ is much greater than that of H^+ as titratable acid (T.A.). We will now attempt to explain these points in light of what is known about the renal regulation of acid-base balance in health.

Acidification and H^+ Excretion. The ability to reduce the pH of urine normally does not necessarily connote a capacity to excrete normal amounts of H^+. This fact is shown in Table 10-3, where in chronic renal failure, less H^+ was excreted even though

Table 10-3
Characteristics of H^+ balance in healthy persons and in patients with moderately severe chronic renal failure

State	GFR (ml/min)	Plasma $[HCO_3^-]$ (mMoles/L)	Urine pH	Urinary Excretion of H^+ (mMoles/day)		
				Total	As T.A.[a]	As NH_4^+
Healthy	120	28	6.17	56[b]	23	37
Chronic renal failure	14	19	5.99	33[b]	18	17

[a]T.A. = titratable acid.
[b]Total urinary excretion of H^+ = T.A. + NH_4^+ − HCO_3^-; hence, total excretion is slightly less than the sum of T.A. and NH_4^+.
Modified from D. P. Simpson, *Medicine* (Baltimore) 50:503, 1971.

the urine pH was actually slightly lower than in the healthy subjects. The point can be further amplified by the following considerations.

The kidneys handle H^+ by the three mechanisms shown in Figure 10-13: (a) the reabsorption of filtered HCO_3^-, (b) the excretion of titratable acid, and (c) the excretion of NH_4^+. To the extent that in the first reaction, the CO_2 that is formed within the tubular lumen diffuses into the cell to form more H^+, there is no *net* secretion of H^+; that is, reaction (a) is a mechanism for reclaiming filtered HCO_3^-, not for excreting H^+. Only through reactions (b) and (c) is H^+ excreted.

In the mild metabolic acidosis of chronic renal failure, the systemic arterial pH might be 7.33 (p. 139). If the plasma HCO_3^- concentration is 19 mMoles per liter (see Table 10-3), the arterial P_{CO_2} would be 38 mm Hg (Fig. 5-4). The P_{CO_2} of urine is usually the same as the arterial P_{CO_2}. Applying this value to the Henderson-Hasselbalch equation (Fig. 10-14a), it can be seen that the urine pH will be about 6.0 when the urinary concentration of HCO_3^- is 1.0 mMole per liter, but the urine pH will be about 5.0 when the urinary concentration of HCO_3^- is about 0.1 mMole per liter. These calculations show that the urine pH can be lowered almost to the minimal value merely by reabsorbing virtually all the filtered HCO_3^-. Since this process involves only mechanism (a), above, in which no *net* secretion of H^+ takes place (Fig. 10-13a), the calculations show that *theoretically,* the urine can be acidified to a minimal value without entailing the excretion of H^+. Actually, this situation does not occur, for as the pH of tubular fluid decreases from 7.33 in Bowman's space to 6.0 at the end of the collecting duct, HPO_4^{2-} is titrated to $H_2PO_4^-$ (Figs. 10-13b and 10-14b), and secreted NH_3 is converted to NH_4^+ (Figs. 10-13c and 10-14b). In both processes, H^+ is excreted. Despite the reactions shown in Figure 10-14b, however, *the amount of H^+ that is excreted will depend not so much on the urinary pH as on the amounts of phosphate and NH_3 that are present in the tubular fluid.* The ordinate of Figure 10-14b shows the amount of H^+ excreted per quantum of HPO_4^{2-} or NH_3 presented for titration; therefore, if, say, five times more HPO_4^{2-} or NH_3 were to traverse the tubular system, the amount of H^+ excreted would rise fivefold without any change in urinary pH.

Even though "urinary acidification" and "urinary excretion of H^+" are not synonymous, they are correlated. Figure 10-15c, which is based on experiments in normal man, shows that at any given rate of phosphate buffer excretion, the rate at which titratable acid is excreted is greater during metabolic acidosis than during normal acid-base status. The probable reason lies in physicochemical reactions. Progressive systemic metabolic acidosis is

TUBULAR LUMEN

PERITUBULAR FLUID

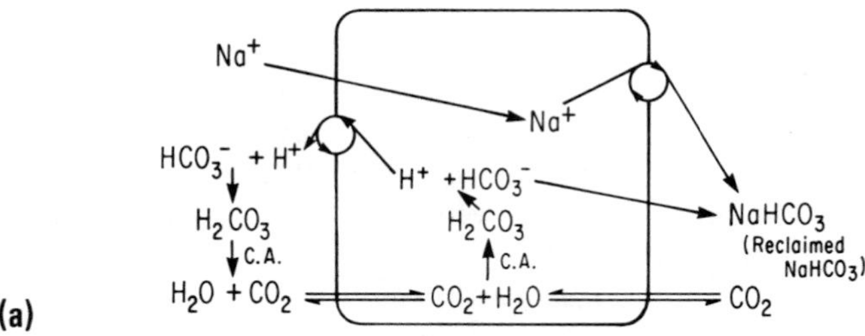

(a)

Na2HPO4
Na+
Na+
NaHPO4- + H+
H+ + HCO3-
H2CO3
C.A.
NaH2PO4 (T.A.)
CO2+H2O
NaHCO3
(New HCO3-)
CO2

(b)

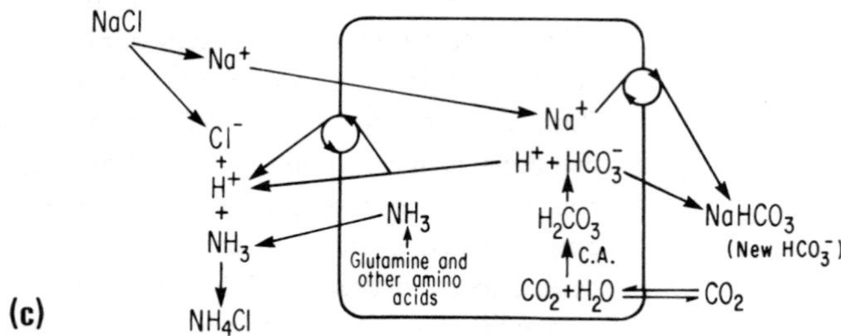

(c)

Figure 10-13
Three mechanisms through which the kidneys handle H^+.

(a) Reclamation of the HCO_3^- that is filtered; in this reaction, little if any H^+ is excreted.

(b) Formation of titratable acid (T.A.).

(c) Formation of NH_4^+.

C.A. = carbonic anhydrase. Modified from H. Valtin, *Renal Function: Mechanisms Preserving Fluid and Solute Balance in Health.* Boston: Little, Brown, 1973.

$$\text{urine pH} = 6.1 + \log\frac{[HCO_3^-]}{P_{CO_2}\cdot 0.03}$$

$$= 6.1 + \log\frac{1\text{mMole/L}}{1.14\text{mMoles/L}}$$

(a)

$$= 6.04$$

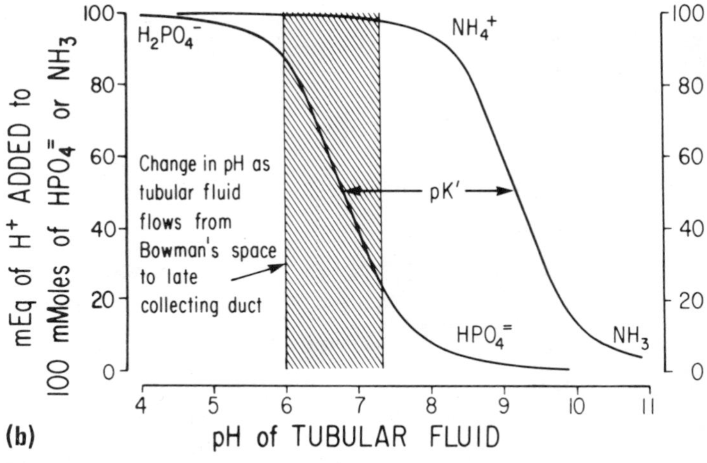

(b)

Figure 10-14
(a) Utilization of the Henderson-Hasselbalch equation to calculate urine pH when the urinary concentration of HCO_3^- is 1 mMole per liter and the P_{CO_2} in urine is 38 mm Hg.

(b) Titration of HPO_4^{2-} and of NH_3 by H^+ as the pH of tubular fluid is decreased from 7.33 in Bowman's space to 6.00 in the late collecting duct. With a p*K'* of about 9.2, the NH_3/NH_4^+ system is a relatively poor buffer in the pH range that ordinarily exists in tubular fluid (approximately the area covered by the shaded rectangle). Nevertheless, in health — although not in chronic renal failure — about two-thirds of total urinary H^+ is excreted as NH_4^+ because the supply of NH_3 is so plentiful.

usually accompanied by a progressive decrease in urinary pH. It can be calculated from the Henderson-Hasselbalch equation that at a urinary pH of 7.40, four times more of the main urinary buffer — phosphate — would exist in the form HPO_4^{2-} than in the form $H_2PO_4^-$ (Fig. 10-14b). As the urine pH is lowered to 6.40, this relationship is reversed, so that 2.5 times more of the phosphate would exist as $H_2PO_4^-$ (which represents H^+ excreted in the form of T.A.; Fig. 10-13b) than as HPO_4^{2-}; further, at a urine pH of 5.40, 25 times more would exist as T.A. (Fig. 10-14b). The sample calculation beneath Figure 10-15c shows that at a urine pH of 5.99 — which is typical of chronic renal failure (Table 10-3) — about 6.5 times more of the urinary phosphate would exist as T.A. than as the HPO_4^{2-} moiety of the buffer. Given a urinary phosphate excretion in chronic renal failure of 5

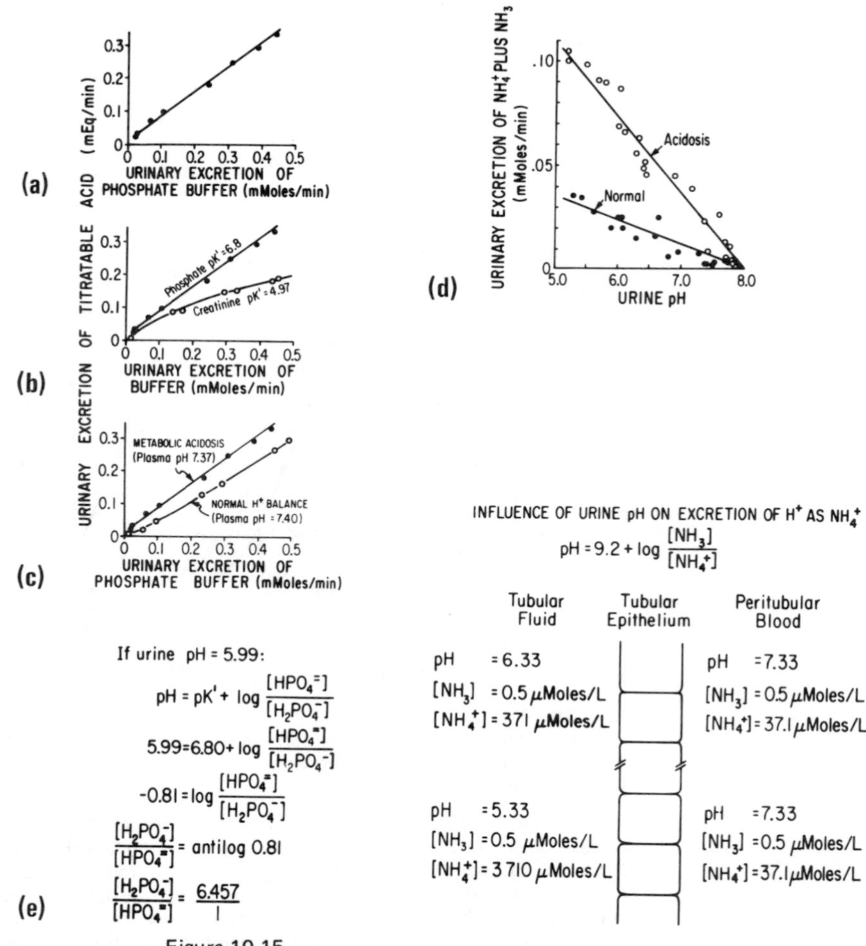

Figure 10-15
Factors that influence the rate of urinary excretion of titratable acid (*left*) and NH_4^+ (*right*).

Other things being equal, the excretion of T.A. rises (a) as more phosphate buffer traverses the tubules, (b) if the pK' of the buffer falls within the pH range of tubular fluid (see Fig. 10-14), and (c) if the urinary pH is lowered, as in metabolic acidosis. From H. Valtin, *Renal Function: Mechanisms Preserving Fluid and Solute Balance in Health.* Boston: Little, Brown, 1973.

(d) Again, other things being equal, the excretion of NH_4^+ rises if metabolic acidosis is present or as the urine pH falls. From R. F. Pitts, *Fed. Proc.* 7:418, 1948.

(e) The latter effect is explained by the phenomenon of nonionic diffusion. Possible reasons for a quantitative discrepancy between (d) and (e) are given in the text. Adapted from D. P. Simpson, *Medicine* (Baltimore) 50:503, 1971.

to 20 mMoles per day, the effect of urinary pH on H^+ excretion as T.A. may amount to only 1 or 2 mMoles of H^+ per day. Although this amount may seem trivial in light of a daily positive balance of about 20 mMoles of H^+ (Table 10-3), this effect may be meaningful over a period of years.

The influence of urinary pH on the excretion of H^+ in the form of NH_4^+ is shown in Figure 10-15d. Either during normal acid-base status or during metabolic acidosis, the urinary excretion of NH_4^+ is greater, the lower the urinary pH. The explanation for this fact lies in the phenomenon of nonionic diffusion, which is illustrated in Figure 10-15e; the slightly acidotic blood pH of 7.33 that is characteristic of chronic renal failure has been used for illustration. Of the two components of the ammonia/ammonium buffer system, the lipid-soluble NH_3 moves easily through epithelial cell membranes and is therefore thought to be in diffusional equilibrium between the urine and the blood. In contrast, transepithelial transport of the water-soluble ionized moiety, NH_4^+, is confined to the aqueous channels of the membranes, which makes the membranes highly impermeable to NH_4^+. As NH_3 is secreted into tubular fluid having a lower pH than peritubular blood, the NH_3 is titrated to NH_4^+ (Fig. 10-14b). By use of the Henderson-Hasselbalch equation, it can be calculated that at equilibrium and a tubular fluid pH or urinary pH of 6.33, the urinary concentration of NH_4^+ will be 10 times higher in the urine than in the blood, and at a urine pH of 5.33, it will be 100 times higher. Since the formation of NH_4^+ is one route by which the kidneys excrete H^+ (Fig. 10-13c), it follows that the greater the acidification of the urine (i.e., the lower the urine pH), the greater the excretion of H^+. (Note that the calculated rise for NH_4^+ in Figure 10-15e exceeds the measured increase as reflected in the slope for "acidosis" in Figure 10-15d. The exact reasons for this quantitative discrepancy are not yet known, but they may involve principally the following: (1) limitation of NH_3 synthesis during acidosis, possibly because of a relative deficiency of substrate; (2) failure of NH_3 to reach equilibrium as it diffuses from the peritubular blood into the tubular fluid; and (3) a decreased supply of blood – and hence of NH_3 – to the distal portions of the nephron where the tubular fluid pH is lowered to the minimal value.)

Titratable Acid (T.A.). The three factors that influence the rate at which T.A. is excreted in health are shown in Figure 10-15a–c; they are the amount of buffer that is available in the tubular fluid to accept H^+, the type (i.e., the pK') of these buffers, and the urinary pH. All three factors tend to be normal in chronic renal failure. Phosphate remains far and away the main urinary buffer, as it is in health. In connection with Figure 10-9, we described the dynamics by which the excretion of phosphate remains at or near the normal value during chronic renal disease; if the patient is on a low protein intake, the value will be somewhat reduced. Further, as shown in Table 10-3, the urinary pH tends to be nearly the same during chronic renal failure as in health. It follows that the excretion of T.A. should be normal or just slightly reduced in chronic renal failure, and this is indeed the case (Table 10-3). Inasmuch as the number of nephrons is greatly diminished, however, the rate of T.A. excretion per nephron is markedly increased, often by as much as fivefold.

Ammonium Ion. One possible explanation for the striking decrease in the urinary excretion of NH_4^+ during chronic renal failure (Table 10-3) is that damaged renal cells cannot generate NH_3 at a normal rate. The results illustrated in Figure 10-3 show, however, that this proposal is not correct, for during stage III the experimental, diseased kidney with a markedly reduced number of nephrons was able to excrete more NH_4^+ than when that same kidney was healthy. In fact, each remaining nephron excreted far more NH_4^+ during uremia than during health, as estimated by the value of $U_{NH_4^+} \cdot \dot{V}/GFR$. And before the onset of uremia during stage II, the value of $U_{NH_4^+} \cdot \dot{V}/GFR$ for the experimental kidney was about the same as it was in the same kidney before its number of nephrons was reduced.

The correct explanation for the decreased total NH_4^+ excretion during chronic renal failure lies, rather, in the loss of nephrons that produce NH_3 and in the decrease of total renal blood flow, which adds NH_3 to the renal pool of this substance. When the reduction in total functioning renal tissue has reached a critical point, the remaining renal cells cannot produce a normal amount of NH_3, even though this capacity per nephron has been greatly stimulated.

Most of the reasons for the stimulation of NH_3 production can be deduced from what we know about the regulation of renal NH_3 production during health. Two of the factors are shown in Figure 10-15d: urine pH and systemic acidosis. Inasmuch as the urine pH tends to be normal in chronic renal failure (Table 10-3), this influence cannot be invoked; in fact, this factor may limit, rather than increase, NH_3 production (see Decreased Flexibility, below). Acidosis, however, is an invariable concomitant of chronic renal failure, and it probably serves as a major stimulant; the mechanisms by which acidosis augments renal NH_3 production are not yet fully understood. A third influence has to do with the difference in pH between the tubular fluid and the peritubular blood. Because the NH_3/NH_4^+ system is subject to nonionic diffusion, the greater the difference in pH between the two fluids, the greater the rate at which the secreted NH_3 is carried off as NH_4^+ (Fig. 10-15e). The consequent larger sink for NH_3 thus increases the rate of NH_3 secretion. In chronic renal failure, the difference in pH between the tubular fluid and blood is usually smaller than in health, so this factor, if anything, tends to retard NH_3 production. The rate of peritubular blood flow may also influence the rate of tubular secretion of NH_3: Under the admittedly unusual circumstances when the urine and blood have the same pH, the greater the blood flow relative to the flow of tubular fluid, the greater the proportion of total NH_3 that diffuses into the blood sink, and hence the smaller the tubular secretion. Inasmuch as the renal blood flow is usually decreased less than the GFR in chronic renal failure, this effect would also tend to retard, rather than augment, renal NH_3 production, although the effect may be vitiated by the enhanced flow rate within each nephron (Table 10-2). Thus, acidosis provides the main explanation. Additionally, however, there is the influence of the uremic environment, which, as discussed in connection with Figure 10-3, raises the rate of renal NH_4^+ excretion even when systemic acidosis is no more severe than in health.

Buffering by Bone. The total excretion of H^+ is less in chronic renal failure than in health (Table 10-3), and this decrease is greater than can be accounted for by a possible reduction in dietary protein and hence a decrease in the production of nonvolatile acids. Patients in chronic renal failure are thus in positive external balance for H^+; nevertheless, they do not manifest progressive acidosis unless there is deterioration of renal function. The reason is that the extra H^+ is buffered by the apatite of bone. In the process, bone is depleted of Ca^{2+} (Fig. 10-12), most of which is excreted in the urine. This effect may contribute importantly to the development of renal osteodystrophy. It can be estimated that if bone buffers 15 mEq of H^+ per day — a not unreasonable estimate in chronic renal failure (Table 10-3) — nearly 50 percent of bone Ca^{2+} might be lost in about three years.

Decreased Flexibility. As chronic renal failure progresses, the various mechanisms reviewed above that prevent serious acidosis approach a maximum capacity. Ultimately, a point is reached when the maximum capacity is exceeded, either by dietary indiscretion that increases the daily production of acid or, much more commonly, by loss of functioning renal tissue to a critical degree. It can be shown, for example, that in some patients with far-advanced chronic renal disease, the production of NH_3 cannot be increased further by supplying additional glutamine as a substrate, as it can in healthy subjects or in patients with less severe renal failure. This failure to increase NH_3 production is probably the main explanation for decreased flexibility. Some nephrologists — though not others — believe that a defect in urinary acidification (see next paragraph) may play an additional role.

Having stressed up to this point that the urine pH tends to be normal in chronic renal failure, we must now seemingly retract that dictum. Whether or not a self-contradiction is involved depends on the meaning that we attach at any one time to the term "normal." If we consider the urinary pH of healthy adult humans eating ad libitum as "normal," then patients with chronic renal failure can acidify their urine normally (Table 10-3). If, however, we ask whether such patients can lower their urinary pH to a value of about 5.00 or less – a value that is seen in healthy adults when they are given a load of acid and ample phosphate buffer – then the answer appears to be no, and in that sense, the patients cannot be said to acidify their urine normally. Even though each nephron of a chronically diseased kidney handles a load of acid and phosphate that is similar to what the nephrons of healthy subjects handle when they are challenged with a load, most patients cannot reduce their urine pH below 6.00. As reviewed above, the influence of urinary pH on the excretion of T.A. and NH_4^+ is such that the inability of patients in chronic renal failure to achieve a minimal urinary pH limits their capacity to excrete H^+. Although this effect may be negligible for phosphate, it is probably not so for the excretion of NH_4^+ by nonionic diffusion.

The main cause for the acidifying defect may be a so-called bicarbonate leak; that is, there is less complete proximal tubular reabsorption of HCO_3^-, which leads to higher urinary concentrations of HCO_3^- in patients with chronic renal failure than in healthy persons (see Acidification and H^+ Excretion, above; also Chap. 12, under Renal Tubular Acidosis). The defect becomes most apparent when the plasma HCO_3^- concentration of patients with chronic renal failure is raised to the normal range. Under these circumstances, the fraction of filtered HCO_3^- that is excreted may rise from the healthy value of < 1 percent to as much as 20 percent. In turn, the cause for the leak is not yet known. If, as some believe, it is the result of increased fractional excretion of Na^+ (Fig. 10-7) or of hyperparathyroidism (Fig. 10-12), it would be another example of the trade-off hypothesis; in this instance, a diminished capacity to excrete H^+ would be the price exacted for the maintenance of Na^+ and phosphate balance.

Glucose

The dynamics for the renal handling of glucose, both in health and disease, can be tested through the glucose titration curve (Fig. 10-16). In this procedure, the filtered load of glucose ($GFR \cdot P_G$) is steadily increased by raising the plasma concentration of glucose, P_G, and the tubular system is titrated to determine the plasma concentration at which the "carrier" for glucose

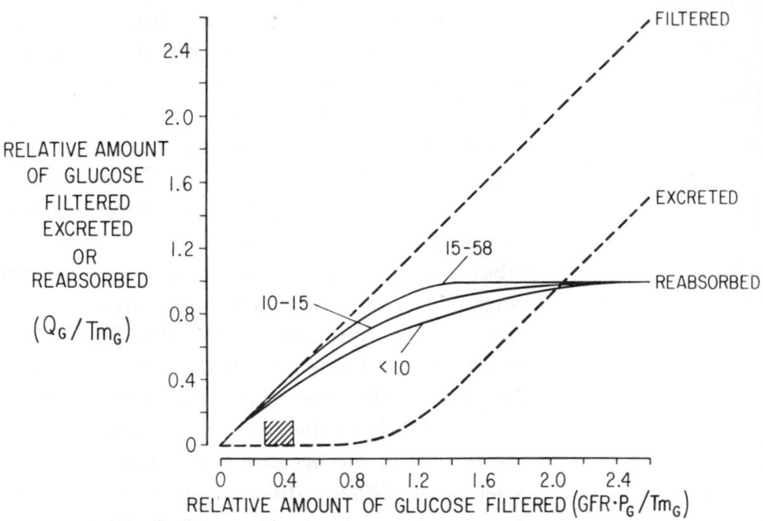

Figure 10-16
Glucose titration curves on 17 patients with some form of chronic glomerulonephritis or chronic pyelonephritis. The patients were divided into three groups: those whose GFR ranged from 15 to 58 ml per minute, those with a GFR of 10 to 15 ml per minute, and those whose GFR was less than 10 ml per minute. The increase in splay with advancing chronic renal failure is apparent. The variables have been expressed in relative amounts in order to permit comparison of data from different patients on the same scale. The shaded area spans the approximate range of GFR $\cdot$ P_G/Tm_G in health. Q_G = amount of glucose filtered, excreted, or reabsorbed; Tm_G = maximal amount of glucose reabsorbed per unit time; P_G = plasma concentration of glucose. Adapted from R. E. Rieselbach et al., *J. Clin. Invest.* 46:157, 1967.

becomes saturated and glucose is spilled in the urine. Normally, maximal reabsorption for glucose, Tm_G, is reached somewhat gradually, and the resultant curve shows what is known as *splay.* The splay is thought to reflect two variables: the affinity of the carrier for glucose and the degree of glomerulotubular balance for glucose.

Glucose titration curves on patients with varying degrees of renal failure due to either chronic glomerulonephritis or chronic pyelonephritis are shown in Figure 10-16. When the GFR ranged between 15 and 58 ml per minute, the degree of splay was almost identical to that of the curve for healthy individuals. In patients whose GFR was more curtailed, however, the degree of splay became increasingly marked. The curves explain why most patients with chronic renal failure do not spill glucose in the urine. In health and at a normal P_G of about 100 mg/100 ml, the balance between the amount of glucose that is presented to the proximal tubules for reabsorption (GFR $\cdot$ P_G) and the maximal capacity of these tubules to transport glucose (Tm_G) ranges between about 0.25 and 0.45. Under these conditions, glucose does not appear in the urine; glucosuria begins only after P_G has been raised to nearly 200 mg/100 ml, that is, when GFR $\cdot$ P_G/Tm_G has a value of about 0.8 (see dashed curve indicating excretion in Fig. 10-16). During progressive chronic renal failure when the P_G remains normal, the increasing splay extends into the normal range for GFR $\cdot$ P_G/Tm_G (Fig. 10-16), that is, into the range where at a normal P_G, the capacity of the tubules to reabsorb glucose just equals the amount of glucose that is presented to the tubules by filtration. Note that this encroachment on the normal range occurs only in far-advanced chronic renal failure when the GFR has been reduced by more than 85 percent. Only in this circumstance, and when the balance between the filtered load and Tm_G is exceeded, does glucose appear in the urine.

A slight shift to the right in the value for GFR $\cdot$ P_G/Tm_G also contributes to the occasional occurrence of glucosuria in chronic renal failure. When estimated per nephron, both the filtered load and the maximal rate of transport for glucose increase but the former increases proportionately slightly more than the latter; consequently, the ratio GFR $\cdot$ P_G/Tm_G rises slightly and the encroachment of the splay on the range where glucose is excreted in the urine may occur somewhat sooner than it would have, had the ratio stayed within the normal range.

There may be several reasons for the increased splay during chronic renal failure. One is competition by uremic toxins or other substances that accumulate in renal failure for the glucose sites on the carrier. This possibility is supported by the finding that in experiments of the types shown in Figures 10-3, 10-7, and 10-8, abnormal splay does not appear until stage III, that is, not until uremia has set in. A second reason may be a trade-off for the decreased fractional reabsorption of Na^+ (Fig. 10-7), for it has been shown experimentally that the reabsorption of glucose may be partly linked in some manner to the reabsorption of Na^+. Increased glomerulotubular imbalance for glucose is a third possibility, which, however, is rendered unlikely by the evidence provided in the types of animal experiments mentioned above. If such imbalance were to arise from the anatomical or functional changes of, say, pyelonephritis, then we would expect to see increased splay in the curves for the diseased kidney before as well as after the onset of uremia; however, increased splay is apparent only in the latter situation, that is, during stage III.

Other Substances

Because the kidneys regulate the balances for a very large number of solutes, this section on the renal handling of water and solutes could be extended considerably. Substances such as Mg^{2+}, uric acid, and protein come to mind. Their handling during chronic renal failure will not be considered in detail here, not necessarily because they are less important or because less is known about them, but because the *principles* by which their renal handling might be analyzed have been covered in the foregoing material. Armed with an understanding of this material, those who are interested can learn more about such other substances by consulting some of the references cited at the end of this chapter.

Nor will we consider further the changes in the renal handling of the various other compounds that may be responsible for many of the abnormalities that comprise the uremic syndrome. For example, the chronic anemia that is typical of chronic renal failure probably results partly from the decreased production of erythropoietin by the ever-diminishing renal tissue. Abnormal renal production of vasoactive compounds may play a role in the hypertension of chronic renal failure (Chap. 14). And both the central and peripheral neuropathy that are seen, as well as the involvement of many other organ systems, may be due at least in part to the accumulation of as-yet-unidentified uremic "toxins."

Treatment

Details about the management of patients in chronic renal failure can be found in a large number of standard treatises. In this chapter, we have restricted the discussion of treatment to those instances where a therapeutic principle could be deduced from an understanding of the pathogenesis. Examples that have been proposed but which are not yet necessarily in routine use include the curtailment of dietary proteins and the substitution of keto-acid skeletons of amino acids to alleviate the problems of H^+, K^+, sulfate, and phosphate balance; the reduction of phosphate intake in proportion to the decrease in GFR in order to prevent the undesirable consequences of hyperparathyroidism; the use of analogues of vitamin D_3, such as 1-α-hydroxycholecalciferol, to compensate for the lack of renal production of 1,25-$(OH)_2$-D_3; and the proportional reduction of Na^+ intake. It also follows from a recognition of the decreased flexibility in the handling of most substances, that any sudden or excessive change in the acquisition of water or solutes should be avoided, and the more advanced the renal failure, the less the latitude for altering intake.

Ultimately, the loss of nephrons is so great that even the most stringent dietary and other measures can no longer sustain life. At this point, many patients can be offered either chronic dialysis or transplantation. The principles of dialysis were discussed in Chapter 9 (Fig. 9-7). Chronic dialysis usually needs to be done three times a week, and the procedure takes about 6 hours; it can be carried out at home or in a dialysis center. Transplantations are performed using either closely related relatives or cadavers as donors. Details about both types of procedures can be found in numerous texts and monographs. Suffice it to sav here that although these measures are gratifyingly lifesaving, they do not assure a normal life span for many patients (Fig. 10-17), and they

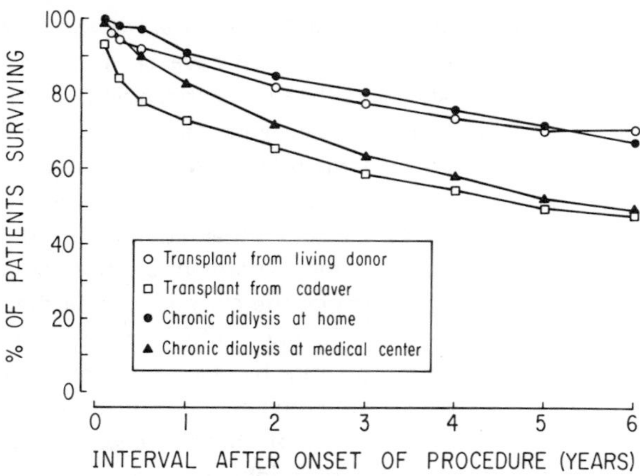

Figure 10-17
Survival of patients with chronic renal failure after they either have received a transplanted kidney or have been started on chronic dialysis. The lower survival of patients who are dialyzed at a medical center compared to those receiving dialysis at home probably reflects the better general condition of the latter group. Data from J. F. Moorhead (ed.), *Dialysis, Transplantation, Nephrology* 10:xxvii, 1973.

are not as simple as most people believe. Both procedures — even a highly successful transplantation — require constant medical vigilance, each entails its own numerous complications, and for many patients the quality of life is far from normal.

Summary

Because the kidney is the major regulatory organ for water and numerous solutes, chronic renal failure poses a serious challenge to external balance. The problem arises essentially from a loss of nephrons rather than from damage to the nephrons. The loss can be induced by a host of very different renal diseases (Table 10-1) that lead to a nearly proportional reduction in both glomerular and tubular function. The GFR declines in rough proportion to the loss of nephrons. Consequently, the GFR (or the plasma creatinine concentration or BUN) can be used to gauge the reduction in the number of nephrons; dividing the value of a given variable (e.g., Na^+ excretion) by the GFR will yield an estimate of that function per nephron.

Chronically diseased kidneys are characterized by a rather astounding concurrence of marked anatomical and functional heterogeneity among nephrons; and yet near-preservation of glomerulotubular balance and external balance for water and solutes is maintained. The term *adaptive nephrons* serves to emphasize this important feature of renal behavior during chronic renal failure.

Patients with even far-advanced chronic renal failure can stay in external balance on a *normal dietary intake.* So long as the balance continues to be regulated principally through urinary excretion, it follows that each nephron must excrete much more water and solute — often as much as 50 times more — during chronic renal failure than in health. The means whereby this feat is accomplished depend upon the mode in which the kidneys normally process a given substance. If the substance is handled by glomerular filtration only (e.g., creatinine) or by filtration and a relatively constant fractional reabsorption (e.g., urea), external balance is reestablished by a rise in the plasma concentration and a consequent increase in the filtered load. If the substance is filtered and reabsorbed (e.g., water, Na^+, or phosphate), an increase in its excretion per nephron is achieved by decreasing the fraction of its filtered load that is reabsorbed. In the case of glucose, which is also filtered and reabsorbed, the problem is different, since normally, virtually all the filtered glucose is reabsorbed. In that case, the Tm_G per nephron is preserved in chronic renal failure, so that, except in rare patients, the capacity of each nephron to reabsorb all the glucose that is filtered into it is maintained. If the substance is filtered and secreted, then external balance is reestablished (e.g., K^+) or approached (e.g., H^+) by increasing the rate at which each nephron secretes the substance. Finally, if a substance is produced by the kidney (e.g., NH_3), there may be an increase in its synthesis per nephron.

The fact that the renal adjustments occur simultaneously for numerous substances and precisely for each substance makes it likely that several different mechanisms are responsible for the adaptations. Such factors may include parathyroid hormone, the postulated natriuretic hormone, the uremic toxins or "middle molecules," and as-yet-unidentified compounds that may accumulate or be depleted in the uremic milieu. In addition, the renal handling of some substances is influenced by an osmotic diuresis per nephron, which is an invariable consequence of chronic renal failure. Finally, it seems likely that in at least some cases, balance for a given compound may be affected adversely by a trade-off; for example, the increased splay in the glucose titration curve as well as the HCO_3^- leak of chronic renal failure may be the undesirable consequences of the need for preserving Na^+ balance.

For some substances, the maintenance of external balance is aided by extrarenal routes. Thus, the production of urea may be decreased to the extent that hepatic protein synthesis, utilizing NH_3 derived from urea, is increased in uremia. Or the fecal excretion of K^+ may rise appreciably. Or, although the external balance for H^+ is not corrected by this mechanism, a drastic change in systemic pH is prevented through the buffering of H^+ by bone. Some of these extrarenal compensations probably come into play mainly when the initial renal adaption has been pressed to its limit. The tubular secretion of K^+, for example, probably cannot be increased beyond approximately 350 percent of the filtered load, and increased fecal excretion becomes evident at about this point. In other instances, however, an extrarenal mechanism is not available, and therefore further decreased flexibility or deleterious consequences may follow when the limits of renal adaptation for these substances are exceeded. Such a state is reached late in renal failure when the fractional reabsorption of Na^+ has been reduced to about 50 percent of the filtered load, or when the fractional reabsorption of phosphate has been reduced to 10 percent so that hyperphosphatemia, hyperparathyroidism, and renal osteodystrophy follow. The handling of H^+ is an exception in that the limits of renal adaptation for it are reached early in renal failure. This is the one substance, therefore, for which external balance is not maintained, and progressive, fatal acidosis is prevented only because the retained H^+ ions are buffered by bone.

Problem 10-1

The following clinical history, abstracted from the *New England Journal of Medicine* (290:793, 1974), was selected to illustrate some important aspects of chronic renal failure and to emphasize that measures such as dialysis and transplantation, which we tend to view as curative, bring their own problems. This patient's history is somewhat atypical, however, in that he was born with only one kidney and required a subtotal parathyroidectomy for persistent hypercalcemia. Lest we give an exaggerated impression of the poor quality of life in chronic renal failure, a more encouraging history is presented in Problem 10-2.

Renal disease was first diagnosed in this patient at age 12, when on routine examination he was discovered to have proteinuria; x-ray examination at that time showed that the right kidney was absent. At age 19, he was admitted to a hospital for treatment of pneumonia, and at that time his BUN was found to be 33 mg/100 ml (Table 10-4). The calyceal system of the left kidney was only indistinctly outlined by intravenous pyelography (I.V.P.). One year later, the patient was readmitted to the hospital because of abdominal pain. Although the cause of the pain was not determined, a repeat I.V.P. showed diminution of renal size, and the laboratory values shown in Table 10-4 were now found. By age 23, the patient was complaining of pruritus, fatigability, and continuing abdominal pain, and he was again hospitalized. The laboratory values reflected further deterioration of renal function and anemia. The patient's blood pressure was now 160/100 mm Hg. Eight months after this hospitalization, dialysis with an artificial kidney was begun, and two weeks later, the patient received a kidney from a sibling. At the time of the transplantation, the

Table 10-4
Representative laboratory values for a patient with chronic pyelonephritis in his only kidney

Age (Years)	BUN/Creatinine (mg/100 ml)	C_{Creat}* (liters/24 hr)	Plasma Ca^{2+} (mg/100 ml)	Plasma Phos (P)* (mg/100 ml)	Hct* (%)
19	33/–	–	–	–	–
20	62/4.4	28	9.8	5.5	–
23	135/14.4	9	9.7	11.1	28
After transplantation:					
24	32/1.3	–	11.2	2.6	–
24½	–/1.3	–	11.6	2.3	–
26	10/1.2	–	–	–	–
28½	–	–	11.0	2.3	–
30	17/1.2	–	10.7	2.2	40
After subtotal parathyroidectomy:					
31	–/1.2	–	9.9	2.9	–

*C_{Creat} = clearance of endogenous creatinine; Phos (P) = phosphate phosphorus; Hct = hematocrit.

patient's left kidney was excised; it was small and, on microscopic examination, showed chronic pyelonephritis, nephrosclerosis, and severe nephrocalcinosis.

Following transplantation, renal function and blood pressure returned to normal, and the anemia was corrected without other specific treatment. Now, however, persistent hyperparathyroidism became a major problem. Hypercalcemia and hypophosphatemia persisted (Table 10-4). At about age 28½ years, the patient developed pain in both wrists, and x-rays revealed calcification of the radial arteries. He then developed further pruritus and epigastric distress that was relieved by antacids. He experienced episodes of dizziness, flushing, and sweating. Emotional problems of long standing appeared to be aggravated and were manifested by anxiety and hypomanic behavior. The serum concentration of PTH was at least twice the normal value.

Because of these continuing difficulties, a subtotal parathyroidectomy was performed at age 30 years. The results of physical and laboratory examination prior to operation were essentially unremarkable save for the hypercalcemia and hypophosphatemia (Table 10-4, Age 30). Four enlarged parathyroid glands were found at operation, and all but about 200 mg of one of these was removed. Microscopically, the glands revealed chief-cell hyperplasia, which is characteristic of either primary or secondary hyperparathyroidism. Within four days after the operation, the serum Ca^{2+} concentration had dropped to 8.8 mg/100 ml. The patient showed steady improvement with regard to the alleviation of the pain in his wrists, the dizzy spells, and especially his emotional status.

1. On the basis of the BUN and serum creatinine concentrations, what would you predict the patient's GFR to have been at ages 20 and 23 years? Are the creatinine clearances in accord with your predictions?
2. What would you estimate the patient's urinary excretion of urea and creatinine to have been at age 20 — about normal, less than normal, or greater than normal?
3. The plasma concentration of phosphate (reported as phosphorus) at age 20 was slightly high (see Table 1-1). Is this fact consistent with the degree of renal failure? About what fraction of the filtered load of phosphate was being reabsorbed at this time? Are you surprised that the serum Ca^{2+} concentration was well within the normal limits at this time?
4. Can you explain the development of persistent hypercalcemia after renal transplantation? (*Hint:* See Figure 10-11.)

Problem 10-2

The following history of a patient whom we have followed since 1966 is presented not as a problem but to illustrate the gratifying results that can be obtained through the measures of dialysis and transplantation.

The patient is the mother of six children, all delivered by cesarean section because of a small pelvic outlet. At age 30, during the seventh month of her last pregnancy, she developed a sore throat, which was followed one month later by gross hematuria and generalized edema. The baby was delivered during the eighth gestational month. Six weeks later, the patient developed a high fever and she passed urine of a reddish-brown tinge. On referral to a medical center, she was found to be mildly hypertensive (140/80 mm Hg), and her urine contained numerous red blood cells, some hyaline casts, and protein. She excreted 12.5 g of protein in 24 hours, and her BUN was 19 mg/100 ml. Chronic glomerulonephritis, possibly poststreptococcal, was diagnosed at that time.

For the next seven and a half years she was followed by her private physician. Her course was characterized by progressive hypertension, proteinuria, and renal failure. Headaches, nosebleeds, and anemia presented increasing problems. At age 37, she suddenly and rapidly became very much worse, and she was again referred to the medical center.

On admission, she was semiconscious and appeared moribund. Her blood pressure was 230/140 mm Hg, her pulse rate 120 per minute, and her temperature 38.6°C. In addition to her appearance, positive findings on physical examination included arteriolar narrowing and flame hemorrhages in the eyegrounds, as well as uremic pericarditis, which was reflected by a loud friction rub and heart failure. She was oliguric, passing about 200 ml of urine per day. Laboratory data showed a Hct of 26 percent, a BUN of 176 mg/100 ml, and the following serum concentrations: Na^+ 131 mEq per liter, K^+ 5.3 mEq per liter, Cl^- 96 mEq per liter, HCO_3^- 16 mEq per liter, phosphate (phosphorus) 11.9 mg/100 ml, Ca^{2+} 8.2 mg/100 ml, uric acid 12.2 mg/100 ml, and total protein 5.5 g/100 ml, with albumin and globulin concentrations of 2.9 and 2.6 g/100 ml, respectively.

Both of the patient's brothers immediately declared themselves eager to donate a kidney (although this possibility was not suggested to them by any physician). The patient was maintained on peritoneal dialysis for a period of two months while arrangements for transplantation were made. She was then transferred to another medical center where, after three further weeks of dialysis with an artificial kidney, the left kidney from one of her brothers was transplanted into the patient's right iliac fossa, and the ureter from the donated kidney was attached to the patient's bladder. The patient's own kidneys were removed at this operation. The postoperative course was characterized by an immediate return of normal urine flow and of normal blood pressure. The BUN concentration was 7 to 12 mg/100 ml, the serum creatinine concentration 0.6 to 0.8 mg/100 ml, and the endogenous creatinine clearance 75 to 115 ml per minute; all other laboratory values, including the Hct, became normal. Azathioprine (Imuran) and prednisone were given to combat the possibility of immunological rejection; the latter drug was gradually discontinued.

The patient returned home nearly five months after she became desperately ill. For about the first year, she was followed very closely, as often as twice a week, but then the visits became less frequent as the likelihood of immunological rejection diminished. Within about six months after the transplantation, the patient gradually resumed full activity, not only in looking after a large household and three chronically ill in-laws, but also in long and arduous hours of helping in the family grocery store.

Even though for at least nine years since the transplantation the patient has been considered to be a well person, her medical history during this period has not been that of a totally healthy woman in her 40s. Her medical records at the original medical center alone have gone into three more volumes since the transplantation. Every time she complained of fever, abdominal pain, bone pain, edema, or other symptoms and signs that might be lightly dismissed in another patient, the worry of a possible immunological rejection or reaction to a drug has arisen. She has had no less than ten hospital admissions since the transplantation was performed. Problems and procedures — the latter of which were performed by "conservative" physicians who ordinarily keep operations and other therapy to an absolute minimum — have included recurrent cystitis and acute pyelonephritis due to stricture of the transplanted ureter, cystoscopies and retrograde urography, cystoureteropyeloplasty for the stricture, arthritis (probably related to the drug treatment), recurrent abdominal pain and lymphedema of the right leg that required sigmoidoscopy and exploratory laparotomy, severe dermatitis and fever resulting from a reaction to an antibiotic, acquired renal tubular acidosis (see Chap. 12 and Problem 12-2), mild congestive heart failure of unknown cause that required treatment with diuretics and a low-salt diet, and a severe overdose with prednisone because of a mix-up in a pharmacist's instructions. Nevertheless, the patient has already enjoyed ten years of life that would have been denied her had dialysis and renal transplantation not been available, and it is possible that she will live a normal life span. When last tested (ten years after transplantation), her serum creatinine concentration was 1.9 mg/100 ml.

Selected References

General

Black, D. A. K. (ed.). *Renal Disease* (3rd ed.). Oxford, Eng.: Blackwell, 1972.

Brenner, B. M., and Rector, F. C., Jr. (eds.). *The Kidney.* Philadelphia: Saunders, 1976.

Bricker, N. S., Klahr, S., and Lubowitz, H. The Kidney in Chronic Renal Disease. In M. H. Maxwell and C. R. Kleeman (eds.), *Clinical Disorders of Fluid and Electrolyte Metabolism* (2nd ed.). New York: McGraw-Hill, 1972.

Bright, R. *Reports of Medical Cases, Selected with a View of Illustrating the Symptoms and Cure of Diseases by a Reference to Morbid Anatomy.* London: Longman, Rees, Orme, Brown, & Green, 1827.
In a sense, these reports might be considered the first published clinicopathological conferences. Certainly, Bright recognized the value of correlating post-mortem findings with the clinical history, for he wrote in his preface: "... it is more particularly my wish to preserve and explain by faithful Engravings the recent appearances of those morbid changes of structure which have been connected with the symptoms ...." Although Bright applied this approach to a wide range of diseases — including those of the lungs, intestines, and brain — the "reports" are most noted for elucidating diseases of the kidneys. The first section of volume I is devoted to "Diseased Kidney and Dropsy," and it is here that Bright presented the evidence that, in his opinion, linked certain instances of edema with renal disease, coagulable urine (shown by his associate, Dr. Bostock, to be due to protein in the urine), and hematuria.

de Wardener, H. E. *The Kidney. An Outline of Normal and Abnormal Structure and Function* (4th ed.). Edinburgh: Churchill/Livingstone, 1973.

Edelmann, C. M., Jr. (ed.). Pediatric nephrology. *Pediatr. Clin. North Am.* 18:347, 1971.
This volume contains, among others, articles on the pathophysiology and treatment of chronic renal failure in patients.

Edelmann, C. M., Jr. (ed.). *Pediatric Kidney Disease.* Boston: Little, Brown, 1978.

Erslev, A. J., and Shapiro, S. S. Hematologic Aspects of Renal Failure. In M. B. Strauss and L. G. Welt (eds.), *Diseases of the Kidney* (2nd ed.). Boston: Little, Brown, 1971.

Fried, W. Erythropoietin. *Arch. Intern. Med.* 131:929, 1973.

Giordano, C. (ed.). Uremia. *Kidney Int.* 7 [Suppl. 3] : S-267, 1975.

Gotch, F. A., and Krueger, K. K. (eds.). Adequacy of dialysis. *Kidney Int.* 7 [Suppl. 2] :S-1, 1975.

This volume covers not only dialysis but also other topics related to chronic renal failure: diet, renal osteodystrophy, hematological disorders, cardiovascular complications, and neurological abnormalities.

Lancet Editorial. Anaemia in chronic renal failure. *Lancet* 1:959, 1975.

Massry, S. G. (ed.). Symposium on kidney and hormones. *Nephron* 15:161, 1975.

Maxwell, M. H., and Kleeman, C. R. (eds.). *Clinical Disorders of Fluid and Electrolyte Metabolism* (2nd ed.). New York: McGraw-Hill, 1972.

Papper, S. *Clinical Nephrology* (2nd ed.). Boston: Little, Brown, 1978.

Raskin, N. H., and Fishman, R. A. Neurologic disorders in renal failure. *N. Engl. J. Med.* 294:143 and 204, 1976.

Ross, E. J. Chronic Renal Failure. In D. A. K. Black (ed.), *Renal Disease* (3rd ed.). Oxford, Eng.: Blackwell, 1972.

Schreiner, G. E., and Maher, J. F. *Uremia. Biochemistry, Pathogenesis and Treatment.* Springfield, Ill.: Thomas, 1961.

Schrier, R. W. (ed.). *Renal and Electrolyte Disorders.* Boston: Little, Brown, 1976.

Seldin, D. W., Carter, N. W., and Rector, F. C., Jr. Consequences of Renal Failure and Their Management. In M. B. Strauss and L. G. Welt (eds.), *Diseases of the Kidney* (2nd ed.). Boston: Little, Brown, 1971.

Strauss, M. B., and Welt, L. G. (eds.). *Diseases of the Kidney* (2nd ed.). Boston: Little, Brown, 1971.

Wills, M. R. *The Biochemical Consequences of Chronic Renal Failure.* Baltimore: University Park Press, 1971.

Anatomical and Functional Changes

Addis, T., and Oliver, J. *The Renal Lesion in Bright's Disease.* New York: Hoeber, 1931.

Allison, M. E. M., Wilson, C. B., and Gottschalk, C. W. Pathophysiology of experimental glomerulonephritis in rats. *J. Clin. Invest.* 53:1402, 1974.

Bank, N., and Aynedjian, H. S. Individual nephron function in experimental bilateral pyelonephritis. I. Glomerular filtration rate and proximal tubular sodium, potassium, and water reabsorption. *J. Lab. Clin. Med.* 68:713, 1966.

Bricker, N. S. On the meaning of the intact nephron hypothesis. *Am. J. Med.* 46:1, 1969.

Bricker, N. S. On the pathogenesis of the uremic state. An exposition of the "trade-off hypothesis." *N. Engl. J. Med.* 286:1093, 1972.

Bricker, N. S., Klahr, S., and Rieselbach, R. E. The functional adaptation of the diseased kidney. I. Glomerular filtration rate. *J. Clin. Invest.* 43:1915, 1964.

Edwards, B. R., Novakova, A., Sutton, R. A. L., and Dirks, J. H. Effects of acute urea infusion on proximal tubular reabsorption in the dog kidney. *Am. J. Physiol.* 224:73, 1973.

Gottschalk, C. W. Function of the chronically diseased kidney. The adaptive nephron. *Circ. Res.* 28 [Suppl. II] : II-1, 1971.

Gottschalk, C. W. (ed.). Jean Redman Oliver: A Festschrift. *Kidney Int.* 5:75, 1974.

This symposium honors Dr. Oliver, a life-long champion of the value and necessity for correlating function with structure, both in health and in disease.

Heptinstall, R. H. *Pathology of the Kidney* (2nd ed.). Boston: Little, Brown, 1974.

Kauker, M. L., Lassiter, W. E., and Gottschalk, C. W. Micropuncture study of effects of urea infusion on tubular reabsorption in the rat. *Am. J. Physiol.* 219:45, 1970.

Kramp, R. A., MacDowell, M., Gottschalk, C. W., and Oliver, J. R. A study by microdissection and micropuncture of the structure and the function of the kidneys and the nephrons of rats with chronic renal damage. *Kidney Int.* 5:147, 1974.

Lubowitz, H., Purkerson, M. L., Sugita, M., and Bricker, N. S. GFR per nephron and per kidney in chronically diseased (pyelonephritic) kidney of the rat. *Am. J. Physiol.* 217:853, 1969.

Oliver, J. R. *Architecture of the Kidney in Chronic Bright's Disease.* New York: Hoeber Med. Division, Harper & Row, 1939.

Platt, R. Renal failure. *Lancet* 1:1239, 1951.

Platt, R. Structural and functional adaptation in renal failure. *Br. Med. J.* 1:1313 and 1372, 1952.

Platt, R., Roscoe, M. H., and Smith, F. W. Experimental renal failure. *Clin. Sci.* 11:217, 1952.

Rapoport, S., Brodsky, W. A., West, C. D., and Mackler, B. Urinary flow and excretion of solutes during osmotic diuresis in hydropenic man. *Am. J. Physiol.* 156:433, 1949.

Rocha, A., Marcondes, M., and Malnic, G. Micropuncture study in rats with experimental glomerulonephritis. *Kidney Int.* 3:14, 1973.

Sawabu, N., Takazakura, E., Handa, A., Shinoda, A., Takada, A., and Takeuchi, J. Intrarenal vascular changes in experimental glomerulonephritis. *Kidney Int.* 1:89, 1972.

Wagnild, J. P., Gutmann, F. D., and Rieselbach, R. E. Functional characterization of chronic unilateral glomerulonephritis in the dog. *Kidney Int.* 5:422, 1974.

Wesson, L. G., Jr., and Anslow, W. P., Jr. Excretion of sodium and water during osmotic diuresis in the dog. *Am. J. Physiol.* 153:465, 1948.

Urea, Creatinine, and Toxins

Clements, R. S., Jr., DeJesus, P. V., Jr., and Winegrad, A. I. Raised plasma-myoinositol levels in uraemia and experimental neuropathy. *Lancet* 1:1137, 1973.

Walser, M. Use of Isotopic Urea to Study the Distribution and Degradation of Urea in Man. In B. Schmidt-Nielsen (ed.), *Urea and the Kidney.* Amsterdam: Excerpta Medica Foundation, 1970.

Welt, L. G., Black, H. R., and Krueger, K. K. (eds.). Symposium on uremic toxins. *Arch. Intern. Med.* 126:773, 1970.

Wrong, O., Houghton, B. J., Richards, P., and Wilson, D. R. The Fate of Intestinal Urea in Normal Subjects and Patients with Uremia. In B. Schmidt-Nielsen (ed.), *Urea and the Kidney.* Amsterdam: Excerpta Medica Foundation, 1970.

Water

Adams, D. A., Kleeman, C. R., Bernstein, L. H., and Maxwell, M. H. An evaluation of maximal water diuresis in chronic renal disease. II. Effect of variations in sodium intake and excretion. *J. Lab. Clin. Med.* 58:185, 1961.

Bank, N., and Aynedjian, H. S. Individual nephron function in experimental bilateral pyelonephritis. II. Distal tubular sodium and water reabsorption and the concentrating defect. *J. Lab. Clin. Med.* 68:728, 1966.

Dorhout Mees, E. J. Role of osmotic diuresis in impairment of concentrating ability in renal disease. *Br. Med. J.* 1:1156, 1959.

Goldberg, M., and Ramirez, M. A. Effects of saline and mannitol diuresis on the renal concentrating mechanism in dogs: Alterations in renal tissue solutes and water. *Clin. Sci.* 32:475, 1967.

Kleeman, C. R., Adams, D. A., and Maxwell, M. H. An evaluation of maximal water diuresis in chronic renal disease: I. Normal solute intake. *J. Lab. Clin. Med.* 58:169, 1961.

Malvin, R. L., and Wilde, W. S. Washout of renal countercurrent Na^+ gradient by osmotic diuresis. *Am. J. Physiol.* 197:177, 1959.

Tannen, R. L., Regal, E. M., Dunn, M. J., and Schrier, R. W. Vasopressin-resistant hyposthenuria in advanced chronic renal disease. *N. Engl. J. Med.* 280:1135, 1969.

Sodium

Allison, M. E. M., Wilson, C. B., and Gottschalk, C. W. Pathophysiology of experimental glomerulonephritis in rats. *J. Clin. Invest.* 53:1402, 1974.

Bank, N., and Aynedjian, H. S. Individual nephron function in experimental bilateral pyelonephritis. I. Glomerular filtration rate and proximal tubular sodium, potassium, and water reabsorption. *J. Lab. Clin. Med.* 68:713, 1966.

Bricker, N. S. Adaptations in chronic uremia: Pathophysiologic "trade-offs." *Hosp. Pract.* 9(7):119, 1974.

Bricker, N. S., Klahr, S., and Lubowitz, H. The Kidney in Chronic Renal Disease. In M. H. Maxwell and C. R. Kleeman (eds.), *Clinical Disorders of Fluid and Electrolyte Metabolism* (2nd ed.). New York: McGraw-Hill, 1972.

Bricker, N. S., Schmidt, R. W., Weber, H., and Bourgoignie, J. The Modulation of Sodium Excretion in Chronic Renal Disease; the Possible Role of a Natriuretic Hormone. In A. F. Lant and G. M. Wilson (eds.), *Modern Diuretic Therapy in the Treatment of Cardiovascular and Renal Disease.* Amsterdam: Excerpta Medica Foundation, 1973.

Danovitch, G. M., Bourgoignie, J., and Bricker, N. S. Reversibility of the "salt-losing" tendency of chronic renal failure. *N. Engl. J. Med.* 296:14, 1977.

Edwards, B. R., Novakova, A., Sutton, R. A. L., and Dirks, J. H. Effects of acute urea infusion on proximal tubular reabsorption in the dog kidney. *Am. J. Physiol.* 224:73, 1973.

Klahr, S., and Rodriguez, H. J. Natriuretic hormone. *Nephron* 15:387, 1975.

Kleeman, C. R., Okun, R., and Heller, R. J. The renal regulation of sodium and potassium in patients with chronic renal failure (CRF) and the effect of diuretics on the excretion of these ions. *Ann. N.Y. Acad. Sci.* 139:520, 1966.

Platt, R. Sodium and potassium excretion in chronic renal failure. *Clin. Sci.* 9:367, 1950.

Platt, R., Roscoe, M. H., and Smith, F. W. Experimental renal failure. *Clin. Sci.* 11:217, 1952.

Schmidt, R. W., Bourgoignie, J. J., and Bricker, N. S. On the adaptation in sodium excretion in chronic uremia. The effects of "proportional reduction" of sodium intake. *J. Clin. Invest.* 53:1736, 1974.

Schrier, R. W., and Regal, E. M. Influence of aldosterone on sodium, water and potassium metabolism in chronic renal disease. *Kidney Int.* 1:156, 1972.

Slatopolsky, E., Elkan, I. O., Weerts, C., and Bricker, N. S. Studies on the characteristics of the control system governing sodium excretion in uremic man. *J. Clin. Invest.* 47:521, 1968.

Wesson, L. G., Jr., and Anslow, W. P., Jr. Excretion of sodium and water during osmotic diuresis in the dog. *Am. J. Physiol.* 153:465, 1948.

Potassium

Hayes, C. P., Jr., McLeod, M. E., and Robinson, R. R. An extrarenal mechanism for the maintenance of potassium balance in severe chronic renal failure. *Trans. Assoc. Am. Physicians* 80:207, 1967.

Platt, R. Sodium and potassium excretion in chronic renal failure. *Clin. Sci.* 9:367, 1950.

Schrier, R. W., and Regal, E. M. Influence of aldosterone on sodium, water and potassium metabolism in chronic renal disease. *Kidney Int.* 1:156, 1972.

Schultze, R. G., Taggart, D. D., Shapiro, H., Pennell, J. P., Caglar, S., and Bricker, N. S. On the adaptation in potassium excretion associated with nephron reduction in the dog. *J. Clin. Invest.* 50:1061, 1971.

Phosphate, Calcium, Parathyroid Hormone, and Vitamin D

Avioli, L. V. Vitamin D, the kidney and calcium homeostasis. *Kidney Int.* 2:241, 1972.

Avioli, L. V., and Teitelbaum, S. L. The Renal Osteodystrophies. In B. M. Brenner and F. C. Rector, Jr. (eds.), *The Kidney.* Philadelphia: Saunders, 1976.

Bone, J. M., Davison, A. M., and Robson, J. S. Role of dialysate calcium concentration in osteoporosis in patients on haemodialysis. *Lancet* 1:1047, 1972.

Brickman, A. S., Coburn, J. W., and Norman, A. W. Action of 1,25-dihydroxycholecalciferol, a potent, kidney-produced metabolite of vitamin D_3, in uremic man. *N. Engl. J. Med.* 287:891, 1972.

DeLuca, H. F. The kidney as an endocrine organ for the production of 1,25-dihydroxyvitamin D_3, a calcium-mobilizing hormone. *N. Engl. J. Med.* 289:359, 1973.

DeLuca, H. F. Recent advances in our understanding of the vitamin D endocrine system. *J. Lab. Clin. Med.* 87:7, 1976.

DeLuca, H. F., and Schnoes, H. K. Metabolism and mechanism of action of vitamin D. *Annu. Rev. Biochem.* 45:631, 1976.

de Wardener, H. E. Some Fresh Observations on Calcium and Phosphate Metabolism in Chronic Renal Failure. In I. Gilliland and J. Francis (eds.), *The Scientific Basis of Medicine Annual Reviews, 1972.* London: Athlone Press, 1972.

Eastwood, J. B., Harris, E., Stamp, T. C. B., and de Wardener, H. E. Vitamin D deficiency in the osteomalacia of chronic renal failure. *Lancet* 2:1209, 1976.

Fraser, D. R., and Kodicek, E. Unique biosynthesis by kidney of a biologically active vitamin D metabolite. *Nature* 228:764, 1970.

Galante, L., MacAuley, S., Colston, K., and MacIntyre, I. Effect of parathyroid extract on vitamin-D metabolism. *Lancet* 1:985, 1972.

Habener, J. F., and Schiller, A. L. Pathogenesis of renal osteodystrophy — A role for calcitonin? *N. Engl. J. Med.* 296:1112, 1977.

Henderson, R. G., Russell, R. G. G., Ledingham, J. G. G., Smith, R., Oliver, D. O., Walton, R. J., Small, D. G., Preston, C., Warner, G. T., and Norman, A. W. Effects of 1,25-dihydroxycholecalciferol on calcium absorption, muscle weakness, and bone disease in chronic renal failure. *Lancet* 1:379, 1974.

Kassirer, J. P. Hyperphosphatemia, hyperparathyroidism and bighead. *N. Engl. J. Med.* 289:1367, 1973.

Kaye, M., Frueh, A. J., and Silverman, M. A study of vertebral bone powder from patients with chronic renal failure. *J. Clin. Invest.* 49:442, 1970.

Kleeman, C. R. (ed.). Divalent ion metabolism and osteodystrophy in chronic renal failure. *Arch. Intern. Med.* 124:261, 1969.

Kodicek, E. The story of vitamin D. From vitamin to hormone. *Lancet* 1:325, 1974.

Massry, S. G. (ed.). Divalent ions in renal failure. *Kidney Int.* 4:71, 1973.

Massry, S. G., and Coburn, J. W. Renal Osteodystrophy. In M. H. Maxwell and C. R. Kleeman (eds.), *Clinical Disorders of Fluid and Electrolyte Metabolism* (2nd ed.). New York: McGraw-Hill, 1972.

Mawer, E. B., Backhouse, J., Taylor, C. M., Lumb, G. A., and Stanbury, S. W. Failure of formation of 1,25-dihydroxycholecalciferol in chronic renal insufficiency. *Lancet* 1:626, 1973.

Norman, A. W., and Henry, H. 1,25-Dihydroxycholecalciferol — a hormonally active form of vitamin D_3. *Recent Prog. Horm. Res.* 30:431, 1974.

Parker, T. F., Vergne-Marini, P., Hull, A. R., Pak, C. Y. C., and Fordtran, J. S. Jejunal absorption and secretion of calcium in patients with chronic renal disease on hemodialysis. *J. Clin. Invest.* 54:358, 1974.

Pellegrino, E. D., and Biltz, R. M. The composition of human bone in uremia. Observations on the reservoir functions of bone and demonstration of a labile fraction of bone carbonate. *Medicine* (Baltimore) 44:397, 1965.

Pierides, A. M., Ellis, H. A., Simpson, W., Dewar, J. H., Ward, M. K., and Kerr, D. N. S. Variable response to long-term 1α-hydroxycholecalciferol in haemodialysis osteodystrophy. *Lancet* 1:1092, 1976.

Raisz, L. G. A confusion of vitamin D's. *N. Engl. J. Med.* 287:926, 1972.

Raisz, L. G. Calcium, Phosphate, Magnesium, and Trace Elements. In M. H. Maxwell and C. R. Kleeman (eds.), *Clinical Disorders of Fluid and Electrolyte Metabolism* (2nd ed.). New York: McGraw-Hill, 1972.

Rasmussen, H., and Bordier, P. The cellular basis of metabolic bone disease. *N. Engl. J. Med.* 289:25, 1973.

Rasmussen, H., and Bordier, P. *The Physiological and Cellular Basis of Metabolic Bone Disease.* Baltimore: Williams & Wilkins, 1974.

Slatopolsky, E., Caglar, S., Gradowska, L., Canterbury, J., Reiss, E., and Bricker, N. S. On the prevention of secondary hyperparathyroidism in experimental chronic renal disease using "proportional reduction" of dietary phosphorus intake. *Kidney Int.* 2:147, 1972.

Slatopolsky, E., Robson, A. M., Elkan, I., and Bricker, N. S. Control of phosphate excretion in uremic man. *J. Clin. Invest.* 47:1865, 1968.

Hydrogen Ion

Goodman, A. D., Lemann, J., Jr., Lennon, E. J., and Relman, A. S. Production, excretion, and net balance of fixed acid in patients with renal acidosis. *J. Clin. Invest.* 44:495, 1965.

Henderson, L. J., and Palmer, W. W. On the several factors of acid excretion in nephritis. *J. Biol. Chem.* 21:37, 1915.

Lemann, J., Jr., Litzow, J. R., and Lennon, E. J. The effects of chronic acid loads in normal man: Further evidence for the participation of bone mineral in the defense against chronic metabolic acidosis. *J. Clin. Invest.* 45:1608, 1966.

Lubowitz, H., Purkerson, M. L., Rolf, D. B., Weisser, F., and Bricker, N. S. Effect of nephron loss on proximal tubular bicarbonate reabsorption in the rat. *Am. J. Physiol.* 220:457, 1971.

Mudge, G. H., Silva, P., and Stibitz, G. R. Renal excretion by non-ionic diffusion. The nature of the disequilibrium. *Med. Clin. North Am.* 49:681, 1975.

Pellegrino, E. D., and Biltz, R. M. The composition of human bone in uremia. Observations on the reservoir functions of bone and demonstration of a labile fraction of bone carbonate. *Medicine* (Baltimore) 44:397, 1965.

Relman, A. S. Renal acidosis and renal excretion of acid in health and disease. *Adv. Intern. Med.* 12:295, 1964.

Robinson, R. R., and Owen, E. E. Intrarenal distribution of ammonia during diuresis and antidiuresis. *Am. J. Physiol.* 208:1129, 1965.

Schwartz, W. B., Hall, P. W., III, Hays, R. M., and Relman, A. S. On the mechanism of acidosis in chronic renal disease. *J. Clin. Invest.* 38:39, 1959.

Simpson, D. P. Control of hydrogen ion homeostasis and renal acidosis. *Medicine* (Baltimore) 50:503, 1971.
A learned, concise exposition of H^+ balance, not only in health but also during chronic renal insufficiency.

Slatopolsky, E., Hoffstein, P., Purkerson, M., and Bricker, N. S. On the influence of extracellular fluid volume expansion and of uremia on bicarbonate reabsorption in man. *J. Clin. Invest.* 49:988, 1970.

Steinmetz, P. R., Eisinger, R. P., and Lowenstein, J. The excretion of acid in unilateral renal disease in man. *J. Clin. Invest.* 44:582, 1965.

Sullivan, L. P. Ammonium excretion during stopped flow: A hypothetical ammonium countercurrent system. *Am. J. Physiol.* 209:273, 1965.

Van Slyke, D. D., Linder, G. C., Hiller, A., Leiter, L., and McIntosh, J. F. The excretion of ammonia and titratable acid in nephritis. *J. Clin. Invest.* 2:255, 1926.

Villamil, M. F., Yeyati, N., Enero, M. A., Alvarez, C. C. P., and Taquini, A. C. Renal excretion of hydrogen ion in chronic renal failure. *Helv. Med. Acta* 30:47, 1963.

Wrong, O., and Davies, H. E. F. The excretion of acid in renal disease. *Q. J. Med.* 28:259, 1959.

Other Substances

Contiguglia, S. R., Alfrey, A. C., Miller, N., and Butkus, D. Total-body magnesium excess in chronic renal failure. *Lancet* 1:1300, 1972.

Fried, W. Erythropoietin. *Arch. Intern. Med.* 131:929, 1973.

Kleeman, C. R. (ed.). Divalent ion metabolism and osteodystrophy in chronic renal failure. *Arch. Intern. Med.* 124:261, 1969.

Lancet Editorial. Anaemia in chronic renal failure. *Lancet* 1:959, 1975.

Massry, S. G. (ed.). Divalent ions in renal failure. *Kidney Int.* 4:71, 1973.

Raisz, L. G. Calcium, Phosphate, Magnesium, and Trace Elements. In M. H. Maxwell and C. R. Kleeman (eds.), *Clinical Disorders of Fluid and Electrolyte Metabolism* (2nd ed.). New York: McGraw-Hill, 1972.

Rieselbach, R. E., Shankel, S. W., Slatopolsky, E., Lubowitz, H., and Bricker, N. S. Glucose titration studies in patients with chronic progressive renal disease. *J. Clin. Invest.* 46:157, 1967.

Shankel, S. W., Robson, A. M., and Bricker, N. S. On the mechanism of the splay in the glucose titration curve in advanced experimental renal disease in the rat. *J. Clin. Invest.* 46:164, 1967.

Steele, T. H., and Rieselbach, R. E. The contribution of residual nephrons within the chronically diseased kidney to urate homeostasis in man. *Am. J. Med.* 43:876, 1967.

Treatment

Alfrey, A. C., LeGendre, G. R., and Kaehny, W. D. The dialysis encephalopathy syndrome. Possible aluminum intoxication. *N. Engl. J. Med.* 294:184, 1976.

Bennett, W. M., Singer, I., Golper, T., Feig, P., and Coggins, C. J. Guidelines for drug therapy in renal failure. *Ann. Intern. Med.* 86:754, 1977.

Berlyne, G. M. (ed.). *Nutrition in Renal Disease.* Baltimore: Williams & Wilkins, 1968.

Blagg, C. R., and Scribner, B. H. Maintenance Dialysis. In D. A. K. Black (ed.), *Renal Disease* (3rd ed.). Oxford, Eng.: Blackwell, 1972.

Bone, J. M., Davison, A. M., and Robson, J. S. Role of dialysate calcium concentration in osteoporosis in patients on haemodialysis. *Lancet* 1:1047, 1972.

Brenner, B. M., and Rector, F. C., Jr. (eds.). *The Kidney.* Philadelphia: Saunders, 1976.
The final section of this authoritative, two-volume work is devoted to the various aspects of treating patients with chronic renal failure: diet, dialysis, transplantation, hypertension, infection, and drugs.

Calland, C. H. Iatrogenic problems in end-stage renal failure. *N. Engl. J. Med.* 287:334, 1972.

Campbell, J. D., and Campbell, A. R. The social and economic costs of end-stage renal disease. A patient's perspective. *N. Engl. J. Med.* 299: 386, 1978.

Chow, K-W., and Walser, M. Substitution of five essential amino acids by their alpha-keto analogues in the diet of rats. *J. Nutr.* 104:1208, 1974.

Evans, D. B. Diseases of the urinary system. Management of chronic renal failure by dialysis and transplantation. *Br. Med. J.* 1:1585, 1977.

Giordano, C. Use of exogenous and endogenous urea for protein thesis in normal and uremic subjects. *J. Lab. Clin. Med.* 62:231, 1963.

Giordano, C., Phillips, M. E., de Pascale, C., de Santo, N. G., Fürst, P., Brown, C. L., Houghton, B. J., and Richards, P. Utilization of keto-acid analogues of valine and phenylalanine in health and uraemia. *Lancet* 1:178, 1972.

Giovannetti, S., and Maggiore, Q. A low-nitrogen diet with proteins of high biological value for severe chronic uraemia. *Lancet* 1:1000, 1964.

Gotch, F. A., and Krueger, K. K. (eds.). Adequacy of dialysis. *Kidney Int.* 7 [Suppl. 2]:S-1, 1975.

This volume covers not only dialysis but also other topics related to chronic renal failure: diet, renal osteodystrophy, hematological disorders, cardiovascular complications, and neurological abnormalities.

Green, H. H., and Appleton, F. Chronic Renal Failure. In H. F. Conn (ed.), *Current Therapy 1975.* Philadelphia: Saunders, 1975.

Korsch, B. M., Fine, R. N., Grushkin, C. M., and Negrete, V. F. Experiences with children and their families during extended hemodialysis and kidney transplantation. *Pediatr. Clin. North Am.* 18:625, 1971.

Lancet Editorial. Synthesis of essential aminoacids. *Lancet* 1:191, 1972.

Lancet Editorial. Dialysis osteodystrophy. *Lancet* 2:451, 1976.

Levy, N. B., and Wynbrandt, G. D. The quality of life on maintenance haemodialysis. *Lancet* 1:1328, 1975.

Lowrie, E. G., Lazarus, J. M., Hampers, C. L., and Merrill, J. P. Cardiovascular disease in dialysis patients. *N. Engl. J. Med.* 290:737, 1974.

Mackey, B. G. (ed.). *Eighth Annual Contractors' Conference.* Artificial Kidney Program of the National Institute of Arthritis, Metabolism, and Digestive Diseases. Washington, D.C.: U.S. Department of Health, Education, and Welfare, 1976.

The proceedings of this conference can be obtained as DHEW Publication No. (NIH) 76-248, from the U.S. Government Printing Office. The annual proceedings are a source of information not only for advances in dialysis but also about problems in chronic renal failure.

Matas, A. J., Simmons, R. L., Kjellstrand, C. M., Buselmeier, T. J., and Najarian, J. S. Increased incidence of malignancy during chronic renal failure. *Lancet* 1:883, 1975.

Merrill, J. P. Present status of kidney transplantation. *D. M.* November 1974.

Milne, M. D. (ed.). Management of renal failure. *Br. Med. Bull.* 27:95, 1971.

Mitch, W. E., Lietman, P. S., and Walser, M. Effects of oral neomycin and kanamycin in chronic uremic patients: I. Urea metabolism. *Kidney Int.* 11:116, 1977.

Nolan, B. Transplantation of the Kidney. In D. A. K. Black (ed.), *Renal Disease* (3rd ed.). Oxford, Eng.: Blackwell, 1972.

Richards, P., Ell, S., and Halliday, D. Direct evidence for synthesis of valine in man. *Lancet* 1:112, 1977.

Rubin, A. L., Stenzel, K. H., and Reidenberg, M. M. (eds.). Symposium on drug action and metabolism in renal failure. *Am. J. Med.* 62:459, 1977.

Shepherd, A. M. M., Stewart, W. K., and Wormsley, K. G. Peptic ulceration in chronic renal failure. *Lancet* 1:1357, 1973.

Stewart, W. K., Fleming, L. W., and Manuel, M. A. Muscle cramps during maintenance haemodialysis. *Lancet* 1:1049, 1972.

Walser, M. Use of Isotopic Urea to Study the Distribution and Degradation of Urea in Man. In B. Schmidt-Nielsen (ed.), *Urea and the Kidney.* Amsterdam: Excerpta Medica Foundation, 1970.

Walser, M., Coulter, A. W., Dighe, S., and Crantz, F. R. The effect of keto-analogues of essential amino acids in severe chronic uremia. *J. Clin. Invest.* 52:678, 1973.

Walser, M., Lund, P., Ruderman, N. B., and Coulter, A. W. Synthesis of essential amino acids from their α-keto analogues by perfused rat liver and muscle. *J. Clin. Invest.* 52:2865, 1973.

11 : Consequences of Urinary Obstruction

Some degree of hindrance to the flow of urine is a rather common clinical problem, and it is important because obstruction, even when partial and mild, may lead to renal dysfunction and to irreversible damage to the kidneys. Urinary obstruction may be acute or chronic (lasting years), partial or complete, unilateral or bilateral, and the consequences will vary depending on which combination exists. Acute, complete, bilateral obstruction (or an acute, complete, unilateral block in a patient who has only one kidney) will be manifested as anuric acute renal failure (Chap. 9), a dramatic event that if reversed in time, can lead to rapid and complete recovery. On the other hand, chronic, partial, unilateral or bilateral obstruction may cause no renal dysfunction or damage if the block is minimal. By far the most common occurrence is a chronic, partial, and bilateral obstruction of such a degree of severity that it leads to slow and progressive anatomical and functional changes as well as to destruction of the renal parenchyma. This chapter deals exclusively with the last form of obstruction.

Definitions

Literally, *hydronephrosis* refers to a process in the kidneys that is characterized by an abnormally large collection of water within them. The term is most commonly used to denote dilatation of those portions of the intrarenal urinary conduits that can be visualized on an intravenous pyelogram (I.V.P.): namely, the minor and major calyces and the renal pelvis (Fig. 11-1). Although there is usually dilatation of the renal tubules as well, this effect is ordinarily not visible on I.V.P.

The term *hydrocalyx* is used to denote dilatation of a single calyx or a few isolated calyces; this is a different and much more rare condition than hydronephrosis, which commonly entails the dilatation of all or most calyces. *Hydroureter* means water within the ureter, and it refers to dilatation of all or part of that structure.

The constellation of anatomical and functional changes in the kidneys that result from obstruction of the urinary passages –

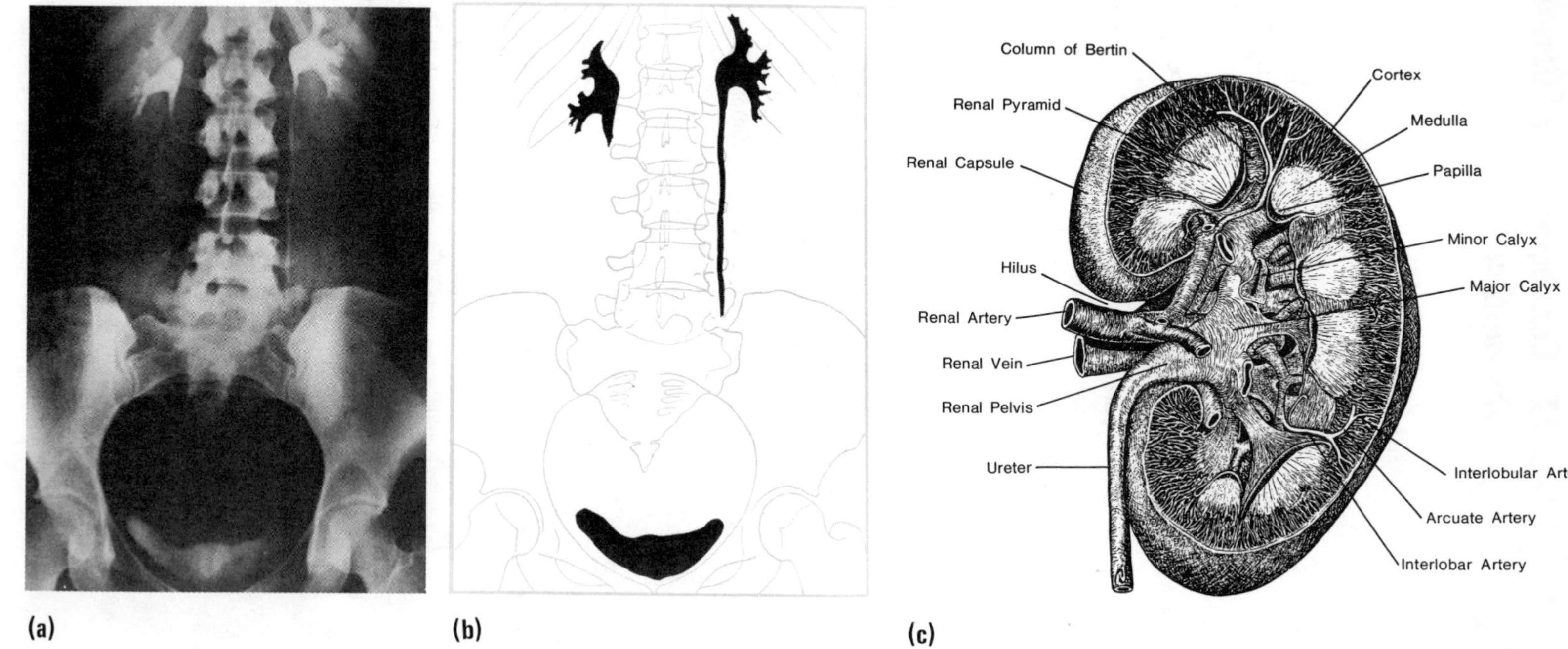
Column of Bertin
Renal Pyramid
Renal Capsule
Hilus
Renal Artery
Renal Vein
Renal Pelvis
Ureter
Cortex
Medulla
Papilla
Minor Calyx
Major Calyx
Interlobular Artery
Arcuate Artery
Interlobar Artery

(a) (b) (c)

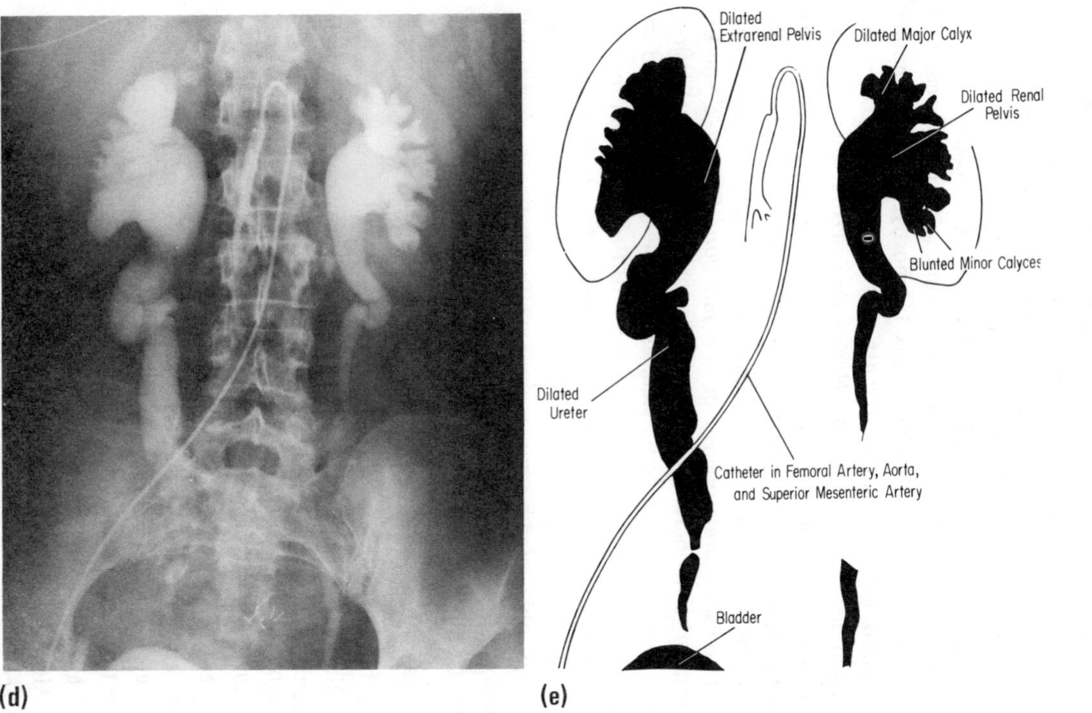

Figure 11-1
(a) and (b) Normal urinary collecting system as visualized by intravenous pyelogram (I.V.P.). From M. Kory and S. O. Waife (eds.), *Kidney and Urinary Tract Infections.* Indianapolis: Lilly Research Labs, 1971.

(c) For orientation, a sagittal section of the human kidney is illustrated. From H. Valtin, *Renal Function: Mechanisms Preserving Fluid and Solute Balance in Health.* Boston: Little, Brown, 1973.

(d) and (e) Severe bilateral hydronephrosis in a 50-year-old woman due to adhesions following pelvic exenteration for cloacogenic carcinoma of the rectovaginal septum. In this instance, the urinary collecting system was visualized coincidentally as part of an arteriogram performed for other than the renal problem. Courtesy of Peter J. Spiegel.

and that form the subject of this chapter — is described by the term *obstructive nephropathy.*

Causes and Sites of Obstruction

Impediment to the flow of urinary fluid can originate anywhere from the proximal tubule to the urethra. Such lesions within the renal tubules, however, do not ordinarily lead to overt renal dysfunction unless numerous or most tubules are involved, as in some forms of acute renal failure when the *initiating* event is not an obstruction. Therefore, obstructive nephropathy may result from blockage occurring anywhere distal to a minor calyx. (There may be exceptions to this rule in that rarely, obstruction of the collecting ducts — as by uric acid stones or myeloma proteins — might also lead to obstructive nephropathy.)

Some of the sites and major causes of obstruction at these sites are shown in Figure 11-2. Normally, the spatial arrangement of muscles and the innervation of the urinary passages from the minor calyx to the urethral meatus assure sequential progression of urine distad and prevent reflux by mostly valve-like (though by some valvular) action at the points of potential obstruction shown in Figure 11-2. (1) *Hydrocalyx* occurs when the exit passage of a minor or major calyx is occluded, for example, by the lodging of a stone at this site (site a of Fig. 11-2). (2) Obstruction at the junction between the ureter and the renal pelvis, the so-called ureteropelvic or *U-P junction* (Fig. 11-2, site b), is most commonly caused by some form of congenital lesion; examples include intrinsic stenosis, external pressure caused by aberrant bands or vessels, and abnormalities of smooth muscles that lead to incoordinated peristalsis. Staghorn calculi are another cause. (3) Blockage along the *ureter* (Fig. 11-2, site c) is most commonly caused by stones; chronic inflammation, such as tuberculosis; injury; developmental abnormalities of the muscles, nerves, or both; and intrinsic or extrinsic tumors. (4) As the ureter enters the bladder at the *ureterovesical junction* (Fig. 11-2, site d), it normally takes an oblique course through the muscular wall of the bladder. The obliquity is essential to the valve-like action at this point, for during micturition, the bladder muscle compresses the ureter and thereby prevents reflux of urine and retrograde transmission of the intravesical pressure along the ureter. It follows that interference with this valve-like action — which is caused mainly by congenital malformations of the ureterovesical junction — will lead to a "functional obstruction" in the sense that both the volume of the urine and the hydrostatic pressure proximal to the junction will be abnormally high. If this condition is allowed to continue (e.g., for years), then secondary changes such as chronic inflammation, fibrosis, and muscular hypertrophy may contribute to an actual obstruction. (5) The final major locus for obstruction is the *neck of the*

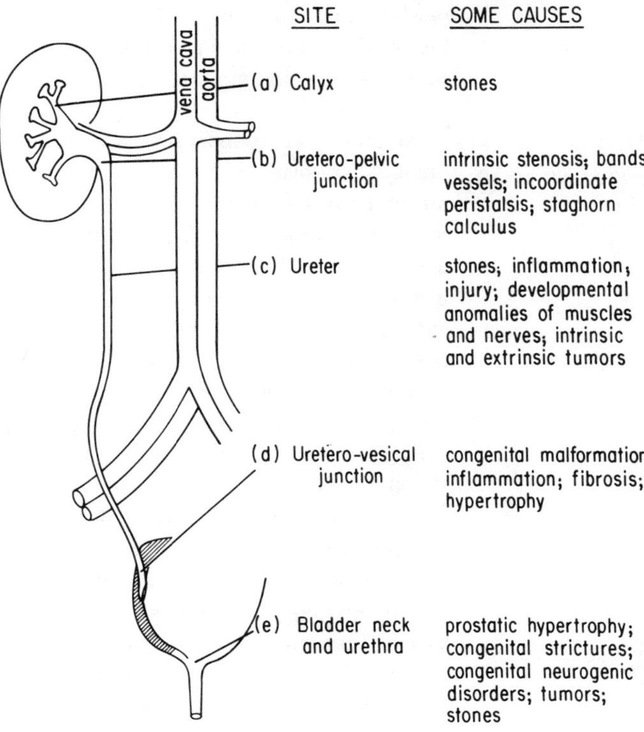

Figure 11-2
Sites of urinary obstruction and some causes of blockage at each site. The normal oblique course of the ureter through the wall of the bladder is shown. Adapted from F. Hinman, Jr., in M. F. Campbell and J. H. Harrison (eds.), *Urology* (3rd ed.). Philadelphia: Saunders, 1970.

bladder and the urethra (Fig. 11-2, site e), where the causes of blockage include benign prostatic hypertrophy, congenital strictures, tumors, and stones.

Influence of Site and Cause on Obstructive Nephropathy

Both the site and the cause of urinary tract obstruction are of obvious importance because some locations and certain lesions are much more amenable to satisfactory therapy than are others. However, there is another, though related, reason why the site and cause are important, and that is the extent to which they influence the development of obstructive nephropathy. This extent is a function of (1) the degree and (2) the duration of obstruction, of (3) the locus of the lesion, and of (4) the magnitude of associated pyelonephritis.

It is self-evident how items (1) and (2) might vary with the type and location of the lesion. The site of obstruction — item (3) above — will in part determine the extent of nephropathy, because the urinary bladder and ureter accommodate to the accumulation of fluid by mechanisms to be described in the next section. This accommodation, which ultimately amounts to minimizing the increase of hydrostatic pressure within the system, can be effected to a much greater degree by the ureter and bladder than by the collecting conduits within the kidney. Other things being equal, therefore, a given degree of obstruction at the ureteropelvic junction (Fig. 11-2, site b) is likely to have more deleterious effects on renal function than a similar blockage at more distal points. As concerns item (4), infection and its extension into the kidneys is a very frequent concomitant of chronic urinary obstruction. Not only does blockage entail some of the classic components for chronic infection — namely, a nidus and poor drainage — but in addition, the diagnostic investigation and the treatment of obstruction usually require instrumentation of the urinary passages. And the type and frequency of instrumentation will vary with the type and location of the lesion. Even though modern urological techniques minimize or prevent trauma and the introduction of bacteria, infection still remains an ever-present risk. In any case, by whatever route the infectious agents get to the kidney, pyelonephritis is often one of the most important contributors to renal dysfunction during urinary obstruction.

Hydronephrosis

Along with pyelonephritis, the major cause of damage to the kidneys during obstruction is hydronephrosis and the transmission of abnormally high hydrostatic pressure to renal structures (see Causes of Impairment, below). Hydronephrosis may result in the accumulation of almost incredible amounts of fluid — in excess of 3 liters and, rarely, as much as 10 to 15 liters — within

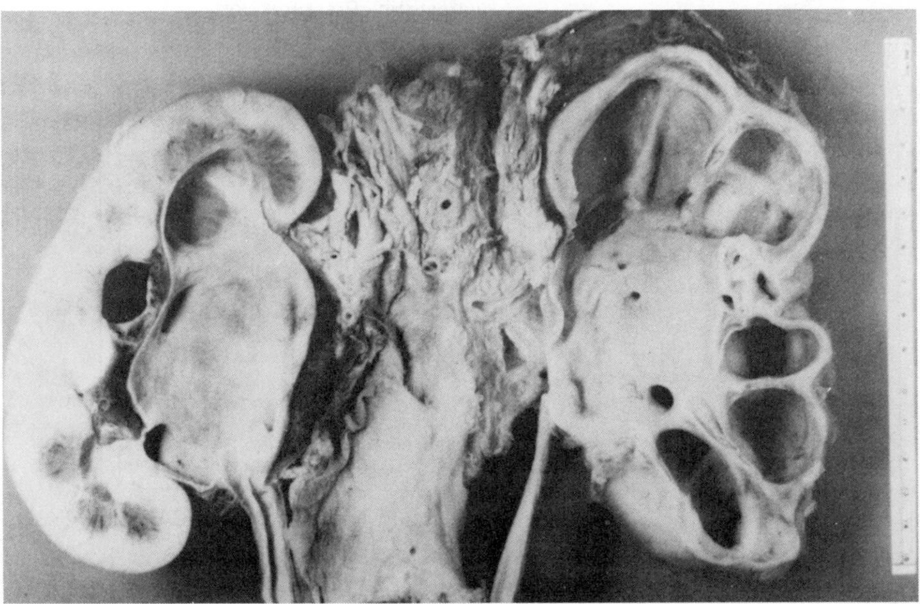

Figure 11-3
Kidneys from a 21-year-old man with bilateral hydronephrosis due to obstruction at the ureteropelvic junctions. In the kidney shown on the left, the renal pelvis and calyces (see Fig. 11-1c) are dilated, but most of the cortical tissue has been preserved. In the kidney on the right, severe hydronephrosis has destroyed virtually all functioning tissue, with only some columns of Bertin (Fig. 11-1c) remaining. From R. H. Heptinstall, *Pathology of the Kidney* (2nd ed.). Boston: Little, Brown, 1974.

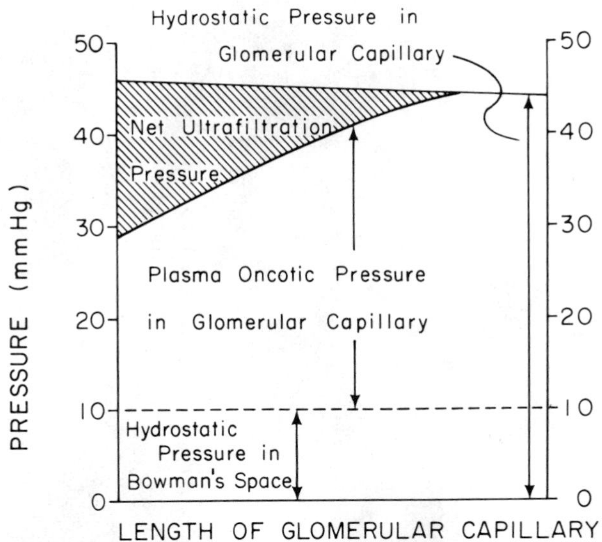

BALANCE OF MEAN VALUES

Hydrostatic pressure in glomerular capillary	45 mmHg
Hydrostatic pressure in Bowman's space	10
Plasma oncotic pressure in glomerular capillary	27
Oncotic pressure of fluid in Bowman's space	0*
Net ultrafiltration pressure	8 mmHg

* *The concentration of protein in Bowman's space fluid is negligibly small; the estimated oncotic pressure is perhaps 0.3 mmHg.*

Figure 11-4
Starling forces involved in glomerular ultrafiltration. Although the results were derived from rats, they are likely to pertain to humans as well. From H. Valtin, *Renal Function: Mechanisms Preserving Fluid and Solute Balance in Health.* Boston: Little, Brown, 1973. Data from B. M. Brenner et al., *J. Clin. Invest.* 50:1776, 1971.

the kidneys. Inasmuch as the kidneys are enveloped by a fairly indistensible capsule, fluid must collect at the expense of the renal parenchyma (Fig. 11-3).

The problem of explaining the pathogenesis of hydronephrosis can best be clarified by reviewing the dynamics of glomerular ultrafiltration (Fig. 11-4). Three of the four Starling forces, which determine the movement of fluid across capillary membranes, are involved (an additional determinant of glomerular filtration, namely, the rate of plasma flow through the glomerular capillaries, is not considered here): (1) the hydrostatic pressure within the glomerular capillaries promotes ultrafiltration out of the capillaries, and this pressure is opposed by (2) the oncotic pressure of plasma within the glomerular capillaries and (3) the hydrostatic pressure in Bowman's space. So long as the sum of the last two forces is less than the first, the net ultrafiltration pressure has a positive value (Fig. 11-4), and the formation of glomerular filtrate continues. At the point where the sum of the second and third pressures equals the value of the first, however, the formation of filtrate stops. Within hours after the onset of urinary obstruction, the pressure within the collecting system can rise by 25 mm Hg or more, and this pressure is transmitted retrograde through the tubules to Bowman's space. An increase of about 25 mm Hg in the hydrostatic pressure in Bowman's space should stop glomerular filtration (Fig. 11-4) and hence prevent the accumulation of fluid proximal to the site of obstruction. Yet, the massive aggregation of fluid that constitutes hydronephrosis (Figs. 11-1d and 11-3) shows that fluid must continue to enter the collecting system during continued obstruction. Normally, the *net* entry of fluid into the nephrons and hence into the more distal conduits occurs exclusively through glomerular filtration. The problem of explaining how hydronephrosis develops is thus one of identifying the mechanisms by which the balance of Starling forces during obstruction again leads to a positive net ultrafiltration pressure (Fig. 11-4) and to the continued production of filtrate, albeit at a lower rate.

Some experimental data that are pertinent to the explanation are shown in Figure 11-5. Figure 11-5a shows the results obtained on rats in which chronic partial obstruction was induced by loosely tying a silk ligature around the upper ureter, just below the ureteropelvic junction. Two to four weeks later, despite a degree of obstruction that reduced the GFR to 18 percent of the control value, the hydrostatic pressure in the proximal tubule (and hence in Bowman's space) was only slightly raised, and the glomerular filtration rate within a single surface nephron (sGFR), far from having ceased, was only moderately reduced. The reasons for this adjustment are reflected in Figure 11-5b and c.

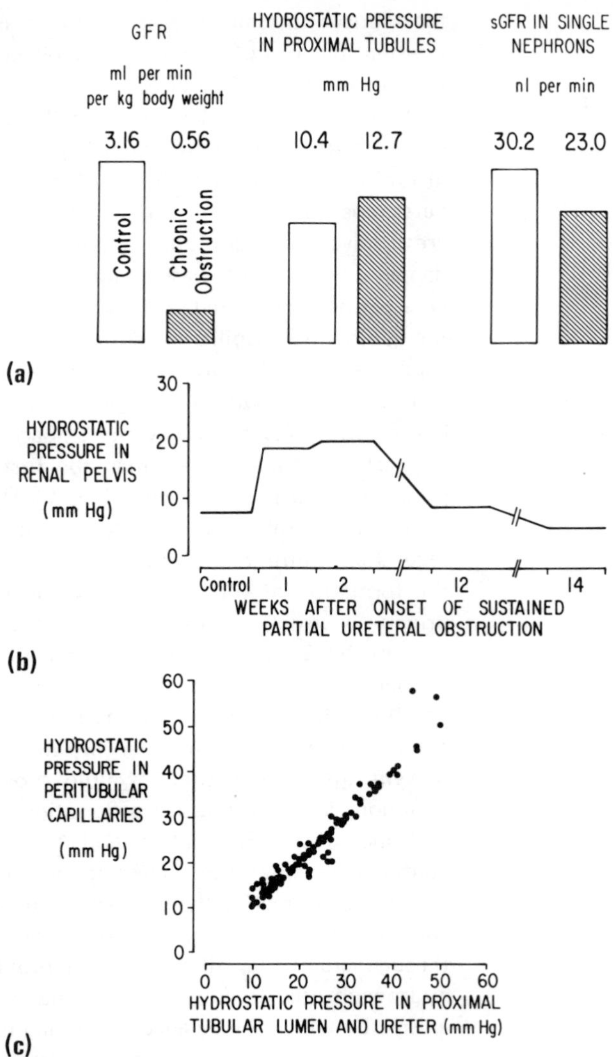
GFR
ml per min
per kg body weight
3.16 0.56
Control
Chronic Obstruction
HYDROSTATIC PRESSURE IN PROXIMAL TUBULES
mm Hg
10.4 12.7
sGFR IN SINGLE NEPHRONS
nl per min
30.2 23.0
(a)
HYDROSTATIC PRESSURE IN RENAL PELVIS
(mm Hg)
0
10
20
30
Control 1 2 12 14
WEEKS AFTER ONSET OF SUSTAINED PARTIAL URETERAL OBSTRUCTION
(b)
HYDROSTATIC PRESSURE IN PERITUBULAR CAPILLARIES
(mm Hg)
0
10
20
30
40
50
60
0 10 20 30 40 50 60
HYDROSTATIC PRESSURE IN PROXIMAL TUBULAR LUMEN AND URETER (mm Hg)
(c)

Figure 11-5
Mechanisms whereby the filtration rate in single nephrons (*sGFR*) is maintained in the face of sustained, partial urinary obstruction.

(a) Data from rats show only a slight rise of proximal intratubular pressure and only a moderate decrease in the sGFR of nephrons at the periphery of the kidney. The fact that the glomerular filtration rate for the entire kidney (*GFR*) decreased proportionately more than the sGFR is probably a reflection not only of a decline in the total number of nephrons but also of greater damage to the nephrons lying in deeper parts of the cortex compared to nephrons in more peripheral locations. Data from D. R. Wilson, *Kidney Int.* 2:119, 1972.

(b) Initial rise and subsequent decline of the intrapelvic pressure of dogs with experimental, chronic, and partial urinary obstruction. Data from N. W. Struthers, *Br. J. Urol.* 41:129, 1969.

(c) Concomitant and equal rise in peritubular capillary pressure as ureteral and proximal tubular pressures are raised *acutely* in rats. Adapted from C. W. Gottschalk and M. Mylle, *Am. J. Physiol.* 185:430, 1956.

Most important is the decline of hydrostatic pressure within the collecting system despite continued obstruction. This effect is shown in Figure 11-5b for the intrarenal pelvis (Fig. 11-1c) of dogs with partial obstruction of the lower ureter; the same phenomenon has been demonstrated in human patients and in other parts of the urinary conduit, such as the ureter and bladder. The fact that the pressure declines even while the volume of the system increases — that is, even while hydronephrosis develops — means that the neuromuscular tone and the force of peristaltic contraction decrease. This is probably the main mechanism by which the GFR is maintained. It also provides the probable explanation why an obstruction at or above the ureteropelvic junction is likely to be more deleterious than an equal degree of blockage at more distal points: the more distal the obstruction, the more abundant and distensible the structures in which a relaxation of the musculature can "buffer" the potential increases in pressure.

The phenomenon shown in Figure 11-5c might also contribute to the maintenance of the sGFR, that is, filtration rate in single nephrons. The results, taken from experiments in rats, show that as the hydrostatic pressure is raised within the collecting system, the pressure in the peritubular capillaries rises equally. Other things being equal, the higher pressure in the capillaries will amount to a greater resistance at the efferent arterioles and might thus lead to an increase of the hydrostatic pressure within the glomerular capillaries, in rough proportion to the increase of pressure in Bowman's space. Although such an effect will tend to maintain the sGFR in the face of obstruction, its pertinence to hydronephrosis is not yet known, because the data in Figure 11-5c show the results of acute obstruction; during chronic obstruction, the return to normal pressure shown in Figure 11-5b may be more relevant.

Under some circumstances, an additional mechanism, which does not involve glomerular filtration, may contribute to the accumulation of fluid in the collecting system. As urine traverses the renal pelvis, ureter, and bladder, many solutes and water diffuse passively in or out of the conduits. It has been shown experimentally in dogs that there is a net movement of water into the ureters and bladder, especially at the low rates of urine flow that might exist during obstruction.

Impairment of Renal Function

Causes of Impairment

In rare instances, mild obstruction may lead merely to a small decrease in the GFR and the renal blood flow (RBF), and the consequent impairment of renal function may be so minimal that it is not detected. Much more commonly, however, sustained partial obstruction leads to a progressive loss of nephrons and therefore to chronic renal failure. Because the forces that destroy renal tissue are transmitted to the kidneys retrograde, there is a tendency for the renal medulla to be affected earlier and more severely than the cortex (Fig. 11-3), and this fact is reflected in the pattern of functional changes described below.

Three major mechanisms contribute to the destruction of nephrons in urinary obstruction: (1) the pressure effects of hydronephrosis, (2) ischemia, and (3) the associated pyelonephritis. As fluid accumulates in the renal pelvis during the development of hydronephrosis, the kidneys may initially swell. This process is limited, however, because the kidneys are surrounded by a relatively indistensible capsule. Consequently, as hydronephrosis progresses, the renal parenchyma is literally crowded out. At first, the pressure effect is exerted mainly on the renal papilla, but eventually virtually all the cortical tissue may be obliterated as well (Fig. 11-3). In addition to the mechanical effects of pressure, there are probably also the injurious influences of decreased blood supply. Total RBF is decreased in obstructive nephropathy. The transmission of increased intratubular pressure to the surrounding vasculature (Fig. 11-5c) results in decreased postglomerular blood flow, and the selective exertion of pressure on the renal papilla might intensify this effect by pressing on the vasa recta. Histological sections of hydronephrotic kidneys also show damage to the preglomerular vessels, a decrease in their number, and elongation, tortuosity, and tearing, especially of the interlobar, arcuate, and interlobular arteries.

Pyelonephritis is so commonly associated with urinary obstruction that the pattern of functional impairment in obstructive nephropathy may be indistinguishable from that of chronic pyelonephritis. Obstruction promotes infection through stasis and often by providing a nidus; in turn, infection tends to promote obstruction through swelling and formation of scar tissue. Thus, urinary obstruction frequently involves a vicious circle in which one process abets the other. So common is the association that urinary obstruction should always be looked for in patients who have unexplained urinary infection, even if those patients have no other symptoms or signs of obstruction.

Pattern of Functional Impairment

In the preceding chapter on chronic renal failure, we pointed out that because of the interdependency of the renal vascular and tubular structures, the functional consequences of nephron damage were by and large identical, no matter what the initiating cause. Although this principle also applies to moderate and severe obstructive nephropathy, the earlier stages represent an exception to the rule. Because there is a predilection for damage to occur to the renal medulla, dysfunctions associated with tubular structures lying in that portion of the kidney appear first and tend to predominate over the other functional changes of chronic renal failure. As shown in Table 11-1, whether urinary obstruction occurs in elderly people or in infants, it almost immediately leads to a defect in the ability to concentrate urine. The defect cannot be corrected with exogenous vasopressin, and it may range in severity from a mild decrease in urine osmolality to marked diabetes insipidus with the excretion of hyposmotic urine. Deficiencies of urinary concentration that cannot be corrected with vasopressin are considered in detail in Chapter 13. Suffice it to say here that in obstructive nephropathy, the deficiency appears to be due to a decrease in the corticopapillary interstitial osmotic gradient (which is normally built up by the loops of Henle) and sometimes additionally to an inability of vasopressin to induce full water permeability in the collecting ducts; that is, the deficiency involves the failure of those portions of the nephron that course through the renal medulla. This conclusion is buttressed by the further observations that the ability to dilute the urine to a minimal osmolality during water diuresis — a function mainly of the cortical structures (site 3, Fig. 7-1) — is preserved until late in obstructive nephropathy and that the sGFR of individual juxtamedullary nephrons is decreased proportionately more than that of the more superficial nephrons (see legend to Fig. 11-5a).

There is disagreement on whether or not the inability to reduce the urinary pH to the normal minimal value reflects selective damage to the medullary collecting ducts. Some investigators

Table 11-1
Major deficiencies of renal function in chronic, partial, bilateral urinary obstruction

State	GFR (ml/min)	Maximal U_{Osm}[a] (mOsm/kg H_2O)	Minimal Urine pH[b]	Maximal $U_{H^+} \cdot \dot{V}$[b] (μEq/min)	Maximal $U_{NH_4^+} \cdot \dot{V}$[b] (μEq/min)
In elderly men with benign prostatic hypertrophy[c]:					
Normal for age	94	≈900	<5.30	>65	>38
Chronic obstruction	57	350	5.78	28	15
In infants and children with congenital obstructions at ureteropelvic junction, ureterovesical junction, bladder neck, and/or urethra[d]:					
Normal (per 1.73 m^2 body surface area)	113	1,089	5.11	119	68
Chronic obstruction	77	578	5.53	87	43

[a]After administration of exogenous vasopressin or water deprivation.
[b]After giving NH_4Cl or in the face of severe metabolic acidosis.
[c]Data from O. Olbrich et al., *Lancet* 1:1322, 1957; G. M. Berlyne, *Q. J. Med.* 30:339, 1961.
[d]Data from W. W. McCrory et al., *Pediatr. Clin. North Am.* 18:445, 1971.

contend that in obstructive nephropathy, this function is impaired out of proportion to the degree of renal failure (Table 11-1) and that it therefore reflects an inability of the collecting ducts to reabsorb filtered bicarbonate or secrete H^+ (or both) at the maximal rates. On the other hand, others have pointed out that only the concentrating defect can be detected in the absence of renal failure, whereas the ability to acidify the urine becomes affected only when the GFR has become reduced. Similarly, it is not yet known whether the lower-than-normal excretion of H^+ as NH_4^+ (Table 11-1) and, possibly, as titratable acid (T.A.; not shown in Table 11-1) might be accounted for simply by the defect in acidification (see Chap. 10, Acidification and H^+ Excretion under Hydrogen Ion), or whether a decrease in number of nephrons must be invoked as an additional explanation.

However these questions are ultimately resolved, the immediate and invariable deterioration of the concentrating mechanism shows that the pattern of functional impairment during the early stages of obstructive nephropathy reflects predominant damage to the renal medullary structures. The fact that the same pattern is observed in patients with unilateral hydronephrosis whose total renal function is normal also speaks for the relative specificity of the changes. Later, as hydronephrosis progresses, the loss of nephrons (Fig. 11-3) determines the pattern of functional impairment, which finally becomes indistinguishable from that of chronic renal failure due to other causes.

Recovery After Relief of Obstruction

That some of the decreased function even in late obstructive nephropathy is due to the effects of transmitted pressure, rather than purely to irreversible destruction of nephrons, is shown by the amount of recovery that can be obtained when the obstruction is removed (Fig. 11-6). In experimental animals, improvement in the affected kidney can occur even after total obstruction of one ureter for one week, and betterment may progress for at least two months after relief of the blockage. Recovery is not invariably seen and when it occurs, its extent will vary with the severity and duration of the preexistent obstruction. But the fact that it may be obtained even years after the onset of partial obstruction (Fig. 11-6) and even after the development of marked hydronephrosis means that correction of the abnormality should almost always be attempted.

Postobstructive Diuresis

In some patients, relief of the obstruction is followed by an osmotic diuresis, which is more intense than would be expected from the degree of renal failure. Postobstructive diuresis occurs predominantly after the relief of bilateral obstruction, and it may be most marked after an acute, complete blockage or at

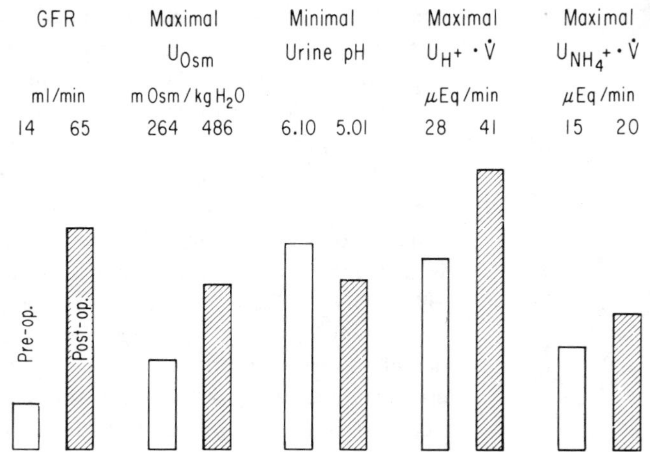

Figure 11-6
Recovery of renal function in elderly men after prostatectomy for benign prostatic hypertrophy. This type of improvement can occur within one to two months after operation, even though partial obstruction has been present for several years. Adapted from G. M. Berlyne, *Q. J. Med.* 30:339, 1961.

least after an acute episode superimposed on a chronic, partial obstruction. The diuresis cannot be ameliorated by giving vasopressin or aldosterone. It may last for a few hours or for several months, and it may be so severe that it will lead to dangerous contraction of the body-fluid volumes unless special care is taken to replace the losses of water and salt.

Some characteristics of postobstructive diuresis are shown in Figure 11-7. In the face of only a moderate reduction in the GFR, there may be an enormous increase in urine flow and in the output of Na^+ and Cl^-. The excretion of urea is increased somewhat less than that of Na^+ and Cl^-, and the changes in K^+ excretion are variable but usually do not contribute a large portion to the total output of solute.

From the results shown in the lower half of Figure 11-7, it may be deduced that failure of salt and water reabsorption in the proximal tubules and loops of Henle contributes importantly to the diuresis (although, as outlined in the next paragraph, decreased reabsorption in more distal segments also contributes). Normally, about 70 percent of the filtered water is reabsorbed in the proximal tubules, 10 to 20 percent in the loops of Henle, and 10 to 15 percent in the distal tubules and collecting ducts. Suppression of reabsorption of the last moiety (as occurs in water diuresis) can thus lead to the excretion of at most 15 percent of the filtered water, and the excretion of as much as 30 percent must therefore reflect decreased reabsorption in the

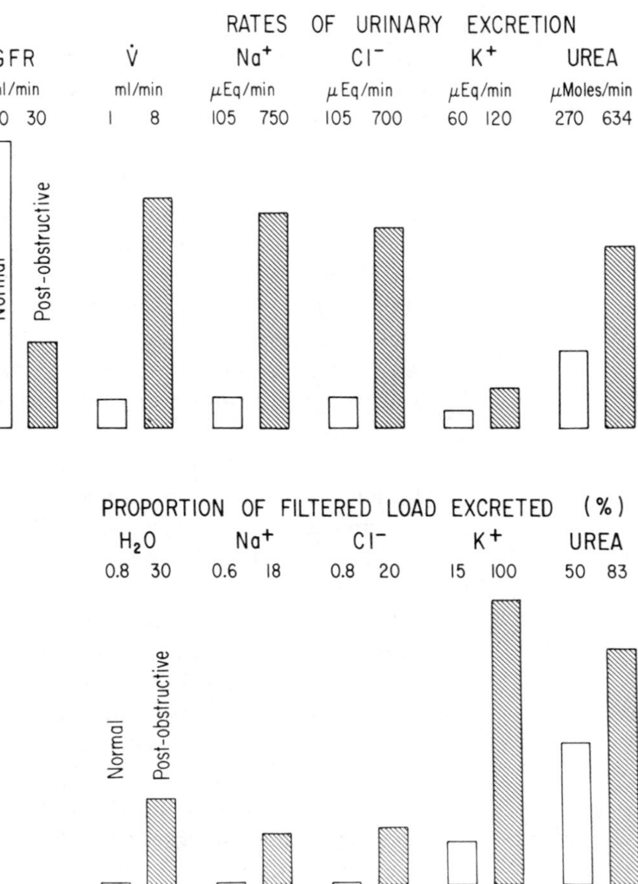

Figure 11-7
Characteristics of postobstructive diuresis in a 60-year-old woman who had experienced intermittent difficulty with uric-acid stones. Six years before the diuresis, her left kidney was removed because of obstruction and chronic pyelonephritis. During the four days prior to the diuresis, a uric-acid stone that had lodged at the right ureteropelvic junction caused the patient to be severely oliguric; the diuresis set in immediately after a catheter was threaded past the obstruction into the renal pelvis. The diuresis subsided during the next 10 days, and the stone was removed 16 days after the onset of diuresis. Data from N. S. Bricker et al., *Am. J. Med.* 23:554, 1957.

segments proximal to the distal tubule. Analogous arguments can be applied to explain the excretion of Na^+ and Cl^-. Normally, no more than 10 percent of the filtered load of these ions is reabsorbed in the distal tubules and collecting ducts (Fig. 7-5); hence, the excretion of twice that proportion (Fig. 11-7) must reflect decreased reabsorption at more proximal sites. Finally, the same reasoning holds for urea. Roughly 50 percent of filtered urea is normally reabsorbed in the proximal tubules, perhaps none from the loops of Henle, virtually none from the distal tubules, and a variable amount from the collecting ducts, depending on the state of diuresis. Elimination of all urea reabsorption from the segments beyond the proximal tubules will usually result in an excretion of no more than 60 percent of the filtered load of urea, and a value as high as 83 percent therefore probably reflects decreased reabsorption of urea from the proximal tubules. (Although the percentage increase in K^+ excretion is impressive, the filtered load of K^+ is so small compared to that of Na^+, Cl^-, and urea that the absolute amount of K^+ excreted contributes relatively little to the total output of solute.)

The above deductions, which are based on the somewhat indirect evidence obtained in man that is shown in Figure 11-7, have been confirmed and extended by more direct approaches, such as the use of micropuncture, microcatheterization, and cross-circulation techniques in experimental animals; these further studies have shown the distal tubules and medullary collecting ducts to be other important sites contributing to the diuresis. During experimental postobstructive diuresis in rats, the rates at which water, K^+, Na^+ (and, by implication, Cl^-) were reabsorbed in the proximal and distal tubules were all much less than in control rats. In loops of Henle, the reabsorptive rates were less for Na^+ (Cl^-) but not for water; there was actual net secretion of Na^+ (Cl^-) in the collecting ducts. Although there is still some disagreement on the mechanisms that effect these changes, there appear to be at least two major causes: (1) Urea, through its osmotic effect, and possibly natriuretic humoral substances, inhibit the reabsorption of NaCl and water in the proximal and distal tubules; and (2) obstruction per se, possibly through increased pressure within the renal pelvis, inhibits the reabsorption of fluid — sometimes to the point of slight secretion — in the medullary collecting ducts.

Some patients develop a positive balance for NaCl and water during the period of obstruction, and such balance may contribute to postobstructive diuresis through various natriuretic influences. A prior positive balance is not, however, prerequisite to the diuresis.

Summary

Obstruction of the urinary passages is a fairly common occurrence, being detectable in about 4 percent of autopsies. It can cover a wide spectrum, ranging from mild blockage having no effect on renal function, to sudden and total blockade eventuating in acute renal failure or to a sustained, partial hindrance that leads to obstructive nephropathy and eventually to chronic renal failure. In this chapter, we have dealt with the last entity.

The major sites of obstruction that can lead to obstructive nephropathy include the outlet of a minor or major calyx, the ureteropelvic junction, the ureter, the ureterovesical junction, and the neck of the bladder and urethra. Certain causes have a predilection for certain sites (Fig. 11-2), and both the type and incidence of the causes may vary with age and sex. Congenital lesions constitute the major cause in both sexes before the age of 20 years, pregnancy and carcinoma of the uterus make obstructive nephropathy more common in women between the ages of 20 and 60, and prostatic hypertrophy, either benign or malignant, raises the incidence of obstruction in males after 60 years of age. Both the type of obstructing lesion and its location may influence the development of obstructive nephropathy by determining the extent of the associated pyelonephritis (a very frequent concomitant of urinary obstruction) as well as the magnitude of the pressure-induced damage to the kidneys; the latter tends to be more severe with lesions near the renal pelvis than at more distal points, because dilatation of conduits outside of the kidneys can attenuate the rise in pressure that follows obstruction.

The development of hydronephrosis presents a puzzle because a rise in pressure proximal to an obstruction would be expected to stop glomerular filtration. Yet, the progressive accumulation of enormous amounts of fluid within the renal pelvis, ureters, and bladder reflects continued filtration in the face of persistent blockage. The production of glomerular filtrate during obstruction is maintained mainly through decreases in the neuromuscular tone and in the force of peristaltic contractions of the urinary passages; the relaxation permits the collecting system to dilate so that a rise of pressure within the system is minimized or prevented. Net movement of water into the ureters and bladder across their walls — not through glomerular filtration — might also contribute to hydronephrosis in some instances of urinary obstruction.

Impairment of renal function during obstruction results from (1) a crowding out of renal parenchyma by the expanding hydronephrosis, (2) decreased nutritive blood supply, and (3) pyelonephritis. The pattern of functional impairment in obstructive nephropathy may be divided into two phases: an early phase, which reflects dominant damage to the renal medullary structures and is characterized by deficiencies in concentrating and acidifying the urine, and a later phase, which is due to the loss of nephrons and may therefore be indistinguishable from chronic renal failure due to other causes. Considerable recovery of renal function may be seen after a blockage is relieved, even though the obstruction has been present for years. This fact makes it imperative that correction of an obstructive lesion be attempted; on the other hand, if the lesion is so mild that it is not affecting function, then "watchful waiting" may be the better policy, since instrumentation carries with it the danger of infection.

Relief of the obstruction – especially of an acute and complete blockage superimposed on a chronic obstruction – is followed in some patients by a severe osmotic diuresis in which NaCl and, to a lesser extent, urea are the main urinary solutes. The diuresis arises from the decreased tubular reabsorption of water, NaCl, and urea. In the proximal and distal tubules, this decreased reabsorption may result mainly from the osmotic effect of urea and possibly from other natriuretic substances; in the medullary collecting ducts, the increased intrapelvic pressure may convert the normal reabsorption of NaCl and water to the secretion of these substances.

Problem 11-1

A 68-year-old man sought help at a hospital because he "didn't feel good." When a more specific history was elicited, the patient stated that for at least two years he had noticed hesitancy in starting urination, as well as a decrease in the caliber and force of the urinary stream. Gradually, the frequency of micturition had increased to hourly during the day and four to five times at night (nocturia), and he had begun to experience urgency incontinence and an occasional loss of urine without warning. The symptoms had become more severe in the month before the patient came to the hospital. During this period, the patient also developed anorexia, lethargy, and intermittent headaches.

Positive findings on physical examination were limited to the following: a blood pressure of 170/90 mm Hg; a midline mass extending from the symphysis pubis to the umbilicus; a broad, firm prostate with an estimated weight of at least 60 g, which contained a firmer nodule at the left base; and two-plus pitting edema in both lower legs, but no signs of heart failure.

The patient was admitted to the Urology Service. When a catheter was passed to the bladder, 1,200 ml of clear urine was obtained and the abdominal mass disappeared. The urine specimen had a specific gravity of 1.006 and a pH of 6.5. It contained 25 white blood cells per high-power field, but no erythrocytes, protein, or glucose; culture of the urine was negative. Other laboratory data included BUN, 86 mg/100 ml; serum creatinine, 7.3 mg/100 ml; serum acid phosphatase, 1.7 units (upper limit of normal, 2.1 units); serum Na^+, 145 mEq per liter; serum K^+, 5.4 mEq per liter; serum Cl^-, 104 mEq per liter; and serum HCO_3^-, 20 mEq per liter. An intravenous pyelogram (I.V.P.) obtained the day after admission showed poor opacification and marked dilatation of both renal pelves and both ureters.

Constant drainage of the urinary bladder was established, and on the first three days in the hospital, the patient's daily urine volumes were 7.5, 5.6, and 5.3 liters, respectively; he lost 10 kg in body weight during this period. On the sixth hospital day, cystoscopic examination performed under spinal anesthesia revealed such severe prostatic enlargement that an open, suprapubic approach would be required in order to remove the gland. A needle biopsy of the prostate was obtained, and it revealed benign hyperplasia. The patient was discharged on the eighth hospital day; he was followed as an outpatient while on constant bladder drainage until he was in better condition for prostatectomy.

After three weeks, the serum creatinine concentration had stabilized at 2.2 mg/100 ml and the serum electrolyte levels were normal. The patient was feeling much stronger, he now had a good appetite, his blood pressure was 120/60 mm Hg, and the headaches and edema had disappeared. On repeat I.V.P. there was improved concentration of the dye within the renal pelvis, much less dilatation of the collecting system, and a large filling defect at the base of the bladder. A suprapubic prostatectomy was performed at this time; all three lobes of the prostate were enlarged, the specimen weighed 85 g and showed benign nodular hyperplasia. When last checked two months later, the patient was voiding clear urine, which was sterile when cultured. He had good control of micturition, and the force of the urinary stream was good.

1. On the basis of the urinalysis done on admission, can you estimate the urine osmolality?
2. How do you explain the urgency incontinence, the hesitancy, the involuntary voiding, and the anorexia, lethargy, and headaches?
3. How do you account for the weight loss of 10 kg during the first three days after admission?
4. Why was prostatectomy not performed immediately on the first admission?

Problem 11-2

At age 13 years this patient was referred by a school nurse to a pediatrician because the patient was lethargic and was suspected of taking drugs. The pediatrician elicited a history of enuresis, polyuria, and polydipsia that had been present for many years, and of a urinary tract infection that had occurred two years earlier. His initial evaluation included a BUN determination (91 mg/100 ml), and he referred the patient to a nephrologist.

On admission to the hospital, the patient was noted to be small, pale, and apathetic, but the physical examination was otherwise unremarkable. Laboratory data confirmed the diagnosis of moderately advanced chronic renal failure: the BUN was 82 mg/100 ml and the serum creatinine concentration, 5.4 mg/100 ml; other findings were metabolic acidosis, anemia, hyperphosphatemia, hypocalcemia, and an elevated plasma concentration of parathyroid hormone. Several urinalyses revealed a specific gravity that was "fixed" at about 1.005 and a protein concentration of 0.05 g/100 ml; the urine did not contain glucose or abnormal amounts of red or white blood cells, and it was sterile when cultured. (Note that obstructive nephropathy – because it affects primarily the renal medullary interstitium – is one of the few causes of renal dysfunction in which the results of urinalysis may be normal or very nearly so.)

Investigations by a urologist included an I.V.P., a voiding cystourethrogram, a cystometrogram, cystoscopy, and retrograde pyelograms, in that order. These tests revealed markedly dilated urinary conduits, including the renal calyces, pelves, both ureters, and the bladder. There appeared to be obstruction at both ureterovesical junctions, which was thought to be due to aperistaltic segments in both ureters. The bladder contracted poorly, and it could not be determined whether this defect resulted from congenital neuromuscular abnormalities or from long-standing polyuria and dilation. Although the patient was at times able to empty her bladder, at other times she could not, and as much as 600 ml of residual urine was sometimes obtained when she was catheterized.

It was obvious that better drainage of the ureters and renal pelves and calyces needed to be established. Consequently, a ureteroneocystostomy was performed 11 days after admission; this procedure consisted of tapering of the lower thirds of both ureters and reimplantation of the ureters into the bladder. Emptying of the bladder remained a problem after the operation, and the patient was therefore taught to express the urine either manually every two hours or by rolling over a ball. Despite these measures, however, her renal function deteriorated, probably because the constant dilation of the bladder was occluding the ureters as they traversed the wall of the bladder. Four months after the operation, her BUN was 103 mg/100 ml, her serum creatinine, 9.9 mg/100 ml, she had developed hypertension of

150/100 mm Hg, her heart had enlarged, and x-rays of the bones showed renal osteodystrophy. The patient was therefore placed on chronic dialysis, after which she received a kidney from her brother; at latest follow-up (14 months later), she was doing well.

Comment. This patient's history has been presented, not as a problem, but to emphasize that if urinary obstruction goes unrecognized and untreated for too long, there may be so much irreversible renal damage that recovery without dialysis or transplantation is impossible. Although chronic renal failure may have been inevitable in this patient (where the cause of the urinary obstruction was probably congenital neuromuscular dysfunction of the bladder and ureters), there can be little doubt that her serious condition could have been diagnosed and treated several years earlier.

Selected References

General

Bricker, N. S., and Klahr, S. Obstructive Nephropathy. In M. B. Strauss and L. G. Welt (eds.), *Diseases of the Kidney* (2nd ed.). Boston: Little, Brown, 1971.

Campbell, M. F., and Harrison, J. H. (eds.). *Urology* (3rd ed.). Philadelphia: Saunders, 1970.

Coe, F. L., and Kavalach, A. G. Hypercalciuria and hyperuricosuria in patients with calcium nephrolithiasis. *N. Engl. J. Med.* 291:1344, 1974.

Glenn, J. F. (ed.). *Urologic Surgery* (2nd ed.). Hagerstown, Md.: Harper & Row, 1975.

Guggenheim, S. J., and Schrier, R. W. Obstructive Nephropathy: Pathophysiology and Management. In R. W. Schrier (ed.), *Renal and Electrolyte Disorders.* Boston: Little, Brown, 1976.

Hinman, F., Jr. The Pathophysiology of Urinary Obstruction. In M. F. Campbell and J. H. Harrison (eds.), *Urology* (3rd ed.). Philadelphia: Saunders, 1970.

Papper, S. *Clinical Nephrology* (2nd ed.). Boston: Little, Brown, 1978.

Smith, L. H., Jr., and Williams, H. E. Kidney Stones. In M. B. Strauss and L. G. Welt (eds.), *Diseases of the Kidney* (2nd ed.). Boston: Little, Brown, 1971.

Williams, H. E. Nephrolithiasis. *N. Engl. J. Med.* 290:33, 1974.

Wilson, D. R. Renal function during and following obstruction. *Annu. Rev. Med.* 28:329, 1977.

Pathogenesis of Hydronephrosis

Blantz, R. C., Konnen, K. S., and Tucker, B. J. Glomerular filtration response to elevated ureteral pressure in both the hydropenic and the plasma-expanded rat. *Circ. Res.* 37:819, 1975.

Bulger, R. E., Lorentz, W. B., Jr., Colindres, R. E., and Gottschalk, C. W. Morphologic changes in rat renal proximal tubules and their tight junctions with increased intraluminal pressure. *Lab. Invest.* 30:136, 1974.

Falchuk, K. H., and Berliner, R. W. Hydrostatic pressures in peritubular capillaries and tubules in the rat kidney. *Am. J. Physiol.* 220:1422, 1971.

Gottschalk, C. W., and Mylle, M. Micropuncture study of pressures in proximal tubules and peritubular capillaries of the rat kidney and their relation to ureteral and renal venous pressures. *Am. J. Physiol.* 185:430, 1956.

Hinman, F., and Hepler, A. B. Experimental hydronephrosis. The effect of changes in blood pressure and in blood flow on its rate of development. II. Partial obstruction of the renal artery: Diminished blood flow; diminished intrarenal pressure and oliguria. *Arch. Surg.* 11:649, 1925.

Hinman, F., and Lee-Brown, R. K. Pyelovenous back flow. Its relation to pelvic reabsorption, to hydronephrosis and to accidents of pyelography. *J. A. M. A.* 82:607, 1924.

Hinman, F., and Vecki, M. Pyelovenous back flow. The fate of phenolsulphonephthalein in a normal renal pelvis with the ureter tied. *J. Urol.* 15:267, 1926.

Kiil, F. *The Function of the Ureter and Renal Pelvis: Pressure Recordings and Radiographic Studies of the Normal and Diseased Urinary Tract of Man.* Philadelphia: Saunders, 1957.

Lawson, J. D., and Tomlinson, W. B. Observations on the dynamics of acute urinary retention in the dog. *J. Urol.* 66:678, 1951.

Levinsky, N. G., and Berliner, R. W. Changes in composition of the urine in ureter and bladder at low urine flow. *Am. J. Physiol.* 196:549, 1959.

Lorentz, W. B., Lassiter, W. E., and Gottschalk, C. W. Renal tubular permeability during increased intrarenal pressure. *J. Clin. Invest.* 51:484, 1972.

Malvin, R. L., Wilde, W. S., and Sullivan, L. P. Localization of nephron transport by stop flow analysis. *Am. J. Physiol.* 194:135, 1958.

Melick, W. F., Karellos, D., and Naryka, J. J. Pressure studies of hydronephrosis in children by means of the strain gauge. *J. Urol.* 85:703, 1961.

Risholm, L., and Öbrink, K. J. Pyelorenal backflow in man. *Acta Chir. Scand.* 115:144, 1958.

Struthers, N. W. The role of manometry in the investigation of pelviureteral function. *Br. J. Urol.* 41:129, 1969.

Wilmer, H. A. The static intrapelvic pressure of the hydronephrotic kidney. *Proc. Soc. Exp. Biol. Med.* 56:52, 1944.

Functional Impairment

Altschul, R., and Fedor, S. Vascular changes in hydronephrosis. *Am. Heart J.* 46:291, 1953.

Berlyne, G. M. Distal tubular function in chronic hydronephrosis. *Q. J. Med.* 30:339, 1961.

Berlyne, G. M., and Macken, A. On the mechanism of renal inability to produce a concentrated urine in chronic hydronephrosis. *Clin. Sci.* 22:315, 1962.

Better, O. S., Arieff, A. I., Massry, S. G., Kleeman, C. R., and Maxwell, M. H. Studies on renal function after relief of complete unilateral ureteral obstruction of three months' duration in man. *Am. J. Med.* 54:234, 1973.

Dorhout Mees, E. J. Reversible water losing state, caused by incomplete ureteric obstruction. *Acta Med. Scand.* 168:193, 1960.

Earley, L. E. Extreme polyuria in obstructive uropathy. Report of a case of "water-losing nephritis" in an infant, with a discussion of polyuria. *N. Engl. J. Med.* 255:600, 1956.

Edvall, C. A. Influence of ureteral obstruction (hydronephrosis) on renal function in man. *J. Appl. Physiol.* 14:855, 1959.

Eknoyan, G., Suki, W. N., Martinez-Maldonado, M., and Anhalt, M. A. Chronic hydronephrosis: Observations on the mechanism of the defect in urine concentration. *Proc. Soc. Exp. Biol. Med.* 134:634, 1970.

Gillenwater, J. Y., Westervelt, F. B., Jr., Vaughan, E. D., Jr., and Howards, S. S. Renal function after release of chronic unilateral hydronephrosis in man. *Kidney Int.* 7:179, 1975.

Guze, L. G., and Beeson, P. B. Experimental pyelonephritis. I. Effect of ureteral ligation on the course of bacterial infection in the kidney of the rat. *J. Exp. Med.* 104:803, 1956.

Guze, L. G., and Beeson, P. B. Experimental pyelonephritis. II. Effect of partial ureteral obstruction on the course of bacterial infection in the kidney of the rat and the rabbit. *Yale J. Biol. Med.* 30:315, 1958.

Hinman, F., and Hepler, A. B. Experimental hydronephrosis. The effect of changes in blood pressure and in blood flow on its rate of development. II. Partial obstruction of the renal artery: Diminished blood flow; diminished intrarenal pressure and oliguria. *Arch. Surg.* 11:649, 1925.

Idbohrn, H., and Muren, A. Renal blood flow in experimental hydronephrosis. *Acta Physiol. Scand.* 38:200, 1957.

Jaenike, J. R., and Bray, G. A. Effects of acute transitory urinary obstruction in the dog. *Am. J. Physiol.* 199:1219, 1960.

Keith, N. M., and Pulford, D. S., Jr. Experimental hydronephrosis. Functional and anatomic changes in the kidney following partial ureteral obstruction. *Arch. Intern. Med.* 20:853, 1917.

Kerr, W. S., Jr. Effect of complete ureteral obstruction for one week on kidney function. *J. Appl. Physiol.* 6:762, 1954.

McCrory, W. W., Shibuya, M., Leumann, E., and Karp, R. Studies of renal function in children with chronic hydronephrosis. *Pediatr. Clin. North Am.* 18:445, 1971.

Olbrich, O., Woodford-Williams, E., Irvine, R. E., and Webster, D. Renal function in prostatism. *Lancet* 1:1322, 1957.

Platts, M. M., and Williams, J. L. Renal function in patients with unilateral hydronephrosis. *Br. Med. J.* 2:1243, 1963.

Roussak, N. J., and Oleesky, S. Water-losing nephritis. A syndrome simulating diabetes insipidus. *Q. J. Med.* 23:147, 1954.

Selkurt, E. E., Brandfonbrener, M., and Geller, H. M. Effects of ureteral pressure increase on renal hemodynamics and the handling of electrolytes and water. *Am. J. Physiol.* 170:61, 1952.

Share, L. Effect of increased ureteral pressure on renal function. *Am. J. Physiol.* 168:97, 1952.

Suki, W., Eknoyan, G., Rector, F. C., Jr., and Seldin, D. W. Patterns of nephron perfusion in acute and chronic hydronephrosis. *J. Clin. Invest.* 45:122, 1966.

Walls, J., Buerkert, J. E., Purkerson, M. L., and Klahr, S. Nature of the acidifying defect after the relief of ureteral obstruction. *Kidney Int.* 7:304, 1975.

Wilson, D. R. Micropuncture study of chronic obstructive nephropathy before and after release of obstruction. *Kidney Int.* 2:119, 1972.

Zetterström, R., Ericsson, N. O., and Winberg, J. Separate renal function studies in predominantly unilateral hydronephrosis. *Acta Paediatr.* (Stockh.) 47:540, 1958.

Postobstructive Diuresis

Bercovitch, D. D., Kasen, L., Blann, L., and Levitt, M. F. The postobstructive kidney. Observations on nephron function after the relief of 24 hr of ureteral ligation in the dog. *J. Clin. Invest.* 50:1154, 1971.

Bricker, N. S., Shwayri, E. I., Reardan, J. B., Kellog, D., Merrill, J. P., and Holmes, J. H. An abnormality in renal function resulting from urinary tract obstruction. *Am. J. Med.* 23:554, 1957.

Buerkert, J., Alexander, E., Purkerson, M. L., and Klahr, S. On the site of decreased fluid reabsorption after release of ureteral obstruction in the rat. *J. Lab. Clin. Med.* 87:397, 1976.

Bulger, R. E., Lorentz, W. B., Jr., Colindres, R. E., and Gottschalk, C. W. Morphologic changes in rat renal proximal tubules and their tight junctions with increased intraluminal pressure. *Lab. Invest.* 30:136, 1974.

Edwards, B. R., Novakova, A., Sutton, R. A. L., and Dirks, J. H. Effects of acute urea infusion on proximal tubular reabsorption in the dog kidney. *Am. J. Physiol.* 224:73, 1973.

Harris, R. H., and Yarger, W. E. The pathogenesis of postobstructive diuresis. The role of circulating natriuretic and diuretic factors, including urea. *J. Clin. Invest.* 56:880, 1975.

Howards, S. S. Post-obstructive diuresis: A misunderstood phenomenon. *J. Urol.* 110:537, 1973.

Jaenike, J. R. The renal functional defect of postobstructive nephropathy. *J. Clin. Invest.* 50:2999, 1972.

Massry, S. G., Schainuck, L. I., Goldsmith, C., and Schreiner, G. E. Studies on the mechanism of diuresis after relief of urinary-tract obstruction. *Ann. Intern. Med.* 66:149, 1967.

McDougal, W. S., and Wright, F. S. Defect in proximal and distal sodium transport in post-obstructive diuresis. *Kidney Int.* 2:304, 1972.

Muldowney, F. P., Duffy, G. J., Kelly, D. G., Duff, F. A., Harrington, C., and Freaney, R. Sodium diuresis after relief of obstructive uropathy. *N. Engl. J. Med.* 274:1294, 1966.

Sonnenberg, H., and Wilson, D. R. The role of the medullary collecting ducts in postobstructive diuresis. *J. Clin. Invest.* 57:1564, 1976.

Vaughn, E. D., Jr., and Gillenwater, J. Y. Diagnosis, characterization, and management of post-obstructive diuresis. *J. Urol.* 109:286, 1973.

Wilson, B., Reisman, D. D., and Moyer, C. A. Fluid balance in the urological patient: Disturbances in the renal regulation of the excretion of water and sodium salts following decompression of the urinary bladder. *J. Urol.* 66:805, 1951.

Wilson, D. R. The influence of volume expansion on renal function after relief of chronic unilateral ureteral obstruction. *Kidney Int.* 5:402, 1974.

Wilson, D. R. Nephron functional heterogeneity in the postobstructive kidney. *Kidney Int.* 7:19, 1975.

Wilson, D. R., and Honrath, U. Cross-circulation study of natriuretic factors in postobstructive diuresis. *J. Clin. Invest.* 57:380, 1976.

Witte, M. H., Short, F. A., and Hollander, W., Jr. Massive polyuria and natriuresis following relief of urinary tract obstruction. *Am. J. Med.* 37:320, 1964.

Yarger, W. E., Aynedjian, H. S., and Bank, N. A micropuncture study of postobstructive diuresis in the rat. *J. Clin. Invest.* 51:625, 1972.

12 : Mechanisms of Discrete Tubular Dysfunction

Definition

This chapter deals with that group of renal diseases in which the defect is limited to one or more tubular transport processes but in which other renal functions, including the GFR, are characteristically normal. Generalized renal failure may intervene in some of these disorders in their later stages; but when it does, it develops as a consequence of generalized tubular damage, which itself will have arisen as a secondary effect of the defect in the primary transport process. Thus, in cystinuria, diminished tubular reabsorption of cystine (Table 12-1) may lead to the formation of cystine stones and ultimately to chronic renal failure due to obstructive nephropathy and infection. Initially, however, the disease is manifested simply by decreased tubular reabsorption and hence increased excretion of cystine, lysine, arginine, and ornithine. Similarly, in renal tubular acidosis, type 1, the defect is initially one of defective tubular secretion of H^+ (Table 12-1), but eventually the patient may develop chronic renal failure from nephrocalcinosis.

Some examples of renal tubular disorders are listed in Table 12-1. A number of features should be noted. (1) Although these conditions are often inherited, many of them can also be acquired. For example, the Fanconi syndrome may have a genetic origin, but it can also be caused by exogenous toxins (e.g., drugs and heavy metals) or endogenous toxins (e.g., copper in Wilson's disease). (2) The conditions may be harmless (as are renal glycosuria or iminoglycinuria), cause morbidity (as do certain forms of cystinuria or vitamin D-resistant rickets), or be fatal in childhood (as are certain types of the Fanconi syndrome). (3) In many instances, the abnormality of transport is not confined to the kidneys, but it may occur as well in other organs, most notably the intestines. Often, in fact, the intestinal defect may be the more important in causing symptoms; such may be the case in vitamin D-resistant rickets and Hartnup disease. (4) In many cases, there is enough overlap of defects to render strict classification impossible. Thus, vitamin D-resistant rickets is sometimes associated with aminoaciduria and renal tubular

Table 12-1
Examples of discrete tubular dysfunctions. The list is by no means exhaustive.

Name (Synonym)	Renal Defect	Comments
Nephrogenic diabetes insipidus (vasopressin-resistant diabetes insipidus; nephrogenic dysfunction of urinary concentration)	↓ Reabsorption of H_2O from distal tubules and collecting ducts due to: ↓ Vasopressin-induced H_2O permeability and/or ↓ Buildup of corticopapillary interstitial osmotic gradient	May be inherited or acquired. When defect is severe, leading to excretion of hyposmotic urine, it is called *diabetes insipidus;* when milder, it is termed a *concentrating defect* (see Chap. 13)
Renal glycosuria	↓ Reabsorption of glucose due to: ↑ Splay and GT imbalance (?) or ↓ Tm_G	Usually discovered on routine examination (e.g., for life insurance); asymptomatic and harmless. Must be distinguished from diabetes mellitus
Renal tubular acidosis (RTA; distal: type 1 or classical RTA; proximal: type 2 RTA)	Proximal type (type 2): ↓ Reabsorption of HCO_3^- Distal type (type 1): ↓ Secretion of H^+	Multiple inherited and acquired causes similar to those listed for Fanconi syndrome
Vitamin D-resistant rickets (familial hypophosphatemia)	↓ Reabsorption of phosphate	Additional inherited defects include abnormal metabolism of vitamin D and deficient absorption of Ca^{2+} from the gut. The latter, by causing secondary hyperparathyroidism (see Fig. 10-11), may be the principal or contributing cause of phosphaturia and hypophosphatemia
Pseudohypoparathyroidism	↑ Reabsorption of phosphate ↓ Reabsorption of Ca^{2+}	An extremely rare, inherited disorder due to partial or complete unresponsiveness of kidneys and bone to parathyroid hormone (PTH)
Cystinuria	↓ Reabsorption of the amino acids cystine, lysine, arginine, and ornithine	May or may not be associated with decreased absorption of the same amino acids from the jejunum
Hartnup disease	↓ Reabsorption of certain aliphatic and ring-structured neutral α-amino acids (glutamine, serine, asparagine,	Named after the first family studied. Associated decreased absorption of tryptophan and other amino acids from

	histidine, threonine, tryptophan) but excluding iminoacids and glycine	jejunum may be more important in causing symptoms (which rarely occur) than the renal defect
Fanconi syndrome (*variants* include, among others, Lignac-Fanconi syndrome, de Toni-Fanconi syndrome, and Lowe's syndrome)	↓ Reabsorption, primarily in proximal tubules, of: Seen early: All amino acids, Phosphate, Glucose Later and variable occurrence: HCO_3^-, K^+, Other substances, Reabsorption of H_2O possibly secondary to hypokalemia and hypercalciuria (see Chap. 13)	May be inherited either as a specific tubular abnormality or as a general metabolic disorder (e.g., cystinosis, Wilson's disease, or glycogen storage disease) that leads to tubular damage. May also be acquired (e.g., in heavy metal poisoning, in multiple myeloma, from usage of outdated tetracyclines, or following renal transplantation). Glucosuria is not seen in Lowe's syndrome
Iminoglycinuria	↓ Reabsorption of proline, hydroxyproline, and glycine	May be associated with decreased intestinal absorption of the same amino acids
Methionine malabsorption	↓ Reabsorption of methionine	Associated with decreased intestinal absorption of methionine (included here mainly to indicate that there is a host of other, mostly discrete aminoacidurias that have not been listed in this table)

acidosis (RTA), possibly as a result of secondary hyperparathyroidism. Similarly, iminoglycinuria may be seen in hyperprolinemia and hydroxyprolinemia, in the Fanconi syndrome, and as a normal phenomenon in babies from newborn up to three months of age. (5) There are many renal tubular defects, and Table 12-1 by no means provides a complete listing. More of these disorders are being described or defined as more precise experimental and diagnostic techniques become available. It is possible, for example, that Bartter's syndrome will eventually be included among these disorders if it should turn out that this disease involves a specific deficiency in the reabsorption of Na^+ in the proximal tubules. (6) It is not necessary to memorize the details of each of these numerous and mostly very rare disorders. What is required is an awareness and a high index of suspicion for the existence of these specific entities. Suspicion should be aroused if any of the following findings in a patient *does not have a ready explanation:* aminoaciduria; polyuria; failure to thrive; mental retardation or other neurological signs (e.g., cerebellar ataxia and hypotonia); rickets, osteomalacia, and bone pain; glycosuria; systemic acidosis with only a weakly acidic urine; and nephrocalcinosis. (7) Because many of the discrete tubular dysfunctions entail an increased excretion of amino acids (Table 12-1), these disorders are sometimes thought of as being identical to the aminoacidurias. This view, however, is incorrect. Increased urinary excretion of amino acids arises perhaps more commonly from the deficient enzymatic breakdown of a given amino acid than from defective tubular transport. An example is phenylketonuria, which arises from a lack of the hepatic enzyme, phenylalanine hydroxylase. There is a consequent elevation in the plasma concentration of phenylalanine and an increase in its filtered load, which then exceeds the tubular capacity for reabsorbing this amino acid. The mechanism for this kind of aminoaciduria – known as the *overflow type* – is thus analogous to that for the glucosuria seen in diabetes mellitus; the analogy can be extended beyond the aminoacidurias to disorders involving other substances, such as L-xylulose in essential pentosuria. Suffice it to say that an overflow type of disorder, of whatever substance, should be distinguished from the discrete renal tubular disorders.

Mechanisms of Defective Tubular Transport

Theoretically, an abnormality of tubular transport may result from one or more of the following four causes: (1) defective reabsorption, (2) defective secretion, (3) defective permeability, or (4) glomerulotubular imbalance. (This classification may be oversimplified or redundant; see next paragraph.) In the following sections, we will describe several specific diseases that exemplify one or more of these mechanisms: cystinuria as a prototype of a discrete reabsorptive defect; the Fanconi syndrome as a generalized abnormality of net reabsorption; renal tubular acidosis, illustrating both a reabsorptive (type 2) and a secretory (type 1) defect; and renal glycosuria, which represents a combination of deficient reabsorption and possibly of glomerulotubular imbalance. Nephrogenic diabetes insipidus will be taken up in the next chapter, where it will be discussed as an example of defective permeability and possibly also of deficient reabsorption.

C. R. Scriver, among others, has presented a functional classification that is based on kinetic analyses of transport. This classification postulates the following defects that, alone or in combination, might account for deficient net reabsorption: (1) decreased uptake at the luminal border; (2) excessive back-flux from the intracellular pool into the lumen; (3) defective intracellular catabolism of the transported species, buildup of that species within the cells, and hence increased back-flux across the luminal membrane; and (4) decreased transport across the peritubular membrane from the cell into the peritubular fluid. Defects of secretion could be explained by the same schema, but with the directions of the fluxes reversed. In this classification, defective permeability and disorders of hormone-mediated transport might be merely special instances affecting one of the four major steps.

Vitamin D-resistant rickets, though an important clinical entity, will not be described in detail in this chapter, because the primary or most important lesion may be deficient transport in the gut rather than in the kidneys. Similarly, no attempt will be made to describe the myriad of discrete tubular disorders, nor even all of those listed in Table 12-1. Only the principles for approaching this type of renal disease will be presented here; the intention is to provide a basis for informed reading about these disorders in the standard textbooks.

Cystinuria: Discrete Reabsorptive Defects

Renal Handling of Amino Acids in Health

Most amino acids are filtered and reabsorbed. Although the details of the handling of amino acids depend on the particular amino acid, certain generalizations hold. The transport process is active (i.e., energy-requiring), probably occurs mainly or solely in the proximal tubules, and is complete for most amino acids, so their concentration in normal urine is zero. At least five different carrier systems have been demonstrated: (1) that for neutral amino acids (e.g., cystine); (2) that for dibasic amino acids (e.g., arginine, ornithine, and lysine); (3) that for dicarboxylic α-amino acids (i.e., aspartic and glutamic acids); (4) that for glycine and the imino acids (proline and hydroxyproline); and (5) that for β-amino acids (e.g., β-alanine and β-aminoisobutyric acid). A transport maximum (*Tm*) can be demonstrated for some amino acids, but the degree of splay in the titration curve may vary widely from the very small splay in the case of lysine, for example, to the very great splay in the case of glycine. In many instances, competitive inhibition by related amino acids can be demonstrated, and most of the carriers show stereospecificity in that the naturally occurring L-amino acids are transported more readily than the D-isomers. In some as-yet-undefined fashion, the transport of certain amino acids depends on the presence of Na^+.

A possible scheme for the active transport of amino acids from the renal tubular lumen into peritubular blood is shown in Figure 12-1. A carrier, C, within the luminal membrane may have affinity for one or more amino acids, A; the chemical nature of the carrier is not yet known, but it may be a specific membrane protein whose production is controlled by a single gene. The dependence of the transport process on Na^+ (which is probably required to produce asymmetry of the carrier) is shown by the formation of a carrier-amino acid-Na^+ complex. By as-yet-unknown mechanisms, this complex "traverses" the luminal membrane, after which the Na^+ and the amino acid are released into the cytoplasm; they then move across the cell, through the peritubular membrane, and into the peritubular fluid and blood. In the process of dissociation of the complex, the carrier, C, undergoes a change to C′, which has a diminished affinity for the

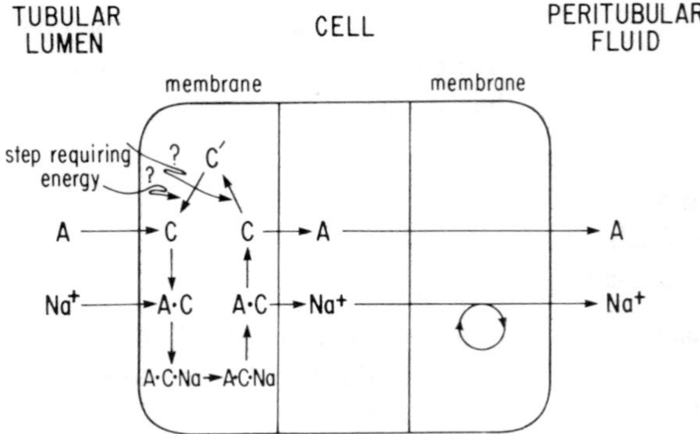

Figure 12-1
Possible scheme for carrier-mediated, active transport of amino acids across the renal tubular epithelium. *A* = amino acid; *Na* = sodium; *C* = carrier with high affinity for A; *C′* = carrier in form with low affinity for A. Adapted from C. R. Scriver and L. E. Rosenberg, *Amino Acid Metabolism and Its Disorders*. Philadelphia: Saunders, 1973.

amino acids and Na^+. The energy-requiring step in active transport is thought to occur either in the transformation of C to C′ or in the reconversion of C′ to C. Although this scheme is hypothetical and although differences in detail undoubtedly exist, the differences may be mainly variations on a theme (e.g., the carrier-mediated transport mechanism might be located in the peritubular rather than the luminal membrane).

Abnormal transepithelial transport of amino acids could theoretically arise from a defect in any one of the steps shown in Figure 12-1, and the ultimate aim of those doing research on the discrete tubular dysfunctions is to pinpoint the defect to a particular step. It can be readily seen that such work will clarify not only a specific and possibly rare disease, but also the general mechanisms of amino acid transport or of other transport systems, be they in the kidneys, the intestines, or other organs. In fact, the significance of the renal tubular disorders rests partly on this wider applicability, which, in the case of a number of disorders, has already taken place.

Defect in Cystinuria

In 1908, A. E. Garrod, in his famous Croonian lectures entitled ***Inborn Errors of Metabolism,*** postulated that cystinuria resulted from an inherited block in the catabolism of cystine. Although the significance of Garrod's highly original proposal of genetically determined failure in metabolism was enormous, he incorrectly classified cystinuria as an overflow type of disorder. It was shown subsequently that decreased catabolism of cystine did not occur in cystinuric patients, a conclusion that must also be drawn from the evidence of C. E. Dent and his associates: that in cystinuria, the increased urinary excretion of cystine – and of three other amino acids, lysine, arginine, and ornithine – takes place in the face of normal or low plasma concentrations of all four amino acids. The defect was defined correctly by Dent, who extended Garrod's concept of inborn errors of peripheral metabolism to "inborn errors of transport."

It was thought originally that since cystine, lysine, arginine, and ornithine share certain structural similarities (most notably the presence of two amino groups), they might all be transported by the same carrier. Subsequent experiments, however, which were performed mainly on renal cortical slices in vitro, made clear that there are two "carriers" for these four amino acids, one for cystine and the other for lysine, arginine, and ornithine. This conclusion has been strengthened by the later finding of cystinuric patients whose excretion of the other three amino acids is normal, as well as of patients who excrete abnormal amounts of lysine, arginine, and ornithine but normal amounts of cystine (so-called hyperdibasic aminoaciduria). One might predict that in classical cystinuria where all four amino acids are excreted at abnormally high rates, there might be demonstrable defects in both carrier systems, whereas in the other types, only one carrier is affected. Although it has not yet been accomplished in classical cystinuria, an abnormality, possibly in the number of carriers, can be demonstrated for the system that transports lysine, arginine, and ornithine; further, a renal tubular defect limited to cystine has been described in at least one pedigree.

In cystinuria, the clearance of cystine can be twice as high as the clearance of inulin, reflecting tubular secretion. It is not yet known, however, what mechanisms underlie this secretory process. Similarly, the mechanisms responsible for the often-associated intestinal defects of amino acid transport have not been unraveled. Suffice it to say that different patterns and degrees of abnormal intestinal transport of the four amino acids have been identified and that there are differences between the renal and the intestinal systems. On the basis of the phenotypic patterns, it has been proposed that there may be as many as nine different genotypes for cystinuria. The disorder is inherited as an autosomal recessive trait, and it can be detected at birth at an incidence of about 1 in 16,000 live births.

The clinical importance of cystinuria arises from the fact that cystine is the least soluble of the naturally occurring amino acids. Its solubility depends on the pH of the solution (Fig. 12-2), and the solubility is particularly low at the pH of normal urine, that is, between pH 5.0 and 6.5. Given the fact that cys-

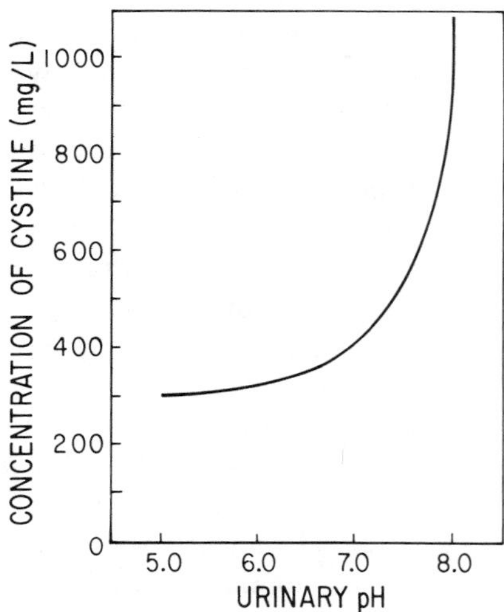

Figure 12-2
Saturating concentrations of cystine in urine at different pH values. Modified from C. E. Dent and B. Senior, *Br. J. Urol.* 27:317, 1955.

tinuric patients commonly excrete 400 to 1,300 mg of cystine in the urine per day (the normal value is 40 to 80 mg per day), it can be seen from Figure 12-2 that these patients are in constant danger of forming cystine crystals and stones, even though cystine can exist in urine in a supersaturated state. The propensity for forming stones is so great that about 50 percent of cystinurics die prematurely from obstructive nephropathy (Chap. 11) and its attendant hazards of infection and urological intervention.

The preventive therapy for cystinuria involves four approaches, only the last two of which have proved really successful: (1) reducing the daily production of cystine through dietary means, (2) increasing the solubility of cystine in urine by raising the urinary pH, (3) increasing the urine volume sufficiently to keep the cystine in solution, and (4) changing the cystine with D-penicillamine to a mixed disulfide, a chemical form that is more soluble than cystine alone. Inasmuch as about 80 percent of the cystine comes from methionine, the dietary approach would have to involve methionine restriction, which brings with it its own serious problems. It is difficult to raise the pH of urine sufficiently to increase the solubility of cystine, mainly because the patient has to take an enormous amount of bicarbonate salts to achieve this goal. A not uncommon dose of $NaHCO_3$ in cystinuric patients is 15 g per day, which, with a standard tablet of 600 mg, involves taking 25 tablets each day. The single most effective measure is to drink enough water to increase the urine volume. If a patient excretes 900 mg of cystine per day on the average, the daily urine volume would have to be at least 3 liters in order to keep the cystine in solution (Fig. 12-2). He would have to drink at least 3 to 4 liters (15 to 20 glassfuls) per day, and this amount would have to be distributed more or less throughout the 24 hours. One usually advises such patients to drink at least 2½ glassfuls when going to sleep. As a result of this intake, the patient will have to arise at least once during the night, at which time he should drink another 2½ glassfuls, and so on. More recently, D-penicillamine has been introduced as chemical therapy. In the reaction shown in Figure 12-3, D-penicillamine undergoes a thiol disulfide exchange to form cysteine-penicillamine mixed disulfide. The latter is much more soluble in urine than is cystine. Both penicillamine and a high fluid intake can not only prevent the formation of new stones but also dissolve existing stones. Unfortunately, penicillamine can have some serious side effects, such as skin rashes, lupus-like arthralgias, nephrotic syndrome, and hematological disorders. It should therefore be used with caution and only when needed. (A clinical history, illustrating the tribulations of a patient with cystinuria, is given as Problem 12-1.)

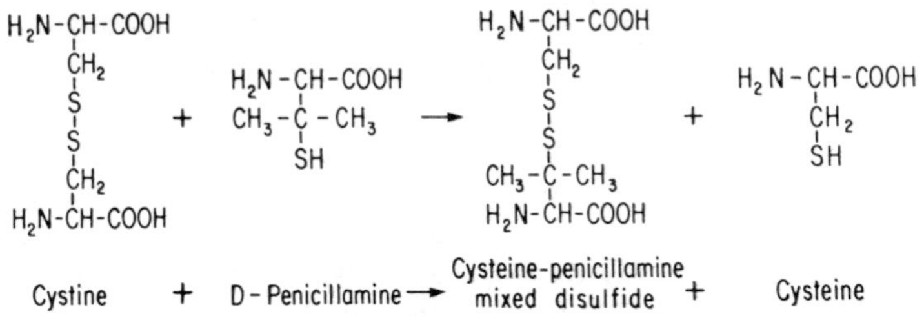

Cystine + D-Penicillamine → Cysteine-penicillamine mixed disulfide + Cysteine

Figure 12-3
Reaction whereby D-penicillamine combines with cystine to form the more soluble cysteine and cysteine-penicillamine mixed disulfide.

Fanconi Syndrome: Generalized Reabsorptive Defect

Phenotypic Picture

Most commonly, the Fanconi syndrome is manifested by increased urinary excretion of virtually all amino acids, glucose, and phosphate. Only the last of these leads to disability; increased phosphate excretion is manifested in children mainly as rickets and a failure to thrive, with death occurring from renal failure, and in adults, as osteomalacia and bone pain. In more severe instances and at later stages, other manifestations and consequences of failure in proximal tubular transport may be seen: increased excretion of HCO_3^- and acidosis, which reflect type 2 RTA (Table 12-1), and increased excretion of K^+ and sometimes of Ca^{2+}, resulting in neuromuscular weakness and nephrogenic diabetes insipidus (Table 12-1 and Chap. 13).

Other phenotypic manifestations depend on the underlying disease, and since the causes are so numerous (Table 12-2), such manifestations can vary from very severe ones (e.g., blindness, mental deficiency, hypotonia, and death before adolescence, as in Lowe's syndrome) to transient hypokalemia, acidosis, and mild renal failure with full recovery after a few weeks (e.g., as in certain types of poisoning).

Defect in Fanconi Syndrome

It is possible, perhaps likely, that all occurrences of the Fanconi syndrome are due to a toxic effect on the renal tubular cells. The toxin can be either exogenous or one that is built up endogenously because of a failure in some metabolic step. (Although there are numerous examples of such endogenous toxins, we shall here cite cystinosis, not only because it is one of the major causes of the Fanconi syndrome, but also to emphasize that it should not be confused with cystinuria. The latter in-

Table 12-2
Causes of the Fanconi syndrome

Hereditary defects in metabolism:
- Cystinosis
- Unknown (so-called idiopathic)
- Lowe's syndrome (oculocerebrorenal syndrome)
- Tyrosinemia
- Galactosemia
- Glycogen storage disease
- Hereditary fructose intolerance
- Wilson's disease (copper toxin)

Exogenous toxins:
- Heavy metals (lead, cadmium, mercury, uranium)
- Drugs (degraded tetracycline, salicylate, tricromyl [3-methylchromone])
- Cresol
- Maleic acid (experimental model in rats)

Others:
- Following renal transplantation
- Multiple myeloma
- Sjögren's syndrome
- Amyloidosis
- Nephrotic syndrome

volves a discrete defect in two renal transport systems; cystinosis, on the other hand, is a generalized metabolic defect that leads to high intracellular concentrations of cystine throughout the body and thereby causes malfunction, including a general failure of renal tubular transport.) That a toxin is probably involved even in the inherited, idiopathic variety of the Fanconi syndrome is suggested by the finding that a 14-year-old boy who had severe chronic renal failure from this form of Fanconi syndrome redeveloped the syndrome within five weeks after receiving a transplanted kidney. The proximal tubular cells may be especially affected, since the toxins may be reabsorbed mainly in this segment of the nephron. Although the kidneys may be particularly susceptible because of the high rate of renal blood flow, other organs are often involved as well, especially the liver, bone marrow, and intestine; in the last, for example, analogous defects in transport are often seen along with the renal defects.

Just how the toxins interfere with proximal tubular transport is not known; since so many exogenous and endogenous substances are implicated (Table 12-2), it is possible that they interfere with transport in different ways. A common thread, however, may be an impairment in the availability of energy that prevents conversion or reconversion of the carrier to its low-affinity or high-affinity forms (Fig. 12-1). Results from the maleic acid-induced experimental model (Table 12-2) of the Fanconi syndrome suggest that the defect in the transport of amino acids does not involve their uptake into the cells and hence does not involve their affinity for the carrier. Rather, the transfer process across the membrane or possibly increased leakage of the amino acids from the cells seems to be implicated. Different steps, however, may be involved with other substances. Whatever the precise defect(s), it leads to an increased excretion of virtually all naturally occurring amino acids (the urinary profile for these acids resembles an ultrafiltrate of plasma), to hyperphosphaturia (because of a low *Tm* for phosphate), and to glucosuria (which results from a low *Tm* for the sugar).

In some instances of the Fanconi syndrome (e.g., in poisoning with certain exogenous compounds, galactosemia, and Wilson's disease), the underlying disease can be treated rather effectively. Beyond that, therapy is aimed at the phenotypic manifestations: phosphate supplementation and the administration of some form of vitamin D for the bone disease, HCO_3^- supplementation for RTA (see below), K^+ supplementation, and often the general management of chronic renal failure (see Chap. 10), which is the immediate cause of death in approximately 50 percent of children and adults with the Fanconi syndrome. Although the excretion of cystine is increased, it is not markedly so; possibly for this reason, the occurrence of renal stones is unusual in the Fanconi syndrome.

Renal Tubular Acidosis (RTA)

Phenotypic Picture

Although as many as seven variants of RTA have been described, the principles of this disorder can be understood by considering the two major forms (Table 12-3): (1) *distal RTA,* also known as *classical RTA* or *type 1* because it was the first to be described, and (2) *proximal RTA,* or *type 2.* We shall here refer to them as the distal and proximal forms, because these designations point to the area of the nephron where the primary defect is thought to be located.

The fundamental defect in RTA is a failure to acidify the urine, but the chain of events that leads to this abnormality differs between the two types of RTA. The normal process of urinary acidification — that is, of the reduction in urinary pH — was described in Chapter 10 in conjunction with Figures 10-13 and 10-14. It was pointed out there that two steps are involved in this process: (1) the reabsorption of virtually all of the filtered HCO_3^-, which occurs mainly in the proximal tubules, and (2) the titration of urinary buffers, principally HPO_4^{2-}, to

Table 12-3
Phenotypic features of renal tubular acidosis (RTA)

Aspect	Distal RTA (type 1 or classical)	Proximal RTA (type 2)
Metabolic acidosis	Present	Present
Urinary HCO_3^- excretion:		
During severe acidosis	Slightly ↑	Nil
With corrected $P_{HCO_3^-}$*	Slightly ↑	Very ↑
Urinary pH:		
During severe acidosis	High	Normally ↓
With corrected $P_{HCO_3^-}$*	High	High
Urinary excretion of T.A.* and NH_4^+:		
During severe acidosis	↓	May be normal
With corrected $P_{HCO_3^-}$*	↓	↓
Therapy	Small amounts of $NaHCO_3$	Relatively large amounts of $NaHCO_3$

*$P_{HCO_3^-}$ = plasma bicarbonate concentration; T.A. = titratable acid.

form titratable acid (T.A.), a process that occurs mainly in the distal tubules and collecting ducts and that requires the secretion of H^+ against fairly large electrochemical gradients. The first step is deficient in proximal RTA. This fact is not immediately apparent from Table 12-3 and Figure 12-4, and requires further explanation with the aid of Figure 12-5.

In the normal state (Fig. 12-5, diagram a), about 85 percent of the filtered HCO_3^- (GFR · $P_{HCO_3^-}$) is reabsorbed in the proximal tubules and most of the remainder in the distal tubules and collecting ducts. Given a normal urinary P_{CO_2} of about 40 mm Hg and a urinary HCO_3^- concentration of less than 1 mMole per liter, the urinary pH will be 5.5 or less (see Fig. 10-14a). In *proximal* RTA, there is a diminution in the rate at which filtered HCO_3^- can be reabsorbed in the proximal tubules. If the plasma HCO_3^- concentration is low, for example, 15 mMoles per liter (Fig. 12-5, diagram b), the filtered load of HCO_3^- will be so reduced that despite the decreased reabsorption in the proximal tubules, the amount of HCO_3^- delivered to the distal nephron is still small enough that virtually all the filtered HCO_3^- can be reabsorbed and practically none is excreted (Fig. 12-4b). Consequently, the urinary pH can still be reduced to about 5.5 (Fig. 12-4a and Table 12-3). However, at lesser degrees of acidosis, as in diagram c of Figure 12-5, the slight increase in the filtered load of HCO_3^- coupled with the defective reabsorption in the proximal tubules now leads to the delivery of more HCO_3^- to the distal nephron than can be reabsorbed from that portion. The resultant excretion of finite

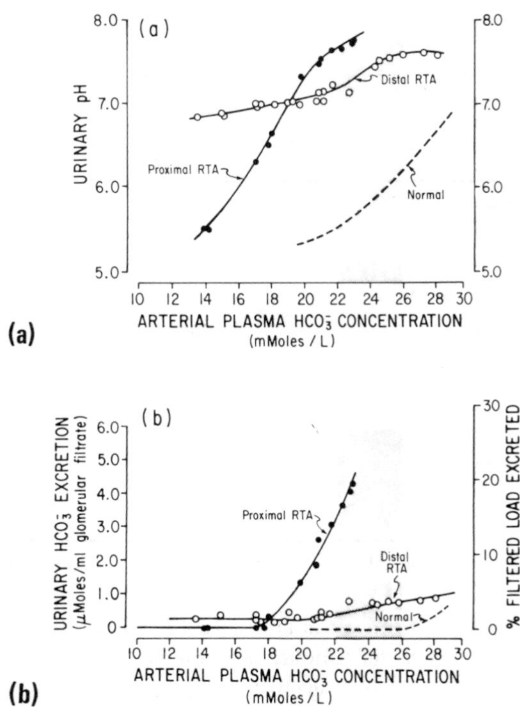

Figure 12-4
Urinary pH (a) and urinary excretion of HCO_3^- (b) in normal subjects and in patients with prototypical distal (type 1) and proximal (type 2) renal tubular acidosis (RTA). Values are shown both during severe acidosis and when the plasma HCO_3^- concentration has been restored to the normal range (shaded area) by giving $NaHCO_3$. In part (b) the left-hand ordinate has been expressed as micromoles per milliliter of plasma filtered in order to correct for different GFRs in different patients; the percentage of the filtered load of HCO_3^- that this excretion rate represents at any GFR is shown on the right. Adapted from A. Sebastian, *Calif. Med.* 116:34, 1972 (May).

amounts of HCO_3^- (Fig. 12-4b) now prevents full reduction of urinary pH (Fig. 12-4a and Table 12-3). This chain of events leads to even greater excretion of HCO_3^- and hence to a higher urinary pH when the plasma concentration of HCO_3^- in patients with proximal RTA is raised to the normal range by $NaHCO_3$ therapy. Under these circumstances (Fig. 12-5, diagram d), as much as 25 percent of the filtered load of HCO_3^- may be excreted, compared to the normal value of less than 0.1 percent.

In *distal* RTA, the defect lies in deficient net H^+ secretion; some investigators believe that this deficiency exists at any urinary pH, whereas others believe that it involves only an inability to pump H^+ against a concentration difference of about 1 to 1,000, which would be required to lower the urinary pH to about 4.5. Inasmuch as in the renal handling of H^+ (Fig. 10-13), one

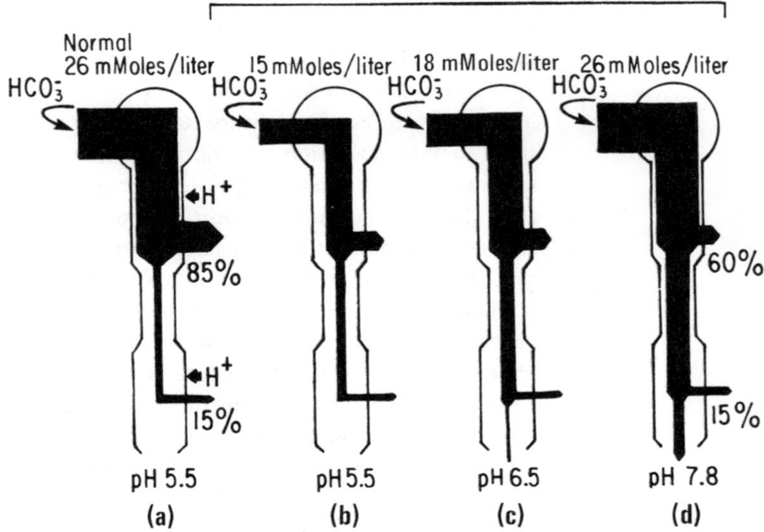

Figure 12-5
Dynamics whereby deficient reabsorption of filtered HCO_3^- in the proximal tubules, as in proximal RTA, can result in minimal urinary pH during severe acidosis (plasma HCO_3^- concentration = 15 mMoles per liter) but abnormally high urinary pH at lesser degrees of acidosis or during normal H^+ balance. Details are described in the text. The normal plasma HCO_3^- concentration of 26 mMoles per liter is slightly higher than the value of 24 mMoles per liter used in this book, which simply reflects the variability between institutions and whether a venous or arterial value is being quoted (see Table 1-1). From R. C. Morris, Jr., *Calif. Med.* 108:225, 1968.

HCO_3^- ion is returned to the blood for each H^+ ion that is secreted, a limitation on the transport of H^+ must necessarily result in an abnormally high excretion of HCO_3^-, no matter how severe the acidosis (Fig. 12-4b); this relation holds even though the defect for secreting H^+ resides in the distal tubules and collecting ducts, since 10 to 20 percent of the filtered HCO_3^- has to be reabsorbed in these segments. Further, once some HCO_3^- appears in the urine – even just 1 to 2 percent of the filtered load – the urinary pH must rise (Fig. 10-14a; also Fig. 12-4a and Table 12-3). Therefore, distal RTA can be distinguished from proximal RTA by the inability to lower urinary pH below about 6.0, no matter how severe the acidosis.

It follows from the above explanations that systemic metabolic acidosis will be seen in both proximal and distal RTA (Table 12-3): in proximal RTA, because the renal threshold for HCO_3^- is decreased (i.e., the plasma concentration at which HCO_3^- appears in the urine is lower than normal; Fig. 12-4b) and in distal RTA, because the deficiency for transporting H^+ necessarily results in renal wastage of HCO_3^- (Fig. 12-4b). It also follows that inasmuch as the urine cannot be acidified normally, the excretion of H^+ in the form of T.A. and as NH_4^+ salts must be diminished (Fig. 10-15; also Chap. 10, under Acidification and H^+ Excretion). The only exception to this consequence is seen in proximal RTA during very severe acidosis (Table 12-3), but since in that condition, the normal minimal urinary pH can be reached only at abnormally low plasma HCO_3^- concentrations (Fig. 12-4a), the resultant, possibly normal rate of H^+ excretion cannot prevent metabolic acidosis. In both types of RTA, the systemic acidosis results from a loss of HCO_3^-, not from the accumulation of some unmeasured anion; consequently, the anion gap is normal in this condition (Table 6-2), and the acidbase abnormality is often referred to as "hyperchloremic acidosis," which may be the first diagnostic clue to RTA.

The aforementioned mechanisms explain why relatively small amounts of $NaHCO_3$ suffice to treat distal RTA, whereas enormous amounts are needed for treating proximal RTA (Table 12-3). As the plasma concentration of HCO_3^- is raised in the former condition, there is little rise in the urinary excretion of HCO_3^- (Fig. 12-4b); consequently, a patient with distal RTA needs only enough HCO_3^- to balance the daily production of fixed H^+, that is, about 1 mEq per kilogram body weight per day in an adult. In proximal RTA, however, the urinary excretion of HCO_3^- rises sharply as the plasma HCO_3^- concentration is raised (Figs. 12-4b and 12-5); therefore, huge amounts of $NaHCO_3$ — for example, 5 to 10 mMoles per kilogram body weight per day or more — will be required to keep the plasma level of HCO_3^- in the normal range.

Complicating phenotypic signs occur relatively rarely in proximal RTA, possibly because these patients can acidify their urine when their plasma HCO_3^- concentration is sufficiently low (Fig. 12-4a) and therefore are not necessarily in positive H^+ balance. The most common feature is retarded growth, which, though its cause is unknown, can be treated satisfactorily with alkali. The disease is often cured spontaneously; if so, treatment can be stopped. Renal wastage of K^+ and hypokalemia are commonly seen, especially when the plasma HCO_3^- concentration is raised through therapy. The most important causes of the kaliuresis probably include the increased flow rate of $NaHCO_3$ in the distal nephron (Fig. 12-5) and an increased electrical potential difference (P.D.) between the interior of the distal tubular cell and the distal tubular lumen.

In contrast to proximal RTA, the distal form is usually accompanied by three major complications: (1) rickets and osteomalacia, as well as retardation of growth in children; (2)

hypercalciuria, renal stones, and nephrocalcinosis; and (3) hypokalemia, which leads to muscular weakness (Chap. 4) and a defect in urinary concentration (Chap. 13). All three complications can probably be ascribed in large part to the positive H^+ balance. As the retained H^+ ions are buffered by bone (Fig. 10-12), the resultant mobilization of Ca^{2+} from bone leads to osteomalacia. The mobilization of Ca^{2+} also leads to hypercalciuria and to the development of renal stones and nephrocalcinosis. These processes may be abetted by a relatively high urinary pH (which decreases the solubility of Ca^{2+}) and by a low urinary excretion of citrate (which ordinarily complexes Ca^{2+}). Hypokalemia results from the increased urinary excretion of K^+, which, however, is due to a different cause than was cited for proximal RTA. Because in the renal handling of H^+, a filtered Na^+ ion is reabsorbed for every H^+ ion that is secreted (Fig. 10-13), the decreased excretion of H^+ in distal RTA leads to an increased flow of Na^+ in the distal tubule, which in turn may lead to the increased excretion of K^+. Often, another consequence of the increased distal flow of Na^+ is an increased urinary excretion of this ion and secondary hyperaldosteronism, which may then also promote increased K^+ excretion.

Defects in RTA

Distal RTA may be seen in a wide variety of clinical conditions: as an isolated renal defect (either acquired or genetic), in association with various inherited or autoimmune systemic disorders, as part of certain generalized renal diseases, with nephrocalcinosis (not as a consequence but as the cause), or with certain forms of intoxication. The ultimate cause for the failure to acidify the urine in distal RTA has not been identified. Possible causes include "weakness" of the active transport system that pumps H^+ into the luminal fluid of the distal tubules and collecting ducts, increased back-diffusion of H^+ from the lumen into the cell or the peritubular fluid (possibly because of abnormal permeabilities of the luminal membrane to H^+ or other ions, such as Cl^-), or a "leak" of HCO_3^- from the proximal nephron to the distal nephron which is insufficient to lead to a marked increase of urinary HCO_3^- excretion (Fig. 12-4b) but enough to maintain a relatively high urinary pH (Fig. 12-4a). In view of the multiple causes of the disorder, it may turn out that different mechanisms, sometimes perhaps in combination, are involved in different states.

Proximal RTA also occurs in a variety of disease states: as a transient idiopathic phenomenon in infants, as an isolated tubular defect (either acquired or genetic), or as part of multiple deficiencies of the proximal tubules, most notably in the Fanconi syndrome. From Figure 12-4b, it is clear that the renal threshold for HCO_3^- (that is, the plasma HCO_3^- concentration at which HCO_3^- appears in the urine) is lower than normal in proximal RTA. If the curves in Figure 12-4b were extended into the supranormal range of plasma HCO_3^- concentration, they would be recognized as HCO_3^- titration curves (see Fig. 12-7). When constructed for patients with RTA, such curves have revealed one group with a low *Tm* for HCO_3^- but a normal splay and a second group with a normal *Tm* but an abnormally large splay; a low renal threshold for HCO_3^- was common to both groups. Just what causes these abnormalities in proximal RTA is not known. Although the issue has not been settled, there is considerable evidence to implicate an abnormal plasma level of PTH, an abnormal renal tubular sensitivity to PTH, phosphate depletion, or some combination of these.

Renal Glycosuria

Definition and Phenotypic Picture

Renal glycosuria is a condition in which glucose is excreted in the urine despite normal blood concentrations of glucose. Because trace amounts of glucose (up to about 300 mg per day) may be excreted by healthy persons, *glycosuria* is here defined as the excretion of >1 g of glucose per day; the excretion rate is variable and may be as great as 100 g per day. Renal glycosuria is considered to be an isolated tubular defect, and it is therefore distinguished from other conditions, notably the Fanconi syndrome, which may be accompanied by glycosuria at normal blood glucose concentrations. The definition is also specific for glucose and thus excludes other so-called melliturias, such as fructosuria, pentosuria, or sucrosuria.

By the above definition, renal glycosuria is a rare condition. If, however, the criteria are relaxed to include any glycosuria occurring in a patient who has a normal glucose tolerance test, the condition is much more common. The disease is usually discovered in the teens upon routine urinalysis, and it is considered by most experts to be benign; it is very important to differentiate it from diabetes mellitus and thereby prevent a patient from being labeled with a chronic and potentially serious disease.

Although there may be several modes of inheritance and a continuum of phenotypic expression, renal glycosuria can be categorized into two major types on the basis of the glucose titration curve (Fig. 12-6; how such curves are obtained was described in conjunction with Figure 10-16). Healthy adults have a maximum rate for the renal tubular transport of glucose, Tm_G, of roughly 325 mg per minute, and their titration curves show relatively small splay. Their renal threshold for glucose — that is,

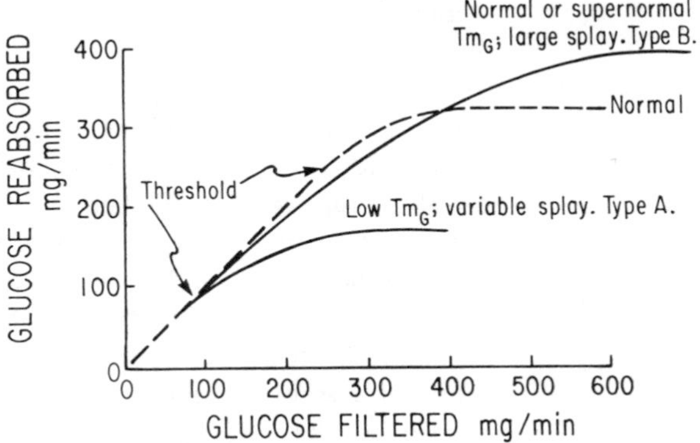

Figure 12-6
Glucose titration curves for healthy young males and for men with the two major types of renal glycosuria. Tm_G = maximum transport rate for glucose. Data from J. J. McPhaul, Jr., and J. J. Simonaitis, *J. Clin. Invest.* 47:702, 1968; graph modified from G. H. Mudge et al., in J. Orloff and R. W. Berliner (eds.), *Handbook of Physiology,* Section 8, Renal Physiology. Washington, D.C.: American Physiological Society, 1973, p. 599.

the plasma concentration of glucose at which the sugar first appears in the urine — is just above 200 mg/100 ml (not to be mistaken for a filtered load for glucose of about 200 mg per minute, as shown in Figure 12-6). One group of patients with renal glycosuria shows a low Tm_G, a low renal threshold for glucose, and a variable degree of splay when expressed in the units shown in Figure 12-6; this group is known as *type A.* A second group shows a normal or supernormal Tm_G and a very large splay that results in a lowered renal threshold; this group has been designated as *type B.* Both types may be found in the same pedigree. Some patients have an associated defect in the jejunal transport of hexoses; this disorder, known as *glucose-galactose malabsorption,* may have a yet different mode of inheritance.

Mechanisms of Renal Glycosuria

Concerning the elucidation of the process of active glucose transport in the kidneys, the intestine, or elsewhere, we are still in the hypothetical stage, much as was outlined for amino acids in Figure 12-1. It follows that until we understand the normal process more fully, it will be difficult or impossible to pinpoint the mechanisms that lead to the abnormal excretion of glucose in renal glycosuria. In the meantime, we can speculate on some possibilities that would be expected to lead to a decrease in the Tm_G or an increase in the splay of the titration curve, either of which might also result in a decreased renal threshold for glucose. Inasmuch as a reduction in Tm_G refers to the transport capacity of all nephrons combined, such reduction could arise, among other possibilities, from (1) a decreased proximal tubular mass, (2) some defect in permeability that prevents the sugar from combining with the active site on the carrier, or (3) a defect in the carrier, such as a reduction in the number of carriers, in the affinity of the carrier for glucose or for Na^+ (glucose transport, as well as amino acid transport, depends in part on Na^+), in the "movement" of the carrier across the membrane, in the utilization of energy, or in a number of other steps (Fig. 12-1). The increased splay may theoretically arise from (1) glomerulotubular (GT) imbalance or (2) a decreased affinity of the carrier for glucose or for some other essential substrate, such as Na^+. The GT imbalance, in turn, could have an anatomical basis (i.e., the volume of absorbing tissue in the proximal tubule may be poorly matched to the filtering surface area of its glomerulus) or a functional basis (e.g., the carriers for glucose may be unevenly distributed among the proximal tubules). There are also numerous other possibilities. To date, despite a number of investigations of the subject, none of the above has been conclusively identified as the major defect in renal glycosuria, although the presence of decreased proximal tubular mass has probably been ruled out as a cause, and some investigators consider GT imbalance to be an unlikely explanation.

Summary

This chapter deals with a group of renal diseases, known as *tubular disorders,* in which epithelial transport is selectively affected, and renal failure is not involved except as a late complication of the primary tubular defect. There is a large variety of these disorders, which may be inherited or acquired. The defects may involve just one transport process (e.g., the reabsorption of glucose in renal glycosuria) or multiple transport systems (e.g., in the Fanconi syndrome), and the consequences of the defects range from harmlessness to death at an early age. Sometimes there are analogous deficiencies of transport in other organs, especially the intestines.

Several prototypes have been described in order to illustrate the principles underlying the renal tubular disorders. Although each condition was chosen to exemplify a particular mechanism of defective transport, there is necessarily overlap in some instances. Thus, although distal RTA has been cited as an example of a defect in tubular secretion, it is possible that the ultimate cause of the deficiency may involve the permeability of the luminal membrane to H^+ or other ions.

Classical cystinuria, in which four amino acids are excreted at abnormally high rates, represents an inborn error in one or possibly two renal reabsorptive systems, namely, in the carrier for lysine, arginine, and ornithine and possibly in the carrier for cystine. Increased urinary excretion of the first three amino acids is probably harmless, but that of cystine usually leads to the formation of renal stones, since cystine is the least soluble of the naturally occurring amino acids. About 50 percent of patients with cystinuria die of obstructive nephropathy. Treatment is aimed at preventing the formation of cystine crystals, mainly by greatly increasing the urine flow and by taking cystine out of solution through the use of D-penicillamine.

In the Fanconi syndrome, nearly all the proximal tubular reabsorptive systems are compromised; those for amino acids, glucose, and phosphate become defective early, and those for HCO_3^-, K^+, and Ca^{2+} usually tend to fail at later stages of the disease. The syndrome has a large number of causes, which may all act ultimately through the same mechanism, namely, toxic interference with the availability of cellular energy. The signs and symptoms as well as the treatability of the Fanconi syndrome can vary widely, depending mainly on the underlying cause.

Renal tubular acidosis (RTA) can be divided into two major forms; in both, there is failure to acidify the urine and to conserve HCO_3^- *when the plasma* HCO_3^- *concentration has been raised to normal.* In one form, proximal RTA, the failure arises from deficient reabsorption of HCO_3^- in the proximal tubules, and in the other, distal RTA, the failure is caused by decreased net secretion of H^+ in the distal tubules and collecting ducts. The proximal type is often seen as part of the Fanconi syndrome. Both types have an array of causes, genetic as well as acquired. Complications are rare in proximal RTA, possibly because patients with this form are not necessarily in positive H^+ balance. However, disabling complications (e.g., osteomalacia, nephrocalcinosis, and K^+ deficiency) are common in distal RTA, where the invariable positive balance for H^+ leads to mobilization of Ca^{2+} from bone. Because the urinary excretion of HCO_3^- rises sharply in proximal RTA as the plasma HCO_3^- concentration is raised, patients with this form require enormous doses of $NaHCO_3$ for treatment; patients with distal RTA can be treated with far less $NaHCO_3$.

Renal glycosuria refers, by definition, to the excretion of more than 1 g of glucose in the urine per day, even though the blood concentration of glucose is normal. Two types of this disorder are distinguished on the basis of the glucose titration curve: one type is associated with a low Tm_G, low renal threshold for glucose, and a variable degree of splay, and the second type occurs in conjunction with a normal or supernormal Tm_G, large splay, and a lowered threshold. The molecular mechanisms underlying the defective transport of glucose remain unknown.

Problem 12-1

This male patient was born in 1932 of parents who were distant cousins. He was in apparently good health until 1957, when he experienced colicky pain in the left flank, which was due to a stone that he passed spontaneously. About two years later, he had further flank pain on the left and passed two more stones spontaneously; these were determined to be cystine stones by chemical analysis. A regimen aimed at a high fluid intake and enough $NaHCO_3$ to keep his urine pH above 7.0 was begun. In 1961, he had yet another calculus on the left, and this time an incision of the renal pelvis (a pyelotomy) was required to remove the stone; chemical analysis again showed cystine. One year later, despite the continuation of the therapeutic regimen, he experienced intermittent pain in the right flank for a period of four months. His urine pH was 6.0 and the urinary sediment contained cystine crystals; the BUN was 15 mg/100 ml. Following an intravenous pyelogram (I.V.P.) that showed a stone in the right ureter and a ureteral stricture, cystoscopy was performed to see if the stone could be dislodged. When this attempt failed, the following operative procedures were performed: the excision of a stone from the renal pelvis (called a pyelolithotomy), the creation of fistulas leading from the renal pelvis to the skin (nephrostomy) and from the ureter to the skin (ureterostomy), and a plastic repair of the right ureter to overcome the stricture (ureteroplasty). A pattern for the urinary excretion of amino acids was obtained, and highly elevated values were found for cystine, lysine, ornithine, and arginine (1,391, 2,337, 535, and 1,253 mg per 24 hours, respectively). The patient was now placed on an oral dose of $NaHCO_3$ for a total of 12 g each day.

In 1965, the patient again had colicky pain in the right flank, but after 3 hours, he spontaneously passed a stone measuring about 0.7 mm in diameter. Approximately one year later, he had 4 hours of severe pain in the right flank; an I.V.P., cystoscopy, and retrograde pyelography showed a stone in the right ureter, and a ureterolithotomy had to be performed. A few days later, an I.V.P. revealed another stone in the right ureter, and this time a second ureterolithotomy was combined with a right nephrostomy. After the second operation, the BUN was 9 mg/100 ml. During the ensuing six months, the patient was watched carefully, and when the urine pH was repeatedly found to be around 6.0, the administration of D-penicillamine (500 mg four times daily) was begun. When, about one month later, the patient developed a skin rash, the use of penicillamine was stopped, but it was then restarted at 500 mg three times daily.

During the following months, intermittent, moderate proteinuria was noted, and eight months after penicillamine therapy was begun, the patient developed swelling in the extremities and abdomen, and he reported having gained about 10 pounds. His BUN at this time was 11 mg/100 ml, the serum creatinine concentration was 1.1 mg/100 ml, and the patient was excreting about 9 g of protein per day. Penicillamine was stopped, the high fluid intake and $NaHCO_3$ administration were continued, and he was placed on a diet without added salt.

The patient's pedigree was studied in 1968. His parents, as stated earlier, were fourth or fifth cousins. The patient had had five siblings, two of whom died in childhood of unknown causes; three siblings appeared well and had no history of renal stones. The patient has seven children, all apparently in good health; urinary excretion rates for cystine, lysine, ornithine, and arginine were normal in all the children.

The patient continues to be followed closely at the hospital where he works as an aide. On a daily intake of $NaHCO_3$ of 6 g, his urine pH (which he tests himself) is about 7.5 or 8.0. He drinks several glassfuls of water before going to sleep, and he is invariably awakened around 2 A.M. with the urge to urinate, at which time he drinks more water. He has no more edema, and the proteinuria has gradually diminished to two-plus or three-plus (see Fig. 8-7). The urinary sediment invariably contains cystine crystals. He passes small calculi several times per year, and although some of these episodes require hospital admissions, he has had no further operations. Periodic intravenous pyelograms show progressive hydronephrosis and hydroureter on the right (see Chap. 11). The BUN and creatinine concentrations have risen gradually to levels (in 1976) of approximately 30 and 2.5 mg/100 ml, respectively.

1. It is often difficult to obtain a comprehensible, chronological story by gleaning a patient's record, especially when the chart runs into several volumes, as in the present instance. Although the above story already represents a rather concise summary of a complicated history, the analysis of the patient's problems — and therefore the management of the illness — would be further aided by a chart, which is kept up to date as part of the patient's record. Construct such a flow sheet.
2. What is the probable mode of inheritance of cystinuria in this patient?
3. Besides cystinuria, what renal disease did the patient contract in 1967? What was its probable cause?
4. When the patient had edema, did it make sense to restrict his dietary intake of Na^+ while treating him with $NaHCO_3$? How much Na^+ was he taking as $NaHCO_3$, and how does this amount compare with a normal dietary intake of Na^+? What alternative might have been used?

Problem 12-2

The patient is the same one whose history was presented in Problem 10-2: a woman who at age 37 received a kidney donated by her brother and who has had excellent results so far as survival of the transplanted kidney is concerned.

About two years after the transplantation, it was noticed that the patient had a mild hyperchloremic acidosis. Typical venous plasma values were Na^+, 140; K^+, 3.8; Cl^-, 108; and HCO_3^-, 21 mEq per liter. The urine pH ranged between 6.4 and 6.6. The BUN at this time was 17 mg/100 ml, the serum creatinine concentration was 1.1 mg/100 ml, and the endogenous creatinine clearance rate was 77 ml per minute. Because renal tubular acidosis (RTA) is known to occur in some patients after renal transplantation, further investigations were carried out to determine whether the patient had RTA, and if so, whether it was of the proximal or distal type. (These tests were done by Dr. Ronald B. Miller and the results are reproduced here with his permission.)

First, a series of plasma HCO_3^- concentrations were correlated with urinary pH values determined simultaneously. In order to save the patient the discomfort and possible complications of repeated arterial punctures, the HCO_3^- concentration was measured as total CO_2 on venous plasma (see Chap. 6, under Chronic Renal Failure). On three occasions, the total CO_2 and the simultaneous urinary pH, respectively, were as follows: 22 mMoles per liter and 6.60, 22 mMoles per liter and 6.50, and 21 mMoles per liter and 6.42.

Next, the patient was given NH_4Cl, 2 mMoles per kilogram of body weight, to see how well she could acidify the urine when challenged with a load of acid. During this test, the plasma HCO_3^- concentration decreased by 5 mEq per liter, and the lowest urinary pH attained during this period was 5.05. The renal threshold for HCO_3^- was 19.6 mMoles per liter.

Finally, the *Tm* for HCO_3^- was determined by means of an intravenous infusion of approximately 450 mMoles of $NaHCO_3$ and the simultaneous measurement of the GFR through determination of the inulin clearance. During this test, the plasma HCO_3^- concentration rose to 37 mMoles per liter, and the *Tm* for HCO_3^-, which was measured during four clearance periods, had an average value of 2.32 mMoles/100 ml of glomerular filtrate. The results of this test, along with the estimation of the renal threshold for HCO_3^-, are graphed in Figure 12-7.

1. Are the laboratory values about two years after transplantation compatible with the diagnosis of RTA?
2. If yes, which type of RTA does the patient have?

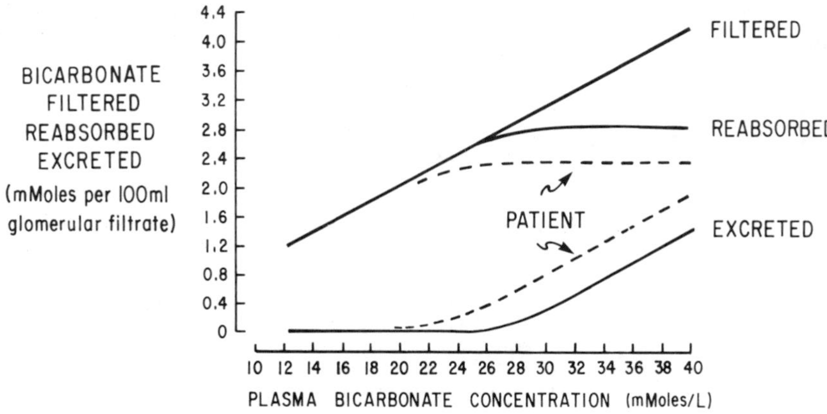

Figure 12-7
Renal handling of HCO_3^- at increasing plasma concentrations of HCO_3^-. The data for normal subjects, portrayed by solid lines, were taken from R. F. Pitts et al., *J. Clin. Invest.* 28:35, 1949. Expressing the ordinate values per unit of glomerular filtrate not only corrects for a changing GFR as $NaHCO_3$ is infused, but also enables comparison among different subjects and patients. The dashed curves, which represent the data for the patient in question (Problem 12-2), were drawn by eye, given the measured renal HCO_3^- threshold of 19.6 mMoles per liter and the measured *Tm* for HCO_3^- of 2.32 mMoles/100 ml of glomerular filtrate.

Selected References

General

de Wardener, H. E. *The Kidney. An Outline of Normal and Abnormal Structure and Function* (4th ed.). Edinburgh: Churchill/Livingstone, 1973. Chap. 18.

Lancet Editorial. Bartter's syndrome. *Lancet* 2:721, 1976.

McKusick, V. A. *Mendelian Inheritance in Man. Catalogs of Autosomal Dominant, Autosomal Recessive, and X-Linked Phenotypes* (4th ed.). Baltimore: Johns Hopkins Press, 1975.

Milne, M. D. Renal Tubular Dysfunction. In M. B. Strauss and L. G. Welt (eds.), *Diseases of the Kidney* (2nd ed.). Boston: Little, Brown, 1971.

Mudge, G. H. Clinical patterns of tubular dysfunction. *Am. J. Med.* 24:785, 1958.

Papper, S. *Clinical Nephrology* (2nd ed.). Boston: Little, Brown, 1978. Chap. 13.

Reynolds, T. B. Renal Tubular Disorders. In M. H. Maxwell and C. R. Kleeman (eds.), *Clinical Disorders of Fluid and Electrolyte Metabolism* (2nd ed.). New York: McGraw-Hill, 1972.

Royer, P. Chronic Tubular Disease. In J. Hamburger, G. Richet, J. Crosnier, J. L. Funck-Brentano, B. Antoine, H. Ducrot, J. P. Mery, and H. deMontera (eds.), *Nephrology.* Philadelphia: Saunders, 1968.

Scriver, C. R., Chesney, R. W., and McInnes, R. R. Genetic aspects of renal tubular transport: Diversity and topology of carriers. *Kidney Int.* 9:149, 1976.

Stanbury, J. B., Wyngaarden, J. B., and Fredrickson, D. S. (eds.). *The Metabolic Basis of Inherited Disease* (3rd ed.). New York: McGraw-Hill, 1972.

This justly famous book contains a number of chapters dealing with the topic of this chapter, especially part 11, entitled "Diseases Manifest Primarily as Transport Disorders."

Woolf, L. I. *Renal Tubular Dysfunction.* Springfield, Ill.: Thomas, 1966.

Aminoacidurias

Crawhall, J. C. Cystinuria – Diagnosis and Treatment. In W. L. Nyhan (ed.), *Heritable Disorders of Amino Acid Metabolism: Patterns of Clinical Expression and Genetic Variation.* New York: Wiley, 1974.

Dent, C. E., and Rose, G. A. Amino acid metabolism in cystinuria. *Q. J. Med.* 20:205, 1951.

Frimpter, G. W. Aminoacidurias due to inherited disorders of metabolism. *N. Engl. J. Med.* 289:835 and 895, 1973.

Garrod, A. E. Inborn errors of metabolism. *Lancet* 2:1, 73, 142, and 214, 1908.

Lee, C. W. G., Yu, J. S., Turner, B. B., and Murray, K. E. Trimethylaminuria: Fishy odors in children. *N. Engl. J. Med.* 295:937, 1976.

Scriver, C. R., and Bergeron, M. Amino Acid Transport in Kidney. The Use of Mutation to Dissect Membrane and Transepithelial Transport. In W. L. Nyhan (ed.), *Heritable Disorders of Amino Acid Metabolism: Patterns of Clinical Expression and Genetic Variation.* New York: Wiley, 1974.
This book also contains a number of other chapters on aminoacidurias.

Scriver, C. R., and Rosenberg, L. E. *Amino Acid Metabolism and Its Disorders.* Philadelphia: Saunders, 1973.

Segal, S. Disorders of renal amino acid transport. *N. Engl. J. Med.* 294: 1044, 1976.

Segal, S., and Thier, S. O. Renal Handling of Amino Acids. In J. Orloff and R. W. Berliner (eds.), *Handbook of Physiology,* Section 8, Renal Physiology. Washington, D.C.: American Physiological Society, 1973.

Silbernagl, S. Renal handling of amino acids – recent results of tubular micropuncture. *Clin. Nephrol.* 5:1, 1976.

Thier, S. O., and Segal, S. Cystinuria. In J. B. Stanbury, J. B. Wyngaarden, and D. S. Fredrickson (eds.), *The Metabolic Basis of Inherited Disease* (3rd ed.). New York: McGraw-Hill, 1972.

Thier, S. O., Segal, S., Fox, M., Blair, A., and Rosenberg, L. E. Cystinuria: Defective intestinal transport of dibasic amino acids and cystine. *J. Clin. Invest.* 44:442, 1965.

Ullrich, K. J., Rumrich, G., and Klöss, S. Sodium dependence of the amino acid transport in the proximal convolution of the rat kidney. *Pflügers Arch. Eur. J. Physiol.* 351:49, 1974.

Fanconi Syndromes

Berliner, R. W., Kennedy, T. J., and Hilton, J. G. Effect of maleic acid on renal function. *Proc. Soc. Exp. Biol. Med.* 75:791, 1950.

Briggs, W. A., Kominami, N., Wilson, R. E., and Merrill, J. P. Kidney transplantation in Fanconi syndrome. *N. Engl. J. Med.* 286:25, 1972.

Fanconi, G., and Bickel, H. Die chronische Aminoacidurie (Aminosäurediabetes oder nephrotisch-glukosurischer Zwergwuchs) bei der Glykogenose und der Cystinkrankheit. *Helv. Paediatr. Acta* 4:359, 1949.

Hunt, D. D., Stearns, G., McKinley, J. B., Froning, E., Hicks, P., and Bonfiglio, M. Long-term study of family with Fanconi syndrome without cystinosis (DeToni-Debré-Fanconi syndrome). *Am. J. Med.* 40:492, 1966.

Lowe, C. U., Terrey, M., and MacLachlan, E. A. Organic-aciduria, decreased renal ammonia production, hydrophthalmos, and mental retardation. *Am. J. Dis. Child.* 83:164, 1952.

Morgan, H. G., Stewart, W. K., Lowe, K. G., Stowers, J. M., and Johnstone, J. H. Wilson's disease and the Fanconi syndrome. *Q. J. Med.* 31:361, 1962.

Morris, R. C., Jr. The clinical spectrum of Fanconi's syndrome. *Calif. Med.* 108:225, 1968.

Otten, J., and Vis, H. L. Acute reversible renal tubular dysfunction following intoxication with methyl-3-chromone. *J. Pediatr.* 73:422, 1968.

Puschett, J. B., Genel, M., Rastegar, A., Anast, C., and DeLuca, H. F. Effects of 25-hydroxycholecalciferol on urinary electrolyte excretion in hypophosphataemic rickets. *Lancet* 2:920, 1974.

Schneider, J. A., and Seegmiller, J. E. Cystinosis and the Fanconi Syndrome. In J. B. Stanbury, J. B. Wyngaarden, and D. S. Fredrickson (eds.), *The Metabolic Basis of Inherited Disease* (3rd ed.). New York: McGraw-Hill, 1972.

Scriver, C. R., and Rosenberg, L. E. *Amino Acid Metabolism and Its Disorders.* Philadelphia: Saunders, 1973. Chap. 10.

Smithline, N., Kassirer, J. P., and Cohen, J. J. Light-chain nephropathy. Renal tubular dysfunction associated with light-chain proteinuria. *N. Engl. J. Med.* 294:71, 1976.

Renal Tubular Acidosis (RTA)

Albright, F., Consolazio, W. V., Coombs, F. S., Sulkowitch, H. W., and Talbott, J. H. Metabolic studies and therapy in a case of nephrocalcinosis with rickets and dwarfism. *Bull. Johns Hopkins Hosp.* 66:7, 1940.

Buckalew, V. M., Jr., Purvis, M. L., Shulman, M. G., Herndon, C. N., and Rudman, D. Hereditary renal tubular acidosis. Report of a 64 member kindred with variable clinical expression including idiopathic hypercalciuria. *Medicine* (Baltimore) 53:229, 1974.

Butler, A. M., Wilson, J. L., and Farber, S. Dehydration and acidosis with calcification at renal tubules. *J. Pediatr.* 8:489, 1936.

Edelmann, C. M., Jr. Renal Tubular Acidosis. In R. W. Winters (ed.), *The Body Fluids in Pediatrics.* Boston: Little, Brown, 1973.

Halperin, M. L., Goldstein, M. B., Haig, A., Johnson, M. D., and Stinebaugh, B. J. Studies on the pathogenesis of type I (distal) renal tubular acidosis as revealed by the urinary P_{CO_2} tensions. *J. Clin. Invest.* 53:669, 1974.

Lancet Editorial. Nephrocalcinosis and renal tubular acidosis. *Lancet* 2:934, 1974.

Morris, R. C., Jr., Sebastian, A., and McSherry, E. Renal acidosis. *Kidney Int.* 1:322, 1972.

Rodriguez-Soriano, J. The renal regulation of acid-base balance and the disturbances noted in renal tubular acidosis. *Pediatr. Clin. North Am.* 18:529, 1971.

Rodriguez-Soriano, J., Boichis, H., and Edelmann, C. M., Jr. Bicarbonate reabsorption and hydrogen ion excretion in children with renal tubular acidosis. *J. Pediatr.* 71:802, 1967.

Rodriguez-Soriano, J., Boichis, H., Stark, H., and Edelmann, C. M., Jr. Proximal renal tubular acidosis. A defect in bicarbonate reabsorption with normal urinary acidification. *Pediatr. Res.* 1:81, 1967.

Sebastian, A., McSherry, E., and Morris, R. C., Jr. Metabolic Acidosis with Special Reference to the Renal Acidoses. In B. M. Brenner and F. C. Rector, Jr. (eds.), *The Kidney.* Philadelphia: Saunders, 1976.

Seldin, D. W., and Wilson, J. D. Renal Tubular Acidosis. In J. B. Stanbury, J. B. Wyngaarden, and D. S. Fredrickson (eds.), *The Metabolic Basis of Inherited Disease* (3rd ed.). New York: McGraw-Hill, 1972.

Taher, S. M., Anderson, R. J., McCartney, R., Popovtzer, M. M., and Schrier, R. W. Renal tubular acidosis associated with toluene "sniffing." *N. Engl. J. Med.* 290:765, 1974.

Tannen, R. L. The response of normal subjects to the short ammonium chloride test: The modifying influence of renal ammonia production. *Clin. Sci.* 41:583, 1971.

Wrong, O., and Davies, H. E. F. The excretion of acid in renal disease. *Q. J. Med.* 28:259, 1959.

Renal Glycosuria

Elsas, L. J., and Rosenberg, L. E. Familial renal glycosuria: A genetic reappraisal of hexose transport by kidney and intestine. *J. Clin. Invest.* 48:1845, 1969.

Krane, S. M. Renal Glycosuria. In J. B. Stanbury, J. B. Wyngaarden, and D. S. Fredrickson (eds.), *The Metabolic Basis of Inherited Disease* (3rd ed.). New York: McGraw-Hill, 1972.

Lindquist, B., Meeuwisse, G., and Melin, K. Glucose-galactose malabsorption. *Lancet* 2:666, 1962.

Marble, A. Renal glycosuria. *Am. J. Med. Sci.* 183:811, 1932.

McPhaul, J. J., Jr., and Simonaitis, J. J. Observations on the mechanisms of glucosuria during glucose loads in normal and nondiabetic subjects. *J. Clin. Invest.* 47:702, 1968.

Monasterio, G., Oliver, J., Muiesan, G., Pardelli, G., Marinozzi, V., and MacDowell, M. Renal diabetes as a congenital tubular dysplasia. *Am. J. Med.* 37:44, 1964.

Mudge, G. H., Berndt, W. O., and Valtin, H. Tubular Transport of Urea, Glucose, Phosphate, Uric Acid, Sulfate, and Thiosulfate. In J. Orloff and R. W. Berliner (eds.), *Handbook of Physiology,* Section 8, Renal Physiology. Washington, D.C.: American Physiological Society, 1973.

Scriver, C. R., Chesdney, R. W., and McInnes, R. R. Genetic aspects of renal tubular transport: Diversity and topology of carriers. *Kidney Int.* 9:149, 1976.

13 : Nephrogenic Dysfunction of Urinary Concentration

Definition, Incidence, and Importance

Many largely unrelated conditions (Table 13-2) can lead to deficiencies of urinary concentration that cannot be corrected with exogenous antidiuretic hormone (ADH or vasopressin) and are therefore called *nephrogenic.* Unlike diabetes insipidus, which by definition (Chap. 2) involves the excretion of large amounts of hyposmotic urine, the pathological states described in this chapter do not necessarily lead to urine that is less concentrated than plasma, although many of them may. We thus define *nephrogenic, or vasopressin-resistant, urinary concentrating defects* as an inability to concentrate urine *maximally,* even though the plasma concentration of ADH is very high. Practically speaking, any patient (except a very young child whose concentrating ability is still developing) who, after water deprivation and exogenous vasopressin administration, is unable to raise the urine specific gravity above 1.020 or the urine osmolality above 700 mOsm/kg H_2O, may be suspected of having a nephrogenic concentrating defect. The definition thus encompasses not only conditions so mild that they may cause no symptoms, but also what is probably the most severe type of diabetes insipidus known (hereditary nephrogenic diabetes insipidus), as well as all degrees of deficiency between these extremes.

Although hereditary nephrogenic diabetes insipidus is a very rare disease, the acquired forms are becoming increasingly prevalent, probably because of the widespread use of drugs (Table 13-2). Lithium, for example, which is used extensively in the treatment of affective disorders, leads to toxic nephrogenic diabetes insipidus in an estimated 12 to 30 percent of patients. The inability to concentrate urine maximally is one of the earliest and commonest manifestations of nephrotoxicity, and it has been suggested that this deficiency might serve as an early diagnostic clue to certain conditions, such as analgesic nephropathy. Sometimes a deficiency of concentration – even though not so severe as to cause problems of water balance – may strengthen a suspected diagnosis, such as one of hypokalemic nephropathy. At other times, it is important for a physician merely to know that a given disease may entail a nephrogenic concentrating defect, so a further, often expensive and unpleasant diagnostic search can be avoided. Finally, apart from their clinical importance, the nephrogenic defects of urinary concentration have served as useful models that have taught us a great deal about the renal countercurrent system and especially about the cellular mode of action of vasopressin.

Effect on Water Turnover

In an adult patient, a defect in concentrating the urine usually does not pose a clinical problem until the urine becomes hypotonic. A quantitative example described earlier (see Chap. 10, under Water) illustrates this point. Suppose an adult on a normal diet takes in (and hence excretes) 600 mOsmoles per day. If that individual concentrates his or her urine maximally to 1,200 mOsm/kg H_2O, the 600 mOsmoles can be excreted in 0.5 liter of urine; if the concentrating ability of that individual is reduced to 600 mOsm/kg H_2O, the required urine volume will be 1 liter; and if the defect has resulted in isosthenuria (i.e., with urine osmolality of about 300 mOsm/kg H_2O), the urine flow will be increased to 2 liters per day if the dietary intake remains the same. This degree of urine flow is unlikely to cause symptoms, except possibly for mild nocturia. The moment, however, that the urine becomes hypotonic with respect to plasma, the diuresis is likely to cause symptoms, since 3 liters of urine per day will be required to excrete 600 mOsmoles at an average urine osmolality of 200 mOsm/kg H_2O, and 6 liters will be required at 100 mOsm/kg H_2O.

In an infant or young child, however, even a mild deficiency of urinary concentration may pose a problem in management for two major reasons: (1) the infant cannot adjust his own intake of water according to thirst and (2) in proportion to size, the infant has a minimal daily requirement for water that is two to three times greater than that of an adult. The reasons for this greater requirement are illustrated in Table 13-1. Energy metabolism is the major determinant of water turnover, because much of the heat produced can be dissipated only with an obligatory loss of water. The metabolic rate, expressed as kilocalories per kilogram of body weight per day, is two to three times greater in infants and young children than in adults, whether it is measured at rest or during activity. In addition, about twice as much of the heat lost is dissipated via insensible water loss in the infant as in the adult, partly because the greater caloric expenditure stimulates respiration and partly because the infant and child have about twice as much surface area per kilogram of body weight as does the adult. The upshot of these differences is that when stressed to conserve water, the very young person

Table 13-1
Determinants of water turnover during growth

Variable	1-Year-Old Child	3½-Year-Old Child	Adult
Body weight (kg)	10	15	70
Surface area (m^2)	0.5	0.65	1.7
Total body water (liters)	7 (68% BW*)	10 (65% BW*)	42 (60% BW*)
Metabolic rate (kcal/kg BW • 24 hr):			
Basal	55	47	23
Active	100	85	35
Insensible water loss (proportion of total heat loss)	50%	—	25%
Water requirement:			
Milliliters per 24 hours	700	1,150	2,000
Proportion of total body water	10%	8%	5%

*BW = body weight.

will deplete his total body water two to three times faster than the adult, and this fact may become consequential in a young child who has only a moderate defect of urinary concentration.

Decreased Corticopapillary Gradient Versus Decreased Water Permeability

The mechanisms by which urine is rendered hypertonic with respect to plasma are summarized in Figure 13-1a. Very briefly, the reabsorption of NaCl, but not of water, from both the thin and thick ascending limbs of Henle initiates countercurrent multiplication by the entire loop of Henle, and this process builds up an osmotic gradient in the medullary interstitium that reaches from the cortex to the papilla, the so-called *corticopapillary gradient.* Vasopressin in the plasma increases the water permeability of the distal tubules and collecting ducts, and as a result of this change, water is transported passively down the osmotic gradient between the tubular fluid and the surrounding interstitium, first out of the distal convolutions into the cortical interstitium (thereby increasing the osmolality of the tubular fluid from hypotonicity to isotonicity) and then out of the collecting ducts (thereby equilibrating the tubular fluid with the hypertonic medullary and papillary interstitium). Therefore, during maximal antidiuresis, the urine osmolality is equal to that of the interstitium at the very tip of the papilla.

According to this process, there can be two fundamental mechanisms that lead to nephrogenic defects of urinary concentration: (1) the failure to build up or maintain a maximal corticopapillary interstitial osmotic gradient or (2) the failure of ADH to increase the water permeability of the distal tubules and collecting ducts, so that osmotic equilibration with the interstitium cannot occur. Experimentally, these mechanisms

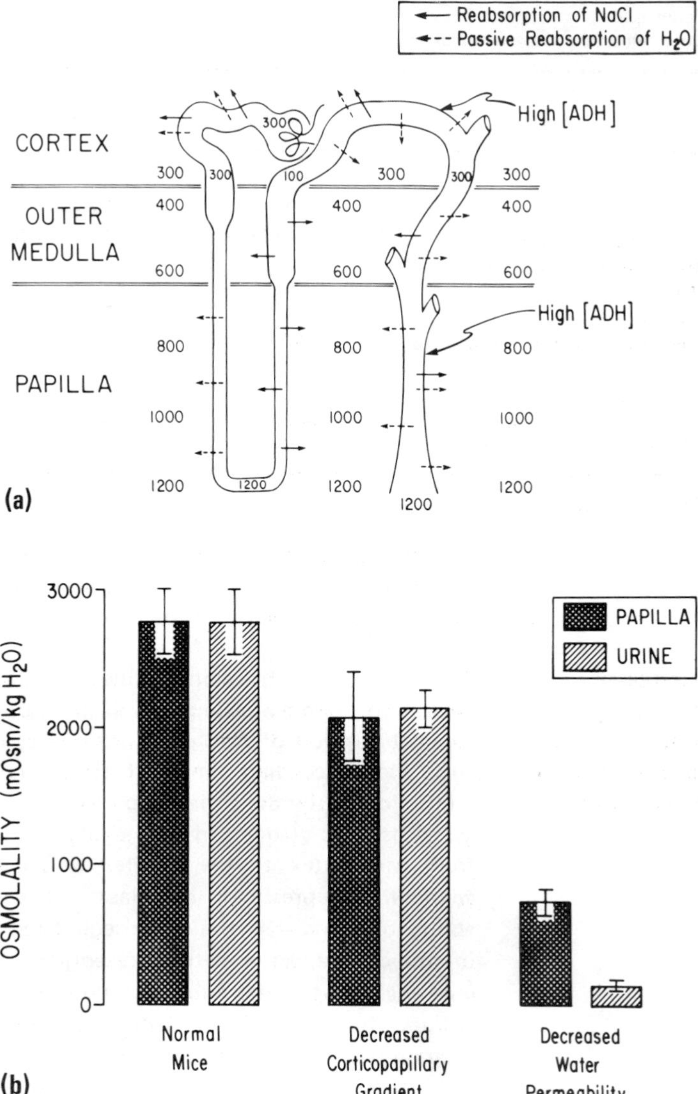

Figure 13-1

(a) Renal countercurrent system for concentrating urine. The numbers denote osmolalities in the tubular fluid and the interstitium; these values are appropriate for a healthy, adult human in maximal antidiuresis. The diagram is greatly simplified in that neither the role of urea nor that of the vasa recta is illustrated. *ADH* = antidiuretic hormone. Modified from H. Valtin, *Renal Function: Mechanisms Preserving Fluid and Solute Balance in Health.* Boston: Little, Brown, 1973.

(b) Osmolalities at the tip of the renal papilla and of the urine in normal mice and in two strains of mice with inherited nephrogenic dysfunction of urinary concentration. All mice were exposed to maximal plasma concentrations of vasopressin (ADH) at the time that the values were determined. The captions at the bottom of the bar graphs denote the *primary* mechanism causing each defect. Data from W. M. Kettyle and H. Valtin, *Kidney Int.* 1:135, 1972.

can be differentiated by measuring the osmolality of the urine (which reflects the osmolality of the fluid at the very end of the collecting ducts) and simultaneously determining the osmolality of the papillary interstitium. Figure 13-1b shows the results of such determinations in normal mice and in two strains with hereditary nephrogenic concentrating defects. In this experiment, normal mice concentrated their urine to about 2,800 mOsm/kg H_2O by equilibrating the fluid in the collecting duct against a papillary interstitium of the same osmolality. The strain of mice shown next has a partial nephrogenic defect of urinary concentration, for even after being given large amounts of ADH, they could reach a urine osmolality of only about 2,100 mOsm/kg H_2O. Inasmuch as their papillary interstitial osmolality was not significantly different from the urine osmolality, one can conclude that the distal tubules and collecting ducts were sufficiently permeable to water to allow osmotic equilibration; hence, the mechanism for the concentrating defect must lie in a decreased corticopapillary gradient. The third strain of mice has hereditary nephrogenic diabetes insipidus, which results in the excretion of enormous volumes of hypotonic urine even when they are given large doses of ADH. The fact that their papillary osmolality is significantly higher than the concurrent urine osmolality reflects the lack of osmotic equilibration of the fluid in the collecting ducts with the interstitium, presumably because vasopressin could not increase the water permeability of the distal tubules and collecting ducts. The finding that the papillary osmolality is lower in these animals than in the normal mice does not necessarily signal the presence of an additional defect; rather, this lowering is a secondary effect of the decreased water permeability and results mainly from the fact that when the flow of tubular fluid in the collecting ducts is very high, virtually no urea is deposited in the medullary interstitium.

It is more difficult to differentiate between the two basic mechanisms in human patients, in whom one cannot measure the papillary osmolality directly. Indirect criteria, the rationale for which was explained in Chapter 7 (under Identifying Sites of Renal Action), can and have been used. For example, adequate delivery of solute to the ascending limbs of Henle for buildup of the corticopapillary gradient can be gauged largely by the C_{H_2O} when vasopressin is absent (Fig. 7-3); or, if the C_{H_2O} is below the normal value because of decreased delivery of solute out of the proximal tubules, C_{H_2O} might be normalized during saline diuresis when more NaCl is delivered to the loops of Henle. Conversely, an increased delivery of isosmotic fluid into the loops of Henle, as when proximal tubular function is affected, might contribute to a concentrating defect by raising the generation of free water. If, by these criteria, the function of the ascending limbs of Henle seems to be normal, then it is assumed by exclusion that the nephrogenic defect in concentration must involve an inability of vasopressin to induce full water permeability in the distal tubules and collecting ducts. Actually, the indirect tests are not done routinely on patients with nephrogenic defects of urinary concentration; they are limited, rather, to research on such patients. Furthermore, most of the evidence that provides the basis for categorizing such patients according to the two major mechanisms (Table 13-2) has been obtained in experimental animals or various preparations in vitro. Often, a combination of the two mechanisms is involved, and the identification of the primary defect may be complicated because of a secondary effect, such as the decrease in the papillary osmolality shown for the third strain of mice in Figure 13-1b.

Cellular Action of ADH

The acronym *ADH* is used advisedly in this section, since there is actually a series of antidiuretic hormones, which vary slightly in structure depending on the species. The structure of arginine-vasopressin, the ADH that is native to most mammals, is shown in Figure 13-2a. In the ADH that normally occurs in *Suina,* lysine has been substituted for arginine in position 8, and this peptide is known as lysine-vasopressin. In amphibians and all other nonmammalian vertebrates, the major ADH is arginine-vasotocin, which differs from arginine-vasopressin only in having isoleucine instead of phenylalanine in position 3.

If it is concluded that a given nephrogenic dysfunction of urinary concentration is due to a deficiency of ADH-induced water permeability, then it may be possible to assign the fault to one or more steps in the chain of events shown in Figure 13-2b. Normally, ADH binds onto a specific receptor located in the basal membrane of cells that can change their permeability in response to the hormone. As hinted above, such cells are located not only in the distal tubules and collecting ducts of mammals, but also in various organs of other species, most notably (for experimental purposes), in the skin of the frog and the urinary bladder of the toad. Depending on the organ and species, the plasma (or cell) membrane that contains the vasopressin receptor is called the basal, basolateral, serosal, or peritubular membrane. Again, depending on the organ and species, the permeability that is altered may involve not only that for water but also those for urea and Na^+; different adenylate cyclases (see below) and different pathways are probably involved in the mediation of each of these permeabilities.

For the present purpose, we will limit the discussion to the permeability of the cell membrane for water. The interaction of ADH with its receptor stimulates the activation of an enzyme,

(a)

$$\begin{array}{ccc} & Phe^{3} - Gln^{4} & \\ & | \quad\quad\quad | & \\ & Tyr^{2} \quad\quad Asn^{5} & \\ & | \quad\quad\quad | & \\ H_2N - & Cys^{1} - S - S - Cys^{6} & - Pro^{7} - Arg^{8} - Gly^{9} - NH_2 \end{array}$$

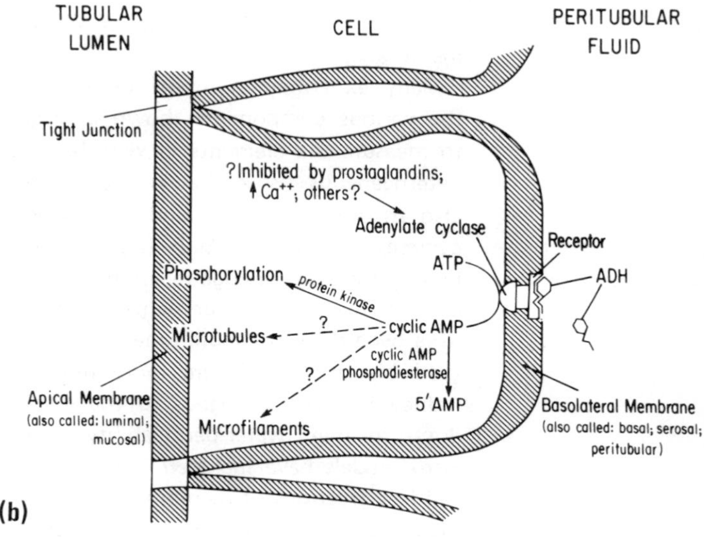

(b)

Figure 13-2
(a) The structure of arginine vasopressin. Numbering begins at the N-terminus.

(b) Chain of events whereby vasopressin (ADH) increases the water permeability of certain epithelial membranes. Although the schema probably applies to all epithelia that change their water permeability in response to ADH, the above diagram is intended to apply especially to cells of the mammalian distal tubule and collecting duct. Note that the receptors for ADH lie in the serosal membrane, whereas the increased permeability is induced in the mucosal membrane. The dashed arrows with question marks indicate that the roles of microtubules and microfilaments in the action of ADH have not yet been defined; the arrows do not necessarily imply a direct effect of cyclic AMP on microtubules and microfilaments. Adapted from T. P. Dousa and H. Valtin, *Kidney Int.* 10:46, 1976.

adenylate cyclase, that catalyzes the formation of cyclic 3′,5′-adenosine monophosphate (cyclic AMP) from adenosine triphosphate (ATP). Cyclic AMP serves as the intracellular mediator or messenger for vasopressin, and its concentration within the cell is controlled not only by its rate of formation from ATP, but also by its rate of breakdown to adenosine 5′-monophosphate (5′-AMP) under the influence of the enzyme, cyclic-AMP phosphodiesterase. Once formed, cyclic AMP induces changes in the apical (also called luminal or mucosal) cell membrane that increase its permeability to water. These changes come about by a series of steps that are just being defined; they probably include the phosphorylation of specific membrane proteins under the influence of an enzyme, protein kinase, and somehow involve the function of microtubules and microfilaments. It is not yet known what the molecular changes are in the apical membrane that increase its permeability to water; it is possible that the changes involve a modification in the secondary and tertiary structure of specific protein(s) at selected sites within the apical membrane.

Many experimental preparations have been used to measure the various components shown in Figure 13-2b. It is difficult to measure the elements in vivo, because the kidney is a highly heterogeneous tissue that is responsive not only to ADH, but also to other hormones and compounds that involve adenylate cyclases and cyclic AMP (e.g., parathyroid hormone). Thus, much of our knowledge regarding the cellular action of ADH has been derived from experiments conducted in vitro. Many studies have been done on anuran membranes, such as the frog skin and toad bladder, which are more homogeneous tissues than the kidney but are analogous to the distal tubules and collecting ducts in their water-permeability response to ADH. Other in vitro models have included isolated cells, fragments of tubules, cell-free fractions of membranes, slices of tissue such as the renal medulla, and isolated, perfused collecting ducts (Fig. 7-4). The preponderance of in vitro experiments is stressed because, although a tremendous amount of useful information has been gained from them, it is not always valid to extrapolate the results thus obtained to a given pathological condition in vivo (Table 13-2).

Clinical Examples

The large variety of conditions that can lead to a nephrogenic deficiency of urinary concentration is reflected in Table 13-2. Again, it should be stressed that although many of these states may eventuate in diabetes insipidus (i.e., in the excretion of large volumes of hyposmotic urine), they often cause only a mild defect of which the patient is not aware. Each state will not be described in detail here; such descriptions can be found in many of the textbooks cited at the end of this chapter.

Table 13-2 includes brief summaries that indicate the type of approach that is being applied for gaining a better understanding of the mechanisms involved and hence for possibly devising new and rational forms of therapy. An attempt has been made to classify each disorder according to its primary defect(s). It is obvious from the number of question marks and dashes in the table that the present state of our knowledge does not permit such strict categorization in many instances. When the primary

Table 13-2
Nephrogenic (vasopressin-resistant) defects of urinary concentration

Condition	Primary Defect*		Comments
	Decreased Corticopapillary Gradient	Decreased Water Permeability	
Due to drugs:			
Lithium	0	+	Acts at steps both proximal and distal to formation of cyclic AMP. May also stimulate thirst, and increases generation of free water by inhibiting reabsorption of isosmotic fluid in proximal tubules. Concentrating defect develops in 12 to 30 percent of patients receiving lithium for affective disorders
Methoxyflurane	?	Probably	May act at step distal to formation of cyclic AMP. Inorganic fluoride, a metabolite of methoxyflurane, may be the offending agent. May influence corticopapillary gradient through vasodilation and washout of solute, not through decreased deposition of solute. Oxalic acid, another metabolite of methoxyflurane, may cause acute renal failure
Demeclocycline	0	+	Severity of concentrating defect is dose-dependent and occurs only at very large doses. Acts at steps both proximal (at higher doses) and distal (at lower doses) to formation of cyclic AMP, possibly by binding to specific membrane protein(s)
Phenacetin and other analgesics	—	—	Usually presents first as sterile pyuria, renal failure, and papillary necrosis. A vasopressin-resistant concentrating defect is always present and might serve as an early clue to the diagnosis. The primary defect has not been identified but is undoubtedly related to ischemic necrosis of the renal papilla
Glyburide and other sulfonylureas	0	?	To be distinguished from other sulfonylureas such as chlorpropamide that have an *anti*diuretic effect (Chap. 2). Inhibit cyclic AMP-mediated water flow in vitro. Increase generation of free water, possibly by inhibiting reabsorption of isosmotic fluid in proximal tubules
Colchicine and vinblastine	0	+	Inhibit antidiuretic action of both vasopressin and cyclic AMP, possibly by disrupting microtubules or preventing the assembly of these cytoplasmic structures. Concentrating defects due to these drugs have not been described in humans

(Continued)

Table 13-2 (Continued)

Condition	Primary Defect*: Decreased Corticopapillary Gradient	Primary Defect*: Decreased Water Permeability	Comments
Amphotericin B, propoxyphene, isophosphamide, and methicillin	—	—	These drugs are unrelated. They have been lumped here, because thus far they appear to be rare causes of nephrogenic concentrating defects in humans. They have been included to suggest that many more drugs are likely to have this toxic potential. The primary defect in each instance is unknown
Due to electrolyte disturbances:			
Potassium deficiency	+	?	Although in most patients, the urine is merely less than maximally concentrated, isosthenuria or hyposthenuria occurs in some patients. The possibility that the defect may be decreased water permeability rests largely on evidence obtained in anuran membranes and from experiments performed in vitro. K^+ deficiency may interfere at steps both proximal and distal to the formation of cyclic AMP. K^+ deficiency may also stimulate thirst
Hypercalcemia	+	?	Calcium, like Na^+, undergoes countercurrent multiplication; accumulation of Ca^{2+} in the renal medulla may therefore cause dysfunction, predominantly of medullary structures. Ca^{2+} inhibits osmotic water flow in anuran membranes as well as vasopressin-stimulated formation of cyclic AMP. Although decreased water permeability in mammals has been demonstrated by some, the possibility that it is an additional primary defect remains controversial. Hypercalcemia may stimulate thirst
Inherited:			
Hereditary nephrogenic diabetes insipidus	—	?	Vary rare but important, because failure to recognize the disease in infants can lead to severe hypertonic volume contraction and cerebral damage. Transmitted as an X-linked recessive trait but with variable expression in some heterozygous females; other modes of inheritance may

			exist. Primary defect is thought to be in one or more steps in the cellular action of vasopressin, but proof is thus far lacking. For treatment, see Chapter 2 (under Causes and Treatment of Diabetes Insipidus) and Answer to Problem 13-1
As part of systemic disorder:			
Sickle-cell anemia	+	—	Urine osmolality is decreased to about 400 mOsm/kg H_2O. Patients with sickle-cell trait show lesser defect. As soon as blood enters the hypertonic renal medulla, erythrocytes containing hemoglobin S will sickle; the relatively low oxygen tension of the renal medulla may contribute to this process. Sickling leads, in turn, to increased blood viscosity and decreased flow in vasa recta. The consequent ischemia interferes with countercurrent multiplication in some as yet undefined way. By the time of adolescence, thrombosis and necrotic destruction of medullary structures may include collecting ducts; at this late stage, decreased water permeability may also be involved
Sjögren's syndrome, amyloidosis, Fanconi's syndrome, sarcoidosis, RTA	—	—	These conditions may rarely present first as disorders of urinary concentration, in which case the impairment may serve as a clue to the underlying disease. Primary defect varies and is unknown in most instances
Malnutrition; anorexia nervosa	+	—	Low protein intake and consequent decreased production of urea lessen concentrating ability by "robbing" the medullary interstitium of urea
Due to disorders of the kidney:			
Chronic renal failure	+	Probably sometimes	Osmotic diuresis per nephron, which decreases interstitial osmolality by mechanisms described in Chapter 10 (see Osmotic Diuresis per Nephron), usually leads to isosthenuria. Hyposthenuria occurs rarely; in that event, decreased water permeability may be involved
Pyelonephritis	—	—	May cause concentrating defect even early in course because initial injury is to renal medulla. Primary defect is not known
Obstructive nephropathy	+	Sometimes	Mechanism(s) discussed in Chapter 11 (see Pattern of Functional Impairment)
Tubulointerstitial diseases: medullary cystic disease, medullary sponge kidney, polycystic disease, transplanted kidney, urate nephropathy, radiation nephritis, Balkan nephropathy	Probably in most instances	Rarely (?)	These relatively rare conditions are characterized by damage to tubules and interstitium, often with a predilection for the renal medulla. Although diminished ability to concentrate the urine is frequently just a minor aspect of a broader syndrome, this deficiency can at times be a major and initial symptom

(Continued)

Table 13-2 (Continued)

Condition	Primary Defect*: Decreased Corticopapillary Gradient	Primary Defect*: Decreased Water Permeability	Comments
Miscellaneous:			
Postobstructive diuresis	+	—	Main defect is decreased reabsorption of solutes from proximal tubules and loops of Henle. (For further description, see Chap. 11, under Postobstructive Diuresis.)
Diuretic phase of oliguric acute renal failure	Probably	Probably 0	Now that careful fluid and solute balance is maintained during the oliguric phase, massive loss of water and solutes after the resumption of urine flow is rarely seen. Occasionally, however, recovery of GFR prior to that of tubular function leads to severe and prolonged osmotic diuresis
Osmotic diuresis: mannitol, other diuretics, and glycosuria	+	—	The detailed mechanisms are described in Chapter 7 (see Osmotic Diuretics; also Ethacrynic Acid and Furosemide). The importance of this and the next two conditions is not so much that they may pose problems in fluid management (except possibly in pediatrics) as that awareness of these entities can explain polyuric states and therefore allay concern that the patient may have some form of diabetes insipidus (Chap. 2)
Prolonged water diuresis	+	—	Surprisingly, the primary defect is almost certainly not in altered water permeability. The decreased corticopapillary gradient results mainly from diminished deposition of urea in medullary interstitium (see Chap. 2, under Types of Diabetes Insipidus, Pitfalls)
Paroxysmal hypertension	—	—	A rare complication of hypertensive disease, in which nocturnal paroxysms of high blood pressure are accompanied by vasopressin-resistant hyposthenuria

*+ = definitely present; 0 = definitely not involved; ? = some, but not conclusive, evidence to implicate this mechanism; dash (—) = no direct evidence for or against the mechanism.

mechanism involves decreased ADH-induced water permeability, an attempt is made to localize the defect further to one of the steps illustrated in Figure 13-2b. It should be stressed that a decrease in the corticopapillary gradient does not necessarily entail faulty functioning of the ascending limbs of Henle; as described above, it could result from deficient delivery of isosmotic fluid out of the proximal tubules, from washout of the gradient by the medullary blood flow following vasodilation, or from decreased deposition of urea, as in malnutrition. In some instances (e.g., lithium intoxication, K^+ deficiency, or hypercalcemia), stimulation of thirst — that is, primary polydipsia (see Chap. 2, under Types of Diabetes Insipidus) — may be an additional primary cause for the disturbance of urinary concentration.

Summary

In this chapter we have dealt with inabilities to concentrate the urine maximally, even in the face of higher than normal plasma concentrations of antidiuretic hormone (ADH). The deficiency may be so mild as not to cause symptoms, or it may be manifested as the most severe form of diabetes insipidus known in human patients, hereditary nephrogenic diabetes insipidus. A large variety of disparate conditions (Table 13-2) can lead to nephrogenic defects of urinary concentration, possibly because diminution in the capacity to concentrate urine is one of the earliest signs of nephrotoxicity. Because of the widespread use of drugs and because of the prevalence of obstructive and infectious nephropathies, these disorders are not rare.

Although mild deficiencies of urinary concentration are unlikely to cause symptoms or pose problems of management in the adult, an infant is more vulnerable. This difference arises from two facts: (1) the infant cannot adjust his own intake of water according to thirst, and (2) the infant's metabolic rate is two to three times higher than that of the adult, so the infant loses relatively more water during evaporative heat loss.

Either of two primary mechanisms can lead to a vasopressin-resistant (or nephrogenic) defect of urinary concentration: (1) a decrease in the corticopapillary interstitial osmotic gradient or (2) a decrease in the vasopressin-induced water permeability of the distal tubules and collecting ducts. In some instances, both causes may be present. A decrease in the corticopapillary gradient may result not only from an intrinsic flaw in the ascending limb of Henle, but also, among other causes, from decreased delivery of fluid out of the proximal tubule, from decreased reabsorption of urea from the medullary collecting ducts, or from an increased rate of blood flow through the medulla. Deficient water permeability in the presence of ADH can result from interference in one or more of the steps that are involved in the cellular action of the hormone (Fig. 13-2b). Because a primary defect in permeability will inevitably diminish the reabsorption of urea from the medullary collecting ducts, it is accompanied by a diminution of the corticopapillary gradient as a secondary effect.

The categorization of nephrogenic concentrating defects according to the two major primary mechanisms given in Table 13-2 is not routinely attempted on human patients but is largely limited to research. Such research, however, is highly pertinent to the management of human illness, since it is based on the axiom that the more we know about the mechanisms that cause a given disorder, the more logical and effective the treatment is likely to be.

Problem 13-1

The following clinical history has been abstracted and slightly modified from R. V. Lee et al. (*N. Engl. J. Med.* 284:93, 1971).

A 54-year-old woman had suffered from manic-depressive episodes for about 25 years. At age 52, she had been started on 1,500 mg of lithium carbonate per day. Within two months thereafter she developed marked thirst and polyuria; she drank water at least every 2 hours throughout the day and night. She did not, however, report these symptoms to her psychiatrist, and she continued taking lithium, from which one might surmise that the medication was otherwise making her feel better.

At age 54, glucose was discovered in her urine, and one month later she was admitted to the hospital with diabetic ketoacidosis, even though she had been placed on a diet and an oral hypoglycemic agent. She stopped taking the lithium three days before this admission. The ketoacidosis was corrected on the first day of admission by measures similar to those described in Chapter 6 (under Uncontrolled Diabetes Mellitus), and the diabetes mellitus was thereafter adequately controlled through dietary means and with insulin.

Because it was felt that the patient still needed treatment for her affective disorder, lithium carbonate (1,500 mg per day) was restarted as soon as the diabetes mellitus was under control. Pertinent laboratory values during the subsequent course are shown in Table 13-3.

Seven days after starting lithium therapy, the patient had severe polyuria and hyposthenuria. She was then deprived of all drinking fluid for 12 hours and was given five units of vasopressin (ADH); the results after this procedure are shown in Table 13-3. Lithium therapy was continued until the twenty-ninth day, when the patient developed neurological signs of lithium intoxication, associated with a toxic level of lithium in

Table 13-3
Selected data for a 54-year-old woman with lithium-induced diabetes insipidus

Variable*	Days on Lithium: 7	Days on Lithium: 8 (H_2O deprivation plus ADH administration)	Days off Lithium: 12 (After ADH administration)	Days off Lithium: 28
Body weight (kg)	77	73.8	–	–
P_{Li} (mEq/L)	0.82	0.69	–	–
BUN (mg/100 ml)	11	–	–	–
$\dot{V}$ (liters/24 hr)	>6	–	–	~2
U_{Osm} (mOsm/kg H_2O)	86	198	293	500
P_{Osm} (mOsm/kg H_2O)	296	342	–	–
U_G (mg/100 ml)	0	0	0	0

*P_{Li} = plasma lithium concentration; BUN = blood urea nitrogen concentration; $\dot{V}$ = urine flow rate; U_{Osm} = urine osmolality; P_{Osm} = plasma osmolality; U_G = urine glucose concentration.

the serum of 3.04 mEq per liter. Lithium therapy was stopped, and the subsequent improvement in the urinary concentrating capacity is shown in Table 13-3.

1. Interpret the water deprivation test. Is it likely that stimulation of thirst by lithium (see Table 13-2) played a major role in producing the increased water turnover? Was the rise in plasma osmolality consonant with the loss of weight during the water deprivation test?
2. Given the fact that lithium produced diabetes insipidus in this patient even when the concentration of lithium in the plasma was not at toxic levels, how might one treat this patient?

Problem 13-2

The following account, freely translated from a report by Gänsslen and Fritz (*Klin. Wochenschr.* 3:22, 1924), dramatizes the desperation of a young man with diabetes insipidus on the field of battle in World War I.

Since earliest youth, he had drunk large amounts of water, and even though his parents punished him severely – even beat him – they had been unable to rid him of the habit. Nowadays he has to drink 10–12 liters per day. This 'addiction' proved particularly annoying while he was at the front from 1915 to 1918. He described in moving words how he suffered from unbearable thirst in the trenches and again later, while a prisoner of war in France; and how he risked grenades and severe punishment when crawling to the nearest puddle in order to quench his thirst with the most questionable fluids. He did not care whether he drank urine or rain water, and he was perfectly willing to risk the danger of infection or even death, in order to satisfy his thirst.

Comment. In a sense, this problem should have appeared in Chapter 2, for the patient described almost certainly had hereditary *hypothalamic,* not nephrogenic, diabetes insipidus. Although the report by Gänsslen and Fritz appeared long before the two types of diabetes insipidus were distinguished, we can make the diagnosis in retrospect, because in the patient in question, the disease was inherited as an autosomal dominant trait, not as an X-linked form, which is almost certainly the case for hereditary nephrogenic diabetes insipidus.

The above history illustrates several important points that a physician must bear in mind: (1) Many parents do not understand this or other illnesses, conclude that the child is just being stubborn, and often express this interpretation and their feelings of guilt for having produced such a child by the use of angry punishment. (2) A patient with any of the three forms of diabetes insipidus may suffer greatly when drinking fluid is withdrawn. For this reason, and because the desperation can lead to surreptitious drinking, a water deprivation test should be started in the morning and run during the day, not as a routine overnight test. (3) Although even patients with severe diabetes insipidus may remain in good health so long as they have access to water, those such as infants and unconscious or confused patients are instantly in a precarious position when they cannot express or satisfy their thirst.

Selected References

General

Berl, T., Anderson, R. J., McDonald, K. M., and Schrier, R. W. Clinical disorders of water metabolism. *Kidney Int.* 10:117, 1976.

Bradley, S. E. (ed.). Symposium on hormones and the kidney. *Kidney Int.* 6:261, 1974.
This compilation includes articles on angiotensin, adrenocortical hormones, catecholamines, vasopressin, parathyroid hormone, thyroid hormone, and estrogens – any of which may influence the urinary concentrating mechanism.

Epstein, F. H. Disorders of renal concentrating ability. *Yale J. Biol. Med.* 39:186, 1966.

Harrington, J. T., and Cohen, J. J. Clinical disorders of urine concentration and dilution. *Arch. Intern. Med.* 131:810, 1973.

Jamison, R. L. Urinary Concentration and Dilution. The Role of Antidiuretic Hormone and the Role of Urea. In B. M. Brenner and F. C. Rector, Jr. (eds.), *The Kidney.* Philadelphia: Saunders, 1976.

Jamison, R. L., and Maffly, R. H. The urinary concentrating mechanism. *N. Engl. J. Med.* 295:1059, 1976.

Kettyle, W. M., and Valtin, H. Chemical and dimensional characterization of the renal countercurrent system in mice. *Kidney Int.* 1:135, 1972.

Miller, M., Dalakos, T., Moses, A. M., Fellerman, H., and Streeten, D. H. P. Recognition of partial defects in antidiuretic hormone secretion. *Ann. Intern. Med.* 73:721, 1970.

Schrier, R. W. (ed.). Symposium on water metabolism. *Kidney Int.* 10:1, 1976.
This symposium contains, among others, articles on thirst, the pro-

duction and actions of antidiuretic hormone, and pathological states of water excretion.

Stern, P. Nephrogenic Defects of Urinary Concentration. In C. M. Edelmann, Jr. (ed.), *Pediatric Kidney Disease.* Boston: Little, Brown, 1978.

Valtin, H. Genetic Models for Hypothalamic and Nephrogenic Diabetes Insipidus. In T. E. Andreoli, J. J. Grantham, and F. C. Rector, Jr. (eds.), *Disturbances in Body Fluid Osmolality.* Washington, D.C.: American Physiological Society, 1977.

Action of Antidiuretic Hormone (ADH)

Andreoli, T. E., Grantham, J. J., and Rector, F. C., Jr. (eds.). *Disturbances in Body Fluid Osmolality.* Washington, D.C.: American Physiological Society, 1977.
This volume contains several useful contributions on the cellular action of ADH.

Andreoli, T. E., and Schafer, J. A. Mass transport across cell membranes: The effects of antidiuretic hormone on water and solute flows in epithelia. *Annu. Rev. Physiol.* 39:451, 1976.

Barnes, L. D., Hui, Y. S. F., Frohnert, P. P., and Dousa, T. P. Subcellular distribution of the enzymes related to the cellular action of vasopressin in renal medulla. *Endocrinology* 96:119, 1975.

Chase, L. R., and Aurbach, G. D. Renal adenyl cyclase: Anatomically separate sites for parathyroid hormone and vasopressin. *Science* 159:545, 1968.

Dousa, T. P. Cellular action of antidiuretic hormone in nephrogenic diabetes insipidus. *Mayo Clin. Proc.* 49:188, 1974.

Dousa, T. P., and Barnes, L. D. Effects of colchicine and vinblastine on the cellular action of vasopressin in mammalian kidney. A possible role of microtubules. *J. Clin. Invest.* 54:252, 1974.

Dousa, T. P., and Valtin, H. Cellular action of antidiuretic hormone in mice with inherited vasopressin-resistant urinary concentrating defects. *J. Clin. Invest.* 54:753, 1974.

Dousa, T. P., and Valtin, H. Cellular actions of vasopressin in the mammalian kidney. *Kidney Int.* 10:46, 1976.

du Vigneaud, V. Hormones of the mammalian posterior pituitary gland and their naturally occurring analogues. *Johns Hopkins Med. J.* 124:53, 1969.

Grantham, J. J. Action of Antidiuretic Hormone in the Mammalian Kidney. In K. Thurau (ed.), *MTP International Review of Science: Kidney and Urinary Tract Physiology.* Baltimore: University Park Press, 1974.

Grantham, J. J., and Orloff, J. Effect of prostaglandin E_1 on the permeability response of the isolated collecting tubule to vasopressin, adenosine 3′, 5′-monophosphate, and theophylline. *J. Clin. Invest.* 47:1154, 1968.

Hays, R. M. Antidiuretic hormone. *N. Engl. J. Med.* 295:659, 1976.

Hays, R. M. Antidiuretic hormone and water transport. *Kidney Int.* 9:223, 1976.

Kachadorian, W. A., Wade, J. B., and DiScala, V. A. Vasopressin: Induced structural change in toad bladder luminal membrane. *Science* 190:67, 1975.

Kokko, J. P. The role of the renal concentrating mechanisms in the regulation of serum sodium concentration. *Am. J. Med.* 62:165, 1977.

Kurtzman, N. A., and Boonjarern, S. Physiology of antidiuretic hormone and the interrelationship between the hormone and the kidney. *Nephron* 15:167, 1975.

Monn, E., Osnes, J. B., and Øye, I. Basal and hormone-induced urinary cyclic AMP in children with renal disorders. *Acta Paediatr. Scand.* 65:739, 1976.

Moses, A. M., and Share, L. (eds.). *Neurohypophysis.* Basel: Karger. 1977.
This symposium, held on the 20th anniversary of the first international

meeting on the neurohypophysis, covers topics on the neurohypophyseal hormones ranging from the association of vasopressin with its receptor to clinical disorders of water balance.

Orloff, J., and Handler, J. The role of adenosine 3′, 5′-phosphate in the action of antidiuretic hormone. *Am. J. Med.* 42:757, 1967.

Rasmussen, H., and Goodman, D. B. P. Calcium and cAMP as interrelated intracellular messengers. *Ann. N.Y. Acad. Sci.* 253:789, 1975.

Robison, G. A., Butcher, R. W., and Sutherland, E. W. *Cyclic AMP.* New York: Academic, 1971.

Roy, C., Barth, T., and Jard, S. Vasopressin-sensitive kidney adenylate cyclase. Structural requirements for attachment to the receptor and enzyme activation: Studies with vasopressin analogues. *J. Biol. Chem.* 250:3149, 1975.

Schwartz, I. L., and Schwartz, W. B. (eds.). Symposium on antidiuretic hormones. *Am. J. Med.* 42:651, 1967.

Singer, S. J., and Nicolson, G. L. The fluid mosaic model of the structure of cell membranes. *Science* 175:720, 1972.

Sutherland, E. W., Jr. The biological role of adenosine-3′, 5′-phosphate. *Harvey Lect.* 57:17, 1961.

Taylor, A., Maffly, R., Wilson, L., and Reaven, E. Evidence for involvement of microtubules in the action of vasopressin. *Ann. N.Y. Acad. Sci.* 253:723, 1975.

Taylor, A., Mamelak, M., Reaven, E., and Maffly, R. Vasopressin: Possible role of microtubules and microfilaments in its action. *Science* 181:347, 1973.

Drugs

Appel, G. B., and Neu, H. C. The nephrotoxicity of antimicrobial agents. *N. Engl. J. Med.* 296:663, 722, and 784, 1977.

Civan, M. M., and Castleman, B. Congestive heart failure with azotemia of six years' duration. *N. Engl. J. Med.* 282:382, 1970.

Cousins, M. J., Mazze, R. I., Kosek, J. C., Hitt, B. A., and Love, F. V. The etiology of methoxyflurane nephrotoxicity. *J. Pharmacol. Exp. Ther.* 190:530, 1974.

Crandell, W. B., and Macdonald, A. Nephropathy associated with methoxyflurane anesthesia. A follow-up report. *J. A. M. A.* 205:798, 1968.

Crandell, W. B., Pappas, S. G., and Macdonald, A. Nephrotoxicity associated with methoxyflurane anesthesia. *Anesthesiology* 27:591, 1966.

De Fronzo, R. A., Abeloff, M., Braine, H., Humphrey, R. L., and Davis, P. J. Renal dysfunction after treatment with isophosphamide (NSC-109724). *Cancer Chemother. Rep.* 58:375, 1974.

Dousa, T. P. Interaction of lithium with vasopressin-sensitive cyclic AMP system of human renal medulla. *Endocrinology* 95:1359, 1974.

Duggin, G. G., and Mudge, G. H. Analgesic nephropathy: Renal distribution of acetaminophen and its conjugates. *J. Pharmacol. Exp. Ther.* 199:1, 1976.

Duggin, G. G., and Mudge, G. H. Phenacetin: Renal tubular transport and intrarenal distribution in the dog. *J. Pharmacol. Exp. Ther.* 199:10, 1976.

Forrest, J. N., Jr., Cohen, A. D., Torretti, J., Himmelhoch, J. M., and Epstein, F. H. On the mechanism of lithium-induced diabetes insipidus in man and the rat. *J. Clin. Invest.* 53:1115, 1974.

Gottlieb, L. S., and Trey, C. The effects of fluorinated anesthetics on the liver and kidneys. *Annu. Rev. Med.* 25:411, 1974.

Hochman, S., and Gutman, Y. Lithium: ADH antagonism and ADH independent action in rats with diabetes insipidus. *Eur. J. Pharmacol.* 28:100, 1974.

Kincaid-Smith, P., Saker, B. M., and McKenzie, I. F. C. Lesions in the vasa recta in experimental analgesic nephropathy. *Lancet* 1:24, 1968.

Lancet Editorial. Methoxyflurane and the kidneys. *Lancet* 1:1168, 1972.

Lancet Editorial. The wages of analgesics. *Lancet* 2:1484, 1973.

Martinez-Maldonado, M., and Opava-Stitzer, S. Distal nephron function of the rat during lithium chloride infusion. *Kidney Int.* 12:17, 1977.

Martinez-Maldonado, M., Stavroulaki-Tsapara, A., Tsaparas, N., Suki, W. N., and Eknoyan, G. Renal effects of lithium administration in rats: Alterations in water and electrolyte metabolism and the response to vasopressin and cyclic-adenosine monophosphate during prolonged administration. *J. Lab. Clin. Med.* 86:445, 1975.

Mazze, R. I., Shue, G. L., and Jackson, S. H. Renal dysfunction associated with methoxyflurane anesthesia. A randomized, prospective clinical evaluation. *J. A. M. A.* 216:278, 1971.

Singer, I., and Forrest, J. V. Drug-induced states of nephrogenic diabetes insipidus. *Kidney Int.* 10:82, 1976.

Singer, I., and Rotenberg, D. Demeclocycline-induced nephrogenic diabetes insipidus. In vivo and in vitro studies. *Ann. Intern. Med.* 79:679, 1973.

Singer, I., and Rotenberg, D. Mechanisms of lithium action. *N. Engl. J. Med.* 289:254, 1973.

Singer, I., Rotenberg, D., and Puschett, J. B. Lithium-induced nephrogenic diabetes insipidus: In vivo and in vitro studies. *J. Clin. Invest.* 51:1081, 1972.

Torp-Pederson, C., and Thorn, N. A. Acute effects of lithium on the action and release of ADH in rats. *Acta Endocrinol.* (Kbh.) 73:665, 1973.

Wallin, J. D., and Kaplan, R. A. Effect of sodium fluoride on concentrating and diluting ability in the rat. *Am. J. Physiol.* 232:F 335, 1977.

Webb, R. K., Woodhall, P. B., Tisher, C. C., and Robinson, R. R. Acute effects of lithium on the renal concentrating mechanism in a primate. *Am. J. Physiol.* 228:909, 1975.

Electrolyte Disturbances

Bennett, C. M. Urine concentration and dilution in hypokalemic and hypercalcemic dogs. *J. Clin. Invest.* 49:1447, 1970.

Buckalew, V. M., Jr., Ramirez, M. A., and Goldberg, M. Free water reabsorption during solute diuresis in normal and potassium-depleted rats. *Am. J. Physiol.* 212:381, 1967.

Epstein, F. H. Calcium Nephropathy. In M. B. Strauss and L. G. Welt (eds.), *Diseases of the Kidney* (2nd ed.). Boston: Little, Brown, 1971.

Finn, A. L., Handler, J. S., and Orloff, J. Relation between toad bladder potassium content and permeability response to vasopressin. *Am. J. Physiol.* 210:1279, 1966.

Gottschalk, C. W., Mylle, M., Jones, N. F., Winters, R. W., and Welt, L. G. Osmolality of renal tubular fluids in potassium-depleted rodents. *Clin. Sci.* 29:249, 1965.

Hollander, W., Jr., and Blythe, W. B. Nephropathy of Potassium Depletion. In M. B. Strauss and L. G. Welt (eds.), *Diseases of the Kidney* (2nd ed.). Boston: Little, Brown, 1971.

Lassiter, W. E., Frick, A., Rumrich, G., and Ullrich, K. J. Influence of ionic calcium on the water permeability of proximal and distal tubules in the rat kidney. *Pflügers Arch. Ges. Physiol.* 285:90, 1965.

Manitius, A., Levitin, H., Beck, D., and Epstein, F. H. On the mechanism of impairment of renal concentrating ability in potassium deficiency. *J. Clin. Invest.* 39:684, 1960.

Relman, A. S., and Schwartz, W. B. The nephropathy of potassium depletion. A clinical and pathological entity. *N. Engl. J. Med.* 255:195, 1956.

Suki, W. N., and Eknoyan, G. Tubulo-interstitial Disease. In B. M. Brenner and F. C. Rector, Jr. (eds.), *The Kidney.* Philadelphia: Saunders, 1976.

Inherited Diabetes Insipidus

Andreoli, T. E., and Schafer, J. A. Nephrogenic Diabetes Insipidus. In J. B. Stanbury, J. B. Wyngaarden, and D. S. Fredrickson (eds.), *The*

Metabolic Basis of Inherited Disease (4th ed.). New York: McGraw-Hill, 1978.

Bode, H. H., and Crawford, J. D. Nephrogenic diabetes insipidus in North America — the *Hopewell* hypothesis. *N. Engl. J. Med.* 280:750, 1969.

Crawford, J. D., and Bode, H. H. Disorders of the Posterior Pituitary in Children. In L. I. Gardner (ed.), *Endocrine and Genetic Diseases of Childhood and Adolescence* (2nd ed.). Philadelphia: Saunders, 1975.

Fichman, M. P., and Brooker, G. Deficient renal cyclic adenosine 3′-5′ monophosphate production in nephrogenic diabetes insipidus. *J. Clin. Endocrinol. Metab.* 35:35, 1972.

Forssman, H. On hereditary diabetes insipidus. *Acta Med. Scand.* [Suppl. 159]:9, 1945.

Williams, R. H., and Henry, C. Nephrogenic diabetes insipidus: Transmitted by females and appearing during infancy in males. *Ann. Intern. Med.* 27:84, 1947.

Miscellaneous Causes

Alleyne, G. A. O., Statius van Eps, L. W., Addae, S. K., Nicholson, G. D., and Schouten, H. The kidney in sickle cell anemia. *Kidney Int.* 7:371, 1975.

Hatch, F. E., Culbertson, J. W., and Diggs, L. W. Nature of the renal concentrating defect in sickle cell disease. *J. Clin. Invest.* 46:336, 1967.

Holliday, M. A., Egan, T. J., Morris, C. R., Jarrah, A. S., and Harrah, J. L. Pitressin-resistant hyposthenuria in chronic renal disease. *Am. J. Med.* 42:378, 1967.

Keitel, H. G., Thompson, D., and Itano, H. A. Hyposthenuria in sickle cell anemia: A reversible renal defect. *J. Clin. Invest.* 35:998, 1956.

Naik, D. V., and Valtin, H. Hereditary vasopressin-resistant urinary concentrating defects in mice. *Am. J. Physiol.* 217:1183, 1969.

Perillie, P. E., and Epstein, F. H. Sickling phenomenon produced by hypertonic solutions: A possible explanation for the hyposthenuria of sicklemia. *J. Clin. Invest.* 42:570, 1963.

Richards, P., and Wrong, O. M. Dominant inheritance in a family with familial renal tubular acidosis. *Lancet* 2:998, 1972.

Roussak, N. J., and Oleesky, S. Water-losing nephritis. A syndrome simulating diabetes insipidus. *Q. J. Med.* 23:147, 1954.

Schrier, R. W., and Berl, T. Nonosmolar factors affecting renal water excretion. *N. Engl. J. Med.* 292:81 and 141, 1975.

Tannen, R. L., Regal, E. M., Dunn, M. J., and Schrier, R. W. Vasopressin-resistant hyposthenuria in advanced chronic renal disease. *N. Engl. J. Med.* 280:1135, 1969.

Welt, L. G., and Lyle, C. B., Jr. The Kidney in Sickle Cell Anemia. In M. B. Strauss and L. G. Welt (eds.), *Diseases of the Kidney* (2nd ed.). Boston: Little, Brown, 1971.

Treatment

Bell, N. H., Clark, C. M., Jr., Avery, S., Sinha, T., Trygstad, C. W., and Allen, D. O. Demonstration of a defect in the formation of adenosine 3′,5′-monophosphate in vasopressin-resistant diabetes insipidus. *Pediatr. Res.* 8:223, 1974.

Crawford, J. D., and Kennedy, G. C. Chlorothiazid in diabetes insipidus. *Nature* 183:891, 1959.

Earley, L. E., and Orloff, J. The mechanism of antidiuresis associated with the administration of hydrochlorothiazide to patients with vasopressin-resistant diabetes insipidus. *J. Clin. Invest.* 41:1988, 1962.

Hillman, D. A., Neyzi, O., Porter, P., Cushman, A., and Talbot, N. B. Renal (vasopressin resistant) diabetes insipidus. Definition of the effects of a homeostatic limitation in capacity to conserve water on the physical, intellectual, and emotional development of a child. *Pediatrics* 21:430, 1958.

Himmelhoch, J. M., Forrest, J., Neil, J. F., and Detre, T. P. Thiazide-lithium synergy in refractory mood swings. *Am. J. Psychiatry* 134:149, 1977.

Jones, N. F., Barraclough, M. A., Barnes, N., and Cottom, D. G. Nephrogenic diabetes insipidus. Effects of 3,5,cyclic-adenosine monophosphate. *Arch. Dis. Child.* 47:794, 1972.

McConnell, R. F., Jr., Lorentz, W. B., Jr., Berger, M., Smith, E. H., Carvajal, H. F., and Travis, L. B. The mechanism of urinary concentration in nephrogenic diabetes insipidus. *Pediatr. Res.* 11:33, 1977.

Moses, A. M., and Miller, M. Drug-induced dilutional hyponatremia. *N. Engl. J. Med.* 291:1234, 1974.

14 : Renal Mechanisms Involved in Hypertension

Incidence and History

Elevation of the systemic arterial blood pressure is one of the commonest signs in clinical medicine. In the United States alone, some 20 to 25 million people have hypertension, which is often associated with serious morbidity; so-called hypertensive cardiovascular disease is one of the leading causes of death among the American population.

Richard Bright was perhaps the first to recognize the possible importance of the kidneys in both causing and maintaining high blood pressure. In his famous reports of medical cases published in 1827, he called attention to the association of contracted kidneys with hypertrophy of the left ventricle. (Measurement of the systemic blood pressure was not yet part of the routine physical examination.) The next major step was the publication in 1892 by C. E. Brown-Séquard and A. d'Arsonval of results of experiments that suggested an endocrine role for the kidneys. R. Tigerstedt and P. G. Bergman combined this suggestion with the earlier observation of Bright, and looked for a substance elaborated by the kidneys that might influence cardiovascular function. In their thorough, lucid, and dramatic report of 1898, they showed that a water-soluble, nondialyzable, heat-labile extract of renal cortex from a healthy rabbit caused a prolonged and striking elevation of blood pressure when injected into the jugular vein of another rabbit. They were convinced that the substance was not one of the known excretory products in the urine, and they proposed that "for the sake of brevity," the substance be called *renin.* In a further cautious and prescient interpretation of their data, they suggested that renin might be indirectly responsible for the cardiac hypertrophy that is seen in some forms of renal disease.

In 1934, H. Goldblatt and his co-workers described an experimental model for hypertension, which is still used extensively today. In devising the model, Goldblatt invoked his observation as a pathologist that hypertension was almost invariably associated with sclerosis of the renal arteries and arterioles, but that some patients with generalized arteriosclerosis, though without involvement of the renal vessels, did not have hypertension. The popular view held at that time was that renal vascular disease occurred secondarily to the hypertension; in contrast, Goldblatt proposed that impairment of the renal circulation might be the causative event, and he supported his thesis with the model that is described in a subsequent section.

During the ensuing years, there has been a great deal of work done on the many factors through which the kidneys might cause hypertension. These factors fall into two general categories: (1) the effects of pressor and depressor agents of renal origin, including renin-angiotensin and certain prostaglandins, and (2) the regulation of the extracellular fluid volume, involving mainly the renal handling of salt and water and the renin-angiotensin-aldosterone system. The regulation of these factors in turn implicates many other variables, including, among others, changes in systemic and renal hemodynamics, the activity of the sympathetic nervous system, the sensitivity of peripheral and renal vessels to vasoactive substances, the intake of salt and water, and the action of vasopressin. With so many inputs contributing to the control of blood pressure, one might predict that different mechanisms underlie the many and various forms of hypertension. Although, in a sense, this view may turn out to be correct, many think that renal function or dysfunction may be the common element that accounts for the vast majority of hypertensive disease, even for so-called essential hypertension, which comprises 80 to 90 percent of all hypertensive disorders and which in former years could be diagnosed only in the absence of *demonstrable* renal dysfunction. It should be stressed, however, that a causative role for the kidneys in essential hypertension — let alone in all forms of essential hypertension — has not yet been proved. Nor should one lose sight of the fact that there are less common causes of hypertension that may not implicate the kidneys: for example, adrenocortical hyperfunction, pheochromocytoma, thyrotoxicosis, brain tumors, and others.

In this chapter, after giving a few definitions, we shall describe the major renal mechanisms that can lead to elevation of the systemic arterial blood pressure and that may at various times be involved in the causation and maintenance of different forms of hypertension. We shall then present a composite of several theories that attempts to combine many of the proposed mechanisms into a unifying schema for the most common form of hypertensive disorder, essential hypertension.

Definitions

Although the kidneys may be the final common pathway in most instances of hypertension, different states of renal function are recognized as particular causes of high blood pressure. These states are described by the following definitions:

Renal or renal parenchymal hypertension: elevation of systemic arterial blood pressure that is seen in association with most states of chronic renal failure (Table 10-1) and with some types of acute renal failure.

Renovascular hypertension: high blood pressure caused by stenosis of the renal artery or one of its main branches. The stenosis is usually due to arteriosclerosis or congenital fibrous dysplasia. Although this entity is probably only a very rare cause of high blood pressure (accounting for <1 to 5 percent of all hypertension), it is particularly important for what it has taught us about the role of renin-angiotensin in hypertension.

Renoprival hypertension: elevation of systemic arterial pressure that is seen in patients who do not have sufficient functioning renal tissue to sustain life and who are therefore on chronic dialysis (Fig. 9-7). Such patients either have shrunken kidneys or both of their kidneys have been removed in preparation for transplantation.

Essential hypertension: all hypertension of unknown cause, excluding, therefore, not only the three categories listed above, but also other forms, such as Cushing's syndrome, primary hyperaldosteronism, pheochromocytoma, thyrotoxicosis, brain tumor, coarctation of the aorta, or any other disorder that is known to be associated with hypertension. Some investigators believe that occult renal parenchymal disorders may underlie as much as 75 percent of even essential hypertension. Thus, as the mechanisms involved in hypertension are unraveled, the incidence of essential hypertension may dwindle or the term may even be dropped.

Renin-Angiotensin-Aldosterone System

The renin-angiotensin-aldosterone system and its relationship to systemic arterial blood pressure are shown in Figure 14-1. *Renin* is secreted by the juxtaglomerular apparatuses (JGA) in the kidney, probably from granular cells that are located mainly or exclusively in the afferent arterioles. Renin is a specific proteolytic enzyme that splits a decapeptide from *angiotensinogen,* an α_2-globulin substrate that is produced by the liver. The decapeptide, *angiotensin I,* may have little physiological action of its own; it is converted to an active principle, *angiotensin II,* through the loss of two terminal amino acids under the influence of *converting enzyme.* The conversion occurs mainly in the lungs, but also in the kidneys and perhaps in other organs as well. Angiotensin II is broken down in the plasma through the catalytic action of several *angiotensinases.* Angiotensin II has two principal actions by which it influences the

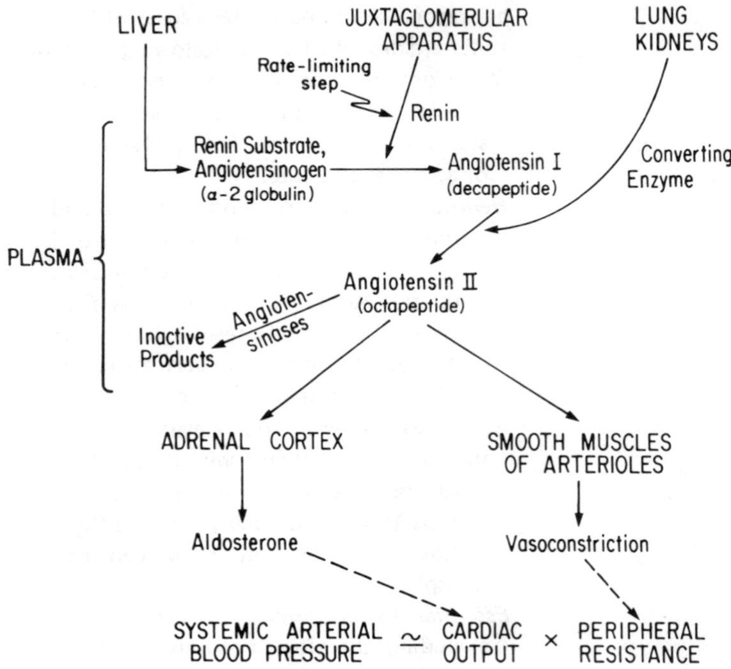

Figure 14-1
Dynamics of the renin-angiotensin-aldosterone system and its possible relation to the systemic arterial blood pressure. Note that the rate-limiting step for the production of angiotensin II is the secretion of renin by the juxtaglomerular apparatus. The converting enzyme has been grouped with the plasma components because the conversion of angiotensin I to angiotensin II occurs mainly in the capillaries of the lungs and partly, perhaps, in the arterioles of the kidneys.

level of the systemic arterial blood pressure. (1) It is an extremely potent vasoconstrictor, and this action when exerted on the smooth muscles of the peripheral arterioles increases the total peripheral resistance. (2) It stimulates the zona glomerulosa of the adrenal cortex to secrete aldosterone, and through this action, it tends to increase the total body Na^+, the extracellular fluid volume, and hence the cardiac output.

Control of Renin Release

The plasma concentration of angiotensin II is controlled primarily by the rate at which renin is released from the JGA (Fig. 14-1). It is therefore of critical importance to understand the feedback system by which the components shown in Figure 14-1 regulate the production of renin (Fig. 14-2). In addition to a direct effect, angiotensin II indirectly regulates the release of renin by three major mechanisms: (1) baroreception in the afferent arterioles, (2) alteration of the amount of NaCl flowing at the macula densa, and (3) the influence of sympathetic nerves on the arterioles of the JGA. Depending on the circumstances, these

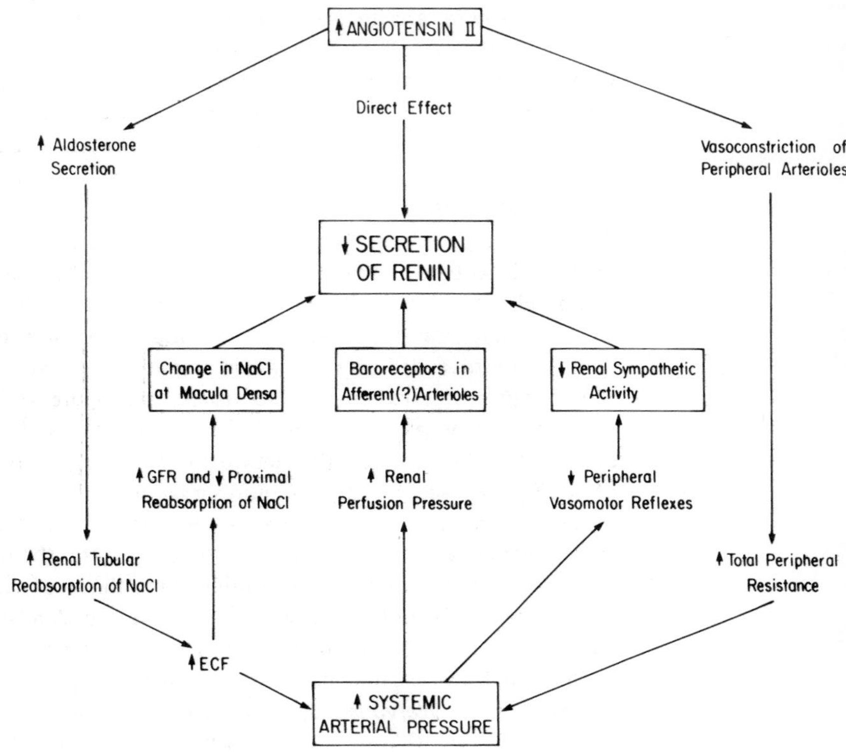

Figure 14-2
Direct and indirect means by which the plasma concentration of angiotensin II exerts negative feedback control on the renal secretion of renin. *ECF* = extracellular fluid volume. Modified from K. M. McDonald and R. W. Schrier, in R. W. Schrier (ed.), *Renal and Electrolyte Disorders.* Boston: Little, Brown, 1976.

three may act together in a coordinated manner, or one or more may predominate over the others.

Baroreceptor Mechanism. Figure 14-2 shows a negative feedback system whereby an increase in renal perfusion pressure decreases the release of renin. The opposite is also true: A decrease in renal perfusion pressure stimulates the release of renin. The presence of a baroreceptor mechanism has been demonstrated by an ingenious, though nonphysiological, model: the nonfiltering kidney. In this model, changes in the flow of NaCl at the macula densa are eliminated by stopping glomerular filtration — but not renal blood flow — through prior renal ischemia plus ureteral ligation; the influence of sympathetic nerves or of catecholamines is excluded in this model through prior renal denervation and adrenalectomy. Even under these circumstances, a decrease in renal perfusion pressure, whether induced by hemorrhage or by constriction of the aorta above the renal arteries, leads to an increase in the release of renin.

Macula Densa Mechanism. Experiments in which the intratubular load of NaCl to the area of the macula densa is varied independently of changes in renal perfusion pressure leave little doubt that NaCl in the region of the JGA can influence the release of renin. Major controversy remains, however, about the details of this mechanism. It is not known whether Na^+, Cl^-, or both are sensed; whether it is their concentration or amount that is sensed; whether their presence within the tubular fluid or in the reabsorbate is the perceived variable; whether the macula densa cells, the lacis cells, or the granular cells are the sensors; and most importantly, whether an increase in NaCl at the macula densa leads to a decrease or an increase in the release of renin. It is because of these unresolved issues that Figure 14-2 speaks only of a "change in NaCl at the macula densa" and does not specify the direction or the nature of the change. The theory of K. Thurau (see Fig. 9-3) requires that increased NaCl at the macula densa leads to an increase in renin secretion, whereas the view championed by A. J. Vander and others states the opposite. It should be noted that Thurau is referring to the *local* generation of angiotensin II within a single nephron, while Vander's reference is more to the peripheral generation of the peptide; this distinction, however, may not be sufficient to resolve the conflict.

Sympathetic Nervous System and Catecholamines. The arterioles of the JGA are innervated by sympathetic nerve fibers. Electrical stimulation of the renal nerves as well as stimulation of β-adrenergic receptors by isoproterenol increase the release of renin, whereas renal denervation and β-adrenergic blockade by propranolol have the opposite effect. It can be shown experimentally that these effects are distinct from those that act via baroreceptors or the macula densa.

Other Influences. At least three other factors, in addition to those shown in Figure 14-2, may play a physiological role in the control of renin release. (1) There is an inverse correlation between the plasma concentration of K^+ and the release of renin. It is possible that this effect is exerted through changes in the delivery of NaCl to the macula densa. (2) Vasopressin, even at physiological doses, inhibits the release of renin. This effect is apparently independent of changes in the three major mechanisms listed above. (3) Prostaglandin E_2 stimulates, and indomethacin (see below) blocks, the production or release of renin.

Role of Renin in Hypertension

Despite the seemingly clear-cut connection between the renin-angiotensin-aldosterone system and the systemic arterial blood pressure that is suggested in Figure 14-1, the role of renin in the maintenance of normal blood pressure and the production of hypertension remains largely unknown. The problem of assigning

Table 14-1
Plasma renin activity (PRA) and systemic arterial blood pressure (B.P.) in various disease states*

Disorder	PRA	B.P.
Cirrhosis	↑	↔ or ↓
Nephrotic syndrome	↑	↔ or ↓
Pregnancy	↑	↔
Preeclampsia	Falls from previous ↑	↑
Renal parenchymal hypertension	↔ or slightly ↑	↑
Renovascular hypertension	↑ in ~65%	↑
	↔ in ~35%	↑
Renoprival hypertension:		
Diseased kidneys still in patient	↔ or slightly ↑	↑
Anephric	Probably 0	↑
Essential hypertension	↔ in ~75%	↑
	↓ in ~25%	↑
	↑ in very few	↑
Primary aldosteronism	↓	↑
Bartter's syndrome	↑	↔ or ↓

*↔ = normal; ↓ = decreased; ↑ = increased.

a causative relationship is illustrated by Table 14-1. Some conditions (e.g., cirrhosis, the nephrotic syndrome, and normal pregnancy) are associated with high plasma levels of renin but normal or low blood pressure, and in preeclampsia, hypertension develops even though the plasma renin level decreases from its previously high value. In some disorders, such as a proportion of renovascular and essential hypertension, the plasma renin levels may be normal or low while the blood pressure is high. And in the patient whose kidneys have been removed and who is being kept alive by dialysis, there may be no renin, although hypertension persists. The inescapable conclusion is that although renin may be responsible for hypertension in some patients, it may play no role or only a minor role in other patients, or at least at that stage of the hypertension when the renin was measured. In fact, despite a tremendous amount of research effort, renin has been assigned an indisputable causative function only in renovascular hypertension, and only in that portion of patients with this disorder whose plasma level of renin is elevated (Table 14-1).

When one recalls that renovascular hypertension is a relatively rare condition that constitutes less than 5 percent of all hypertensive disease, the problem of the causative role of renin is placed in perspective. That is not to say that renin is unimportant in other forms of hypertension, but rather that the interrelationships of the many factors that contribute to hypertension are so

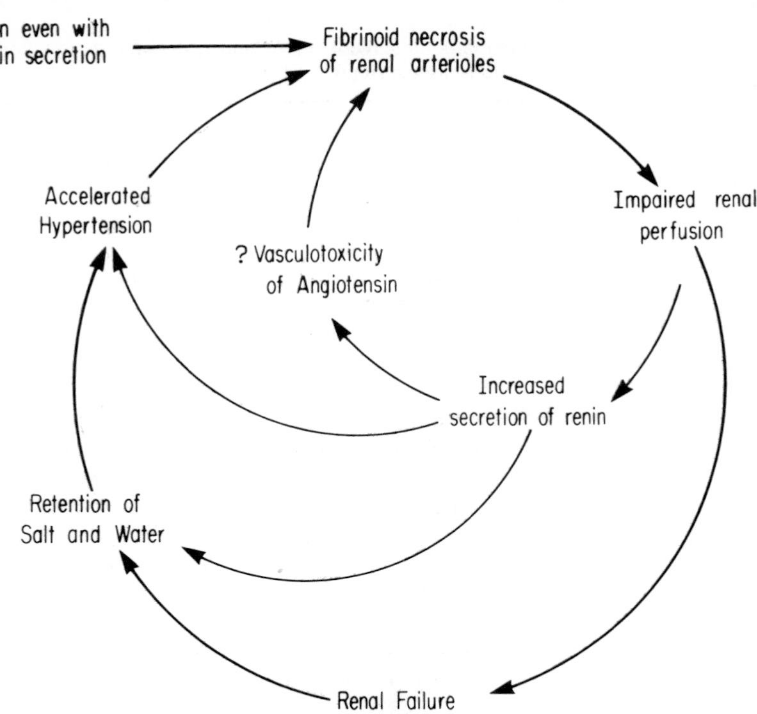

Figure 14-3
Vicious circle of malignant hypertension. Although most commonly the cycle begins with essential hypertension, other forms of high blood pressure can also initiate the chain of events. The question mark indicates that it is not yet settled whether angiotensin directly causes damage to vessels. Modified from K. M. McDonald, in R. W. Schrier (ed.), *Renal and Electrolyte Disorders.* Boston: Little, Brown, 1976.

complex that it is difficult to define the contribution of each factor in many instances, at least at the present state of our knowledge. Such factors include not only those that are discussed in subsequent sections, but also additional effects, such as an inverse relationship between the Na^+ balance and vascular sensitivity to angiotensin II, a possible shift in the set point for the feedback action of aldosterone on renin secretion, as well as others.

The essential difficulty with any substance that, like renin, is produced by the kidney is illustrated in the vicious circle of malignant hypertension (Fig. 14-3): High blood pressure of any cause may lead to fibrinoid necrosis of the renal arterioles and impaired renal perfusion; the latter causes an increase in renin secretion, which in turn aggravates the high blood pressure, causes further damage to the renal arterioles, and so on. (This chain of events is not in conflict with the schema of Figure 14-2, where increased blood pressure is shown to lead to decreased release of renin; in arteriolar nephrosclerosis, the damage to the renal vessels is such that despite increased blood pressure, renal perfusion and the GFR are decreased.) Once the vicious circle has begun, it is difficult to say whether the high plasma concentration of renin is the cause or the result of the hypertension; this dilemma applies to virtually every hypertensive condition in which a high plasma concentration of renin has been measured. Hope for solving the riddle is held out by experimental or therapeutic agents that specifically inhibit renin, converting enzyme, or angiotensin II: If high renin levels contribute to a given hypertension, then the blood pressure should be lowered as the inhibitor is given (Fig. 14-1). Despite considerable work along these lines, the explanation for various forms of hypertension is not yet at hand, probably because most forms involve a variety of causative elements or because different elements may predominate at different stages of even the same form of hypertension.

Evaluation of Plasma Renin Levels. Figure 14-2 reflects other interdependent variables — namely, the state of Na^+ balance, aldosterone secretion, and the volume of extracellular fluid — that can influence not only the blood pressure but also the rate at which renin is elaborated. Since these variables can differ widely from one hypertensive patient to another, *each measurement of the plasma renin level must be evaluated in light of the concurrent Na^+ intake.* In order to ease this problem in clinical practice, graphs have been devised in which the rate of urinary Na^+ excretion is used to reflect the state of Na^+ intake (Fig. 14-4). Other factors that must be considered in assessing the possible functional meaning of a given plasma renin level are (1) the patient's posture at the time the blood sample was taken, for renin activity is usually higher when the patient is in the upright rather than in the resting supine position; (2) the administration of diuretic agents, which are commonly used in the treatment of hypertension and most of which tend to increase the release of renin; (3) the age of the patient, since renin levels are considerably lower in older than in younger patients; and (4) diurnal fluctuations.

In summary, the difficulty of assigning a causative role for renin in the various forms of hypertension has at least three roots: (1) the fact that renin secretion is governed by many factors, which themselves can influence blood pressure; (2) the fact that some of these factors may in part determine the reactivity of the arterioles to angiotensin II; and (3) the fact that a given rise in the plasma level of renin might be the result, rather than the cause, of high blood pressure.

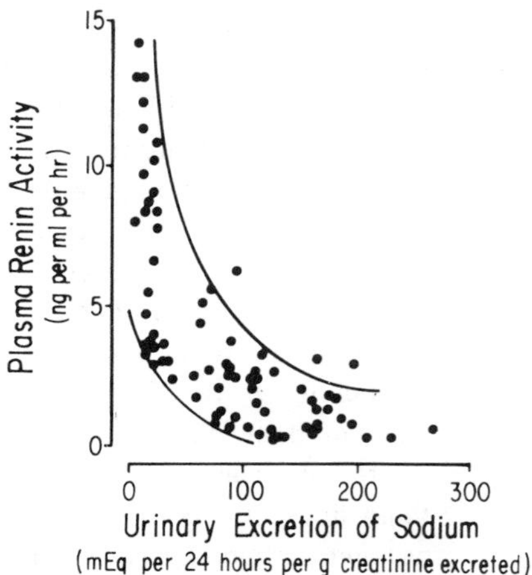

Figure 14-4
Influence of the daily intake of sodium (as reflected in the 24-hour total excretion of the ion) on the activity of renin in the plasma. The values for sodium have been adjusted according to the amount of creatinine excreted in order to account for individuals of varying sizes and skeletal muscle mass (see comment regarding creatinine in Table 1-3). Modified from K. M. McDonald, in R. W. Schrier (ed.), *Renal and Electrolyte Disorders.* Boston: Little, Brown, 1976.

Prostaglandins

The renin-angiotensin-aldosterone system is a mechanism of renal origin that tends to raise the systemic blood pressure; there are also substances produced within the kidneys that tend to lower the blood pressure. This fact was established in a series of experiments by several investigators working independently. In 1947, E. Braun-Menéndez and U. S. von Euler showed that the removal of both kidneys from rats can lead to high blood pressure, so-called renoprival hypertension; obviously, this hypertension could not be caused by the presence of renal substances, such as renin, but it might have been the consequence either of the action of an extrarenal compound that is normally metabolized by the kidneys, of the absence of a renal vasodilator substance, or of the uremic state. The last possibility was rendered unlikely when it was shown by A. Grollman and his associates that the production of uremia in dogs through the diversion of urine into the vena cava (i.e., by eliminating the excretory functions of the kidneys but not their endocrine role) did not necessarily lead to hypertension. These workers therefore proposed that the anephric type of renoprival hypertension is caused not by the liberation of a pressor substance, but by the absence of an anti-pressor activity of renal origin. Subsequently, it was demonstrated that such activity could be found in extracts of renal medulla. Although the activity may be due to several substances (e.g., bradykinin, antihypertensive neutral lipids, or the prosta-

Table 14-2
Influence of furosemide or indomethacin, given alone or in combination, on systemic arterial blood pressure and on components influencing the blood pressure*

	Systemic Arterial Blood Pressure	Urinary Na^+ Excretion	Plasma Renin Activity	Urinary Aldosterone Excretion
Furosemide	↓	↑	↑	↑
Indomethacin	↑	↔	Slight ↓	↓
Furosemide plus indomethacin	↔	↑	Slight ↑	↑

*↑ = greater than control; ↓ = less than control; ↔ = approximately the same as control.
Data from R. V. Patak et al., *Prostaglandins* 10:649, 1975.

glandins), most attention has been focused recently on the prostaglandins, so named because they were first extracted, in the early 1930s, from semen.

The prostaglandins are fatty acids with virtually ubiquitous occurrence and numerous functions; one of the earliest biological effects to be identified was a profound lowering of the systemic arterial blood pressure. These compounds appear in three series of very similar chemical structure: prostaglandin E (PGE), prostaglandin F (PGF), and prostaglandin A (PGA). The PGEs and PGFs are very rapidly and extensively metabolized during a single passage of blood through the lungs, whereas the PGAs are degraded more slowly by the lungs. This fact has led to the suggestion that the first two types are local mediators, whereas the last may be a circulating hormone. (The proposal is stated cautiously, because there is major disagreement on this point, arising mainly from the methodological difficulties in measuring prostaglandins, especially in plasma.) Prostaglandin E has vasodilator effects, and it has been found in high concentrations at two sites within the kidney where it is probably synthesized in specialized interstitial cells: the juxtamedullary area and the inner medulla.

Effects Related to Blood Pressure

The observation that the prostaglandins can lower systemic blood pressure, both in experimental animals and in normotensive and hypertensive humans, has led to the suggestion that the prostaglandins may act as physiological modulators of blood pressure. Based on the kinds of results shown in Table 14-2, it has been proposed that this regulatory function *may* be exerted not only through antagonism of various constrictor effects, but also through influencing Na^+ balance and the extracellular fluid volume.

Much of the information regarding the effects of prostaglandins has been gained by use of an inhibitor of prostaglandin synthesis, indomethacin. The results shown in Table 14-2 were obtained on four normotensive human subjects and six patients with essential hypertension; all were tested in the steady state while ingesting 150 mEq of Na^+ per day. Many diuretic agents, including furosemide, are used in the treatment of hypertension. In both normotensive and hypertensive subjects, furosemide decreased the mean arterial blood pressure and increased the urinary excretion of Na^+ and aldosterone, as well as the plasma activity of renin. When indomethacin alone was given to the same subjects — which presumably resulted in a diminution of the levels or absence of the prostaglandins — the opposite changes were observed. And when furosemide and indomethacin were given together, the changes resembled an algebraic sum of the two effects.

It is not yet clear how the prostaglandins bring about some of the changes shown in Table 14-2; their influence on urinary Na^+ excretion, for example, may result from altering the intrarenal distribution of blood flow or the Starling forces at the peritubular capillaries (see Chap. 3, under Regulation of Na^+ Balance in Health). Also, solutions to some of the seeming paradoxes — for example, increased urinary excretion of Na^+ in the face of increased aldosterone levels or decreased blood pressure with increased renin levels — seen with furosemide administration have not been worked out. The results *suggest* that the solutions to these problems may involve the modulating action of the prostaglandins. The present state of the art does not justify extension beyond this cautious speculation, and Table 14-2 is presented mainly to show that the prostaglandins may play a physiological and pathological role in the regulation of blood pressure and that this role may involve complex interactions with the many other elements that influence the blood pressure.

Extracellular Fluid Volume (ECF)

The role of the volume of ECF in the regulation of systemic arterial blood pressure has been hinted at in Figure 14-1: *Other things being equal,* the greater the ECF, the larger the cardiac output and the higher the blood pressure. That illustration, however, as well as Figures 14-2 and 14-3 intimate that the influence of the ECF on the blood pressure is mediated mainly through the renin-angiotensin-aldosterone system. That the ECF can exert this control in the absence of renin is perhaps most clearly shown in patients with renoprival hypertension. Figure 14-5 shows the results on three patients with chronic renal failure from whom both kidneys were removed and who were being kept alive through continuous dialysis with an artificial kidney; these patients, being anephric, probably had no renin (Table 14-1). During the control period, when the patients had a normal ECF, their mean arterial pressures were normal. The ECF was then

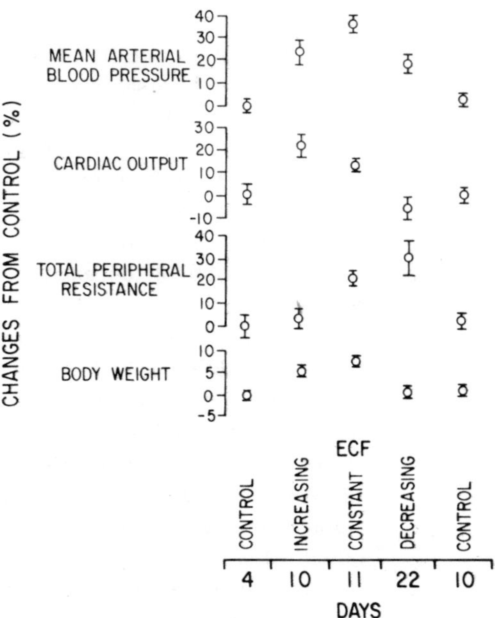

Figure 14-5
Results on three anephric patients in whom extracellular fluid volume was deliberately expanded, as reflected by the gain in body weight. Shown are the effects on the systemic arterial blood pressure and on its two major determinants, cardiac output and peripheral resistance. Number of days denotes the duration of each period. Modified from G. T. Coleman et al., *Circulation* 42:509, 1970.

deliberately expanded over a period of 10 days by regulating the dialysis so that the daily rate of fluid intake exceeded the output; this expansion was accompanied by an increase in systemic blood pressure, which was due mainly to an increased cardiac output. During the next 11 days, the patients were maintained at the expanded ECF; the blood pressure rose even more, but the cardiac output actually decreased while the peripheral resistance increased. During the 22-day period when the expansion of the ECF was corrected, the blood pressure declined even though the peripheral resistance increased further; the cardiac output was therefore decreased to below the control level during this period.

These results have been interpreted as follows. At first, the increased ECF raises the cardiac output and hence the blood pressure. The latter change calls forth autoregulation, not only in the kidneys but also in many other organs. Consequently, both the renal resistance and the total peripheral resistance rise, and this increase sustains the hypertension during the steady state of ECF expansion; the rise in resistance may also cause a decrease in the return of venous blood to the heart and thus account for the concurrent decrease in cardiac output. As the ECF is again decreased, cardiac output and hence blood pressure fall, even though the peripheral resistance increases further, possibly because the autoregulatory mechanisms have been "revved up" and can decrease only with time.

There are several reasons why it is often difficult to demonstrate the role of the ECF in hypertension: (1) When renal function is normal, an expansion of the ECF is very quickly followed by a natriuresis (Fig. 3-2) known as *pressure diuresis,* which returns the ECF to control values. The pressure diuresis probably results partly from an increased filtered load of NaCl but mainly from the decreased tubular reabsorption of salt and water, which involves aldosterone and changes in the Starling forces (see Chap. 3, under Regulation of Na^+ Balance in Health). (2) With the kidneys in situ, activation of the renin-angiotensin-aldosterone system and possibly of the prostaglandins may obscure the influence of changes in the ECF. Paradoxically, this fact is even reflected in a few patients with renoprival hypertension, that is, those in whom the diseased kidneys are still in the body. Some of these patients manifest severe and unrelenting hypertension that can be corrected only through bilateral nephrectomy, which is effective presumably through the removal of renin (see Answer to Problem 14-2). (3) Normally, the baroreceptor mechanism very quickly returns the systemic blood pressure nearly to normal; an appreciable rise in blood pressure may occur only when prompt natriuresis cannot rapidly restore the ECF to normal.

Other Evidence for Role of ECF

Total Exchangeable Sodium. In anephric patients maintained on dialysis, the blood pressure is higher, the greater the amount of Na^+ in the body. This finding is only another means of expressing the phenomenon shown above in Figure 14-5, for according to Equation 3-1 (Chap. 3), the size of the ECF will be a direct function of the amount of Na^+ aboard. It is at least partly for this reason that most diuretics have an antihypertensive effect; some diuretic agents, however, lower the blood pressure because they *may* also influence vascular tone.

It is also a consistent observation that certain populations who eat much salt, such as the people living in northern Japan, have a higher incidence of hypertension than do other populations. It is possible that a genetic predisposition of the kidneys to retain salt is a prerequisite to this phenomenon. This possibility is suggested by the existence of a strain of rats whose blood pressure rises on a high intake of salt. The susceptibility can be lessened (although not abolished) by transplanting kidneys from normal rats into the sensitive ones; conversely, the propensity for hypertension can be transferred by transplanting kidneys from the sensitive animals into normal rats.

Acute Renal Failure. Although the high blood pressure in this condition may have a number of causes (e.g., high levels of renin), the expansion of the ECF is often an important causative element. Patients in oliguric acute renal failure are especially prone to expansion of the ECF (Chap. 9), and their hypertension can often be corrected by reducing their ECF through reduced intake or dialysis.

Sensitivity to Vasoconstrictors. Both in experimental animals and in patients, the arterioles are much more sensitive to angiotensin II and catecholamines in salt-loaded individuals than in salt-depleted ones.

Primary Aldosteronism. Along with the anephric patient (Fig. 14-5), the prototype of volume-expansion hypertension is primary aldosteronism, because in this condition, renin secretion is suppressed (Fig. 14-2 and Table 14-1). In this relatively rare condition (which may account for perhaps 1 percent of all hypertension), autonomous, and hence "primary," overproduction of aldosterone leads to the renal retention of NaCl and thus to the expansion of the ECF and to hypertension, the last being a sine qua non to the diagnosis.

Goldblatt Kidney

The classic work by H. Goldblatt, which involved the production of renovascular hypertension in dogs, was performed long before many of the elements discussed in the preceding sections had been identified. Nevertheless, the Goldblatt experiments are described here because these experiments can be more clearly interpreted in light of the subsequent work that has just been discussed. Although "Goldblatt hypertension" mimics renovascular hypertension (which only accounts for less than 5 percent of all hypertensive disease in humans), the import of Goldblatt's studies extends far beyond that of providing an analog of the human disease; the model continues to provide insights into the causation of most forms of high blood pressure, including essential hypertension.

The following description is not limited to Goldblatt's original experiments; it also includes modifications and facts that have been introduced subsequently.

Two-Kidney and One-Kidney Models

The two types of approaches that are used in the experimental production of renovascular hypertension are shown in Figure 14-6. In the *two-kidney type,* the renal artery of one kidney is partially constricted and the opposite kidney is left untouched. High blood pressure ensues over a period of weeks; the rate of rise and the duration required to reach a stable level of hypertension vary with the species and the precise procedure used. In

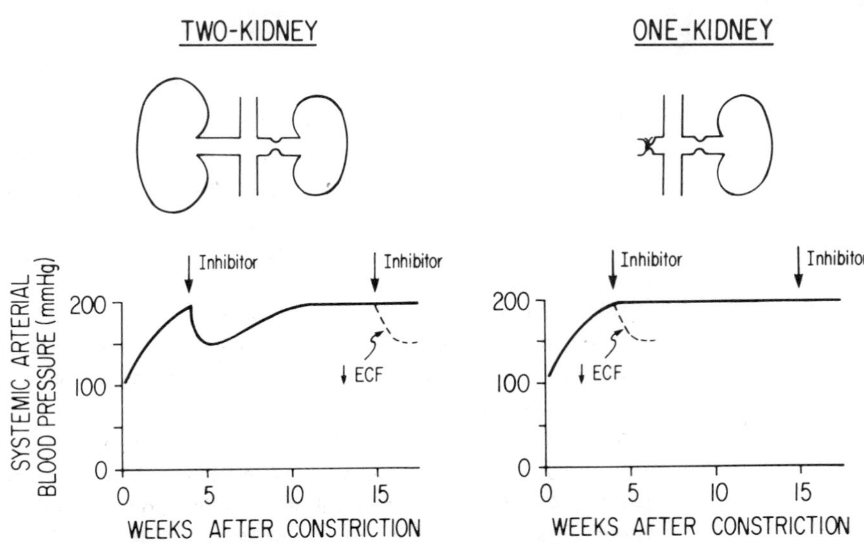

Figure 14-6
Goldblatt hypertension of the two-kidney and one-kidney types. The solid curves represent the results that are usually obtained; the dashed curves, results that are seen after salt restriction and reduction in the volume of extracellular fluid (ECF). In these experiments on rats, an inhibitor of angiotensin II was used. Analogous results have been obtained both in other species, including man, and with inhibitors of other components of the renin-angiotensin system (see Fig. 14-1). Based on H. Gavras et al., *Science* 180:1369, 1973; H. Gavras et al., *Science* 188:1316, 1975.

order to test the role of the renin-angiotensin system in the production of hypertension, various inhibitors are now most commonly employed. The usual observation in the two-kidney model is that in the early phase, an inhibitor of, say, angiotensin II will reduce the blood pressure, whereas later on, it will not. Such results have been interpreted to mean that stimulation of the renin-angiotensin system by the baroreceptor mechanism as well as possibly through the macula densa (Fig. 14-2) is the major cause of the hypertension initially. During this phase, the untouched kidney, being perfused by a higher pressure, undergoes a pressure natriuresis (see next section), which may result in negative Na^+ balance. As hypertension continues, however, it causes changes in the untouched kidney, which then begins to retain salt and H_2O (Fig. 14-8; also Fig. 14-3). Ultimately, it is thought, a point is reached where the resulting expansion of the ECF depresses the secretion of renin (Fig. 14-2) and becomes itself the major cause of the high blood pressure. This interpretation is strengthened by the finding that in the later phase — what is known as the *maintenance phase* — of two-kidney Goldblatt hypertension, an inhibitor of the renin-angiotensin system will not lower the blood pressure unless the

ECF is first reduced and renin secretion stimulated through salt restriction (Fig. 14-4).

In the *one-kidney model,* one kidney is first removed and the renal artery is partially constricted in the opposite kidney (Fig. 14-6). Hypertension again ensues, but now, most commonly, an inhibitor of the renin-angiotensin system does not cause a fall in blood pressure. This finding has been interpreted to mean that in the one-kidney model, the impossibility of producing a pressure diuresis and negative Na^+ balance immediately leads to expansion of the ECF as the predominant cause of the hypertension, a situation that is comparable to the dynamics of the maintenance phase in the two-kidney model. Again, the interpretation is strengthened by the finding that prior salt restriction will cause a reduction in blood pressure in response to an inhibitor in the early phase of even the one-kidney model; it should also be stressed that some investigators have demonstrated an effect of inhibitors during the first week of one-kidney Goldblatt hypertension, even when salt was not restricted.

Therapeutic Implications. Often in clinical medicine, the discovery of a causative agent in a specialized circumstance leads to an overly enthusiastic application to more generalized situations; such was the case with Goldblatt hypertension. The demonstration of the role of renin in the two-kidney model aroused the suspicion that renal production of renin might be responsible for much of human hypertensive disease. The resulting surge of uninephrectomies performed during the ensuing 20 years had largely disappointing results, which we can now better understand. The maintenance phase of two-kidney Goldblatt hypertension (Fig. 14-6) is analogous to the one-kidney model in the sense that the "removal" of the opposite kidney through fibrinoid necrosis and renal failure (Fig. 14-3) has led to the point where salt and water retention and the expansion of the ECF have resulted in a normal or even decreased renin level and have therefore replaced the renin-angiotensin mechanism as the cause of the sustained high blood pressure. Removal of a kidney at this stage is more likely to aggravate than to cure the problem, since it may lead to yet further expansion of the ECF. This reasoning is now appreciated, and nephrectomy for the treatment of hypertension, even when the stenosis of a renal artery is demonstrated, is performed only when the concentration of renin is approximately twice as high in the renal vein of the affected kidney as in that of the opposite kidney, that is, only if it seems likely that overproduction of renin by the diseased kidney is the major cause of the hypertension and that production of renin by the untouched kidney is still being inhibited by the high perfusing pressure and by the high levels of angiotensin (Fig. 14-2).

Since in the two-kidney model, hypertension damages the opposite, untouched kidney, it also follows that the constricted kidney must be removed or repaired early, that is, before the untouched kidney has begun to fail. Given these limitations, it now seems likely that nephrectomy or repair of a renal artery can only cure less than 1 percent of all human hypertensive disease.

Theories of Essential Hypertension

Far and away the most common form of human hypertensive disease is essential hypertension. By its definition, this term denotes a wastebasket category; it encompasses all high blood pressure for which the cause has not been identified. We have just reviewed the known major mechanisms for high blood pressure and we have seen that while they can be shown to play a causative role in some disease states at certain times, their influence cannot be demonstrated in all instances and specifically not in all patients with essential hypertension (see Table 14-1). Nevertheless, the common thread of the role of the kidneys runs through all the mechanisms: renin-angiotensin-aldosterone, prostaglandins, extracellular fluid volume, and Goldblatt hypertension. This fact has given rise to the view that renal function or dysfunction underlies even essential hypertension, or at least a majority of the instances thereof. In the past, a number of investigators have proposed theories for the pathogenesis of hypertension that have sought to take into account the complicated interplay of the numerous influences on blood pressure. What follows is the exposition of one *theoretical schema* that incorporates many of the suggestions advanced by others.

Pressure Natriuresis

Central to the theories is the phenomenon of pressure natriuresis (Fig. 14-7) referred to above (under Extracellular Fluid Volume). When the systemic arterial pressure and hence the renal perfusing pressure are raised, there results an increased urinary excretion of NaCl and water. Since autoregulation largely prevents an increase in the GFR under these circumstances, the natriuresis is due to decreased tubular reabsorption of NaCl and water, probably mainly as a consequence of an increase in the hydrostatic pressure within the peritubular capillaries (Fig. 3-2). It is an experimental observation that in hypertension of many causes, including essential hypertension, the curve for pressure natriuresis is shifted to the right, giving rise to a family of curves (Fig. 14-7); this shift is known as the *resetting of pressure natriuresis.* The mechanism for the resetting is not yet known, but it may be related mainly to an increase in the filtration fraction. This increase means that more plasma than normally is skimmed from the blood that courses through the glomerular capillaries. The consequent rise in the oncotic pressure of plasma in the

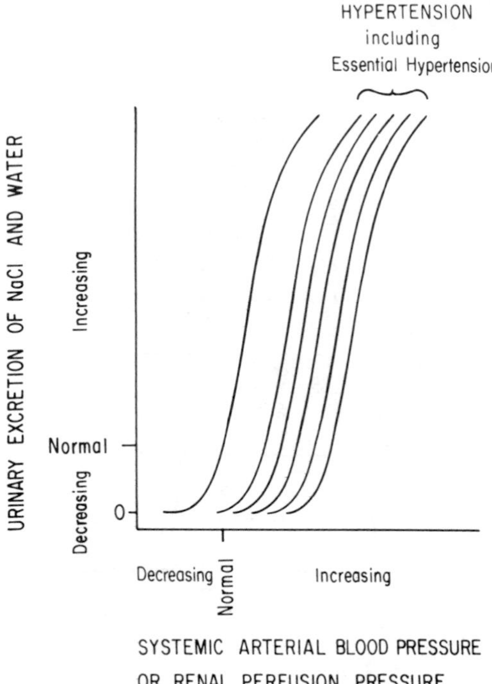

Figure 14-7
Pressure natriuresis as demonstrable in man and in various experimental preparations, including the isolated, perfused kidney. The same relationship is obtained if salt intake, rather than blood pressure, is altered primarily. Resetting of pressure natriuresis is reflected in the family of curves labeled "Hypertension." Adapted from J. J. Brown et al., *Lancet* 2:320, 1974, and A. C. Guyton et al., *Chest* 65:328, 1974; also based on the findings of numerous investigators.

peritubular capillaries will increase the tubular reabsorption of salt and water, and it may thus counterbalance the opposite influence that arises from increased peritubular hydrostatic pressure (Fig. 14-8).

It can be seen from Figure 14-7 that *once resetting has occurred,* a higher than normal blood pressure will be required to maintain balance for NaCl; that is, the urinary NaCl excretion reflects a steady-state intake and this amount of salt can be excreted only at a higher blood pressure. This fact illustrates two major and related features of theories for hypertension: (1) the dilemma of the chicken and the egg and (2) the division of most forms of hypertensive disease into an early phase that starts the high blood pressure and a later phase that maintains it (Fig. 14-8). As it stands, Figure 14-7 implies that systemic arterial pressure is the independent and initiating event, since the blood pressure is graphed on the abscissa. Some investigators, however, would switch the coordinates in Figure 14-7, thereby making

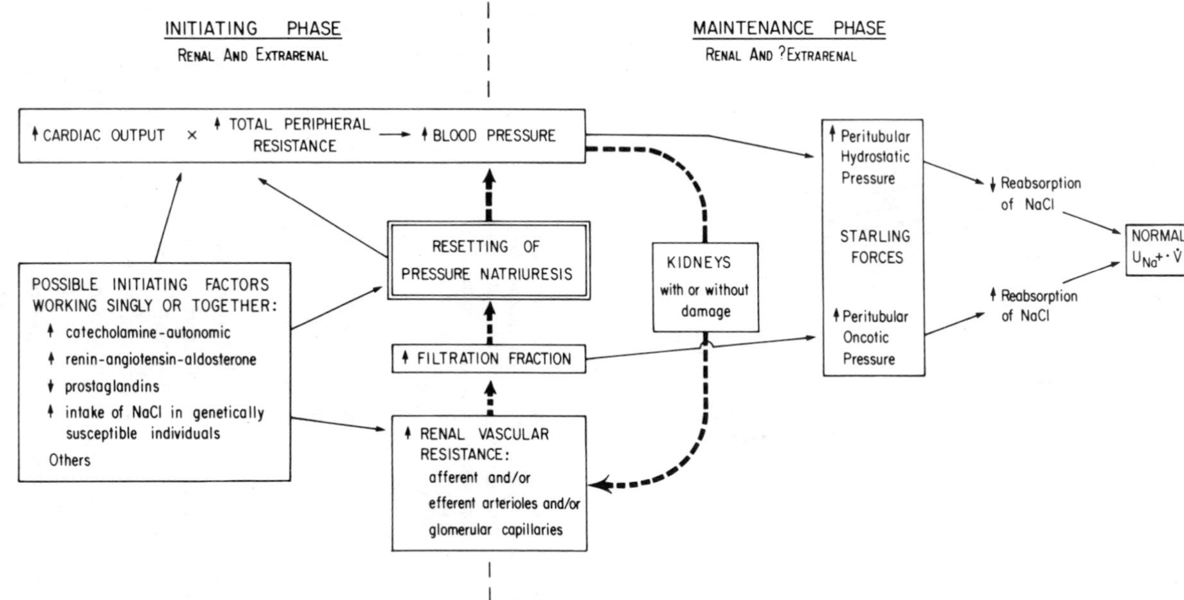

Figure 14-8
Composite of several theories for the pathogenesis of essential hypertension. The renal factors involved in the maintenance phase are outlined by the heavy dashed lines and constitute a self-perpetuating cycle. There is also evidence for the action of extrarenal factors in the maintenance phase, possibly through the resetting of carotid baroreceptors. Finally, there is debate whether an increase in peritubular hydrostatic pressure occurs. $U_{Na^+} \cdot \dot{V}$ = rate of urinary NaCl excretion. Although many investigators have contributed to these theories, this schema is based mainly on the views of A. C. Guyton et al., *Chest* 65:328, 1974, and J. J. Brown et al., *Lancet* 1:1217, 1976.

urinary salt excretion the independent variable and implying that an inability of the kidneys to excrete a given salt load at a normal blood pressure is the change that starts the hypertension.

Theoretical Schema

A composite of some of the theories for essential hypertension that have been proposed is shown in Figure 14-8. Note that the resetting of pressure natriuresis — that is, the elevation of the blood pressure at which a given salt load can be excreted (Fig. 14-7) — is placed at the center, half in the initiating phase and half in the maintenance phase, to indicate that it may play a pivotal role both in starting and maintaining essential hypertension. High blood pressure, increased renal vascular resistance, and an increased filtration fraction have been placed in similar positions because, through the self-perpetuating cycle indicated in the figure by the heavy dashed lines, they might also both start and maintain essential hypertension.

Initiating Phase. It is likely that eventually the single category of essential hypertension will be subdivided into several types according to the initiating abnormality. The primary event might be hyperactivity of the catecholamine-autonomic nervous system, increased renin-angiotensin levels, a change in other humoral substances that influence the cardiovascular system, an abnormal response to a salt load, or a number of other factors, both known and possibly not yet identified. Depending on which element comes first, the initial rise in blood pressure might be caused mainly by an increase in cardiac output, by an increase in the total peripheral resistance, or both. Note also that these two determinants of the blood pressure might be influenced either directly by the primary element (in which case the initiating phase could be extrarenal) or indirectly by increasing renal vascular resistance or somehow resetting pressure natriuresis (in which case the initiating phase would be at least partly renal in origin). There is no doubt, however, that renal vascular resistance is increased once essential hypertension has been established.

Maintenance Phase. Once the blood pressure has been elevated, several events occur that will not only maintain hypertension but aggravate it with time. One is the influence of high blood pressure on the kidneys. This effect will not necessarily lead to overt renal failure and malignant hypertension (as shown in Figure 14-3), but it may involve much more subtle changes that decrease the renal blood flow but not the GFR and that would therefore not be recognized, in the conventional sense, as failure of renal function. (The vicious circle shown in Figure 14-8 by the heavy dashed lines is therefore not necessarily the same as the cycle shown in Figure 14-3.) Such changes, however, will elevate the filtration fraction, which is a constant finding in essential hypertension and which, as mentioned above, may lead to a resetting of pressure natriuresis. As explained earlier, the increase in the filtration fraction, by counterbalancing Starling forces, might also account for the fact that NaCl balance and the ECF tend to be normal in most patients with established essential hypertension. It is not yet known which of the elements in the self-perpetuating cycle shown in Figure 14-8 are causes and which are consequences, and it is possible that these elements change roles depending on the type and duration of essential hypertension. The maintenance phase might also involve extrarenal factors that involve the resetting of carotid baroreception.

Summary

A possible major role for the kidneys in the causation of high blood pressure was suspected at least 150 years ago when Richard Bright called attention to the association of renal disease and left ventricular hypertrophy. Since then, several renal mechanisms have been identified. They fall into two general categories: (1) those involving the action of vasoactive compounds and (2) those involving the regulation of the extracellular fluid volume (ECF).

Renin, which is secreted by the juxtaglomerular apparatuses (JGA), controls the production of angiotensin II, a most potent vasoconstrictor, and in part the production of aldosterone, which is an important regulator of the ECF. The secretion of renin, in turn, is controlled by three major factors: (1) baroreception in the afferent arterioles, (2) sensing of NaCl at the macula densa, and (3) sympathetic activity at the JGA.

The prostaglandins are fatty acids that are classified into several types, depending on their molecular structure. The prostaglandins of the E series (PGE) can lower blood pressure through vasodilation, and they are synthesized by specialized interstitial cells in the kidneys.

Although renin may play a role in the regulation of the ECF through its influence on aldosterone, the blood pressure can also be affected through changes of the ECF in the absence of renin. This fact can be most clearly demonstrated in anephric patients on dialysis, who probably have no renin. Expansion of the ECF through infusion of saline in these patients leads to an elevation of blood pressure, which at first is due to an increase in cardiac output, and then to an increase in the total peripheral resistance that occurs while the cardiac output falls to normal (Fig. 14-5).

The roles of some of the above elements are illustrated in so-called two-kidney Goldblatt hypertension (Fig. 14-6), a model that was actually devised before many of the facts about the renin-angiotensin-aldosterone system and the role of the ECF were known. Stimulation of renin-angiotensin activity is probably the major cause of the high blood pressure seen during the early phase of this model. Later, however, continued hypertension causes functional and structural changes in the untouched kidney, which lead to salt and water retention and expansion of the ECF. At this point, renin activity is often suppressed, and an increased ECF then becomes the cause of the sustained high blood pressure.

The Goldblatt model illustrates several further points: (1) Most hypertensive disorders probably can be divided into an initial, induction phase when one or more mechanisms may predominate and a second, maintenance phase when one or more other mechanisms may assume the major role. (2) Often in clinical medicine when a new phenomenon is discovered, there follows a vigorous therapeutic application based on concepts derived from this phenomenon, which, at first surprisingly, fails. Thus, the identification of the role of renin in Goldblatt hypertension led for nearly 20 years to a spate of nephrectomies that proved very disappointing, because, as we now know, renin may be the main, direct cause of high blood pressure only at certain stages and in certain types of hypertension. (3) Although the clinical analog of the Goldblatt model, namely, renovascular hypertension, accounts for less than 5 percent of high blood pressure in humans, the model – with its induction phase and a maintenance phase – probably has much wider applicability; it may extend even to essential hypertension, which accounts for 80 to 90 percent of human hypertensive disease (Fig. 14-8). Similarly, primary aldosteronism has assumed much greater importance than its rarity would imply, since it provides a prototype of ECF-expansion hypertension with low plasma concentrations of renin.

Considering that the kidneys have been implicated in hypertension for at least 150 years, that renin was discovered before the twentieth century, and that the prostaglandins and the Goldblatt mechanism were studied in the early 1930s, it may seem that progress in this field has been slow. The main reason for the delay lies in the fact that systemic arterial blood pressure is determined by the interplay of numerous renal and extrarenal factors. Some factors predominate in some forms of high blood pressure, other factors prevail in other forms, and a given factor may play a major causative role at one stage of a single type of hypertension but not at another stage of the same disorder. Consequently, hypertension is undoubtedly not a single entity, but rather it represents an assortment of different disorders. It may well turn out that the kidneys embody the final common pathway for virtually all high blood pressure, even for essential hypertension. The basis for this assertion is reflected in Figure 14-8, which attempts to invoke the numerous elements that determine blood pressure into a unifying theory.

Problem 14-1

A mother of two was in apparently excellent health until age 41 when she volunteered to donate blood. She had done so several times previously, the last time about one year earlier. On the present occasion, it was noted that the blood pressure in both arms while she was sitting was approximately 210/115 mm Hg. She was referred to her private doctor who, in addition, noted an abnormality on the intravenous pyelogram (I.V.P.); the right kidney, though within normal limits in size, was smaller than the left, and it showed delayed opacification of the calyceal system. There was no evidence of renal failure, and chlorothiazide administration had little effect on the blood pressure, reducing it to about 180/110 mm Hg.

The doctor then referred the patient to a specialty center, where the previous findings were quickly confirmed. Without medication, the patient's blood pressure averaged 190–200/110–115 mm Hg. The results of physical examination were normal except for slight arteriolar narrowing in the eyegrounds and the presence of a high-pitched, to-and-fro bruit in the right upper quadrant. An I.V.P. examination employing both rapid-sequence and delayed films again revealed a smaller right kidney with delayed nephrogram and delayed excretion on that side, findings that were confirmed by aortography (Fig. 14-9). An electrocardiogram (ECG) showed questionable hypertrophy of the left ventricle. Other laboratory tests, all of which were normal, included complete blood count; urinalysis; BUN and serum creatinine concentrations; serum Na^+, K^+, Cl^-, and HCO_3^- concentrations; 24-hour urinary excretion of vanillylmandelic acid (VMA); and x-ray of the chest. A renal arteriogram, performed by injecting contrast medium into the right renal artery, revealed a stenotic lesion in the middle third of the main renal artery, characteristic of fibrous dysplasia (Fig. 14-9). At the same procedure, blood was obtained by means of a catheter from both renal veins and from the inferior vena cava. Analysis of these samples for renin showed: sample from left renal vein, 36.4 nanograms of angiotensin II generated per milliliter of plasma per hour; sample from right renal vein, 35.3 ng/ml per hour; and sample from vena cava, 23.7 ng/ml per hour (normal value, 0.8 to 2.8 ng/ml per hour).

The standard criterion for operating on this type of stenotic lesion is that the renal venous activity for renin should be at least 1.5 times greater on the affected side than on the opposite side. Nevertheless, surgical correction was advised in this patient because she was relatively young, her hypertension was of recent onset, and the plasma renin values were so high. Accordingly, the stenotic lesion was removed, and the resulting gap in the artery was covered with a patch graft from a saphenous vein.

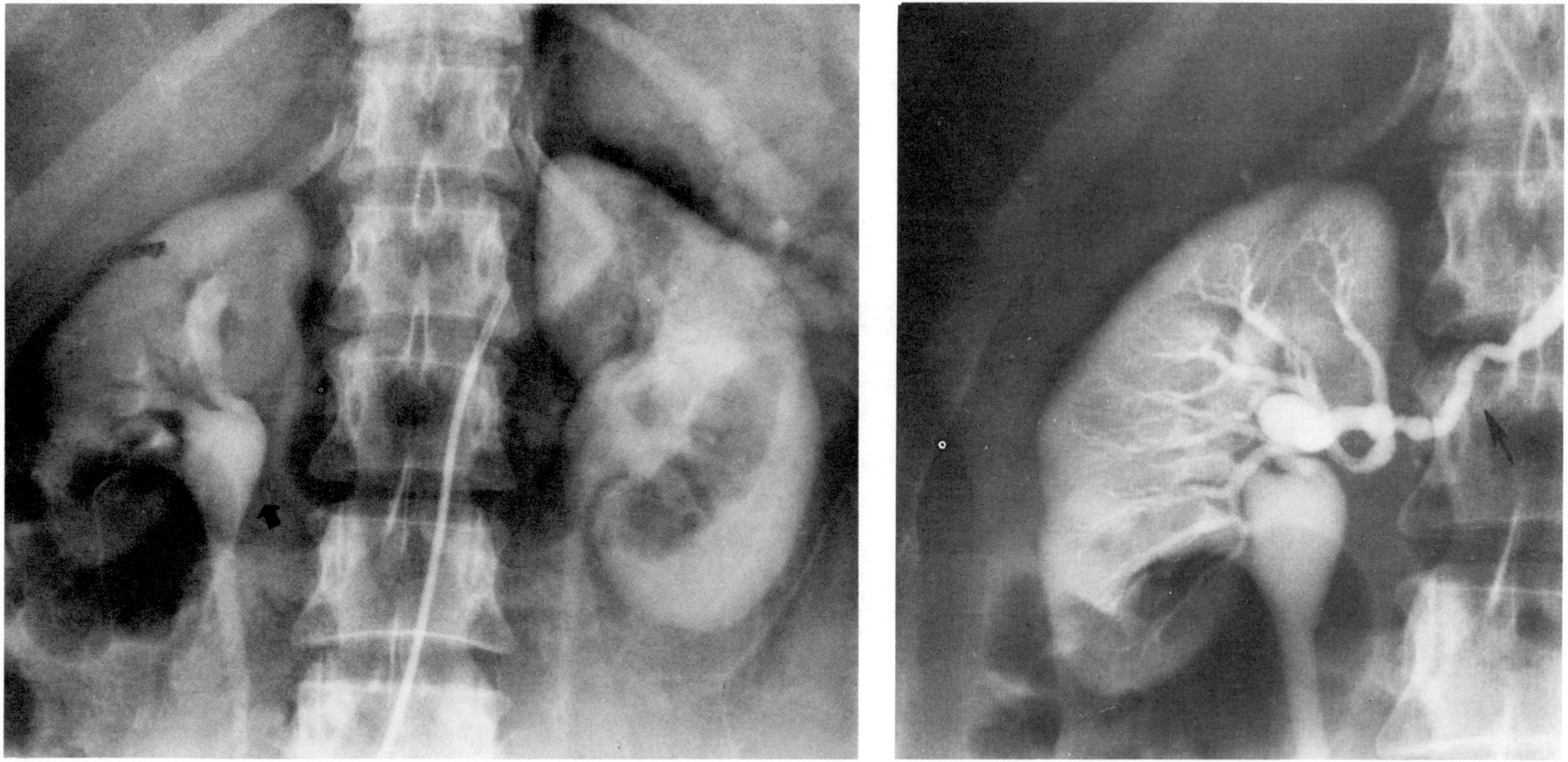

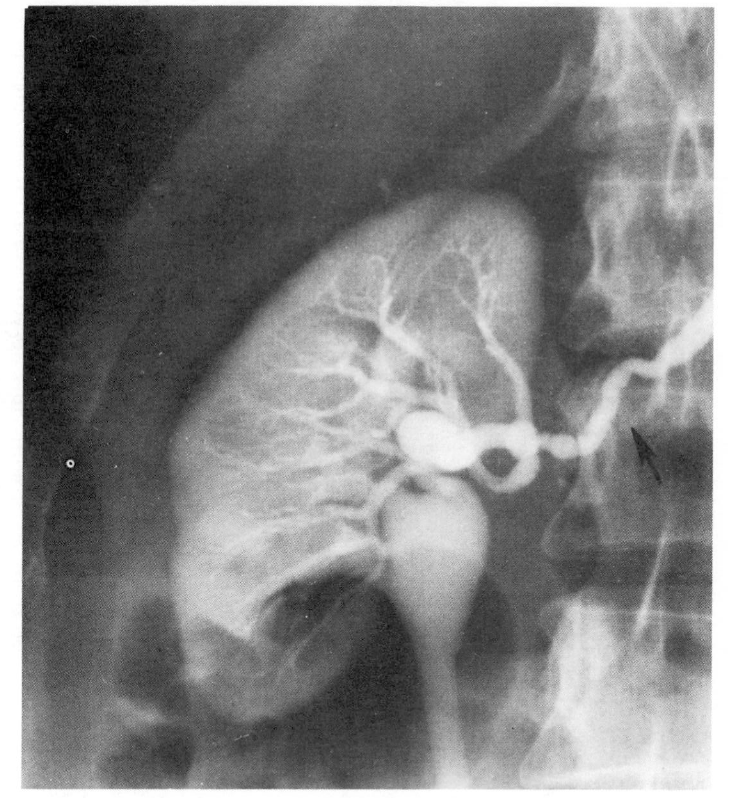

Figure 14-9
X-rays of the kidneys of a 41-year-old woman with hypertension. Contrast agent was injected (*left*) into the aorta (opacified catheter); the film shows delayed excretion and hyperconcentration (*arrow*) of the contrast medium in the right kidney, which is smaller than the left. The renal arteriogram (*right*) reveals a stenotic lesion (*arrow*) in the middle third of the main right renal artery. Courtesy of Peter J. Spiegel.

The patient's blood pressure returned to normal levels during the first three postoperative days, but then it rose again to about 180/100 mm Hg on the fifth day. The patient was discharged, and hydralazine hydrochloride and chlorothiazide were prescribed. During the ensuing two months, the blood pressure declined again, hydralazine therapy was discontinued and the dosage of chlorothiazide reduced, and by mid-April of 1970, the hypertensive medications were stopped entirely. The patient has been followed carefully for seven years, during which time her blood pressure has averaged 135/75 mm Hg. Her only regular medication is phenobarbital (15 mg three times daily), which is given because she is a somewhat hyperactive person.

1. Which of the various experimental models of hypertension described in this chapter does this patient's disorder resemble? Why was it important to know that the patient had only recently developed high blood pressure? Was it foolish to operate on this patient when an important criterion for renal venous renin activity was not met?
2. What are the special features of an I.V.P. done for the evaluation of hypertension? How do you explain the findings in this test? Knowing what you do about renal physiology and given the fact that the contrast medium for intravenous pyelography is handled like inulin, would you predict that at some point the medium in the kidney with the stenosis will appear more or less concentrated than in the opposite kidney?

Problem 14-2

We turn once more to the patient described in Problems 10-2 and 12-2, the woman with chronic renal failure who underwent renal transplantation at age 37. After essential hypertension, the renal parenchymal form of hypertension is one of the commonest causes of high blood pressure, and we shall here concentrate on that problem.

At age 30 when renal disease was first diagnosed in this patient, her blood pressure was already mildly elevated at 140/80 mm Hg. During the next seven years, one of the chief problems was progressive hypertension, and when, at age 37, she was admitted to the hospital with terminal renal failure, the blood pressure was repeatedly recorded in the range of 220/140 mm Hg. Her eyegrounds at that time revealed arteriolar narrowing and flame-shaped hemorrhages. During the 2½ months while her life was sustained by peritoneal dialysis and then by machine dialysis, the high blood pressure persisted at values around 160/90 mm Hg, despite the administration of large doses of reserpine and then methyldopa. At one point during this period, she was given two units of packed cells, because some of the doctors attending her were worried about severe anemia. Although she had lost weight steadily throughout the dialysis, she went into pulmonary edema before the transfusion could be completed. Her blood pressure during that episode rose again to a high of 230/120 mm Hg.

Just before transplantation and while the patient was on extracorporeal dialysis and methyldopa, her blood pressure was 200/140 mm Hg. At the same operation when she received a kidney from her brother, both of her own kidneys were removed; on microscopic examination they showed, among other changes, severe thickening of the arterial and arteriolar walls. Immediately after this operation, even while she was still in the postanesthesia room, her blood pressure was recorded at 110/70 mm Hg. The blood pressure has remained in that range during the nine years since transplantation, and hypertension has not been a problem since that procedure.

1. Interpret the findings in the patient's eyegrounds at the time when she was in terminal renal failure.
2. What do you think was the mechanism(s) for her severe hypertension during the three months prior to transplantation?

Selected References

General

Bianchi, G., Fox, U., DiFrancesco, G. F., Bardi, U., and Radice, M. The hypertensive role of the kidney in spontaneously hypertensive rats. *Clin. Sci. Mol. Med.* 45 [Suppl. 1]; 135s, 1973.

Blumenthal, S. (chairman). Report of the task force on blood pressure control in children. *Pediatrics* 59:797, 1977.

Bright, R. *Reports of Medical Cases, Selected with a View of Illustrating the Symptoms and Cure of Diseases by a Reference to Morbid Anatomy.* London: Longman, Rees, Orme, Brown, & Green, 1827.

Brown-Séquard, C. E., and d'Arsonval, A. Des injections sous-cutanées ou intraveineuses d'extraits liquides de nombre d'organes, comme méthode therapeutique. *C. R. Acad. Sci.* (Paris) 114:1399, 1892.

Butler, A. M. Chronic pyelonephritis and arterial hypertension. *J. Clin. Invest.* 16:889, 1937.

Dahl, L. K., and Heine, M. Primary role of renal homografts in setting chronic blood pressure levels in rats. *Circ. Res.* 36:692, 1975.

de Wardener, H. E. *The Kidney. An Outline of Normal and Abnormal Structure and Function* (4th ed.). Edinburgh: Churchill/Livingstone, 1973. Chap. 11.

Genest, J., and Koiw, E. (eds.). *Hypertension — 1972.* Berlin: Springer, 1972.

Hollenberg, N. K., and Adams, D. F. The renal circulation in hypertensive disease. *Am. J. Med.* 60:773, 1976.

Kincaid-Smith, P., and Maxwell, M. H. (eds.). Hypertension and the kidney. *Kidney Int.* 8 [Suppl. 5]:S-151, 1975.

Lancet Editorial. Hypertension in pregnancy. *Lancet* 2:487, 1975.

Laragh, J. H. (ed.). *Hypertension Manual.* New York: Dun-Donnelley, 1973.

Laragh, J. H. (ed.). Symposium on hypertension. *Am. J. Med.* 60:733, 1976.
This symposium includes, among other topics, articles on the renin-angiotensin system, prostaglandins, the autonomic nervous system, and the role of the kidneys.

McDonald, K. M. The Kidney in Hypertension. In R. W. Schrier (ed.), *Renal and Electrolyte Disorders.* Boston: Little, Brown, 1976.

McNeil, B. J., and Adelstein, S. J. Measures of clinical efficacy. The value of case finding in hypertensive renovascular disease. *N. Engl. J. Med.* 293:221, 1975.

McNeil, B. J., Varady, P. D., Burrows, B. A., and Adelstein, S. J. Measures of clinic efficacy. Cost-effectiveness calculations in the diagnosis and treatment of hypertensive renovascular disease. *N. Engl. J. Med.* 293: 216, 1975.

Okamoto, K. Spontaneous hypertension in rats. *Int. Rev. Cytol.* 7:227, 1969.

Page, I. H., and McCubbin, J. W. (eds.). *Renal Hypertension.* Chicago: Year Book, 1968.

Peart, W. S. Hypertension and the Kidney. In D. A. K. Black (ed.), *Renal Disease* (3rd ed.). Oxford, Eng.: Blackwell, 1972.

Pickering, G. W. *High Blood Pressure* (2nd ed.). London: Churchill, 1968.

Rance, C. P., Arbus, G. S., Balfe, J. W., and Kooh, S. W. Persistent systemic hypertension in infants and children. *Pediatr. Clin. North Am.* 21:801, 1974.

Schambelan, M., and Biglieri, E. G. Hypertension and the Role of the Renin-Angiotensin-Aldosterone System in Renal Failure. In B. M. Brenner and F. C. Rector, Jr. (eds.), *The Kidney.* Philadelphia: Saunders, 1976.

Stason, W. B., and Weinstein, M. C. Allocation of resources to manage hypertension. *N. Engl. J. Med.* 296:732, 1977.

Walworth, C. C., and Charman, R. C. Industrial hypertension program in a rural state. *J. A. M. A.* 237:1942, 1977.

Renin-Angiotensin-Aldosterone System

Barajas, L. Renin secretion: An Anatomical basis for tubular control. *Science* 172:485, 1971.

Blaine, E. H., Davis, J. O., and Witty, R. T. Renin release after hemorrhage and after suprarenal aortic constriction in dogs without sodium delivery to the macula densa. *Circ. Res.* 27:1081, 1970.

Boyd, G. W. An inactive higher-molecular-weight renin in normal subjects and hypertensive patients. *Lancet* 1:215, 1977.

Case, D. B., Wallace, J. M., Keim, H. J., Weber, M. A., Sealey, J. E., and Laragh, J. H. Possible role of renin in hypertension as suggested by renin-sodium profiling and inhibition of converting enzyme. *N. Engl. J. Med.* 296:641, 1977.

Davis, J. O. (ed.). Symposium: Advances in our knowledge of the renin-angiotensin system. *Fed. Proc.* 36:1753, 1977.

Davis, J. O., and Freeman, R. H. Mechanisms regulating renin release. *Physiol. Rev.* 56:1, 1976.

Davis, J. O., Freeman, R. H., Johnson, J. A., and Spielman, W. S. Agents which block the action of the renin-angiotensin system. *Circ. Res.* 34:279, 1974.

Dunn, M. J., and Tannen, R. L. Low-renin hypertension. *Kidney Int.* 5:317, 1974.

Esler, M., Zweifler, A., Randall, O., Julius, S., Bennett, J., Rydelek, P., Cohen, E., and DeQuattro, V. Suppression of sympathetic nervous function in low-renin essential hypertension. *Lancet* 2:115, 1976.

Ferguson, R. K., Turini, G. A., Brunner, H. R., Gavras, H., and McKinstry, D. N. A specific orally active inhibitor of angiotensin-converting enzyme in man. *Lancet* 1:775, 1977.

Gavras, H., Ribeiro, A. B., Gavras, I., and Brunner, H. R. Reciprocal relation between renin dependency and sodium dependency in essential hypertension. *N. Engl. J. Med.* 295:1278, 1976.

Granger, P., Dahlheim, H., and Thurau, K. Enzyme activities of the single juxtaglomerular apparatus in the rat kidney. *Kidney Int.* 1:78, 1972.

Hollenberg, N. K., Williams, G. H., Burger, B., Ishikawa, I., and Adams, D. F. Blockade and stimulation of renal, adrenal, and vascular angiotensin II receptors with 1-Sar,8-Ala angiotensin II in normal man. *J. Clin. Invest.* 57:39, 1976.

Lancet Editorial. Propranolol and plasma-renin. *Lancet* 1:243, 1973.

Laragh, J. H., and Sealey J. E. The Renin-Angiotensin-Aldosterone Hormonal System and Regulation of Sodium, Potassium, and Blood Pressure Homeostasis. In J. Orloff and R. W. Berliner (eds.), *Handbook of Physiology,* Section 8, Renal Physiology. Washington, D.C.: American Physiological Society, 1973.

Mahony, J. F., Storey, B. G., Gibson, G. R., Stokes, G. S., Sheil, A. G. R., and Stewart, J. H. Bilateral nephrectomy for malignant hypertension. *Lancet* 1:1036, 1972.

McDonald, K. M., and Schrier, R. W. Disorders of the Renin-Angiotensin-Aldosterone System. In R. W. Schrier (ed.), *Renal and Electrolyte Disorders.* Boston: Little, Brown, 1976.

Miller, E. D., Jr., Samuels, A. I., Haber, E., and Barger, A. C. Inhibition of angiotensin conversion and prevention of renal hypertension. *Am. J. Physiol.* 228:448, 1975.

Moore, S. B., and Goodwin, F. J. Effect of beta-adrenergic blockade on plasma-renin activity and intractable hypertension in patients receiving regular dialysis treatment. *Lancet* 2:67, 1976.

Oparil, S., and Haber, E. The renin-angiotensin system. *N. Engl. J. Med.* 291:389 and 446, 1974.

Padfield, P. L., Beevers, D. G., Brown, J. J., Davies, D. L., Lever, A. F., Robertson, J. I. S., Schalekamp, M. A. D., Tree, M., and Titterington, M. Is low-renin hypertension a stage in the development of essential hypertension or a diagnostic entity? *Lancet* 1:548, 1975.

Peach, M. J. Renin-angiotensin system: Biochemistry and mechanisms of action. *Physiol. Rev.* 57:313, 1977.

Peart, W. S. Renin-angiotensin system. *N. Engl. J. Med.* 292:302, 1975.

Schalekamp, M. A., Beevers, D. G., Briggs, J. D., Brown, J. J., Davies, D. L., Fraser, R., Lebel, M., Lever, A. F., Medina, A., Morton, J. J., Robertson, J. I. S., and Tree, M. Hypertension in chronic renal failure. An abnormal relation between sodium and the renin-angiotensin system. *Am. J. Med.* 55:379, 1973.

Stein, J. H., and Ferris, T. F. The physiology of renin. *Arch. Intern. Med.* 131:860, 1973.

Stokes, G. S., and Edwards, K. D. G. (eds.). *Drugs Affecting the Renin-Angiotensin-Aldosterone System. Use of Angiotensin Inhibitors.* Basel: Karger, 1976.

Streeten, D. H. P., Anderson, G. H., Freiberg, J. M., and Dalakos, T. G. Use of an angiotensin II antagonist (Saralasin) in the recognition of "angiotensinogenic" hypertension. *N. Engl. J. Med.* 292:657, 1975.

Thurau, K., and Mason, J. The Intrarenal Function of the Juxtaglomerular Apparatus. In K. Thurau (ed.), *Kidney and Urinary Tract Physiology.* Baltimore: University Park Press, 1974.

Thurston, H., and Swales, J. D. Low renin hypertension. *Lancet* 2:930, 1976.

Tigerstedt, R., and Bergman, P. G. Niere und Kreislauf. *Skand. Arch. Physiol.* 8:223, 1898.

Vander, A. J. Control of renin release. *Physiol. Rev.* 47:359, 1967.

Williams, G. H. Measurement of renin activity — When is it useful? *N. Engl. J. Med.* 294:1176, 1976.

Williams, G. H. Angiotensin-dependent hypertension — potential pitfalls in definition. *N. Engl. J. Med.* 296:684, 1977.

Prostaglandins and Other Hormones

Bergström, S., Ryhage, R., Samuelsson, B., and Sjövall, J. The structure of prostaglandin E, F_1 and F_2. *Acta Chem. Scand.* 16:501, 1962.

Bradley, S. E. (ed.). Symposium on hormones and the kidney. *Kidney Int.* 6:261, 1974.

Braun-Menéndez, E., and von Euler, U. S. Hypertension after bilateral nephrectomy in the rat. *Nature* 160:905, 1947.

Brown-Séquard, C. E., and d'Arsonval, A. Des injections sous-cutanées ou intraveineuses d'extraits liquides de nombre d'organes, comme méthode therapeutique. *C. R. Acad. Sci.* (Paris) 114:1399, 1892.

Dunn, M. J., and Hood, V. L. Prostaglandins and the kidney. *Am. J. Physiol.* 233:F 169, 1977.

Fisher, J. W. *Kidney Hormones.* New York: Academic, 1971.

Frölich, J. C., Sweetman, B. J., Carr, K., Hollifield, J. W., and Oates, J. A. Assessment of the levels of PGA_2 in human plasma by gas chromatography-mass spectrometry. *Prostaglandins* 10:185, 1975.

Grollman, A., Muirhead, E. E., and Vanatta, J. Role of the kidney in pathogenesis of hypertension as determined by a study of the effects of bilateral nephrectomy and other experimental procedures on the blood pressure of the dog. *Am. J. Physiol.* 157:21, 1949.

Haack, D., and Möhring, J. Vasopressin-mediated blood pressure response to intraventricular injection of angiotensin II in the rat. *Pflügers Arch. Eur. J. Physiol.* 373:167, 1978.

Kaley, G. (ed.). Symposium: The role of prostaglandins in vascular homeostasis. *Fed. Proc.* 35:2358, 1976.

Kuehl, F. A., Jr., Cirillo, V. J., and Oien, H. G. Prostaglandin-Cyclic Nucleotide Interactions in Mammalian Tissues. In S. M. M. Karim (ed.), *Prostaglandins: Chemical and Biochemical Aspects.* Baltimore: University Park Press, 1976.

Lee, J. B., Patak, R. V., and Mookerjee, B. K. Renal prostaglandins and the regulation of blood pressure and sodium and water homeostasis. *Am. J. Med.* 60:798, 1976.

Massry, S. G. (ed.). Kidney and hormones. *Nephron* 15:161, 1975. This symposium includes, among other topics, articles on renin, adrenocortical hormones, prostaglandins, and catecholamines.

McGiff, J. C., and Vane, J. R. Prostaglandins and the regulation of blood pressure. *Kidney Int.* 8 [Suppl. 5]:S-262, 1975.

Möhring, J., Möhring, B., Petri, M., and Haack, D. Vasopressor role of ADH in the pathogenesis of malignant DOC hypertension. *Am. J. Physiol.* 232:F 260, 1977.

Muirhead, E. E., Jones, F., and Stirman, J. A. Antihypertensive property in renoprival hypertension of extract from renal medulla. *J. Lab. Clin. Med.* 56:167, 1960.

Muirhead, E. E., Leach, B. E., Byers, L. W., Brooks, B., Daniels, E. G., and Hinman, J. W. Antihypertensive Neutral Renomedullary Lipids (ANRL). In J. W. Fisher (ed.), *Kidney Hormones.* New York: Academic, 1971.

Padfield, P. L., Brown, J. J., Lever, A. F., Morton, J. J., and Robertson, J. I. S. Changes of vasopressin in hypertension: Cause or effect? *Lancet* 1:1255, 1976.

Tobian, L., and O'Donnell, M. Renal prostaglandins in relation to sodium regulation and hypertension. *Fed. Proc.* 35:2388, 1976.

Zusman, R. M., Caldwell, B. V., Mulrow, P. J., and Speroff, L. The role of prostaglandin A in the control of sodium homeostasis and blood pressure. *Prostaglandins* 3:679, 1973.

Extracellular Fluid Volume (ECF)

Coleman, T. G., Bower, J. D., Langford, H. G., and Guyton, A. C. Regulation of arterial pressure in the anephric state. *Circulation* 42:509, 1970.

Lancet Editorial. Salt and hypertension. *Lancet* 1:1325, 1975.

Möhring, J., Möhring, B., Näumann, H.-J., Philippi, A., Homsy, E., Orth, H., Dauda, G., Kazda, S., and Gross, F. Salt and water balance and renin activity in renal hypertension of rats. *Am. J. Physiol.* 228:1847, 1975.

Stumpe, K. O., Lowitz, H. D., and Ochwadt, B. Fluid reabsorption in Henle's loop and urinary excretion of sodium and water in normal rats and rats with chronic hypertension. *J. Clin. Invest.* 49:1200, 1970.

Vertes, V., Cangiano, J. L., Berman, L. B., and Gould, A. Hypertension in end-stage renal disease. *N. Engl. J. Med.* 280:978, 1969.

Goldblatt Kidney

Brown, J. J., Cuesta, V., Davies, D. L., Lever, A. F., Morton, J. J., Padfield, P. L., Robertson, J. I. S., Trust, P., Bianchi, G., and Schalekamp, M. A. D. Mechanism of renal hypertension. *Lancet* 1:1219, 1976.

Gavras, H., Brunner, H. R., Thurston, H., and Laragh, J. H. Reciprocation of renin dependency with sodium volume dependency in renal hypertension. *Science* 188:1316, 1975.

Goldblatt, H. Experimental hypertension induced by renal ischemia. *Harvey Lect.* 33:237, 1937–38.

Goldblatt, H., Lynch, J., Hanzal, R. F., and Summerville, W. W. Studies on experimental hypertension. I. The production of persistent elevation of systolic blood pressure by means of renal ischemia. *J. Exp. Med.* 59:347, 1934.

Kaufman, J. J. (ed.). Symposium on management of renovascular hypertension. *Urol. Clin. North Am.* 2:215, 1975.

von Knorring, J., Fyhrquist, F., Ahonen, J., Lindfors, O., and von Bonsdorff, M. Renin/angiotensin system in hypertension after traumatic renal-artery thrombosis. *Lancet* 1:934, 1976.

Marks, L. S., Maxwell, M. H., and Kaufman, J. J. Non-renin-mediated renovascular hypertension: A new syndrome? *Lancet* 1:615, 1977.

Theories

Brown, J. J., Lever, A. F., Robertson, J. I. S., and Schalekamp, M. A. Renal abnormality of essential hypertension. *Lancet* 2:320, 1974.

Brown, J. J., Lever, A. F., Robertson, J. I. S., and Schalekamp, M. A. Pathogenesis of essential hypertension. *Lancet* 1:1217, 1976.

Guyton, A. C., Cowley, A. W., Jr., Coleman, T. G., DeClue, J. W., Norman, R. A., and Manning, R. D. Hypertension: A disease of abnormal circulatory control. *Chest* 65:328, 1974.

Koch-Weser, J. Sympathetic activity in essential hypertension. *N. Engl. J. Med.* 288:627, 1973.

Lancet Editorial. Hypertension — The chicken and the egg. *Lancet* 1:345, 1976.

Lee, J. B., and Mookerjee, B. K. The renal prostaglandins as etiologic factors in human essential hypertension: Fact or fantasy? *Cardiovasc. Med.* 1:302, 1976.

Louis, W. J., Doyle, A. E., and Anavekar, S. Plasma norepinephrine levels in essential hypertension. *N. Engl. J. Med.* 288:599, 1973.

Möhring, J., Möhring, B., Petri, M., and Haack, D. Plasma vasopressin concentrations and effects of vasopressin antiserum on blood pressure in rats with malignant two-kidney Goldblatt hypertension. *Circ. Res.* 42:17, 1978.

Padfield, P. L., Brown, J. J., Lever, A. F., Morton, J. J., and Robertson, J. I. S. Changes of vasopressin in hypertension: Cause or effect? *Lancet* 1:1255, 1976.

Selkurt, E. E., Womack, I., and Dailey, W. N. Mechanism of natriuresis and diuresis during elevated renal arterial pressure. *Am. J. Physiol.* 209:95, 1965.

Thompson, J. M. A., and Dickinson, C. J. Relation between pressure and sodium excretion in perfused kidneys from rabbits with experimental hypertension. *Lancet* 2:1362, 1973.

Answers to Problems

Problem 1-1

Inorganic phosphate exists in the serum in two forms: $H_2PO_4^-$ and HPO_4^{2-}. The atomic weight of phosphorus (P) is 31 (see Table 1-7); therefore 1 mMole of phosphate (whether it is monovalent or divalent) contains 31 mg of phosphorus. Furthermore, 6.2 mg/100 ml of P equals 62 mg of P per liter. Therefore,

$$\frac{31 \text{ mg phosphorus}}{1 \text{ mMole phosphate}} = \frac{62 \text{ mg/L}}{x \text{ mMoles/L}}$$

$$x = 2 \text{ mMoles phosphate/L}$$

At a normal venous pH of 7.43, and even at the more acidotic values often found in renal failure, most of the phosphate exists as HPO_4^{2-} (see Fig. 10-14). Hence, for the purposes of this problem, we will assume the phosphate to have a valence of -2. Thus,

$$\frac{31 \text{ mg phosphorus}}{2 \text{ mEq phosphate}} = \frac{62 \text{ mg/L}}{x \text{ mEq/L}}$$

$$x = 4 \text{ mEq phosphate/L}$$

Note that the conversion to millimoles per liter is exact, whereas that to milliequivalents per liter is approximate, since it depends on the actual proportions of total phosphate that exist in the monovalent and divalent forms.

The elevation of the serum phosphate concentration in renal failure illustrates some important concepts in balance. The dynamics in an adult human are illustrated in Figure 1-A. In health, this person ingests about 20 mMoles of phosphate per day as phospholipids. With a normal glomerular filtration rate (GFR) of 180 liters per day (125 ml per minute) and a normal plasma phosphate concentration of 1.2 mMoles per liter (3.7 mg/100 ml), the filtered load of phosphate is $180 \times 1.2 = 216$ mMoles per day. About 90 percent or more of this load is nor-

	HEALTH	RENAL DISEASE (Early)		RENAL DISEASE (Late)	
	(a) Steady State:	*(b) Hypothetical:*	*(c) Actual:*	*(d) Transient:*	*(e) New Steady State:*
	Balance	*Positive Balance*	*Balance*	*Positive Balance*	*Balance*
INTAKE OF PHOSPHATE (mMoles/Day)	20	20	20	20	20
GFR (L/Day)	180	90	90	10	10
PLASMA PHOSPHATE CONCENTRATION (mMoles/L)	1.2	1.2	1.2	1.2	2.2
FILTERED LOAD OF PHOSPHATE $GFR \cdot P_P$ (mMoles/Day)	216	108	108	12	22
PHOSPHATE REABSORBED (mMoles/Day) [Fractional Reabsorption]	196 [91%]	98 [91%]	88 [82%]	1 [10%]	2 [10%]
PHOSPHATE EXCRETED $\dot{V} \cdot U_P$ (mMoles/Day)	20	10	20	11	20
MECHANISM BY WHICH BALANCE IS ATTAINED			Decreased Fractional Reabsorption		Increased P_P and hence increased Filtered Load

Figure 1-A
Dynamics of phosphate balance during progressive renal failure. This depiction is somewhat simplified in that it ignores fecal excretion of phosphate, binding of phosphate to plasma proteins, the Donnan factor, and correction of the phosphate concentration to plasma water rather than whole plasma. Ordinarily, however, these corrections would introduce refinements that are quantitatively negligible. Data adapted from E. Slatopolsky et al., *J. Clin. Invest.* 47:1865, 1968.

mally reabsorbed, mainly or exclusively in the proximal tubules. Hence, about 20 mMoles of phosphate per day is excreted, and, since the daily intake equals the daily output, the person is in phosphate balance.

The person now sustains renal disease, which initially decreases the GFR to one-half of the normal value. At a normal plasma concentration, the filtered load of phosphate is therefore reduced to 108 mMoles per day (Fig. 1-A, column b). If the so-called fractional reabsorption of phosphate *were* to remain at the healthy level of 91 percent, the urinary excretion of phosphate would be reduced to 10 mMoles per day; the patient would then be in positive phosphate balance, and the plasma concentration of phosphate would have to rise. This, however, is a hypothetical situation that may or may not occur early in renal disease. Actually, there is a regulatory adjustment that reduces the fraction of the filtered phosphate that is reabsorbed (Fig. 1-A, column c); that is, less phosphate is reabsorbed, 20 mMoles per day of phosphate is still excreted, and the patient remains in phosphate balance on a normal phosphate intake and at a normal plasma phosphate concentration.

This situation obtains so long as the fractional reabsorption of phosphate can be reduced. The limit of this reduction is about 10 percent of the filtered load of phosphate, and this limit is reached when the GFR is decreased to about one-fifth of the healthy value. When the GFR is decreased further, the patient on a normal intake of phosphate inevitably goes into positive phosphate balance, so the plasma phosphate concentration must rise (Fig. 1-A, column d). A new steady state late in renal disease is reached (Fig. 1-A, column e) when the plasma level of phosphate has risen to a value where the filtered load of phosphate minus the amount of phosphate reabsorbed – that is, the amount of phosphate excreted – again equals the intake of phosphate.

Problem 1-2

The chemical formula for urea is $CO(NH_2)_2$. The atomic weight of nitrogen is 14; hence, there are 28 mg of nitrogen in each millimole of urea. Furthermore, 14 mg of urea nitrogen per 100 ml of blood (i.e., a BUN, or *blood urea nitrogen,* of 14 mg/100 ml) equals 140 mg of urea nitrogen per liter of blood. Since urea is highly diffusible across cell membranes, the concentration of urea is virtually the same in blood cells and in plasma and hence is the same in whole blood. Therefore, a BUN of 140 mg of urea nitrogen per liter of whole blood reflects a concentration of 140 mg of urea nitrogen per liter of plasma.

Given the above facts, one can set up the following proportionality:

$$\frac{28 \text{ mg urea N}}{1 \text{ mMole urea}} = \frac{140 \text{ mg urea N}}{x \text{ mMoles urea}}$$

$$x = 5 \text{ mMoles urea}$$

Urea is a nonelectrolyte, having a negligible osmotic coefficient at the concentrations in which it exists in plasma. Therefore, 5 mMoles of urea per liter of plasma is equivalent to an osmolality of 5 mOsm/kg H_2O.

The solution for the contribution to osmolality of blood glucose is analogous. The molecular weight of glucose is 180; therefore each millimole of glucose contains 180 mg. Since 80 mg of glucose per 100 ml equals 800 mg of glucose per liter,

$$\frac{180 \text{ mg glucose}}{1 \text{ mMole glucose}} = \frac{800 \text{ mg glucose}}{x \text{ mMoles glucose}}$$

$$x = 4.4 \text{ mMoles glucose}$$

Again, the osmotic coefficient for glucose at these concentrations is negligible. Rounding off,

$$4.4 \text{ mMoles glucose/L} \approx 4 \text{ mOsm/kg } H_2O$$

Problem 2-1

Using the assumptions given, the values at the beginning of the test are as shown in the first line of Table 2-A. By the end of the test, 3 percent of the initial weight, or approximately 2.3 liters of H_2O, has been lost. Consequently, the new body weight is 72.7 kg and TBW has been reduced to 42.7 liters. This H_2O, lost as urine and insensibly in the breath and from the skin, disappears initially from the plasma. The resulting increase in plasma osmolality "instantly" causes H_2O to shift from the interstitial space into the plasma compartment, and the consequent rise in interstitial osmolality causes a shift of H_2O out of the intracellular compartment. These shifts continue until osmotic equilibrium among the compartments has been reestablished; that is, a loss of H_2O without solute will be shared by all the compartments in proportion to their original size. The loss of ICW will be 2.3 liters $\times$ 30/45 = 1.5 liters; the loss of ECW, 2.3 liters $\times$ 15/45 = 0.8 liter.

Table 2-A
Water deprivation test in an adult patient

State	Body Weight (kg)	TBW (liters)	ICW (liters)	ECW (liters)	P_{Osm} (mOsm/kg H_2O)	P_{Na^+} (mEq/L)
Beginning of test	75.0	45.0	30.0	15.0	290	140
End of test	72.7	42.7	28.5	14.2	306	148

TBW = total body water; ICW = intracellular water; ECW = extracellular water.

The amount of solute in the extracellular space at the beginning of the test was 15 $\times$ 290 = 4,350 mOsm. The assumption is made that only H_2O, not solute, was lost; hence at the end of the test, the same amount of solute will be dissolved in 14.2 liters, and the new plasma osmolality will be 4,350/14.2 = 306 mOsm/kg H_2O. By analogy, the amount of Na^+ in the extracellular compartment at the beginning of the test will be 2,100 mEq, and the plasma Na^+ concentration at the end of the test will be 148 mEq per liter.

Problem 2-2

Sweating athletes drink according to their thirst, and by this mechanism, they rather precisely restore the *total* volume of their body fluids. However, inasmuch as sweat (compared to distilled water) contains fairly large amounts of Na^+ and Cl^- (Table 1-4) that come from the extracellular space, the loss of sweat reduces the extracellular compartment relatively more than the intracellular compartment; that is, it leads to internal as well as external imbalance (see Chap. 3, under Importance of Na^+ Balance). Restoration of the fluid volumes with water only would not correct the internal imbalance, whereas simultaneous replenishment with NaCl will correct both the internal and external imbalances.

Problem 2-3

Theoretically, a castaway at sea could derive some benefits from drinking a limited amount of seawater. Seawater has an osmolality of approximately 1,000 mOsm/kg H_2O, and under conditions of severe thirst, a castaway might concentrate his urine to 1,400 mOsm/kg H_2O. If he ingests 500 ml of seawater each day and excretes all the solutes ingested therein (namely, 500 mOsm) at a concentration of 1,400 mOsm/kg H_2O, he will excrete 357 ml of urine and would therefore gain 143 ml of free H_2O each day. This gain could prolong his survival by several days.

There are at least two problems, however, that probably render the benefit more theoretical than real. Foremost among these is the fact that seawater acts as a cathartic and is nauseating, at least when taken in excess of 500 ml per day. The resulting diarrhea and possible vomiting would quickly cause the loss of more free H_2O than would be gained. Second, solutes are not excreted in urine in the same proportions as they exist in seawater; thus, imbalances of certain electrolytes will result.

Rather than drink seawater, a castaway at sea can probably help his economy of H_2O most by drinking rainwater when it is available and by minimizing evaporative heat loss through the following measures: (1) sit in the shade when possible, (2) utilize all breeze for convective heat loss, (3) promote conductive heat loss by periodic and short immersions in the sea, and (4) keep the clothing wet, thereby substituting vaporization of seawater for vaporization of body water.

This problem has been engagingly discussed in J. L. Gamble, *Companionship of Water and Electrolytes in the Organization of Body Fluids.* Palo Alto, Calif.: Stanford University Press, 1951, Chap. 3.

Problem 3-1

The patient's status in "health" (i.e., before he developed a cold and the diabetes mellitus went out of control) is shown in the first line of Table 3-A. In this state, about 60 percent of the body weight, or 42 liters, is H_2O; about 40 percent of the body weight, or 28 liters, is intracellular H_2O; and about 20 percent of the body weight is extracellular H_2O. We assume that the plasma Na^+ concentration was normal at this time, and we use the round figure of 140 mEq of Na^+ per liter (Table 1-1). With a nearly normal blood glucose concentration and a normal blood urea concentration (which we may assume because the BUN was

Table 3-A
Development of hyponatremia during uncontrolled diabetes mellitus

State	Body Weight (kg)	TBW* (liters)	ICW* (liters)	ECW* (liters)	Plasma Concentrations: Glucose (mg/100 ml)	Osmolality (mOsm/kg H_2O)	Na^+ (mEq/L)
Healthy	70	42	28	14	126	300	140
Hypothetical transient state	69	41	27.3	13.7	"126" (hypothetical)	307	143
New steady state	69	41	26.3	14.7	756	319	133

*TBW = total body water; ICW = intracellular water; ECW = extracellular water.

normal even when the patient was ill), the plasma osmolality was presumably also normal (Table 1-1), and we use the round value of 300 mOsm/kg H_2O. (If we used the rule of thumb given in Table 1-2 and hence a plasma osmolality of 280 mOsm/kg H_2O, the final answer for this problem would be about the same.)

During the transient, unsteady state, the patient loses 1 liter of fluid, as reflected in the weight loss of 1 kg. We next assume that since this fluid loss was mainly insensible (due to the fever) and partly urinary (because of an osmotic diuresis), it was composed exclusively of H_2O and not of electrolytes. (This assumption is not accurate, but it represents a reasonable estimate.) The total body H_2O is therefore reduced to 41 liters and is distributed between the intracellular and extracellular fluids in proportion to the original volumes of these compartments: ICW = 41 $\times$ 28/42; ECW = 41 $\times$ 14/42. On the assumption that only H_2O, but no Na^+, was lost from the extracellular fluid compartment, the plasma Na^+ concentration would have increased to 143 mEq per liter (140 $\times$ 14/13.7) and the plasma osmolality, to 307 mOsm/kg H_2O (300 $\times$ 14/13.7).

The new steady state can be evaluated as follows. A blood glucose concentration of 756 mg/100 ml adds 35 mMoles to each liter of plasma over the previous state when the blood glucose concentration was 126 mg/100 ml (see Answer to Problem 1-2). As the osmolality of extracellular fluid is raised through the addition of glucose, H_2O is shifted from the intracellular to the extracellular compartment; consequently, the volume of ICW will go from 27.3 to 27.3 − x liters, and the volume of ECW will go from 13.7 to 13.7 + x liters. The amount of glucose added to the extracellular space in the new steady state will therefore be 35(13.7 + x) mMoles. At this point we do not know the value of x, but it can be shown that whether we assume it to be 1 liter or as much as 5 liters, the ultimate solution to this problem will not be very different. We shall therefore take the ECW volume as being equal to 13.7 liters and calculate the amount of glucose added as being 35 × 13.7, or 480 mMoles.

In the transient state, the solute content of the total body H_2O was 41 × 307 = 12,587 mOsm; to this, 480 mOsm of glucose were added, and the new total of 13,067 mOsm was dissolved in 41 liters, giving a new plasma osmolality (at osmotic equilibrium in the new steady state) of 319 mOsm/kg H_2O. In the transient state, the intracellular compartment contained 8,381 mOsm (27.3 × 307), and none of these was lost from this compartment. As the new steady state was attained, however, H_2O was withdrawn from the intracellular compartment, and its new volume can be calculated from the knowledge of the new osmolality of 319 mOsm/kg H_2O: 27.3 × 307/319 = 26.3 liters. Since 1 liter of H_2O was shifted from the intracellular to the extracellular compartment, the new volume of the latter will be 14.7 liters. (It is coincidence that the patient lost 1 liter of TBW and that the internal shift of H_2O was also 1 liter.)

Given the approximation that there was no net loss of Na^+ from the body, the extracellular compartment contained 1,960 mEq of Na^+ (14 × 140 or 13.7 × 143). This amount of Na^+ is now distributed in 14.7 liters of extracellular fluid, yielding a plasma Na^+ concentration of 133 mEq per liter in the new steady state.

Thus, the low plasma Na^+ concentration can be accounted for by the hyperglycemia and the consequent alteration in internal balance. This problem has been oversimplified. In practice, theoretical calculations seldom yield a value for the plasma Na^+ concentration that agrees precisely with the measured value, although the two are often very close. Also, we assumed that there had been no net change in external Na^+ balance, whereas the osmotic diuresis of uncontrolled diabetes mellitus is usually accompanied by a slightly negative Na^+ balance. The major lesson to be learned from this problem is that hyponatremia can and does occur merely from internal shifts of H_2O and in the absence of either a negative external Na^+ balance or a positive external H_2O balance.

There is a slightly more complicated — and mathematically more correct — way of solving this problem, in which x is calculated. Although this method would be more accurate, the numerical answers are very close to the ones derived above. Many formulas have been devised for estimating the decrease in plasma Na^+ concentration that can be anticipated from a given rise in plasma glucose. One rule of thumb states that the plasma Na^+ concentration will fall 1.6 mEq per liter for each increase in glucose concentration of 100 mg/100 ml.

Problem 3-2

The dietary allotment of Na^+ is commonly quoted as so many "grams per day" without specifying whether the amount refers to sodium or to sodium chloride. The purpose of this question is twofold: (1) to emphasize the importance of specifying whether the amount quoted refers to Na^+ or to NaCl and (2) to give some ball-park values.

A normal intake for an adult is 6 to 15 g of salt (i.e., NaCl) per day. One millimole of NaCl is equivalent to 58 mg (see Table 1-7); therefore

$$\frac{58 \text{ mg}}{1 \text{ mMole}} = \frac{6{,}000 \text{ mg}}{x}$$

$$x = 103 \text{ mMoles}$$

Each millimole of NaCl contains 1 mEq of Na^+ and 1 mEq of Cl^-. Thus, the normal daily intake of sodium should be quoted as follows: 6 to 15 g of NaCl (or table salt), or 103 to 259 mMoles of NaCl, or 103 to 259 mEq of Na^+.

If the use of salt at the table is omitted, the daily intake can be reduced to 4 to 7 g of NaCl, which is 69 to 120 mMoles per day or 69 to 120 mEq of Na^+ per day.

If, in addition to eliminating salt at the table, added salt during cooking is also omitted, the daily intake is reduced to 3 to 4 g of table salt (52 to 69 mMoles of NaCl or 52 to 69 mEq of Na^+ per day).

A therapeutic low-salt diet (e.g., as prescribed for congestive heart failure) contains about 2 g of table salt per day, that is, 34 mMoles of NaCl or 34 mEq of Na^+. If the intake is reduced below this value, the variety of foods that may be eaten is very limited, and the food becomes unpalatable. Furthermore, the concurrent use of diuretic agents makes such severe restriction unnecessary.

Ball-park values: It is useful to memorize the following average values, realizing that the range of normality is great.

Normal daily intake: 10 g NaCl; 200 mEq Na^+

Low-salt diet: 2 g NaCl; 35 mEq Na^+

One level teaspoon contains: 6 g NaCl; 100 mEq Na^+

Problem 3-3

One can analyze this problem by calculating the plasma Na^+ concentrations that would result from two hypothetical conditions and comparing these concentrations to the measured value on admission, namely, 160 mEq of Na^+ per liter. This analysis is outlined in Table 3-B.

Just prior to the illness, the baby weighed 8 kg. In a 9-month-old infant, about 70 percent of the body weight is H_2O and

Table 3-B
Sequential analysis for the cause of hypernatremia in infant diarrhea

State	Body Weight (kg)	Volume of Body Fluids TBW* (ml)	ICW* (ml)	ECW* (ml)	P_{Na^+} (mEq/L)
Healthy	8	5,600	3,200	2,400	140
Hypothetical loss of 1 liter H_2O	7	4,600	2,630	1,970	171
Hypothetical loss of 1 liter isotonic NaCl	7	4,600	3,200	1,400	140
Actual loss	7	4,600	2,800	1,800	160

*TBW = total body water; ICW = intracellular water; ECW = extracellular water.

about 40 percent is intracellular fluid (ICW). Subtracting 3,200 ml of ICW from a total body water (TBW) of 5,600 ml yields a volume for extracellular fluid (ECW) of 2,400 ml. We assume a normal plasma Na^+ concentration in health of 140 mEq per liter.

During a relatively acute illness of three days' duration, it may be assumed that all the weight loss that occurs represents loss of H_2O, even though the baby's caloric intake has been poor (Chap. 1, under Clinical Criteria of Fluid and Solute Balance). Hence, the TBW will equal 4,600 ml on admission. The net effect of losing 1 liter of fluid (mainly as diarrhea) and having the electrolyte loss replaced (i.e., by supplemental NaCl in the formula) might have been the loss of 1 liter of pure H_2O. In that event, the H_2O would have been lost from the ICW and ECW in proportion to the relative sizes of these compartments in health (see Answer to Problem 2-1). Therefore, the ICW would have shrunk by $1{,}000 \times 3{,}200/5{,}600 = 570$ ml, and the ECW would have decreased by $1{,}000 \times 2{,}400/5{,}600 = 430$ ml. The amount of Na^+ in the ECW during health was 0.140 mEq/ml $\times$ 2,400 ml = 336 mEq. Since no Na^+ would be lost in the first hypothetical state, this amount of Na^+ would now be diluted in an ECW volume of 1,970 ml: that is, 336 mEq/1.97 liters = 171 mEq per liter. Since this is higher than the measured value of 160 mEq per liter (see Problem 3-3), it is clear that the net effect of the first three days of illness has been a loss not only of H_2O but also of Na^+.

If the loss had been of isotonic saline (see Fig. 1-6), the plasma Na^+ concentration would have remained at 140 mEq per liter. This was obviously not the case, and it is clear, then, that the actual loss consisted of relatively more H_2O than Na^+. Furthermore, an isotonic deficit comes entirely from the ECW, and with a new ECW volume of 1,400 ml, the baby probably would have been in shock. The contrast between these two hypothetical examples emphasizes the fact that for a given total fluid loss, the signs and symptoms of volume contraction are less severe when relatively more H_2O than Na^+ is lost, compared to the effects when the opposite proportionality prevails.

Knowing that the actual loss was of H_2O and Na^+ and knowing the plasma Na^+ concentration on admission, we can estimate the size of the fluid compartments after three days of illness. As relatively more H_2O than Na^+ leaves the ECW, the extracellular compartment becomes hyperosmotic; consequently, H_2O will be withdrawn from the intracellular space until osmotic equilibrium has been reestablished. More hyposmotic fluid will then be lost from the ECW, which will shift more H_2O from the ICW to the ECW. That is, the intracellular space will decrease in proportion to the rise in extracellular osmolality (i.e., in proportion to the rise in the plasma Na^+ concentration). Therefore, the new ICW will be 3,200 $\times$ 140/160 = 2,800 ml, and the new ECW will be 4,600 - 2,800 = 1,800 ml.

Problem 3-4

The first impulse might be to reason that since exchangeable Na^+ resides almost exclusively in extracellular fluid, one calculates the amount needed to correct the hyponatremia by multiplying the deficit of 20 mEq per liter by the ECW. If the ECW were estimated simply as 20 percent of the body weight of 53 kg, the answer — 20 mEq per liter times 10.6 liters — would represent a *gross underestimate.* The reason is that as the infusion of NaCl raises the osmolality of the extracellular fluid, H_2O shifts out of the intracellular space until osmotic equilibrium between the two compartments is reestablished. In this way, the NaCl that is being added to the extracellular compartment is continuously being "diluted," and therefore much more NaCl must be added than was calculated above. When the new steady-state value of 132 mEq of Na^+ per liter is reached, the intracellular fluid will have the same higher osmolality as the extracellular. That is, the intracellular compartment will have participated fully in the change, but without the addition of intracellular solute. Hence, NaCl must be added *as if it were distributed throughout the intracellular as well as extracellular space,* and the amount that needs to be added is therefore calculated by multiplying the deficit of 20 mEq per liter by the total body water. If the TBW is estimated as 60 percent of body weight, then 636 mEq of Na^+ (20 mEq/L $\times$ 31.8 liters) need be given to the patient.

From Figure 1-6, we see that 5% NaCl contains 856 mEq of Na^+ per liter. Therefore, the patient should be given 743 ml of this solution; in practice, one would write an order for 750 ml of 5% saline. Because it is wise to correct imbalances slowly (Chap. 7, under Guidelines), most physicians might aim to err on the low side by prescribing 500 ml of 5% saline. The complete history for this patient is given in Problem 7-2, and the actual treatment, which differed somewhat from what has been calculated here, is analyzed in the answer to that problem.

Problem 4-1

The history is typical of progressive congestive heart failure in an elderly person. The patient was lucky to be under the close surveillance of a physician who kept the patient comfortable and active by means of few and simple measures and drugs.

The loss of appetite before admission was probably due to the heart failure. The patient's gain in weight despite a curtailed food intake reflected accumulation of edema fluid. This finding emphasizes the importance of the body weight as a simple and accurate gauge of fluid balance, not only in heart failure but also as a guide to the efficacy of diuretic therapy. The simple measure of weighing the patient daily – preferably first thing in the morning, nude, and after having voided – is a far better method of assessing fluid balance than the cumbersome and usually inaccurate measuring of the 24-hour "intake and output."

The ECG pattern on admission was compatible with a digitalis effect. The slightly low serum Na^+ and Cl^- concentrations probably reflect the free water retention that is seen in cardiac failure, especially when it is combined with diuretic therapy (Fig. 2-6 and Table 3-3). The low serum K^+ concentration may reflect partly the water retention, but mainly it raises the suspicion of K^+ deficiency resulting from prolonged use of chlorothiazide without K^+ supplementation. This effect may have been aggravated shortly before admission, because the patient's food intake was so poor. Although most physicians would prescribe K^+ supplements when giving chlorothiazide to a patient who is also on digitalis, the necessity for such supplements is not accepted by all.

The patient's signs and symptoms on the third hospital day – nausea, vomiting, weakness, and irregularities of cardiac conduction – almost certainly signified digitalis toxicity, which was precipitated by K^+ deficiency. The marked diuresis induced by furosemide, which accounted for a loss of about 12 liters of edema fluid as reflected in a reduction in body weight of 12 kg, may have been accompanied by urinary K^+ excretion amounting to several hundred milliequivalents. And this kaliuresis, when superimposed on the K^+ deficiency occasioned by prolonged chlorothiazide treatment, precipitated overt K^+ deficiency and digitalis toxicity. The patient's serum K^+ concentration on the morning of the third hospital day was, in fact, 2.4 mEq per liter.

If the patient had shown dangerous cardiac arrhythmias, he would have been treated with K^+ intravenously. In the present situation, however, KCl was given orally, digitalis therapy was stopped for two days, and diuretic therapy was stopped altogether, which sufficed to reverse the picture. KCl was given as a 10% solution, which contains about 6.5 mEq of K^+ per teaspoonful (about 5 ml), and the patient received 20 ml of this solution four times daily for four days (total of about 420 mEq K^+). By that time, the nausea had disappeared, and the patient's normal food intake then slowly corrected the remaining K^+ deficit.

Problem 4-2

This patient illustrates the point that the development of life-threatening hyperkalemia usually requires the concurrence of two abnormalities: (1) decreased renal excretion and (2) increased input of K^+, either exogenous or endogenous. The treatment of acute leukemia creates the constant threat of the development of both conditions. Prednisone, vincristine, and daunorubicin cause the rapid breakdown of lymphocytes, and their use thereby leads to the release of K^+ and nucleoproteins from the destroyed cells. The metabolism of nucleoproteins to uric acid causes the profound rise in the plasma uric acid concentration that was seen in this patient; in fact, the use of cytolytic agents is probably the commonest cause of severe hyperuricemia, especially in children with acute leukemia. Generally, the more severe the neoplastic infiltration, the greater the rise in uric acid as treatment is carried out. Thus, in the present patient, in whom marked hepatosplenomegaly probably reflected heavy leukemic involvement, the severe hyperuricemia was anticipated, and that is why allopurinol was given. This drug inhibits the synthesis of uric acid. It is important to minimize the formation of uric acid, because its elevation in the plasma, especially if marked, is known to cause acute renal failure.

In this patient, despite precautions, the acute oliguric renal failure was probably due to hyperuricemia. The resultant inability to excrete K^+, coupled with the overproduction of K^+ due to increased destruction of cells, led to the hyperkalemia (Table 4-2). Further K^+ may have been given to the patient in the blood transfusion; even though fresh blood was given, the continuing death of cells as blood is stored releases K^+ into the plasma. In addition, the destruction of erythrocytes within hematomas and other collections of blood added more K^+ to the extracellular fluid.

Although it is difficult to identify the immediate cause of death in a patient as ill as this one, the course suggests ventricular arrest from hyperkalemia. In retrospect, it might therefore have been wiser to add intravenous infusions of Ca^{2+}, glucose, and insulin (Table 4-3) to the measures designed to reverse the hyperkalemia and its effects. Often, however, a serum K^+ concentration of 8 mEq per liter does not pose an immediate threat, and the electrocardiographic pattern in this patient was not so alarming (Fig. 4-4) that heroic measures seemed called for. Although possible errors of medical judgment should not be rationalized, it must be emphasized that retrospective reasoning is easier than prospective, and that severely ill patients often have multiple problems (e.g., constant bleeding and impending heart failure in the present patient) that require simultaneous attention.

A few other points, some of which will become clearer in subsequent chapters, might be commented on. The slightly low serum Na^+ and Cl^- concentrations probably reflected an excess intake of fluid relative to the decreased capacity to excrete water during oliguria. The acid-base imbalance was a metabolic acidosis with an increased anion gap, almost certainly due to renal failure (Table 5-3; also Chap. 6, under Metabolic Acidosis). The BUN/creatinine ratio usually has a value of about 10; this ratio was exceeded in this patient because gastrointestinal bleeding with increased protein metabolism led to a disproportionate rise of urea as compared to creatinine (Chap. 8).

Problem 5-1

1. Both the calculation and the method of estimation used in this example are described in the section Conversion of pH to $[H^+]$, on page 115.
2. Calculation of P_{CO_2}:

$$\text{pH} = 6.10 + \log \frac{[HCO_3^-]}{0.03P_{CO_2}}$$

$$7.32 = 6.10 + \log \frac{15}{0.03P_{CO_2}}$$

$$1.22 = \log \frac{15}{0.03P_{CO_2}}$$

$$\frac{15}{0.03P_{CO_2}} = \text{antilog}\,1.22$$

$$\frac{15}{0.03P_{CO_2}} = 16.60$$

$$P_{CO_2} = \frac{15}{16.60 \times 0.03}$$

$$P_{CO_2} = 30.1 \text{ mm Hg}$$

Estimation of P_{CO_2}:
Equation 5-3 states:

$$[HCO_3^-] = 25 \frac{P_{CO_2}}{[H^+]}$$

By estimation, the $[H^+]$ corresponding to a pH of 7.32 is 48 nEq/L (40 + 8). Therefore, from Equation 5-3:

$$15 = 25 \frac{P_{CO_2}}{48}$$

$$P_{CO_2} = \frac{15 \times 48}{25}$$

$$P_{CO_2} = 28.8 \text{ mm Hg}$$

3. Both the calculation and the estimate for this example are given in the section Estimation of $[HCO_3^-]$, in Chapter 5.
4. Calculation of pH from $[H^+]$:

$$\begin{aligned} pH &= -\log [H^+] \\ &= -\log 65 \text{ nEq/L} \\ &= -\log(65 \times 10^{-9}) \text{Eq/L} \\ &= -\log(6.5 \times 10^{-8}) \text{Eq/L} \\ &= 8.00 - \log 6.5 \\ &= 8.00 - 0.8129 \\ pH &= 7.19 \end{aligned}$$

Estimation of pH from $[H^+]$:

$$65 \text{ nEq/L} = 40 \text{ nEq/L} + 25 \text{ nEq/L}$$

$$pH = 7.40 - 0.25$$

$$pH = 7.15$$

The values and units that were requested in Problem 5-1 are shown in italics in Table 5-A.

Table 5-A
Tabulated solutions to questions asked in Problem 5-1

	pH		$[H^+]$ (*nEq/L*)		P_{CO_2} (*mm Hg*)		$[HCO_3^-]$ (*mMoles/L*)	
	Calc.	Est.	Calc.	Est.	Calc.	Est.	Calc.	Est.
(1)	7.40	—	*40*	*40*	40	—	24	—
(2)	7.32	—	—	—	*30*	*29*	15	—
(3)	7.55	—	—	—	44	—	*37*	39
(4)	*7.19*	*7.15*	65	—	75	—	28	—

Problem 5-2

The history of vomiting when the patient was at the other hospital, in conjunction with the volume contraction that the patient showed on physical examination and the report of a high plasma $[HCO_3^-]$, raised the suspicion of a metabolic alkalosis. When the values on admission, listed in Table 5-B, were plotted on Figure 5-2, it turned out that the point fell within the confidence band in Figure 5-2a but below the band in Figure 5-2b. This discrepancy, which is also apparent if the values are plotted on Figure 5-1a and b, is impossible, because both parts of Figures 5-1 and 5-2 are based on the same mathematical relationship, the Henderson-Hasselbalch equation. The physician thus knew immediately that a laboratory error had been made. (Even allowing the $[HCO_3^-]$ in *venous* plasma to be 2 to 3 mMoles per liter higher than in arterial plasma would not eliminate the discrepancy.)

Checking the Henderson-Hasselbalch relationship by arithmetic approximation confirmed the presence of a laboratory error. Using the reported pH of 7.51 and a $[HCO_3^-]$ of 42 mMoles per liter (as the approximate arterial value), the arterial P_{CO_2} was estimated to be 49 mm Hg: First, pH 7.51 corresponds approximately to a $[H^+]$ of 29 nEq per liter; then, according to Equation 5-3,

$$[HCO_3^-] = 25 \frac{P_{CO_2}}{[H^+]}$$

$$42 = 25 \frac{P_{CO_2}}{29}$$

$$P_{CO_2} = \frac{42 \times 29}{25}$$

$$P_{CO_2} = 48.7 \text{ mm Hg}$$

Alternatively, using the reported pH of 7.51 and P_{CO_2} of 34 mm Hg, the $[HCO_3^-]$ for arterial plasma was estimated from the

Table 5-B
Results of laboratory tests on a 61-year-old woman immediately on admission to the hospital and three hours later

Test	On Admission	Three Hours After Admission
Arterial blood:		
pH	7.51	7.48
P_{CO_2} (mm Hg)	34	55
Venous plasma:		
$[HCO_3^-]$ (mMoles/L)	45	42
$[Cl^-]$ (mEq/L)	98	–
$[Na^+]$ (mEq/L)	152	–
BUN (mg/100 ml)	82	–
Creatinine (mg/100 ml)	3.1	–

above equation to be 29 mMoles per liter:

$$[HCO_3^-] = \frac{25 \times 34}{29}$$

$$[HCO_3^-] = 29.3 \text{ mMoles per liter}$$

The physician therefore asked for repeat laboratory determinations, the results of which are listed in the final column of Table 5-B. In the meantime, however, he had already concluded on the basis of the following reasons that the patient almost certainly had a metabolic alkalosis and that the P_{CO_2} was therefore most likely to be the erroneous value: (1) there was a history of vomiting, (2) a high $[HCO_3^-]$ had been determined at the other hospital, and (3) the anion gap was low normal. His deduction was borne out by the repeat measurements (Table 5-B).

Armed with this new information, the physician sought a cause for the metabolic alkalosis. It had been suspected that the patient might have the so-called milk-alkali syndrome, because of the prior history of unexplained hypercalcemia, a BUN/creatinine ratio that had repeatedly exceeded 10 and hence suggested a very high protein intake (Chap. 8), and a history of a "strange personality" and possible food fads. On further questioning, it was learned that the patient had indeed for years drunk 4 to 5 liters of milk daily. When this pattern was ended, she recovered.

It should be emphasized that this is a true history, that laboratory errors do occur, but that by considering all the values in the light of the patient's history and physical findings, a correct diagnosis can nevertheless be ascertained. The chronic renal failure in this patient may have resulted from chronic infection, as had been suspected, or it might have been due to the milk-alkali syndrome itself. In either case, patients who ingest large amounts of alkali are more likely to develop severe metabolic alkalosis if they have concurrent renal failure (Table 6-5).

Problem 6-1

This problem is considered in order to illustrate H^+ balance in the CSF and some of the clinical consequences of the differences between balance in this fluid and that in systemic blood. The key to understanding these differences lies in the following facts: (1) CO_2 diffuses readily across the blood-brain barrier and hence tends to equilibrate quickly between the blood and the CSF; (2) HCO_3^- does not diffuse readily across the barrier and is in fact autonomously regulated in the CSF, possibly by active transport; and (3) CSF contains relatively little nonbicarbonate buffer; thus, in contrast to blood, it is a poor buffer for CO_2.

This patient had a severe systemic metabolic acidosis, with compensatory hyperventilation lowering the P_{CO_2} of arterial blood to 11 mm Hg. Because of the high diffusibility of CO_2 across the blood-brain barrier, the P_{CO_2} of the CSF was lowered almost simultaneously, but not as far as 11 mm Hg (Table 6-A). This difference in P_{CO_2} arises because the CSF is probably in equilibrium with venous rather than arterial blood. The $[HCO_3^-]$ of the CSF, however, was considerably higher than would be predicted from the arteriovenous difference alone, since it is independently regulated. Consequently, the ratio $[HCO_3^-]/0.03P_{CO_2}$ of the Henderson-Hasselbalch equation (Eq. 5-2) was 9 in arterial blood and 13 in CSF, resulting in the much higher pH of the CSF.

Using Equation 5-2 and a pK' of 6.13, it can be calculated that with a P_{CO_2} of 20 mm Hg and a $[HCO_3^-]$ of 3 mMoles per liter, the pH of the CSF would have been 6.83. Deterioration of mental status can be correlated quite closely with the degree of acidosis within the CSF. Hence, at a CSF pH of 6.83, the patient probably would have been in coma and perhaps dead. In that sense, the homeostasis of CSF bicarbonate – which in this instance resulted in the $[HCO_3^-]$ being 5 mMoles per liter higher in the CSF than in arterial blood – may be viewed as a life-sustaining function.

The decline in the patient's mental status after 7 hours of treatment is explained by the further lowering of the CSF pH despite the correction of the arterial pH (Table 6-A). This lowering occurred because the $[HCO_3^-]$ of the CSF rose more slowly than the arterial $[HCO_3^-]$, while at the same time, the P_{CO_2} of the CSF rose simultaneously with the arterial P_{CO_2}. The patient probably could have been aroused by slight, assisted hyperventilation; even lowering the P_{CO_2} in the CSF to 30 mm Hg would have raised the pH to 7.29, given a $[HCO_3^-]$ for the CSF of 13 mMoles per liter. The attending physicians, however,

Table 6-A
Acid-base status of arterial blood and cerebrospinal fluid (CSF) in a 44-year-old man before, during, and after treatment for diabetic ketoacidosis

Test	On Admission	After 7 Hours of Treatment	After 22 Hours of Treatment
Arterial blood:			
pH	6.99	7.39	7.42
P_{CO_2} (mm Hg)	11	31	35
$[HCO_3^-]$ (mMoles/L)	3	18	22
CSF*:			
pH	7.25	7.14	7.30
P_{CO_2} (mm Hg)	20	41	43
$[HCO_3^-]$ (mMoles/L)	8	13	19

*Normal values for CSF: pH = 7.29 to 7.32; $[HCO_3^-]$ = 20 to 24 mMoles/L; P_{CO_2} = 45 to 50 mm Hg; p*K*′ for Henderson-Hasselbalch equation in CSF = 6.13.
Modified from J. B. Posner, A. G. Swanson, and F. Plum, *Arch. Neurol.* 12:479, 1965.

understanding the cause of the patient's obtunded state, elected instead to await further equilibration of the HCO_3^- in the CSF with that in arterial blood. When this occurred, the CSF pH, and hence the mental condition, returned to normal.

There is one seeming contradiction in this problem, which those well versed in respiratory physiology will notice. The main determinant of alveolar ventilation is the pH of CSF; yet, after 7 hours of treatment, the arterial P_{CO_2} rose even though the pH of the CSF fell. The explanation is that HCO_3^- diffuses slowly to the site where the CSF was *sampled;* in the region of the medullary chemoreceptor, the $[HCO_3^-]$, and hence the pH, were almost certainly higher than is reflected in the lumbar CSF values at 7 hours.

Regarding the questions at the end of Problem 6-1, the patient with acute respiratory acidosis and an arterial pH of 7.20 will have an arterial P_{CO_2} of about 70 mm Hg (Fig. 5-1a). Since the P_{CO_2} in the CSF will also be about 70 mm Hg, but the $[HCO_3^-]$ in this fluid will be in the normal range or just a little higher, the CSF pH will probably be between 7.10 and 7.15 (Fig. 5-4).

On the other hand, the patient with metabolic acidosis and an arterial pH of 7.20 will have an arterial $[HCO_3^-]$ of about 10 mMoles per liter (Fig. 5-2a) and an arterial P_{CO_2} of about 20 mm Hg (Fig. 5-2b). The P_{CO_2} in his CSF will therefore be about 20 mm Hg, but the HCO_3^-, being slow to diffuse across the blood-brain barrier, will be higher than 10 mm Hg. Hence, the CSF pH in this patient will be higher than that of his arterial blood.

Table 6-B
Results of laboratory tests on a 63-year-old man with chronic bronchitis, emphysema, and heart failure

Test	On Admission	After 20 Minutes of Hyperventilation
Arterial blood:		
pH	7.29	7.64
P_{CO_2} (mm Hg)	64	28
$[HCO_3^-]$ (mMoles/L)	30	29
P_{O_2} (mm Hg)	41	89
Venous plasma:		
$[Na^+]$ (mEq/L)	142	–
$[Cl^-]$ (mEq/L)	88	–
$[K^+]$ (mEq/L)	4.5	–
$[HCO_3^-]$ (mEq/L)	33	–

Therefore, the patient with acute respiratory acidosis is more likely to show an abnormal mental state.

Problem 6-2

On admission (Table 6-B), the patient had a chronic respiratory acidosis. With a P_{CO_2} of 64 mm Hg and a $[HCO_3^-]$ of 30 mMoles per liter, the arterial point falls below the confidence band in Figure 5-1b. This means that there was more to the acid-base disturbance than an uncomplicated chronic respiratory acidosis. If this had been all there was to the patient's illness, the renal compensation of reabsorbing more filtered HCO_3^- would have raised the plasma $[HCO_3^-]$ to about 35 mMoles per liter. The fact that it was slightly lower than this value means that there was probably an associated metabolic acidosis. The cause of the acidosis was almost certainly a slight degree of lactic acidosis, which was occasioned by tissue hypoxia and which is reflected in the elevated anion gap.

The $[HCO_3^-]$ was high, because renal compensation for respiratory acidosis had increased the reabsorption of filtered HCO_3^-. The $[HCO_3^-]$ was higher in venous than in arterial blood partly because the laboratory method whereby plasma "HCO_3^-" is measured usually entails the determination of total CO_2 (i.e., HCO_3^- + dissolved CO_2 + H_2CO_3) and partly because the P_{CO_2} and consequent production of HCO_3^- within erythrocytes is higher in venous than in arterial blood.

The plasma $[Cl^-]$ was low, mainly because the renal adaptation to chronic hypercapnia is accompanied by increased renal excretion of Cl^-. The mechanisms of this chloruresis are not fully understood. In this patient, Cl^- depletion was abetted by the low-salt diet and the administration of diuretics.

The use of assisted ventilation in this patient inadvertently led to hyperventilation that lowered the P_{CO_2} to 28 mm Hg (see Table 6-B). Because renal compensations for respiratory disturbances do not set in for several days, the [HCO_3^-] was not lowered simultaneously. Consequently, a severe alkalosis ensued. This alkalosis, in turn, caused a decrease in the plasma concentration of ionized Ca^{2+}, which led to tetany.

The appearance of tetany is an emergency situation, since it can progress to dangerous convulsions. The key to stopping the tetany is to lower the pH of the blood, thereby increasing the plasma concentration of ionized Ca^{2+}. This change can be accomplished most quickly by ventilating the patient less vigorously. Some physicians, however, prefer to effect the acidification by giving NH_4Cl. (In fact, many would have anticipated the development of tetany, and they would have given NH_4Cl prophylactically before beginning assisted ventilation; see Chap. 5, under *Note* in section Confidence Bands.)

Giving NH_4Cl has the further advantage of simultaneously replenishing Cl^-, a prerequisite to the renal excretion of HCO_3^- and the final correction of the alkalosis. The importance of replenishing the Cl^- deficit (which, in situations less urgent than that of the present patient, can also be accomplished by giving NaCl or KCl) was emphasized earlier in Chapter 6 (under Metabolic Alkalosis). The mechanisms by which administration of Cl^- permits the renal excretion of HCO_3^- are not fully understood; they may involve an expansion of the extracellular fluid volume.

Problem 7-1

During the control period (Table 7-A), all the patient's plasma values were normal, even though he was in positive Na^+ and H_2O balance, as indicated by the edema and gain in body weight. His urine output was low, probably because he was drinking little; similarly, the low urinary excretion rates for Na^+ and Cl^- being steady-state values, reflected the very low salt intake.

During three days on fairly high doses of ethacrynic acid, his urine flow exceeded 3 liters per day, and the urine contained mainly Na^+ and Cl^-, some K^+, and essentially no HCO_3^-. Inasmuch as the urinary losses accounted for virtually all of the negative balance of these ions, and since we know from the change in body weight that the patient lost about 4.5 liters of fluid, we can estimate the composition of the fluid that was lost. For Cl^-, it must have been the average daily loss of 266 mEq multiplied by 3 days and divided by 4.5 liters, that is, fluid with a Cl^- concentration of about 175 mEq per liter. The approximate composition of the fluid and the consequences of this loss on the ECF are shown in Figure 7-A.

Since the fluid that was lost had about the same Na^+ concentration as the extracellular fluid during the control periods,

Table 7-A
Results of balance studies on a 62-year-old man with arteriosclerotic cardiovascular disease maintained on a diet containing 5 mEq of Na^+ and of Cl^- per day

							Plasma Concentrations					
		Urinary Excretion					Venous			Arterial		
Period	Body Weight (kg)	$\dot{V}$ (ml/day)	Na^+ (mEq/day)	K^+ (mEq/day)	Cl^- (mEq/day)	HCO_3^- (mEq/day)	Na^+ (mEq/L)	K^+ (mEq/L)	Cl^- (mEq/L)	HCO_3^- (mEq/L)	pH	PCO_2 (mm Hg)
Control	94.0	410	2	42	2	0.1	137	4.6	98	23	7.42	38
Therapy (with ethacrynic acid, 50 mg 4 times daily for 3 days)	89.5	3,108	233	64	266	1.1	135	3.9	87	29	7.50	39

Modified from P. J. Cannon, H. O. Heinemann, M. S. Albert, J. H. Laragh, and R. W. Winters, *Ann. Intern. Med.* 62:979, 1965.

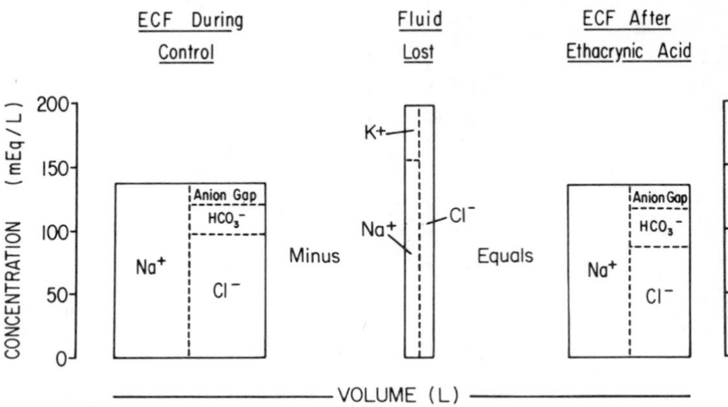

Figure 7-A
Dynamics for the development of contraction alkalosis during diuretic therapy. The solutes are separated by dashed lines to show that they are actually evenly distributed throughout each volume.

the ECF was reduced by 4.5 liters, but with essentially no change in Na^+ concentration. The Cl^- concentration of the lost fluid, however, was much higher than that of the ECF; consequently, the Cl^- concentration in the ECF was reduced after three days of treatment. The HCO_3^- concentration increased reciprocally. The mechanism for the reciprocal change is not fully understood; it may be that Na^+ balance is regulated primarily while that of Cl^- and HCO_3^- follows secondarily, and when sufficient Cl^- is not available to "accompany" the Na^+ as it is transported, the other most available anion, namely HCO_3^-, takes its place (Chap. 6, under Metabolic Alkalosis). Note that this change occurred without a significant alteration in the anion gap.

The alkalosis seen after therapy is thus due to an increase in $[HCO_3^-]$, and it is therefore a primary metabolic alkalosis, essentially unaccompanied by respiratory compensation (i.e., rise in P_{CO_2}). This impression is supported by the fact that the arterial values (see Table 7-A) fall within the confidence bands in Figure 5-2.

Can the rise in $[HCO_3^-]$ be accounted for fully by the reduction in ECF, or was there also an increased loss of H^+ and retention of HCO_3^- during therapy? The answer to this question can be approximated by calculating the $[HCO_3^-]$ that *would be expected* if the sole cause were the reduction in the ECF. If this were the case, then the amount of HCO_3^- in the ECF should not have changed between the control and final state. Hence,

$$ECF_1 \times [HCO_3^-]_1 = ECF_2 \times [HCO_3^-]_2 \qquad (7\text{-}1)$$

where ECF_1 and $[HCO_3^-]_1$ refer to the control period, and ECF_2 and $[HCO_3^-]_2$ refer to the status after therapy. If we estimate that the patient's ECF constituted 25 percent of the body weight when he was edematous, then ECF_1 equals 23.5 liters, and hence ECF_2, after the loss of 4.5 liters, equals 19.0 liters. Substituting these values in Equation 7-1 yields:

$$23.5 \times 23 = 19.0 \times [HCO_3^-]_2$$

$$[HCO_3^-]_2 = \frac{23.5 \times 23}{19}$$

$$[HCO_3^-]_2 = 28.4 \text{ mMoles/L}$$

Since the measured $[HCO_3^-]_2$ was 29 mMoles per liter (Table 7-A), all but 2 percent of the rise can be accounted for merely by the contraction of the ECF. It is for this reason that the metabolic alkalosis that follows vigorous diuretic therapy is called *contraction alkalosis.*

Problem 7-2

The presence of severe hyponatremia – when there is no other obvious cause for a generalized seizure, such as hypoglycemia, history of grand mal epilepsy, or abnormal neurological findings – makes it likely that the seizure was due to hyposmolality of the extracellular fluid (Chap. 2, under Causes and Treatment of SIADH). In the absence of cardiac, hepatic, renal, or adrenal insufficiency (Table 3-3), the first diagnostic suspicion raised by the combination of hyponatremia, plasma hyposmolality, and hyperosmotic urine, all in a patient drinking large amounts of fluid (Fig. 2-5), is SIADH. The history, however, disclosed that three times before, the patient had developed an identical disorder while on diuretics, which made it more likely that furosemide had caused the hyponatremia (Table 3-3), perhaps mainly through salt depletion and secondary retention of water (see below; also Fig. 3-6). For this reason – and because on prior occasions the patient had been treated successfully with infusions of isotonic or hypertonic saline – the patient was treated similarly on the present admission. She was given normal saline (Fig. 1-6) at a rate of 100 ml per hour intravenously, to which some KCl was added (about 120 mEq in 24 hours). The response to this therapy is shown in Table 7-B.

There may be at least two mechanisms through which diuretics cause hyponatremia. This patient illustrates one of them, which, though less common than the other, occurs with sufficient frequency to be an important complication of diuretic therapy. It is seen typically in patients who, like this one, are not edematous but often "self-administer" diuretics for cosmetic reasons or weight reduction, and especially ones who have concurrent polydipsia. Following treatment in the emergency room, the present patient was studied in a controlled setting in a metabolic research ward; understanding of the dynamics of the generation and cor-

Table 7-B
Laboratory data obtained on a 47-year-old woman at the time of admission to the emergency ward and after 18 hours and 34 hours of intravenous infusion of normal saline and KCl supplements

Test	On Admission	After 18 Hours of Treatment	After 34 Hours of Treatment
Venous blood or plasma:			
Na^+ (mEq/L)	112	119	132
K^+ (mEq/L)	3.1	3.7	4.1
Cl^- (mEq/L)	69	79	91
HCO_3^- (mMoles/L)	29	21	25
BUN (mg/100 ml)	10	—	9
Creatinine (mg/100 ml)	0.7	—	—
Sugar (mg/100 ml)	147	—	—
Osmolality (mOsm/kg H_2O)	232	242	277
Urine:			
$\dot{V}$ (ml/min)	0.7	4	5
Osmolality (mOsm/kg H_2O)	600	221	133
Glucose	0	—	—

rection of her hyponatremia are based in part on this subsequent study.

Note that the serum Na^+ concentration rose nearly to normal by giving isotonic saline (Table 7-B). By the reasoning used in the Answer to Problem 3-4, and given a body weight for the patient of 53 kg, it could be calculated that a positive balance of 636 mEq of Na^+ would have been required to raise the patient's plasma concentration from 112 to 132 mEq per liter. The actual balance, however, showed a net gain of only 338 mEq. From this fact it may be concluded that part of the rise in the serum Na^+ concentration must have been due to a loss of H_2O from the extracellular compartment, and this is reflected in the increased excretion of hyposmotic urine. In many such patients, however, the loss of H_2O (as gauged by a decrease in body weight) plus the positive Na^+ balance cannot fully account for the rise in serum Na^+ concentration. In these patients, it is postulated that there is a concomitant rise of intracellular solute, causing H_2O to shift from the extracellular into the intracellular compartment. Although the K^+ supplements may have had this effect in the present patient, they probably played a small role; the effect of K^+ is often much greater in other patients with diuretic-induced hyponatremia.

From this chain of events for the correction of hyponatremia, the probable mechanisms for its induction may be inferred (Fig. 7-B, pathway A). Initially, the diuretic causes a loss of Na^+ and H_2O, that is, an isosmotic contraction. This change may

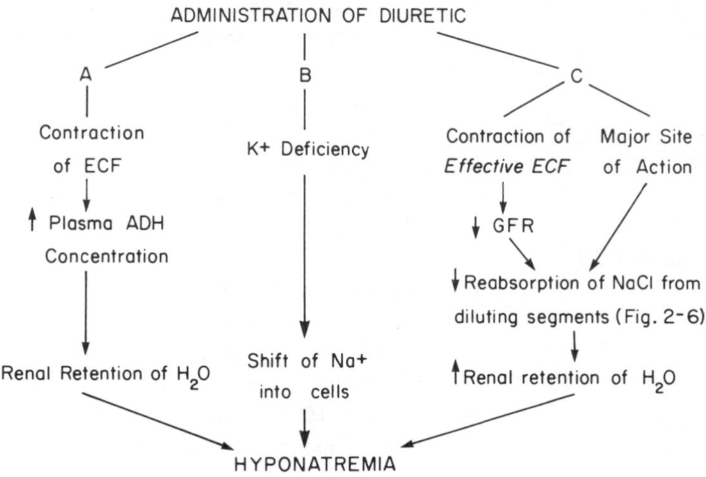

Figure 7-B
Chain of events by which administration of diuretics can lead to hyponatremia. Modified from R. W. Schrier and T. Berl, in R. W. Schrier (ed.), *Renal and Electrolyte Disorders.* Boston: Little, Brown, 1976.

stimulate the secretion of antidiuretic hormone (ADH) via volume receptors, and this effect may have been more pronounced in the present patient, who often experienced postural hypotension after she had had a sympathectomy. The presumed high plasma concentration of ADH, especially when combined with a high intake of fluid, then leads to retention of free water and the development of hyponatremia. Consistent with this chain of events is the finding that the patient appeared well hydrated when she was admitted to the emergency room, and that her GFR, as reflected in the BUN and serum creatinine concentrations (Chap. 8), was normal or even a little increased. The hyponatremia may be aggravated by diuretic-induced K^+ deficiency, which causes Na^+ to shift into the cells (Fig. 4-2; also Fig. 7-B, pathway B).

Except for the role of K^+, this chain of events is reminiscent of that leading to SIADH (Fig. 2-5). The essential difference lies in the continuous, autonomous production of ADH in that syndrome. Because of this autonomy, plasma levels of ADH are not reduced when the ECF of patients with SIADH is further expanded by infusing isotonic saline; consequently, the abnormality cannot be corrected. In contrast, the patient with diuretic-induced hyponatremia may inhibit the secretion of ADH when the ECF is expanded and excrete large volumes of hyposmotic urine (Table 7-B); thereby, the hyponatremia can be corrected with saline infusions.

More commonly, and perhaps sometimes in association with the mechanisms shown in pathways A and B, diuretics will cause hyponatremia according to the dynamics shown in pathway C (Fig. 7-B). Here, a direct effect of the diuretic on the diluting segments of the nephron, plus volume contraction and the chain of events shown in Figure 2-6, lead to a positive balance of H_2O and hence to hyponatremia. Inasmuch as these events are seen in edematous patients whose ECF is expanded, the critical contraction presumably involves the *effective* volume.

Problem 8-1

1. Although most patients come to the attention of a physician at an earlier stage and with a more definite history suggestive of renal impairment than the patient considered here, the story is not that rare. Since the BUN and creatinine concentrations are three times the normal value on repeated testing and since their ratio is 10:1, it can be concluded that the GFR has been reduced to about one-third the normal value, that is, to approximately 30 or 40 ml per minute for an adult man.

2. Of the four questions posed at the beginning of this chapter, the nephrologist can immediately answer two: He can say that the patient has renal disease, since he shows no extrarenal causes of a decreased GFR (e.g., dehydration), and he can estimate the extent of renal impairment. He should now try to establish the cause of the renal disease and its rate or progression.

Given the patient's history, the most likely cause is some form of glomerulonephritis, and in view of the frequent sore throats, it might be of the poststreptococcal variety. The nephrologist should attempt to confirm this impression by personally examining the sediment from several freshly voided urine specimens, for if he can detect erythrocyte casts, that finding will greatly strengthen the diagnosis of glomerulonephritis. He should also look for abnormal serum titers of streptococcal antibodies and complement. These tests fall more in the fields of pathology and clinical medicine; the rationale for the tests is therefore not considered further in this book. (Although it is agreed that streptococcal infections can cause acute glomerulonephritis, there is currently considerable controversy on whether or not they can cause chronic glomerulonephritis.)

A general question to be settled immediately is related to the progression of the disease: Does the patient have acute glomerulonephritis, contracted perhaps during the previous month, or has he for many years had glomerulonephritis that has not caused major symptoms? A third possibility is that he has had mild chronic glomerulonephritis for many years but now has a different, superimposed acute process. It is important to settle these questions not only to give some estimate of prognosis, but also because the treatment of certain acute glomerulonephritides differs in some respects from that of the chronic disease, and because it might be possible to eliminate a superimposed acute process, which might quickly improve the GFR. These points are best investigated through ultrasonographic examination or by some radiological technique that will reveal the size of the kidneys and often offer clues to other possibilities, such as obstruction. If the patient has chronic disease that is causing relentless progression of renal impairment (as does the patient described in connection with Fig. 8-2), then the intravenous pyelogram (I.V.P.) will probably show both kidneys to be small with reduction in the width of the renal cortex.

Almost certainly, the nephrologist would also order some other tests, but this answer has been directed toward the crucial tests of renal function that were considered in this chapter. He would probably not, however, ask for a 24-hour endogenous creatinine clearance test, since it would add no further information, nor is he likely to measure the 24-hour protein excretion, at least not immediately. The patient has a moderate amount of proteinuria, which is compatible with any of the processes mentioned above, and quantitation of the proteinuria is likely to be of greatest help later while following the progression of the disease (see Fig. 8-2).

3. The stableness of the patient's weight and of the BUN and serum creatinine concentrations suggests that he is in a steady state. Therefore, with the patient eating a normal diet (as reflected in his continuing good appetite), his urinary excretion of urea would be in the normal range.

Problem 8-2

This is a striking example of how a high intake of protein can selectively increase the BUN. A normal protein intake is about 1 g of protein per kilogram of body weight per day. Thus, this patient ingested about eight times the normal amount. The elevation of her protein intake can therefore fully account for the BUN of 70 mg/100 ml. In view of this reasoning and the normal findings on serum creatinine determination and urinalysis, one would predict that she has normal renal function. This conclusion is bolstered by the lack of anemia, since patients in whom renal disease has caused the BUN to rise to 70 mg/100 ml are usually anemic.

On the basis of the normal serum creatinine concentration and the patient's small body size, one would predict her GFR to be at the lower limits of normal. This prediction was borne out by the result of the 24-hour endogenous creatinine clearance test, which averaged 82 ml per minute.

There are some other important lessons to be derived from the example of this patient. Despite a large pool of urea in renal failure, urea metabolism is not increased in this condition, and this phenomenon has sometimes been ascribed to the effect of unidentified toxins that a failing kidney cannot fully excrete. The finding in this woman – namely, that without renal failure, urea metabolism was also not increased despite a large urea pool – argues against this explanation. The patient's general well-being when her BUN was so high also shows that the signs and symptoms of renal failure are apparently not due to urea.

Although the patient's intake of Na^+ was exceedingly low over a long period of time (see Answer to Problem 3-2), the conservation of Na^+ by her normal kidneys was so efficient that she did not develop Na^+ deficiency or volume contraction. She was in good health and had normal blood pressure, and her plasma volume was measured to be slightly greater than normal. That her kidneys were attuned to avidly conserving Na^+ (in response to the low-Na^+ diet) is shown by the fact that on two occasions when the patient increased her intake of Na^+, she developed ankle edema (see Fig. 3-1, days 26 through 32).

Problem 8-3

The important questions to be answered regarding this patient are whether he has hypertension, and if so, what its cause is. In view of the history of a renal injury and the finding of proteinuria on two samples, it is important to determine whether the patient has renal disease, which itself could be the cause of hypertension (Chap. 14).

To establish whether the patient has hypertension, his blood pressure was taken on several more occasions. A week after the initial checkup, the values were equivocal: 150/64 and 130/64 mm Hg in the right and left arms, respectively; 150/80 mm Hg in the right leg. Subsequent values, taken at intervals of three months, were: 120/60, 124/64, and 118/62. The electrocardiogram (ECG), a roentgenogram of the chest, and an intravenous pyelogram (I.V.P.) were all normal. The BUN and serum creatinine concentrations were 18 mg/100 ml and 0.8 mg/100 ml, respectively. Since these are "high normal" values, a 24-hour endogenous creatinine clearance test was done next, and in order to quantitate the proteinuria, the 24-hour protein excretion was determined on the same specimen. The creatinine clearance rate was 109 ml per minute, and no protein whatsoever could be detected in the 24-hour urine specimen.

For the time being, therefore, it was concluded that the patient had neither hypertension nor renal failure. The mild proteinuria on two specimens remains unexplained; it may have been due to laboratory error or to some nonspecific cause, such as postural proteinuria (Table 8-4). Similarly, there is no clear explanation for the apparent high blood pressure, but in view of the repeatedly normal levels on subsequent occasions, further tests did not seem justified.

All this is not to assert that the suspicious abnormalities on the initial examination were in error. It does mean, however, that the wisest course is to reassure the patient and his parents and to follow him fairly closely; in this way, time is likely to solve the diagnostic problem. The patient is now being seen at six-month intervals.

Problem 9-1

1. By definition, in adults a urine output of between 50 and 400 ml per day is oliguric while an output of less than 50 ml per day is anuric; therefore, the patient was anuric. This fact may not have been clear-cut on the first day of illness when catheterization yielded 50 ml of urine, because it was not known over what period of time that urine had been formed; however, the distinction became obvious subsequently.

It is important to discriminate between oliguria and anuria, because the latter is a relatively uncommon condition and it arouses suspicion that one of three general entities may be present: obstruction, some type of acute glomerulonephritis, or vascular disease (in order of frequency of occurrence). Thus, the presence of anuria greatly narrows the differential diagnosis.

2. Even though methods for inserting and maintaining urinary catheters have been improved, there is still a potential hazard of starting an infection every time a foreign object is introduced into the urinary passages. Further, the hazard is probably greater when a catheter is kept within the urethra than when it is passed momentarily a number of times. In addition, an indwelling catheter, even if kept within the urethra for only a few hours, can cause extremely uncomfortable urinary urgency and burning on urination that can last for days. Thus, although the topic remains controversial, many physicians advocate intermittent catheterization.

3. Once it had been established that the patient was anuric, the most likely diagnosis was obstruction of the urinary tract. The presence of a mass in the middle of the lower abdomen increased this likelihood. It was therefore imperative to rule out an obstruction, especially since its correction, had it been present, would have removed the cause of the acute renal failure. Not infrequently, a mass such as this is the bladder distended with urine. As it turned out, it was the uterus, which had been enlarged by three leiomyomas.

A second reason for the attention to the abdominal mass was that in a woman of childbearing age, such a mass always raises the possibility of pregnancy. This possibility assumed special importance in this patient, because microangiopathic hemolytic anemia is seen in association with various disorders of pregnancy, as well as with the use of oral contraceptives. The importance of ruling out pregnancy in this patient is reflected in the performance of a dilatation and curettage, which showed a menstrual endometrium.

4. During cystoscopy and retrograde pyelography, not only is an instrument passed through the urethra into the bladder, but a catheter is also threaded up the ureter to "feel" for obstruction and to introduce radiopaque material. Although invaluable when needed, this procedure represents instrumentation of the urinary passages, which should be avoided if possible. Alternative methods for ruling out the presence of obstruction, which obviate such instrumentation, include ultrasonographic examination and sometimes intravenous pyelography, especially when the contrast agent is given as an infusion rather than as a bolus. In the present patient, however, where at least initially, obstruction seemed to be a likely cause for the acute renal failure, many physicians would have elected to use the same course that was followed here. Not only did the cystoscopy and retrograde pyelography conclusively exclude obstruction (for which information the doctors at the second hospital were no doubt grateful), but the procedure would also have treated the obstruction had it been found.

Because retrograde pyelography has the potential of causing complications, the procedure should be limited to one kidney if possible. If the side that is examined is clear (as was the case here), then obstruction cannot be the cause of the anuria, since a single kidney can produce ample urine. If, on the other hand, the side that is examined is found to be blocked, then obstruction should also be looked for in the other kidney.

5. Management of patients often entails decisions that are based on the balance between risks and benefits. This fact is illustrated in the present patient. Although cystoscopy and retrograde pyelography carry a small incidence of complications, these eventualities are seldom, if ever, so serious that they destroy the kidney or require nephrectomy. Hence, it was not essential to be assured of the presence of two kidneys before the procedures were carried out. Closed renal biopsy, however, does involve a finite, albeit small, risk of serious bleeding, which might require nephrectomy. For this reason, and partly to localize the kidney for closed biopsy, both kidneys were visualized by ultrasonography prior to biopsy. Had it been established that only one kidney was present (which occurs in about one in 800 persons), the biopsy might not have been performed, or a so-called open biopsy, in which the kidney is visualized directly through a small incision, might have been carried out instead.

6. During oliguria, if the metabolic rate is normal, the BUN can be expected to rise by about 20 mg/100 ml per day and the serum creatinine concentration by approximately 2.5 mg/100 ml

(Table 1-5). In the present patient, the calculated BUN and serum creatinine concentrations after six days of anuria (about 135 and 16 mg/100 ml, respectively) conform reasonably well to the measured values of 95 and 11.2 mg/100 ml. It is important to consider this point, because deviations from the expected values might lead to the detection of complications (e.g., hemorrhage) or furnish valuable diagnostic clues (see Table 8-3).

Problem 10-1

1. On the basis of a normal value for the BUN of 12 mg/100 ml (Table 1-1), the BUN at age 20 was elevated by a factor of about five (Table 10-A). Hence, the GFR was reduced by roughly the same factor, so assuming that the healthy value for the GFR was 125 ml per minute (see Table 1-5), the GFR in the patient at age 20 was approximately 25 ml per minute. Taking a normal value for the serum creatinine concentration of 1.2 mg/100 ml, analogous computations predict the GFR at age 20 to have been about one-quarter of normal, or approximately 30 ml per minute. In this patient, the creatinine clearance was determined on a 24-hour urine sample; dividing 28 liters by 1,440 minutes yields a value of 19.4 ml per minute. This figure is in reasonably good agreement with the estimates of 25 and 30 ml per minute based on the BUN and creatinine concentrations, respectively. The agreement again serves to emphasize the fact that when the BUN and serum creatinine concentrations are grossly elevated, a creatinine clearance determination adds no useful information (see Chap. 8, under Clearance of Endogenous Creatinine). At

Table 10-A
Representative laboratory values for a patient with chronic pyelonephritis in his only kidney

Age (Years)	BUN/Creatinine (mg/100 ml)	C_{Creat}* (liters/24 hr)	Plasma Ca^{2+} (mg/100 ml)	Plasma Phos (P)* (mg/100 ml)	Hct* (%)
19	33/–	–	–	–	–
20	62/4.4	28	9.8	5.5	–
23	135/14.4	9	9.7	11.1	28
After transplantation:					
24	32/1.3	–	11.2	2.6	–
24½	–/1.3	–	11.6	2.3	–
26	10/1.2	–	–	–	–
28½	–	–	11.0	2.3	–
30	17/1.2	–	10.7	2.2	40
After subtotal parathyroidectomy:					
31	–/1.2	–	9.9	2.9	–

*C_{Creat} = clearance of endogenous creatinine; Phos (P) = phosphate phosphorus; Hct = hematocrit.

age 23, the agreement was as good, yielding values for the GFR of 11.1 and 10.4 ml per minute on the basis of the BUN and creatinine concentrations, respectively, and of 6.3 ml per minute on the basis of creatinine clearance.

2. At age 20, the patient was on a normal diet and his production of urea, arising mainly from the metabolism of dietary protein, was therefore normal. Furthermore, we know that patients with much more severe renal failure than the present patient stay in external balance for urea; by definition, therefore, this patient's urinary excretion of urea was normal.

The same arguments are applied to predicting that the patient's urinary excretion of creatinine was normal, provided the main source of endogenous creatinine – namely, the skeletal muscle mass – had not decreased. Not only is this prediction not in conflict with a decreased creatinine clearance, but the prediction can be verified using the data in Table 10-A. Recall that the creatinine clearance refers to the amount of plasma from which all creatinine is removed. At age 20, this process occurred at the rate of 28,000 ml per day, and since each 100 ml contained 4.4 mg of creatinine, a total of 28,000 × 0.044 or 1,232 mg of creatinine was removed from the plasma during each 24 hours. Moreover, once it is removed from the plasma by glomerular filtration, all the creatinine is excreted in the urine. Note that the value of 1,232 mg falls within the normal range for urinary creatinine excretion in men (Table 1-3).

Finally, if despite deteriorating renal function, the patient's lean body mass did not change, the urinary creatinine excretion should have been roughly the same at age 23 as at 20. Again, utilizing the values for creatinine clearance and serum creatinine concentration given in Table 10-A, one can calculate that 9,000 × 0.144 or 1,296 mg of creatinine per day was removed from the plasma and hence excreted in the urine.

3. The plasma concentration of phosphate (reported as phosphorus) begins to rise at that point in chronic renal failure where the fractional reabsorption of phosphate has been reduced to the minimal value of about 10 percent of the filtered load (see Fig. 10-9), for it is at this point that a positive external balance for phosphate sets in. In adult patients, these events occur when the GFR has been reduced to about 25 ml per minute. Thus, the slight elevation of serum phosphate concentration could be expected in the patient at age 20 when his GFR was approximately 20 ml per minute. It is also consistent with the renal handling of phosphate that the plasma phosphate concentration rose further as renal function deteriorated (age 23) and that it fell within the normal range when normal renal function had been restored through transplantation (Table 10-A).

Ordinarily, there is a reciprocal relationship between the serum concentration of phosphate and that of Ca^{2+}. In most instances of advanced renal failure, one therefore sees hyperphosphatemia associated with some degree of hypocalcemia. The fact that this was not the case at ages 20 and 23 years argues strongly for the presence of secondary hyperparathyroidism prior to renal transplantation, an impression borne out by the severe nephrocalcinosis in the diseased kidney, by the calcification of the radial arteries (which may have antedated the transplantation), as well as by other possible symptoms of hyperparathyroidism, such as pain in the bones and abdomen, pruritus, fatigability, and emotional distress.

4. The development of hypercalcemia after transplantation can be explained through the mechanisms shown in Figure 10-11. Central to the explanation is the hyperfunction of the parathyroid glands mentioned above and confirmed by the microscopic finding of chief-cell hyperplasia. With hyperparathyroidism and now *normal renal function,* the following events occur (Fig. 10-11): decreased tubular reabsorption of phosphate and hence mild hypophosphatemia; reciprocal hypercalcemia, abetted by increased tubular reabsorption of Ca^{2+} and mobilization of Ca^{2+} from bone; and stimulation of the renal production of $1{,}25\text{-}(OH)_2\text{-}D_3$, which in turn raises the extracellular pool of Ca^{2+} by increasing its intestinal absorption and the mobilization of Ca^{2+} from bone.

In the vast majority of patients, the hypercalcemia is only transient, because, through normal feedback mechanisms, the hypercalcemia causes involution of the previously hyperplastic parathyroid glands. It is not known why this feedback signal fails to reverse the hyperparathyroidism in some patients. On the other hand, one reason why persistent hypercalcemia is not seen more commonly may be that many surgeons perform subtotal parathyroidectomy prior to renal transplantation precisely in order to avoid the turn of events that was seen in the present patient.

Problem 11-1

1. This question was asked in order to emphasize my conviction that in the vast majority of patients, the determination of urine or serum osmolality does not provide useful additional information over what is already known about the patient. Although the measurement of osmolality is an invaluable tool for research, it is only rarely required for the optimal management of patients. Exceptions include the differential diagnosis of diabetes insipidus (Figs. 2-2 to 2-4) and possibly a quick screening test for drunkenness in emergency rooms, because intake of alcohol is the commonest cause of serum hyperosmolality in the United States.

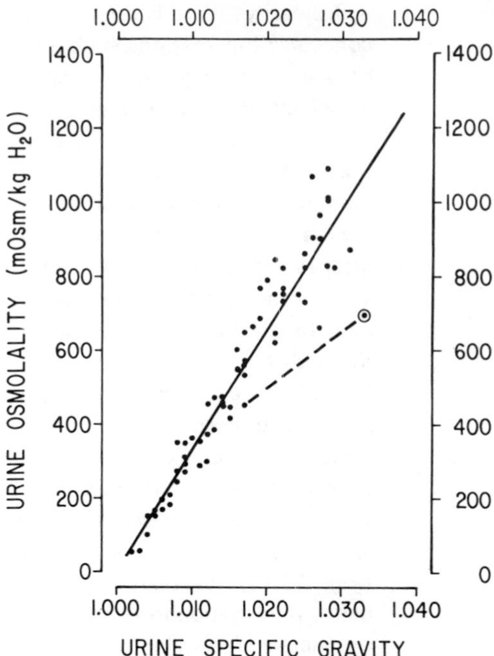

Figure 11-A
Specific gravity (as determined by refractometry) and osmolality (as measured by depression of freezing point) in random urine samples from hospitalized patients. The encircled point is from a sample that contained 4,200 mg of glucose per 100 ml of urine; the dashed line extends to the point that would represent this urine sample if the glucose were removed. A rule of thumb is to subtract 0.004 in specific gravity for every 1,000 mg of glucose per 100 ml of urine. The line was computed by the method of least squares, excluding the encircled point. It is uncommon to have so much protein in the urine that it causes a deviation from the line. This graph is very similar to one published by B. E. Miles et al. (*Br. Med. J.* 2:901, 1954), which was based on normal urine specimens.

Many physicians would cite other examples. But in most patients a sufficiently accurate estimate of the serum osmolality can be made from other laboratory data that are almost invariably already in the chart, namely, the serum concentrations of Na^+, urea, and glucose (see rule of thumb in Table 1-2). Furthermore, except in very rare instances, the urine osmolality can be estimated from a knowledge of the urine specific gravity (Fig. 11-A).

Each point in Figure 11-A shows the specific gravity and osmolality determined on each of 67 urine specimens that were picked at random from samples in a hospital laboratory over a 14-day period. The samples encompassed the gamut of abnormalities, including mild to moderate proteinuria and glycosuria. Only the encircled point to the right in the figure deviates obviously from the solid line; this point represents a urine specimen that contained very large amounts of glucose (4,200 mg/100 ml of urine). Glucose, being a heavier molecule than most of the solutes in urine (Fig. 1-4 and Table 1-7), tends to cause a greater increase in the specific gravity than in the osmolality. It is true that the scatter of the points is such that at any given specific gravity, the estimated osmolality may be off by as much as ±150 or even ±200 mOsm/kg H_2O. Rarely, however, is greater accuracy critical to the optimal management of a patient.

2. As obstruction of the urethra or bladder neck develops, the muscles in the wall of the bladder hypertrophy. In addition, there is often infection, which may irritate the bladder. These factors may cause a sudden, uncontrollable, and forceful contraction of the bladder when the urge to urinate appears, that is, *urgency incontinence* or *involuntary voiding.* The latter may also result when a markedly distended bladder leads to overflow leakage. In the same patient, however, there may at other times be a delay in starting the urinary stream, called *hesitancy,* which results from the time required to generate a force of contraction sufficient to overcome the obstruction. (After prolonged obstruction, as in the patient presented in Problem 11-2, dilatation of the bladder will result in weakness of the muscles, so emptying of the bladder becomes difficult even if there is no blockage to flow distal to the bladder.)

The anorexia, lethargy, and headaches probably represent nonspecific symptoms of the uremic state. Hypertension sometimes accompanies urinary obstruction; it may be related to the often associated expansion of the extracellular fluid volume (Chap. 14), an explanation that is supported by the fact that the blood pressure frequently reverts to normal after the obstruction is relieved. Although the patient's headaches might have been due to the hypertension, it is the current view that hypertension as a cause of headaches has been overstressed.

3. The weight loss of 10 kg during the first three hospital days probably means that the patient had had about 10 liters of excess fluid aboard when he was admitted; this was mainly extracellular fluid, which was reflected in the presence of edema and the loss thereof after the obstruction was relieved. The physician often finds himself in a quandary when managing postobstructive diuresis: Each day he gives many liters of intravenous fluid in order to replace the urinary loss on the preceding day. On each subsequent day, the patient may continue to excrete several liters of urine, and very soon the physician begins to wonder whether his vigorous replacement therapy is causing the high urine flow, or whether the flow represents continuing, obligatory postobstructive diuresis. The issue is best resolved by following the body weight. Most patients and their close relatives

know the patient's approximate normal body weight. Once this weight has been reached, intravenous replacement can be cut down to see if the diuresis will subside.

4. If the condition for which an operation is contemplated will not get worse by waiting, a surgeon prefers to postpone the operation until the patient's condition has improved. In the case of urinary obstruction, catheterization will not only improve the patient's general condition by reversing the uremia, but it may also improve specific urinary functions (e.g., contractions of the ureters and bladder) that may be critical to rapid and satisfactory postoperative recovery.

Problem 12-1

1. A sample flow sheet has been constructed as Table 12-A. Patients often relate a history by referring to the date of a given occurrence, and the physician's record is usually kept by date rather than by age. As a clinical history, however, the age is often more meaningful. A chart like this, periodically brought up to date and kept in the patient's record, can be an invaluable aid and time-saver.

2. Analysis of the pedigree is consistent with an autosomal inheritance, which is the recognized form of transmittance in cystinuria. There may be as many as three mutant alleles, and a number of different genotypes can be recognized on the basis of their urinary excretion of cystine, lysine, ornithine, and arginine. It is unlikely that the patient's two siblings died of cystinuria, since such patients usually succumb later in life as a result of obstructive nephropathy and chronic renal failure.

3. In 1967, at age 35, the patient had the nephrotic syndrome (Table 12-A), which almost certainly occurred as a result of the penicillamine therapy. This disease is a recognized complication of such therapy; the syndrome usually subsides over a number of years.

4. At age 35 when the patient developed the nephrotic syndrome, he was taking 12 g of $NaHCO_3$ per day. The molecular weight for this salt is 84 (Table 1-7); 12 g therefore contains 143 mMoles, and since each millimole has 1 mEq of Na^+, 12 g of $NaHCO_3$ represents a daily surcharge of 143 mEq of Na^+. Since this amount is equal to a normal daily intake of Na^+ (see Answer to Problem 3-2), it does not really help to restrict the salt that the patient may add to his food. An alternative would have been to give the patient $KHCO_3$, for he almost certainly could have excreted that amount of K^+ and remain in balance. The option that was chosen was to give the patient a thiazide diuretic, a means that is now commonly resorted to in order to permit a patient the pleasures of a normal diet.

Table 12-A
Clinical history of a man with cystinuria

Age (Years)	Event	Urine: pH	Urine: Excretion of Amino Acids (mg/24 hr)	Urine: Excretion of Protein (g/24 hr)	BUN/ Creatinine (mg/100 ml)	Procedures and Treatment	Comments
25	Stone in left ureter, passed spontaneously	–	–	–	–/–	–	–
27	Two stones in left ureter, passed spontaneously	–	–	–	–/–	Urine flow increased to 2.5 liters in 24 hours; urine pH > 7.0 with oral $NaHCO_3$	Stones are cystine by chemical analysis
29	–	–	–	–	–/–	Pyelotomy	Cystine composition confirmed
30	Right flank pain for 4 months	6.0	Cys 1,391 Lys 2,337 Orn 535 Arg 1,253	–	15/–	I.V.P., cystoscopy, pyelolithotomy, nephrostomy, ureteroplasty, all on right; $NaHCO_3$ increased to 3 g four times a day	Cystine crystals in urine; stricture of right ureter
33	Stone on right, passed spontaneously	–	–	–	–/–	–	–
34	Severe pain in right flank	–	–	–	–/–	I.V.P., cystoscopy, retrograde, ureterolithotomy	–
		5.8 6.2	–	–	9/–	Repeat I.V.P. and ureterolithotomy plus nephrostomy; D-penicillamine, 500 mg four times a day	–
35	Skin rash	–	–	+++ 0 ++	11/–	D-Penicillamine stopped for 3 days; then restarted at 500 mg three times a day	–
35	Edema (gained 10 lbs.)	–	–	8.6 8.9	11/1.1	Stopped D-penicillamine	Nephrotic syndrome

(Continued)

Table 12-A (Continued)

Age (Years)	Event	Urine			BUN/ Creatinine (mg/100 ml)	Procedures and Treatment	Comments
		pH	Excretion of Amino Acids (mg/24 hr)	Excretion of Protein (g/24 hr)			
36	—	—	—	—	–/–	—	Genetic history: consanguineous parentage; 2 siblings died in childhood, 3 well; 7 children all well, with normal urinary amino acid excretion
37	Occasionally passes small stones spontaneously	7.5	—	++ 8.8	18/1.1	$NaHCO_3$, 1.5 g four times daily. Tests own urine pH; usually 7.0	—
38	—	8.0	—	+++	–/–	—	—
39 to 44	Passes small stones spontaneously	—	—	++	30/2.5	I.V.P.: progressive hydronephrosis and hydroureter on right	Urinary sediment always contains cystine crystals

Problem 12-2

1. In Chapter 6 (under *Comment,* pp. 139-140) we pointed out that HCO_3^- concentration in venous plasma, when determined as total CO_2 content, is 2 to 4 mMoles per liter higher than the arterial value. We may therefore conservatively estimate that the arterial plasma HCO_3^- concentration in the patient was 19 mMoles per liter. It is clear from Figure 12-4a that the urinary pH of a normal individual with a plasma $[HCO_3^-]$ of 19 mMoles per liter would be below 5.5; the fact that the patient's urinary pH was 6.5 is therefore consistent with the diagnosis of RTA. The same arguments apply to the series of three determinations of plasma HCO_3^- concentration and urinary pH done subsequently. Other features that speak for the possibility of RTA are the normal renal function and the normal anion gap of 11 mEq per liter. In a patient like this, immunological rejection leading to renal failure is a constant danger; if that were the cause of acidosis, one should see an elevated anion gap.

2. The acidification test with NH_4Cl showed that the patient could lower the urinary pH to a minimal value when she became sufficiently acidotic. During this test, her total venous CO_2 content dropped from 21 to 16 mMoles per liter; her arterial plasma HCO_3^- concentration was therefore in the range of 13 or 14 mMoles per liter. According to Figure 12-4a, the concurrence of a urinary pH of 5.05 at this plasma HCO_3^- concentration rules out distal RTA. The results of this test emphasize the fact that the ability to lower urinary pH to the minimal value does not eliminate the possibility of RTA, only of distal RTA (Table 12-3); whether or not a patient who can decrease urinary pH below 6.0 has a defect of acidification must be judged *in light of the plasma* HCO_3^- *concentration at which the minimal pH is reached* (Fig. 12-4a). The finding that the renal threshold for HCO_3^- was lowered to about 19 mMoles per liter shows that the patient had proximal RTA. The further finding of an abnormally low *Tm* for HCO_3^- (Fig. 12-7) is consistent with this conclusion.

The patient showed very slight evidence of other proximal tubular deficiency. She excreted approximately 300 mg of glucose in a 24-hour period (for normal amount, see Table 1-3), and she was reabsorbing only 77 percent of the filtered phosphate; however, other proximal tubular functions (e.g., the reabsorption of amino acids) were normal. The RTA has never presented a problem in management of this patient. Ten years after the transplantation, she still has a tendency toward a high serum Cl^- concentration and a low serum HCO_3^- concentration, but, if anything, the tendency is less now than when RTA was first diagnosed in her. The anion gap remains normal, as does the serum K^+ concentration.

The above patient represents an instance of very mild RTA. Other examples, especially of distal RTA and of patients in whom clinical complications have arisen, can be found in the following sources: A. M. Butler et al. *J. Pediatr.* 8:489, 1936; F. Albright et al. *Medicine* (Baltimore) 25:399, 1946; K. L. Pines and G. H. Mudge. *Am. J. Med.* 11:302, 1951; O. Wrong and H. E. F. Davies. *Q. J. Med.* 28:259, 1959; J. Otten and H. L. Vis. *J. Pediatr.* 73:422, 1968; A. Sebastian. *Calif. Med.* 116:34, May, 1972; V. M. Buckalew, Jr., et al. *Medicine* (Baltimore) 53:229, 1974; S. M. Taher et al. *N. Engl. J. Med.* 290:765, 1974; N. Smithline et al. *N. Engl. J. Med.* 294:71, 1976.

Problem 13-1

1. The water deprivation test (Table 13-A) can be interpreted by referring to Figure 2-3. After 12 hours of fluid withdrawal and after the injection of five units of ADH intramuscularly (Table 13-A, 8 Days on Lithium), the urine osmolality had risen to only 198 mOsm/kg H_2O. This value falls on the curve for nephrogenic diabetes insipidus in Figure 2-3. The slight rise in urine osmolality during water deprivation can probably be explained by a decrease in extracellular fluid volume and consequent decrease in the GFR, and then by the chain of events described in Figure 2-6. If lithium-induced thirst (Table 13-2) had played a major role in the concentrating defect — that is, if thirst were an initiating event, not one occurring secondarily to an obligatory high urine flow — then one would have expected the urine osmolality during water deprivation to rise higher than it did, at least to above the osmolality of plasma. In some patients, one can also identify primary polydipsia as a major mechanism by observing a gain in body weight as the patient is challenged with lithium and develops diabetes insipidus.

As in all patients who complain of polyuria and polydipsia, an osmotic diuresis due to uncontrolled diabetes mellitus had to be considered in this patient, especially since she had just been in diabetic ketoacidosis. This possibility was excluded by the repeated absence of glucose from the urine. Note that this patient developed nephrogenic diabetes insipidus on standard therapeutic doses of lithium carbonate that resulted in subtoxic plasma concentrations of lithium (Tables 13-A and 1-1). It is not possible to say whether the presence of diabetes mellitus contributed to her exquisite susceptibility to lithium; the normal BUN value (Table 13-A) at least indicates that the patient did not have advanced diabetic glomerulosclerosis.

The patient lost approximately 4 percent of her body weight during the water-deprivation test, which is exactly the degree of weight loss that one aims for (Chap. 2, under Types of Diabetes Insipidus). During the short interval of 12 hours, such weight loss

Table 13-A
Selected data on a 54-year-old woman with lithium-induced diabetes insipidus

	Days on Lithium		Days off Lithium	
Variable*	7	8 (H_2O deprivation plus ADH administration)	12 (After ADH administration)	28
Body weight (kg)	77	73.8	—	—
P_{Li} (mEq/L)	0.82	0.69	—	—
BUN (mg/100 ml)	11	—	—	—
$\dot{V}$ (liters/24 hr)	>6	—	—	~2
U_{Osm} (mOsm/kg H_2O)	86	198	293	500
P_{Osm} (mOsm/kg H_2O)	296	342	—	—
U_G (mg/100 ml)	0	0	0	0

*P_{Li} = plasma lithium concentration; BUN = blood urea nitrogen concentration; $\dot{V}$ = urine flow rate; U_{Osm} = urine osmolality; P_{Osm} = plasma osmolality; U_G = urine glucose concentration.

in this patient should reflect a loss of water without solute, and one can therefore calculate by how much the plasma osmolality should have risen. Before the start of the test, the patient's total body solute can be estimated as the product of the total body water (TBW, which, in this obese woman, was estimated as 55 percent of the body weight, or approximately 42.4 liters) and the plasma osmolality: 42.4 × 296 = 12,550 mOsm. At the end of the test, the TBW was 42.4 - 3.2 = 39.2 liters. Since she presumably lost very little solute during the test, 12,550/39.2 = new P_{Osm} = 320 mOsm/kg H_2O; that is, the P_{Osm} at the end of the test should have been about 320 mOsm/kg H_2O. For the purposes of this test, the measured P_{Osm} of 342 mOsm/kg H_2O (Table 13-A) is a sufficiently satisfactory check to provide assurance that the test was run properly and that the rise in P_{Osm} was more than ample to stimulate the release of ADH from the posterior pituitary gland.

2. The therapeutic dilemma that arises from improving the affective disorder but at the same time producing diabetes insipidus is not uncommon. Cautious use of thiazide diuretics is often helpful in these situations. When combined with a moderate restriction of salt intake (e.g., 4 g NaCl daily), the administration of 0.5 to 1.0 g chlorothiazide per day can reduce the urine flow to 3 to 4 liters per day and increase the urine osmolality slightly, say, to the level of about 200 mOsm/kg H_2O. The mechanism of this *anti*diuretic effect of diuretic agents is not fully understood

(Chap. 2, under Causes and Treatment of Diabetes Insipidus). Part of the effect is achieved through decreased generation of free water, because chlorothiazide inhibits NaCl transport at site 3 of Figure 7-1. The most important element, however, may be some degree of NaCl depletion, which results in greater fractional reabsorption of isosmotic fluid in the proximal tubules, decreased generation of free water, and decreased urine flow, that is, the type of events shown in Figure 2-6. Depletion of NaCl has a further consequence that can spell either danger or benefit. The reabsorption of lithium as well as of Na^+ is enhanced under these conditions. Consequently, the plasma concentration of lithium will rise when a combination of thiazides and lithium is used. Although this rise can lead to lithium toxicity, it often improves the psychiatric status. In fact, treatment with chlorothiazide may be advisable in patients whose serum concentration of lithium does not rise into the therapeutic range when they are given ordinary dosages of lithium carbonate.

Problem 14-1

1. The patient's illness mimicked the two-kidney model of Goldblatt hypertension (Fig. 14-6). Although probably less than 1 percent of all patients with elevated diastolic blood pressure can experience the gratifying surgical cure that this patient obtained, the problem nevertheless has broad implications for the majority of hypertensive disorders. Once it has been determined that a person has high blood pressure, it *may* be important to move quickly. This point is self-evident in renovascular hypertension, which, as in this patient, is often abrupt and severe in onset and which may quickly induce irreversible and self-perpetuating changes in the unstenosed, "unprotected" kidney. It is therefore important to know that the onset of hypertension was recent, because surgical intervention may work only in the early phase when renin-angiotensin activity plays the major causative role. The necessity for early treatment is not so obvious with other forms of high blood pressure, not only because the rise in pressure is usually much more subtle and gradual, but also because the existence of a reversible initiating phase still rests only on theoretical grounds (Fig. 14-8). Nevertheless, many experts urge prompt treatment of even mild essential hypertension on the supposition that the induction of the self-perpetuating cycle of Figure 14-8 might thereby be prevented. This possibility points up what is possibly one of the most important features of routine physical examinations, since most patients with high blood pressure do not develop symptoms until possibly irreversible changes in the kidneys, heart, and other organs have set in.

It is not justified to sample renal venous blood for renin or to perform renal arteriograms on all patients with high blood pressure on the outside chance that one might effect a surgical cure. A strong suspicion that renovascular hypertension is present is often aroused by several points, which were also seen in the present patient: the abrupt onset of fairly severe hypertension, a bruit in the upper lateral abdomen, and delayed opacification of the calyces as well as a difference in the size of kidneys on I.V.P. The fact that this patient responded so well to the operation even though the renin activity from both kidneys was equally high illustrates that there are few absolutes in clinical medicine, especially in the field of hypertension. Each patient should be treated individually. Although, in retrospect, it was not foolish to operate on the present patient, it must be emphasized that it would be wrong to ignore the criterion in most patients.

2. In an I.V.P. examination for the evaluation of hypertension, more films than normally are taken during the period immediately following the injection of the contrast medium, usually at 30 seconds, at 1, 3, and 5 minutes, and at 20 minutes (the last, to observe delayed washout of the medium). This test is requested in order to investigate the possibility of a stenotic lesion in the renal artery. The stenosis causes enough reduction in renal blood flow to result not only in decreased size of the kidney (not necessarily from ischemic damage but possibly just from a decrease in total renal blood volume), but also in decreased delivery of the contrast medium to the affected kidney. Consequently, the filling of the tubular system with contrast medium – recognized as a nephrogram and seen early – is delayed. Possibly because of the decreased GFR and the sluggish flow of tubular fluid, the nephrogram often persists in the affected kidney long after it has disappeared from the other kidney.

A stenosis in the renal artery decreases the GFR of that kidney, and the decreased GFR in turn often leads to a change in the ability to excrete free water even when overt renal failure has not set in (Fig. 2-6). Whether there is a decrease or an increase in maximal urine osmolality depends on the extent of the reduction in the GFR. When the reduction is mild – as in the present patient, whose BUN and serum creatinine concentrations remained in the normal range – the decreased generation of free water may raise urine osmolality. Hence the contrast agent, like inulin, will be concentrated more in the tubules of the affected kidney, and this fact is reflected by increased opacification on that side (Fig. 14-9). On the other hand, if the GFR is reduced beyond a critical point, decreased reabsorption of NaCl from the ascending limbs of Henle (site 2 in Fig. 7-1) will lead to decreased reabsorption of free water from the collecting ducts and hence to decreased concentration of the medium.

Problem 14-2

1. The decrease in the caliber of the retinal arterioles reflects vasospasm. Whereas normally the retinal arteries are almost as broad as the veins, in severe hypertension they may be only one-fifth as wide. The narrowing is observed even though the walls of the vessels may be sclerosed; thus, there is no conflict between the narrowing seen in vivo and the thickening of the vessel walls (e.g., in the kidneys) reported on microscopy. If the retinal arteriolar spasm is sufficiently severe, it leads to hypoxia, which in turn causes hemorrhages, exudates, and, when most severe, papilledema. Note that in the patient described in Problem 14-1 who responded so well to surgery, there were only minimal changes in the retinas. Examination of the eye-grounds is an important tool in assessing hypertension, as it is indeed for evaluating many other systemic diseases; it is, in many ways, a "noninvasive biopsy." Even severe retinal abnormalities can often be reversed when the blood pressure is lowered, and such was the case in the present patient.

2. The high blood pressure in this patient just before transplantation probably had two major causes: increased ECF and increased renin activity. The first is suggested by the episode of pulmonary edema while she was receiving a blood transfusion, as well as by the decrement in pressure after dialysis was started. The aim throughout the 2½ months of dialysis was to keep the patient at her "dry weight"; in fact, she ate so poorly that she lost weight during this period. Just before the transfusion, however, the peritoneal dialysis had not gone well technically, and it was estimated that the patient had 2 to 3 liters of extra fluid aboard. The administration of packed cells on top of this overload apparently overexpanded the vascular volume enough to precipitate pulmonary edema and to aggravate the hypertension through the mechanism shown in Figure 14-5. As soon as fluid was removed by phlebotomy and further dialysis, the blood pressure fell into the range of 160/90 mm Hg.

Even though renin activity was not measured in this patient, several points suggest that high plasma concentrations of renin played a role in her hypertension: (1) Her high blood pressure persisted despite vigorous therapy with drugs and adequate dialysis, which kept her ECF at the normal level or even slightly lower. (2) The blood pressure instantly fell into the normal range on the day of transplantation, and it has remained there without drug treatment. Inasmuch as the dialysis was considered to have been adequate, the implantation of the normal kidney is unlikely to have lowered the blood pressure by altering the ECF. It might have done so by releasing prostaglandins, but it is more likely that the blood pressure was normalized so promptly because the sources of the high renin levels – namely, both diseased kidneys — were removed at the same operation. This explanation cannot be verified in the case of the present patient, but it has been shown to be valid in other patients with end-stage renal disease where either bilateral nephrectomy or pharmacological inhibition of the renin-angiotensin system has cured an otherwise refractory hypertension. Such patients constitute perhaps 10 to 15 percent of all renoprival hypertension. These aspects of the causation of high blood pressure in terminal renal failure are discussed in the following references as well as in many others: V. Vertes et al. *N. Engl. J. Med.* 280:978, 1969; S. B. Moore and F. J. Goodwin. *Lancet* 2:67, 1976; and D. H. P. Streeten et al. *Prog. Biochem. Pharmacol.* 12:214, 1976.

Index